Atopic Dermatitis:
Inside Out or Outside In?

Atopic Dermatitis: Inside Out or Outside In?

Lawrence S. Chan, MD, MHA, FAAD

Dr. Orville J. Stone Endowed Professor,
Department of Dermatology,
University of Illinois College of Medicine,
Chicago, IL;
Department of Medicine,
Captain James Lovell FHCC,
North Chicago, IL

Vivian Y. Shi, MD, FAAD

Associate Professor,
Department of Dermatology,
University of Arkansas for Medical Sciences,
Little Rock, AR

ELSEVIER

Elsevier
1600 John F. Kennedy Blvd.
Ste 1800
Philadelphia, PA 19103-2899

ATOPIC DERMATITIS: INSIDE OUT OR OUTSIDE IN   ISBN: 9780323847445

Library of Congress Control Number: 2021944556

Senior Content Strategist: Charlotta Kryhl
Senior Content Development Manager: Somodatta Roy Choudhury
Publishing Services Manager: Deepthi Unni
Project Manager: Sindhuraj Thulasingam
Design Direction: Amy Buxton

Printed in India

Last digit is the print number: 9   8   7   6   5   4   3   2   1

Working together
to grow libraries in
developing countries

www.elsevier.com • www.bookaid.org

Contributors

Divya J. Aickara, MS

Julia Arzeno, MD

Smita Awashti, MD

Safiyyah Bhatti, MD

Paul Blackcloud, MD

Lawrence S. Chan, MD, MHA.

Colleen Cotton, MD.

Lawrence Eichenfield, MD.

Kayla Fourzali, MS

Jennifer Fernandez, RD

John Frew, MBBS (Hons) MMed MSc PhD FACD

Rachel Shireen Golpanian, BA

David Grand, MD

Takashi Hashimoto, MD

Jason Ezra Hawkes, MD, MS

Aleksi Hendricks, BS

Penelope Hirt, MD

Marcia Hogeling, MD

Jennifer Hsiao, MD

Victor Huang, MD

Jonwei Hwang, BS

Joanna Jaros, MD

Yana Kost, BA

Christina Kursewicz, BS

Dylan E. Lee, MD

Griffin R. Lee, BS

Hadar Lev-Tov, MD, MAS

Peter Lio, MD

Mary E Logue, MD

Haruyo Nakajima-Adachi, PhD

Jennifer Ornelas, MD

Daniela Sanchez, BS

Vivian Y. Shi, MD

Michiko Shimoda, PhD

Raja Sivamani, MD, MS, AP.

Aimee Caroline Smidt, MD (FAAD, FAAP).

Kyle Tegtmeyer, BS

Alexis Tracy, MD

Khiem Tran, MD, PhD

Dr. Masako Toda, PhD.

Marta Turowski, MD, MBA

Michelle Vy, MD

Claire Wilson, BS

Peggy A Wu, MD, MPH

Hera Wu, BA

Joseph Yardman-Frank, MPH

Gil Yosipovitch, MD.

Jeffrey Zhao, BA

Tian Hao Zhu, MD

Tian Ran Zhu, MD

Preface

Atopic dermatitis, a chronic, itchy, inflammatory skin disease, has caught the attention of the medical community in recent years due to the disease's significant increase in prevalence over the last decades, particularly in the developed nations. As a result, a substantial amount of investigations, in both clinical and laboratory aspects, have been conducted in search for answers of reasons underlying such increase of prevalence to occur and for optimal therapeutic options. While many factors have been viewed as contributors to the development of the disease, some seem to be on the opposite spectrum of the others, no single root cause has been identified. On one hand, defect in certain skin barrier protein, like filaggrin, has been found in some patients affected by atopic dermatitis, pointing to external factors that penetrate the internal weakness of the skin to cause skin inflammation. On the other hand, explicit altering of the skin immune milieu by artificially expressing a prominent Th2 cytokine interleukin-4 in the basal epidermis results in the skin barrier-intact interleukin-4-transgenic mice with a disease phenotype that fulfills the clinical diagnostic criteria of human atopic dermatitis, pointing to triggering internal factors of immune dysregulation.

In *Atopic Dermatitis: Inside Out or Outside In?* we attempt to analyze this burdensome disease from a distinct perspective. The clinical and laboratory evidence in support of internally initiated factors and those in support of externally triggered causes are delineated separately. We aim to develop better understanding of the different components that may influence the initiation, progression, and sustainment of this inflammatory disorder. The ultimate goal of this book is to help clinicians who care for atopic dermatitis to develop a therapeutic strategy consistent with the knowledge resulted from the most updated evidence.

Specifically, this book is organized into four sections. After introducing the topic of "atopy" in Section I, Section II of this book is devoted to discussions of external factors, including skin barrier, microbiome and dysbiosis, immunogens, nutrition, environmental pollution, and clinical evidence supporting external factors. In Section III, internal factors such as keratinocytes, microvasculature, humoral and cellular factors, skin-gut-lung permeability, neuro-sensory mechanisms, epigenetics, and clinical evidence in support of internal factors are delineated. Section IV concludes the book by providing therapeutic recommendations for targeting internal factors, external factors, and internal/external combined factors.

With the disease statistic showing a continuing increase of prevalence of atopic dermatitis in a worldwide dimension, we sincerely hope this book will come at a timely manner to assist the physicians and the medical researchers who devote their career in search for the underlying pathophysiology and better therapeutic solutions.

Lawrence S. Chan
Vivian Y. Shi

Foreword

Atopic dermatitis is one of the most common—and most burdensome—skin disorders, well recognized for its impact on quality of life. While topical steroids have been the mainstay of treatment for many years, with systemic immunosuppressants or phototherapy reserved for the more severely affected patients who are recalcitrant to topicals, improved understanding of the disease and, though this understanding, improved treatment have been a huge unmet need. Fortunately, in just the past 15 years there has been an explosion of research related to atopic dermatitis, including more than 2000 articles published in 2019 alone, as cited in PubMed. This multifaceted research has greatly changed our concepts about the underlying pathogenesis, subphenotypes of disease, comorbidities, and new directions for more targeted therapy. Growing interest in atopic dermatitis and moving advances forward has spawned collaborative networks to foster education and research, such as the International Eczema Council and the International Society for Atopic Dermatitis, in addition to greatly increasing the membership in and impact of patient organizations focused on atopic dermatitis worldwide.

As such, it is fitting that Drs. Chan and Shi, with contributions from other experts, have written this new text on atopic dermatitis, with a focus on the tightly intertwined environmental/environment sensing factors (external factors) and response components (internal factors) that are thought to be pathogenic for this disorder. While the text begins with historical perspectives and how they have evolved, it chronicles the progress with copious detail and numerous references. Topics range from the complexities of the skin barrier, which goes beyond the genetic and cytokine-induced deficiency of filaggrin; the potential role of the microbe in protecting against exacerbation of microbial alterations in driving disease; the uniform skewing toward a type 2 immunophenotype in skin but variations that may reflect age, race, ethnicity, and severity; the relationship between cytokines and itch; and the great progress made in interventions from generation and testing of targeted therapies.

Drs. Chan and Shi are to be congratulated for their outstanding accomplishment in editing this up-to-date textbook. The book provides a reference guide for state-of-the-art understanding of a highly prevalent skin disorder as we start a new decade of discovery and patient support in 2020.

Amy S. Paller, MD
Walter J Hamlin Professor and Chair of Dermatology
Professor of Pediatrics
Northwestern University Feinberg School of Medicine
Chicago, IL, United States

Acknowledgment

The editors would like to thank many basic scientists and clinical investigators for their dedicated works in atopic dermatitis. The results of their works collectively provide the backbone of contents for this book. National Eczema Association and eczema patient support groups deserve our special recognition. Furthermore, the editors would also like to thank dermatopathologist Dr. Wenhua Liu for providing many outstanding histopathologic photos of atopic dermatitis. Certainly, the editors would like to thank all the contributing authors who committed to the writing of this book. In addition, the editors would like to thank our family members who have supported us throughout these writing and editing processes. Finally, the editors would like to thank University of Illinois College of Medicine and Captain James Lovell Federal Healthcare Center (Dr. Chan) and University of Arkansas for Medical Sciences and University of Arizona, Tucson (Dr. Shi) for their generous support of our academic endeavors.

*Cover art is courtesy of Catherine Ludwig, Vivian Y. Shi, and Lawrence S. Chan

Contents

Contents

1

Historic Perspective

JEFFREY ZHAO, KYLE TEGTMEYER, AND PETER A. LIO

KEY POINTS

- From the historic perspective, atopic dermatitis has gone through several evolutionary periods of understanding and development.
- From ancient times to the 18th century, medical communities started to recognize a type of itchy skin disease. Although the term *eczema* had been used, no unified concept had been developed and no understanding of its underlying pathophysiology was established.
- The 19th century witnessed the rapid development of dermatology as a specialty, with the effort of classifying skin diseases based on clinical findings, and the recognition of acute and chronic forms of eczema, the infant onset of eczema, and the systemic link between atopy of skin and atopy of the respiratory system.
- By the 20th century, the dermatology community formed a unified concept of atopic dermatitis from divergent hypotheses under the framework of the cutting-edge science of the immune system to explain the pathophysiology of disease, leading to the coining of the term *atopic dermatitis* to establish a set of diagnostic criteria and a link between skin atopy and allergic mechanisms.
- From the historic perspective, the approach of managing eczema has gone through multiple modifications as disease pathophysiology became more well delineated.

Introduction

To introduce the subject of historic perspective on eczema, the following quote serves nicely:

> *Eczema has been rightly called the keystone of dermatology, and he who fully masters its management is not only skilled in regard to treating one of the most common and distressing of all cutaneous diseases, but has acquired a knowledge of the principles of dermatologic practice which will assist in the treatment of many, if not all, other maladies of the skin.*
>
> **L. DUNCAN BULKLEY** (*Eczema and its management: A practical treatise based on the study of three thousand cases of the disease*, 1881)

As early as 1881, the medical community recognized the importance of eczema as a skin disease of high impact in medicine and in society. In this chapter we discuss the history of eczema from the perspectives of three historical time frames: ancient times through the 18th century, the 19th century, and the 20th century. We then discuss the historical approach to eczema treatment.

Ancient history and middle ages, through the 18th century

Eczema has presumably afflicted humans since well before the advent of written language. Healers and historians of antiquity have documented pruritic rashes and their remedies with great accuracy and astonishing classification systems. Unfortunately, interpretation of these ancient writings is often difficult and contentious at times. Though the first accepted report of a medical condition resembling atopic dermatitis (AD) is commonly cited as Suetonius' account in *The Twelve Caesars*, it is important to note the centuries of pre-Roman medical accounts of pruritic dermatoses that afflicted these early civilizations and examine the practices surrounding the treatment of these conditions (Mier, 1975).

The Ebers Papyrus, a compilation of hieratic writings dating to 1500 B.C.E., describes accounts of many skin ailments and popular Egyptian remedies of the time. Several portions of the 65-foot-long scroll depict eczema affecting the scalp, which likely were manifestations of seborrheic dermatitis (Bhattacharya, Strom, & Lio, 2016). Many topical remedies for cutaneous conditions were described in these writings, including modalities such as emollients, physical abrasives, lactic acid, the first descriptions of phototherapy with coingestion of the weed *Ammi majus*, and "heliotherapy" applied to the lesion (Brodsky, Abrouk, Lee, & Kelly, 2017; El-Domyati & Attia, 2015). A shard of Egyptian pottery from the Toronto Museum depicts a case of copper-induced contact dermatitis, with a secondary infection of weeping eczema productive of an odor resembling rotten fish eggs (Liddell, 2006). While the ancient Egyptians described numerous different cutaneous conditions, no specific reference to AD or eczema as a distinct entity has been identified.

Across the Red Sea, the civilizations of Mesopotamia also documented many dermatologic lesions in cuneiform tablets from the first millennium B.C.E. Unfortunately, the inhabitants of ancient Mesopotamia failed to preserve their deceased as well as their Egyptian counterparts did, thus precluding any correlative approach to understanding Akkadian words representing ailments of the skin. This has created contention among Akkadian scholars over the correct translations of medical terms. Adamson (1988) argues that the moist lower extremity skin lesion known as "rułibłu" describes a weeping eczema found in both children and adults. Scurlock and Andersen (2010) note in their review of writings from Ashur, Babylon, and Nineveh that the quantity of descriptors used to classify skin lesions in Mesopotamian works far dwarfs those of any other organ system of the body, thus reflecting an ancient appreciation for the diverse ailments of the skin. "KURAšTU" is commonly translated as eczema by cuneiformists, though Scurlock and Andersen more recently favor a translation of ringworm based on descriptions of clinical features. Given the difficulty of ensuring accurate understandings of Mesopotamian descriptions of these skin lesions it is not surprising that few texts on the history of AD have confidently included these pre-Roman accounts in their historical canon of ancient dermatologic literature.

Roman historian Suetonius described the first entity truly matching our modern concept of AD in his annals of the Julio-Claudian dynasty. Several family members, including Emperors Augustus and Claudius, were afflicted with a syndrome that appears to have features of the atopic triad (Ring, 1985). Notably, Augustus suffered from bouts of asthma, rhinitis, and eczema; Claudius developed a horse dander allergy and recurrent attacks of rhinoconjunctivitis. In 543 C.E. the Byzantine physician Aëtius of Amila used the term *eczema* to describe "hot and painful phlyctenae which do not ulcerate" (Wigley, 1953) and was credited with being the first to associate the word with descriptions of "eruptions consisting of small pustules, accompanied by burning sensation and pain, which sometimes spread to the whole body" (Friedman, 1930).

Medicine during the second millennium C.E. in Europe owed much to the works of Persian physician and scholar Abu 'Ali al-Husayn Ibn Sina, known as Avicenna. His encyclopedia, *The Canon of Medicine*, was translated into Latin in the 12th century and became standard reading for medieval era medical students in Europe and the Islamic world until the 17th century (Avicenna, 1973). Sir William Osler considered this text "a medical bible for a longer time than any other work" (Atarzadeh, Heydari, Sanaye, & Amin, 2016). Mentions of eczema are found in his sections on swellings, of which there are watery, gaseous, and papular subtypes. He classifies "certain forms of eczema" as papular inflammatory swellings. Inflammatory swellings are due to a "corporeal change showing that material has been removed from one tissue to another" known as a "catarrh" (Avicenna,

1973). This latter term would appear many times in the literature through the 19th century.

Eczema as a term originated from the Greek word meaning "to bubble, to boil over, or to burst," and it was used by Hippocrates in his writings on disorders of the skin (460–377 B.C.E.), including the *Corpus Hippocraticum* (Alsaidan et al., 2015). Hippocrates had a remarkably advanced understanding of physical exam findings as external manifestations of systemic diseases, including recognition of finger clubbing as a sign of occult lung cancer (Alsaidan et al., 2015). One of his well-cited accounts of an Athenian man "taken by itching over his whole body, but especially on his testicles and forehead" who then developed "lepra (white scale) to the view" and passed away is referred to by some dermatologic historians as a possible instance of AD. Others, however, contend that this case report is more consistent with a presentation of scabies in light of his prescribed regimen of a sulfur bath and subsequent development of "dropsy" or generalized edema and a rapid-onset fulminant outbreak (Norton, 2007; Tilles, Wallach, & Taïeb, 2007).

Italian physician Girolamo Mercuriale (1530–1606 C.E.) published the first modern book on dermatologic conditions, *De Morbis Cutaneis*, which featured accounts of infantile pruritic disorders of the head and neck resembling infantile eczema (Sulzberger, Wise, & Wolf, 1935). In 1763, François Boissier de Sauvages de Lacroix (1706–1767) coined the term *tinea lactea* to describe this skin condition of newborns, and Jean-Louis Alibert further described *teigne muqueuse, achor muqueuse* as precursors to the modern clinical entities of AD and seborrheic dermatitis (Kramer, Strom, Ladizinski, & Lio, 2017). These early French dermatologists adopted an understanding of skin disease in line with Hippocrates' humoral theory in which patients would sometimes be advised that no treatment was necessary because rapidly altering a patient's equilibrium state could do more harm than good.

The 19th century

The 19th century was a time of rapid development in dermatology. In 1801, the opening of the Hôpital Saint-Louis gave way to a wave of influential French dermatologists, including Ernest Henri Besnier who would become the medical director. Besnier coined the term *prurigo diathésique* (Besnier, 1892). A major innovation in the field was the development of a schema for classifying lesions by Robert Willan and Thomas Bateman. Prior to the 19th century, F. B. de Sauvages of Lyon created a simple system of symptom-based features (de Sauvages, 1771). Antoine Charles Lorry (1726–1783) expanded upon this by following in the footsteps of Carl Linnaeus in developing a taxonomic approach to skin lesions using morphology. J. J. R. von Plenck created a system of 14 classes also based on symptoms but without a detailed stratification of subclasses within each larger grouping (von Plenck, 1796). By this point there was much disagreement within the literature as to how to name and classify AD, as no one standard system had yet been agreed upon. As New York dermatologist L. Duncan Bulkley noted: "It is true…the fact that no less than one hundred and twenty Latin names are associated with eczema, by different writers, while the total designations applied to this eruption exceeds one hundred and eighty!" (Bulkley, 1900).

The advent of the Bateman and Willan system and its adoption by dermatologists across the globe allowed for a shared language through which scholars in the field would be able to communicate their findings in a universal manner. Eczema belonged to the "vesicular" or bullous genera in this schema and was defined as an "eruption of minute vesicles, non-contagious, crowded together" in an anatomic distribution that covers the thighs, axilla, and perianal surfaces. Another entity in the Bateman and Willan system that resembles modern AD is *porrigo larvalis willani* (Bateman & Willan, 1817). Literally translated, this term describes a crusted mask that covers the face of the infant. These descriptions are rather fitting as the erythematous and crusting facial lesions of children with the disorder from Bateman and Willan's time accurately depict facial AD as we know it today. Bateman and Willan believed the stimulus for these eruptions was external rather than internal, citing reports of chemicals and sunlight triggering vesicular outbreaks. It is here that their contemporaries would note the broad class of eczema encompassed a distinct entity that 20th-century dermatologists would call dermatitis venenata, or contact dermatitis. One such author, Pierre Rayer, pointed to the "ease and a rapidity" that the lesions we now know as contact dermatitis would abate after removal of the stimulant (Rayer, 1845).

Rayer was the first scholar to distinguish acute and chronic forms of eczema within the Bateman and Willan scheme. He describes three forms of acute eczema (eczema simplex, eczema rubrum, and eczema impetiginodes) as well as chronic eczema (Rayer, 1845). Rayer's eczema simplex featured small clusters of vesicles with red patches covering large surfaces of the body. He distinguishes eczema simplex from the similarly appearing lichen simplex by noting that eczema simplex vesicles are filled with serum that oozes when punctured rather than the more solid lesions of lichen simplex that are productive of blood. Eczema rubrum is a "more intense" eruption with prominent erythema, erysipelas, red serum contained within vesicles, and irregular "jagged border." He paints vivid descriptions of warmth and redness emanating from lesions, with the local inflammation providing a furnace for the eruptions that recur and relapse.

Tormented by pruritus of the most violent description, patients thus affected talk of nothing but heat of blood, inward fires… They cannot forget themselves in sleep; their sufferings, lulled for an instant, often return suddenly and without appreciable cause; nothing can then prevent or moderate the energy with which they begin to scratch themselves; a bloody serum flows from the torn surface of the skin; but, nothing assuaged, the pruritus continues as unbearable as before, particularly when the perineum, orifice of the vagina, or verge of

the anus is the part affected; when left to itself, this cruel state often continues for months and even for years
RAYER (1845)

One of Rayer's principal contributions to the understanding of eczema was the description of natural history of the disease. He describes the scabbing of chronic eczema after vesiculopustular eruptions as well as the intriguing relapsing-remitting pattern in patients (Rayer, 1845). Absent, however, from Rayer's characterization of the disease is any mention of associated asthmatic comorbidities.

Sir Erasmus Wilson, a contemporary of Rayer who also recognized the importance of the acute and chronic nature of eczema, hinted at a link between the skin findings of the disease and other elements of the atopic triad. He lectured on the association between eczema and respiratory conditions, including bronchitis. Records from a prominent American botanical remedy journal on treatments for dermatologic conditions cite lectures from Wilson near the end of the 19th century that demonstrate an understanding of the link between eczema and asthmatic conditions: "Eczema…is not infrequently associated with a similar inflammation of the mucous membrane of the air-passages of the lungs, giving rise to bronchitis" (Wilson, 1871). The "sudden increase of the cutaneous inflammation relieving the mucous membrane, and *vice versa;* and this association of bronchitis and eczema is sometimes maintained during the entire lifetime of the individual" (Wilson, 1871).

Wilson also contributed to a better understanding of infantile eczema, noting that children developed lesions that commonly affected "the scalp, the eyelids, the ears, particularly the backs of the ears, the integument around the mouth, the armpits, the groins, and the ends of elbows, wrists, knees, and ankles" (Wilson, 1871). He defines eczema as "a chronic inflammation attended with desquamation, exudation, and pruritus," with the pruritic skin lesions becoming thick and forming "condensation of the integument" in a manner similar to the scaly lesions of psoriasis. In fact, Wilson lectured on his interpretation of psoriasis as a natural progression of eczema known as "chronic eczema squamosum" (Wilson, 1871). Wilson also considered pityriasis a chronic form of "exhausted eczema" after a change in the quality of skin tissue to form "excessive abundance of minute micaceous scales, and excessive pruritus" (Wilson, 1871). For Wilson, "nothing can be more obvious in practice than the transition of an eczema from its more active stages into the chronic condition of a psoriasis on the one hand, or of a pityriasis on the other; and only by violence can their separation be accomplished" (Wilson, 1871).

In Austria, the young dermatologist Ferdinand von Hebra conducted the first modern experiments establishing that a subtype of eczema developed after chemical or mechanical irritation of the skin (Finnerud, 1952). He demonstrated that stimulation of the pubic region with the *Arnica* plant could yield eruptions on the face and distant regions. A passionate teacher, von Hebra also sought to train a future generation of physicians specialized in dermatology and requested the Austrian government to appoint him the title of lecturer on skin disease. He founded the Vienna General Hospital's dermatologic service and trained multiple prominent dermatologists, including Heinrich Köebner, Carl Auspitz, and Moritz Kaposi. Dissatisfied with Bateman and Willan's lack of an etiologic basis for classification of disease, he sought to understand the mechanisms of common skin ailments. His first great accomplishment was the publication of a paper establishing the *Sarcoptes* mite as the infectious cause of scabies. von Hebra was noted to state: "Never abandon a case as hopeless, but continue to study it on the basis of knowledge of its pathology and etiology until you find some way to help." As a result of his investigations into the nature of eczema, von Hebra introduced the term *mycosis sive eczema exurarum* into the literature (Finnerud, 1952). This term was not adopted in his era, but later 20th-century dermatologists would continue to explore a link with fungal infections. von Hebra's "constitutional prurigo" featuring an infantile disease of urticarial rash with pruritic papules closely approximated contemporary accounts of infantile eczema but differed in subtle yet controversial ways. von Hebra maintained that his eponymous prurigo affected extensor surfaces as well as flexural ones, generating debate for decades about the proper place of this disease entity in the annals of dermatologic literature (Zavaleta & Mom, 1948), noting that "…in people affected by prurigo, few of the lower extremities are especially pointed in the direction of extension; it is to a lesser degree on the side of the flexion and by no means in the articular folds the pigmentation is pronounced in intense prurigo, it is not very marked in light prurigo" (von Hebra & Kaposi, 1872). He also associated this form of skin disease to certain social classes, namely the poor, the Jewish, and those of lower social rungs.

In 1885, Chicago physician Henry T. Byford proposed an understanding of infantile eczema pathogenesis related to ineffective waste processing by the liver in a case series of children in the rash (Byford, 1885). This theory was popular in the literature, with Chicago physician L Duncan Bulkley noting the infantile eczema rash was not linked to common irritating agents that infants commonly are exposed to, such as "irritating diaper-linen, harsh bandages" since "the disease very frequently does not get well upon removal of these irritants" (Bulkley, 1881). Bulkley believed there was a psychosomatic trigger to outbreaks of eczema, classifying "neurotic eczema" as a subtype seen in many of his patients.

An unmarried lady, aged 53 years, was the executive officer of a charitable institution, and her duties were arduous and exacting. On Tuesday of each week she was particularly tried on account of the weekly meeting and inspection of a board of lady visitors, and that night was often sleepless. Her eczema of the face and hands was always aggravated on the succeeding morning; indeed, the eruption, which would often yield very satisfactorily to treatment during the week would burst out afresh on the Wednesday morning succeeding the visit

BULKLEY (1891)

He also wrote of the link between eczema and asthma, noting that the comorbidity of bronchial hyperreactivity disorders in his dermatology patients suggested there was "a condition of the pulmonary mucous tract similar to that found on the skin in eczema" (Bulkley, 1881). Importantly, he also evaluated his patients for an association between eczema and diseases of the lung parenchyma and concluded that "lung diseases cannot be said to be associated with eczema in any important manner…patients with eczema are as a rule free from lung trouble; except the asthmatic complications before alluded to" (Bulkley, 1881). Like other 19th-century dermatologists, he distinguished between the "simple inflammation of the skin, as from heat, poison ivy, etc." known at the time as "dermatitis" from true eczema based on history and cessation of the skin eruption with removal of the stimulus. He noted that masquerading lesions that had been used interchangeably in earlier dermatologic literature, including prurigo, which less often involves the flexural surfaces compared to eczema and seldom features "sharp, inflammatory character, and irregular distribution of papules" (Bulkley, 1881). Bulkley's works shed light on prognosis of different forms of eczema, with accounts of easily treatable acute vesicular eruptions and recalcitrant forms of eczema that involved the palms. Though eczema shared features of other forms of dermatitis caused by scabies and irritants, there were constitutional features Bulkley could not pinpoint that hinted at a systemic illness similar to "gout and rheumatism" rather than merely a local inflammatory reaction of the skin (Bulkley, 1881). This final point was controversial in the literature, as an opposing school of thought held that eczema in all forms derived from a local infection of the skin rather than a systemic illness.

The mid-to-late 19th century saw the emergency of the "toxin principle" and the theory that AD was a manifestation of internal disease—much like the Hippocratic view of disease popular throughout much of Europe. Proponents of this theory, including Philippe Gaucher, believed that eczema was the manifestation of the body trying to eliminate toxins that caused various internal diseases, and attempts to treat it could lead to "driving in the disease" (Morris, 1894). He believed that treatment of AD in children was especially dangerous. Louis-Anne-Jean Brocq, a French contemporary, thought it dangerous to treat lesions in those who are "aged, gouty, arthritic, or asthmatic," noting that "in treating their eczema too energetically one may, indeed, determine the appearance of the gravest pulmonary or even cerebral congestions" (Van Harlingen, 1889). Proponents of this school of thought held the prevailing opinion that AD should not be treated in most cases. However, not all contemporaries of Gaucher and Brocq agreed. Wilson (1871) opined that "eczema infantile, when left to itself, has no natural tendency to resolution or spontaneous cure; on the contrary, it merges progressively into a chronic form."

Near the end of the 19th century some physicians were starting to place more emphasis on determining the cause and exact etiology of AD. Morris thought of AD as having either a parasitic or neurologic etiology, and he noted that the field needed to investigate the true cause of AD to guide therapeutic choices. In 1891, Brocq and Lucien Jacquet introduced "neurodermite diffuse" into the literature to describe what would become known in the English literature as the neurodermatoses. In modern medical literature these are closer to the skin-picking disorders in the *Diagnostic and Statistical Manual of Mental Disorders*, Fifth Edition. Brocq describes the lesions as lichenified plaques that appear at flexural aspects of the knees and elbows. They presented in two forms: disseminated and localized. Features that were characteristic of this disease of the nervous and cutaneous organ systems included neuropsychiatric symptoms such as mood lability, depression, and hyperesthesia (Rudikoff, 2014). Later, 20th-century dermatologists, including Fred Wise, note that these lesions are not histologically or morphologically consistent with true eczema and that some of Brocq's descriptions are more in line with outbreaks of psoriasis and pityriasis rubra pilaris (Wise & Wolf, 1938). Nonetheless, neurodermatitis and associated terms would be used interchangeably in the literature with descriptions of various eczematous disorders by prominent authors until the consolidation of terminology in the mid-20th century.

German physician Paul Gerson Unna ended the century with a histopathologic approach to the study of cutaneous disease that sought to link all clinical features with microscopic and laboratory findings. Through histologic assessments of AD, he determined that "the essential cause of [AD] is the inoculation of a germ" (Stelwagon, 1891). Unna differentiated AD into two entities: the first resembling the rash of "staphylogenic impetigo" pathologically driven by "bacteria—the morococci of eczema" and the second appearing as "much more multiform" and due to "ever-increasing congestion of leucocytes and serous transudation" (Unna & Walker, 1896). Remarkably, these findings occurred a century before the field reexamined the role of *Staphylococcus aureus* colonization and AD.

The 20th century

The early 20th century saw the continued exploration of old ideas and a slow convergence of overlapping definitions of AD with emerging theories of a new pathophysiology grounded in advances in allergy and immunology. Dermatologist L. Duncan Bulkley (mentioned earlier) led the American clinical research efforts with his case series of thousands of patients with the affliction. He defined "true eczema" in a 1901 manuscript as "an acute or chronic, noncontagious, inflammatory, polymorphous, constitutional disease of the skin, accompanied with itching and burning" that was distinct from the features of simple dermatitis caused by identifiable irritants such as poison ivy or mechanical abrasion (Jamieson, 1901).

Bulkley's theories on neurotic eczema persisted into the new century, with several investigators continuing to explore neuropsychiatric manifestations of the disease. A narrative study of 88 patients seen at Massachusetts General Hospital, including 32 with AD, found "patients with atopic dermatitis show psychoneurotic symptoms more frequently than do the patients with lupus erythematosus or normal controls" though less than the psychoneurotic group in frequency (Greenhill & Finesinger, 1942). The authors noted a "definite correlation between events which evoked feelings of anger and depression and exacerbations of the eruption in the patients with atopic dermatitis" (Greenhill & Finesinger, 1942).

Arthur Hall published the first major 20th-century treatise on infantile eczema in his 1905 thesis and later 1907 *British Journal of Dermatology* manuscript. These pieces reviewed the major theories of etiology, including the digestive school of thought, the external irritant theory, traumatic origins of eczema, the "external irritants of infancy," the neurocutaneous theory, and "eczema as a (protective) cutaneous reaction" (Hall, 1905). Hall appeared to be most intrigued by the gastrointestinal theory, noting that cases of eczema seldom occurred during the summer months when diseases of the gastrointestinal tract flourished. He drew attention to the trend of eruptions of skin irritation in his patients predominantly during the winter months. "What is generally called eczema, whether it occurs in infants or adults, is a form of reaction or response of the neurocutaneous apparatus to external irritation," noted Hall. Chicago physician Samuel Feinberg further explored possible associations with seasonal changes, publishing a report on patients who presented with symptoms during the "mold season" between June and November (Feinberg, 1939). Many of these patients also were allergic to several species of pollen and fungi.

At this point, the field was crowded with competing classifications and disease mechanisms, with Sutton aptly stating in his 1928 textbook, "[T]he fact remains that eczema is only a sort of dermatological scrap-heap out of which, from time to time, certain diseases that present a characteristic and definite symptomatology are extracted." This quickly changed after a series of innovations in the emergent field of allergy and immunology, which as a term was first introduced by Von Pirquet in 1911. An important development was the creation of the patch test assay by Joseph Jadassohn in 1895, first presented at the Fifth Congress of the German Society of Dermatology (Lazzarini, Duarte, & Ferreira, 2013).

The first major paper in the field of allergy and eczema was a case series by Towle and Talbot (1912) showing association between eczema and indigestion. The authors noted a close relationship between outbreaks of skin findings and changes in stool consistency as determined by gross and microscopic analysis. In most cases, the skin changes were very prototypical vesicular eczematous eruptions primarily affecting the head and lower abdomen. These eruptions came in two types (exudative-predominant and nonexudative processes) with the time span between prodromal symptoms and full eruptions varying from patient to patient. American pediatrician Kenneth Blackfan was inspired by these experiments and the work of Felix Mendel and Henry Lee Smith. He applied Mendel's previously developed skin antigen assay to study whether animal proteins generated an allergic response in eczema patients. In a landmark 1916 paper, Blackfan put his theory of an eczema protein "idiosyncracy" to the test. Of subjects exposed to cutaneous injections of various animal proteins, only 1 of 43 test subjects without a history of eczema demonstrated a positive protein antigen response compared to 22 of 27 patients with eczema. He noted that "a history of eczema in early life is nearly always the rule with patients who are unable to take different foods, such as eggs, shell-fish, pork, etc., on account of urticaria and edema and sometimes asthma" whereas patients without a history of eczema rarely had positive reactions to protein antigen exposure. Chandler Walker demonstrated in 1918 that this association between eczema and allergic responses was not limited to food protein but also applied to proteins obtained from horse dandruff, ragweed, and pollen. Walker (1918) noted that a small amount of externally or internally applied proteins paradoxically improved the disease symptoms in eczema patients, though past a certain threshold exposure to increasing amounts of protein exacerbated the disease.

Coca and Cooke (1923) first adopted the term *atopy* in the medical literature after consulting philologist Edward Perry for help in describing a pathologic entity that was appropriately deemed "strange" in Greek terms. They explicitly defined several features of the peculiar nonanaphylactic type of hypersensitivity reaction known as atopy, including the characteristic of being "greatly lessened but not completely removed by the suitable injection of the active substance." Though atopy shared features with anaphylaxis and infectious hypersensitivity, all three types of reactions were clearly distinct from "non-antigenic" reactions of dermatitis venenata caused by irritants such as poison ivy (Coca & Cooke, 1923).

Sulzberger and Wise developed the first modern definition of AD. Nine features listed by the authors included a family history of atopy, prior infantile eczema, locations of skin lesions at the elbow and knee flexural folds as well as neck, chest, and face, gray-brown lesions, no true vesicles, irritability with vasomotor agitation, negative patch test results, positive prick tests and intradermal tests, and serum positivity (Wise & Sulzberger, 1933). Five years later Osborne and Walker (1938) developed their own list of diagnostic criteria, including family history of allergy, association with reaction to specific foods, age at onset, and stereotypical location of skin lesions that included ankles, wrists, and cheeks. These pioneering experiments demonstrated that certain substances could provoke the eczematous reaction in individuals with a predisposition. In a 1939 review, Feinberg declared "atopic dermatitis" was now the commonly accepted term in the literature for what had formerly been known by a variety of names ranging from neurodermatitis to eczema. Wise and Wolf (1938) published lectures contained very familiar descriptions of the disease entity appearing first in infants and affecting the antecubital and popliteal fossa, wrists, and face all with positive responses to the Prausnitz-Küstner antibody test. Interestingly, Wise and Wolf continued to use separate terms to define infantile eczema from AD despite noting that the two disease forms only differ in subtle ways while sharing the same broad clinical and histologic traits.

Toward the latter 20th century, researchers strived to develop precise and replicable methods of diagnosing AD. The fruit of these labors was a set of criteria from Hanifin and Rajka published in 1980 that defined AD as requiring at least three of the following major features: pruritus, flexural lichenification or linearity in adults, facial and extensor involvement in children, chronic or chronically relapsing dermatitis, and a personal or family history of atopy. It required at least 3 of 23 originally defined minor features as well (Hanifin, 1980). These criteria were further honed by the UK Working Party in 1994, who validated their diagnostic criteria through a study of patients from nine centers. Their criteria required itchy skin in addition to three of the following five criteria: history of involvement of the flexor skin folds, personal history of atopy (asthma or allergic rhinitis), generally dry skin in the last year, visible flexural eczema, and onset under the age of 2 years (for children ≥4 years) (Williams, Burney, Pembroke, & Hay, 1994). The UK Working Party's criteria have been validated in other populations (Brenninkmeijer, Schram, Leeflang, Bos, & Spuls, 2008) and have since become the de facto standard for diagnosis of AD today.

Historical approaches to the treatment of eczema

Hippocrates approached treatment of dermatologic disease with the philosophy that the opposite of what the lesion's characteristics were should be applied as a counterbalance (e.g., for moist lesions he would prescribe a drying agent and for dry he would suggest an emollient) (Alsaidan et al., 2015). Hippocrates was also a proponent of the humoral approach to medicine (i.e., the theory that human disease is the result of imbalance of the four humors: blood, phlegm, yellow bile, and black bile). Practitioners of the humoral theory believed that AD was the body's attempt to right any imbalances in the four humors, and thus interventions could only interfere with the healing process. This theory continued to influence many 19th-century dermatologists, particularly French physicians such as Alibert, Brocq, and Gaucher (Stelwagon, 1916). The French school of dermatology viewed treatment of eczema as "constitutional," involving multiple modalities, including but not limited to medicine, diet, and exposure to the outdoors (Stelwagon, 1916).

Erasmus Wilson was an early advocate of treatment of AD and other cutaneous pathologies, breaking from the humoral approach to medicine that was popular in his time. He differentiated cutaneous diseases into acute and chronic forms, providing different treatments for these different forms. For chronic AD, he applied his "law of treatment of cutaneous disease," which contained three key principles for the treatment of infantile eczema: "elimination, restoration of power, and alleviation of local distress" (Wilson, 1871). For elimination, he recommended a solution of calomel (see later for discussion) with white sugar or milk; for alleviation of local distress, he recommended "benzoated ointment of the oxide of zinc"; and he recommended arsenic as a last step for the somewhat oddly termed "restoration of power." von Hebra was another early advocate of treatment of AD; he suggested the use of treatments such as "oily or fatty [emollients]" and would add "mercury, zinc, lead, copper, iodine, arsenic, sulphur... [or] tar in cases of eczema" (von Hebra, Fagge, Pye-Smith, Kaposi, & Tay, 1866). Though tar was used by many 19th- and early 20th-century dermatologists dating back two millennia to Dioscorides, it was not systematically studied as a treatment modality until Downing and Bauer's landmark 1948 paper characterizing 600 subjects receiving tar for eczema and psoriasis. They compared coal tars of different types and manufactured at different temperatures, noting that all performed with roughly similar clinical efficacy (Downing & Bauer, 1948). By the mid-20th century, tar was deemed to be an effective adjunct treatment for AD. Tar was viewed favorably for subtypes of "dry sluggish" eczema and continued to be prescribed well into the modern era.

Around the same time, Rayer (1845) developed a three-fold principle of treatment with the components of "regimen, rest, and time." He was rather conservative with prescribing medication, noting that many mild cases of eczema simply resolved after "changing the nurse" who was attending the patient on the ward or following a sudden change in a person's diet (Rayer, 1845). Rather skeptical of many concoctions used by his contemporaries, he appeared to adopt a "do no harm" strategy for mild cases. Among his treatment arsenal were emollients for localized lesions, soothing ointments such as oxide of zinc and protochloride of mercury for "furfuraceous" or flaky lesions, and blood-letting for severe eruptions of eczema rubrum (Rayer, 1845). Byford (1885) describes a case series of infantile eczema eruptions of the scalp treated with topical calomel. Calomel, or mercury(I) chloride, was popular in 19th-century medicine in the United States and England for a variety of illnesses, including syphilis, gout, tuberculosis, and malignancy. Unfortunately, high doses of oral calomel led to severe side effects of mercury poisoning, including stomatitis and gastrointestinal complaints of vomiting and bloody diarrhea (Bufford & Lane, 1915). In the tradition of the French school of dermatology, Byford (1885) also noted that in many cases "a properly regulated diet is necessary, and in some cases is all that need be recommended."

At the start of the 20th century, dermatologic textbooks contained lengthy lists of tinctures and remedies for controlling symptoms of AD. Arsenic was a popular agent used in severe cases of infantile eczema. Bulkley (1900) noted the "almost specific control which arsenic will have over eczema in small children," but also noted "it seems to have less effect on the disease after the age of 5 years." Bulkley (1900) stated a "tumblerful of milk, slightly warmed, one

hour before each meal, followed if possible, by a rest of half an hour in a darkened room" was efficacious for AD, and particularly in neurotic eczema. He also wrote of topical, "local" treatments, including Lassar paste (composed of zinc oxide) and gelatin-glycerin preparations, which were often added to camphor, salicyclic acid, or resorcinol—common therapies used in many cutaneous ailments at the time. Other topical compounds such as picric acid and potassium permanganate were noted to provide relief of pruritus with AD (Bulkley, 1900).

Later works by Morris contradicted Bulkley's work, stating "[one must] clear one's mind of the notion that arsenic or any other drug is specific" to AD (Morris, 1894). He categorized treatments as internal remedies or local therapies and recommended tailoring treatments to the individual's disease rather than the use of static treatment regimens for all patients. Among internal treatments, Morris (1894) recommended antimony, calomel, quinine, strychnine, ergot, belladonna (atropine), and sedatives such as opium, along with light clothing and "complete rest, both of mind and body." For local treatments, he recommended the use of creams and pastes containing ingredients such as salicylic acid, zinc oxide, and petroleum jelly, only after the "removal of all crusts and scales that prevent the free access of the remedy to the seat of the disease" (Morris, 1894). Other physicians, such as Henry Boenning, recommended the use of topical treatments for AD. He detailed a case of a young patient successfully treated with "sulphur ointment with carbonic acid to be applied twice daily over the thickened skin and the papules, preceding the application by a hot bath" (Boenning, 1882). For pruritus refractory to arsenic, Wise and Wolf (1938) recommended exposing the afflicted lesion to roentgen rays as a last resort.

Despite 20th-century progress in understanding the link between allergy and eczema, food and antigen-based treatment modalities were noted by early dermatologists to be ineffective. Wise and Wolf (1938) conceded that "little can be done to influence the atopic state" by targeting specific allergens that triggered disease flares in patients. Feinberg (1939) wondered if this puzzling nonresponse phenomenon suggested a missing link in the atopy theory as a whole, asking "is it not logical to assume that the general concept of allergy is probably correct but that the specific exciting cause is missed?"

Summary

Despite a careful examination of the history of eczema, it remains unclear whether many of the trends over the centuries in classification reflect changes in nosology and disease understanding rather than actual changes in the entity itself. It is possible that, like cultures, languages, and species, diseases undergo alterations over time, such that our modern version of eczema may differ significantly from what was described millennia ago. It may also be the case that with changes in lifestyle and available therapies, the contemporary milieu significantly alters the presentation and natural history of some diseases.

Regardless, an undeniable—if bumpy at times—progression toward a broader and deeper understanding of eczema is now evident. Particularly in the past few decades, we have witnessed an explosion in both scientific understanding and therapeutic innovations, built on the long and fascinating history of this persistent, itchy malady.

Further readings

Bhattacharya, T., Strom, M. A., & Lio, P. A. (2016). Historical perspectives on atopic dermatitis: Eczema through the ages. *Pediatric Dermatology, 33*(4), 375–379.

Everett, M. A., Loser, C., Plewig, G., & Burgdorf, W. H. (2013). *Pantheon of dermatology: Outstanding historical figures.* Springer-Verlag.

Kramer, O. N., Strom, M. A., Ladizinski, B., & Lio, P. A. (2017). The history of atopic dermatitis. *Clinics in Dermatology, 35*(4), 344–348.

References

Adamson, P. B. (1988). Some infective and allergic conditions in ancient Mesopotamia. *Revue d'Assyriologie et d'Archeologie Orientale, 82*(2), 163–171.

Alsaidan, M., Simmons, B. J., Bray, F. N., Falto-Aizpurua, L. A., Griffith, R. D., & Nouri, K. (2015). Hippocrates' contributions to dermatology revealed. *JAMA Dermatology, 151*(6), 658.

Atarzadeh, F., Heydari, M., Sanaye, M. R., & Amin, G. (2016). Avicenna—A pioneer in dermatology. *JAMA Dermatology, 152*(11), 1257. https://doi.org/10.1001/jamadermatol.2016.0026.

Avicenna. (1973). In O. C. Gruner (Ed.), *The canon of medicine.* AMS Press.

Bateman, T., & Willan, R. (1817). *Delineations of cutaneous diseases: Exhibiting the characteristic appearances of the principal genera and species comprised in the classification of the late Dr. Willan and completing the series of engravings begun by that author.* Longman, Hurst, Rees, Orme, and Brown.

Besnier, E. (1892). Première note et observations préliminaires pour servir d'introduction à l'étude des prurigos diathésiques (dermatites multiformes prurigineuses chroniques exacerbantes et paroxystiques, du type du prurigo de Hebra). *Annals of Dermatology Syphilis, 3,* 634–648.

Bhattacharya, T., Strom, M. A., & Lio, P. A. (2016). Historical perspectives on atopic dermatitis: Eczema through the ages. *Pediatric Dermatology, 33*(4), 375–379. https://doi.org/10.1111/pde.12853.

Blackfan, K. D. (1916). Cutaneous reaction from proteins in eczema. *American Journal of Diseases of Children, 11*(6), 441–454.

Boenning, H. C. (1882). A case of prurigo. *Philadelphia Medical Times, 12,* 519.

Brenninkmeijer, E. E. A., Schram, M. E., Leeflang, M. M. G., Bos, J. D., & Spuls, Ph. I. (2008). Diagnostic criteria for atopic dermatitis: A systematic review. *British Journal of Dermatology, 158*(4), 754–765. https://doi.org/10.1111/j.1365-2133.2007.08412.x.

Brocq, L., & Jacquet, L. (1891). Notes pour servir à l'histoire des névrodermites. Du lichen circumscriptus des anciens auteurs, ou lichen simplex chronique de M. le Dr E. Vidal. G. Masson.

Brodsky, M., Abrouk, M., Lee, P., & Kelly, K. M. (2017). Revisiting the history and importance of phototherapy in dermatology. *JAMA Dermatology, 153*(5), 435.

Bufford, J. H., & Lane, C. G. (1915). Calomel poisoning: A case of some value to our fellow practitioners. *The Journal of the American Medical Association, 65*(2), 161.

Bulkley, L. D. (1881). *Eczema and its management: A practical treatise based on the study of 2,500 cases of the disease.* GP Putnam's Sons.

Bulkley, L. D. (1891). *On the relation of eczema to disturbances of the nervous system, the medical news.* Henry C. Lea's Son.

Bulkley, L. D. (1900). Recent advances in dermatology which are of service to the general practitioner. *The Journal of the American Medical Association, 36*(13), 853–858.

Byford, H. T. (1885). Observations on the cause and treatment of infantile exzema and allied eruption. *The Journal of the American Medical Association, 12,* 317–318.

Coca, A. F., & Cooke, R. A. (1923). On the classification of the phenomena of hypersensitiveness. *The Journal of Immunology, 8*(3), 163–182.

de Sauvages, F. B. (1771). Nosologie méthodique: Dans laquelle les maladies sont rangées par classes, suivant le système de Sydenham, et l'ordre des botanists (vol. 2). chez Hérissant.

Downing, J. G., & Bauer, C. W. (1948). Low and high temperature coal tars in the treatment of eczema and psoriasis: A clinical investigation and evaluation. *Archives of Dermatology and Syphilology, 57*(6), 985–990.

El-Domyati, M., & Attia, E. (2015). The history of dermatology, venereology and dermatopathology in different countries—Egypt. *Global Dermatology, 2,* S34–S38.

Feinberg, S. M. (1939). Seasonal atopic dermatitis: The role of inhalant atopens. *Archives of Dermatology and Syphilology, 40*(2), 200–207.

Finnerud, C. W. (1952). Ferdinand von Hebra and the Vienna School of Dermatology. *AMA Archives of Dermatology and Syphilology, 66*(2), 223–232.

Friedman, R. (1930). Eczema—To be or not to be. *Archives of Dermatology and Syphilology, 22*(2), 244–267.

Greenhill, M. H., & Finesinger, J. E. (1942). Neurotic symptoms and emotional factors in atopic dermatitis. *Archives of Dermatology and Syphilology, 46*(2), 187–200.

Hall, A. J. (1905). *An enqiry into the etiology of infantile eczema.* University of Cambridge.

Hanifin, J. M., & Rajka, G. (1980). Diagnostic features of atopic dermatitis. *Acta Dermato-Venereologica, 92(Suppl),* 44–47.

Jamieson, W. A. (1901). Eczema, with an analysis of eight thousand cases. *Edinburgh Medical Journal, 10*(5), 460.

Kramer, O. N., Strom, M. A., Ladizinski, B., & Lio, P. A. (2017). The history of atopic dermatitis. *Clinics in Dermatology, 35*(4), 344–348.

Lazzarini, R., Duarte, I., & Ferreira, A. L. (2013). Patch tests. *Anais Brasileiros de Dermatologia, 88*(6), 879–888.

Liddell, K. (2006). Skin disease in antiquity. *Clinical Medicine, 6*(1), 81.

Mier, P. D. (1975). Earliest description of the atopic syndrome? *British Journal of Dermatology, 92*(3), 359.

Morris, M. A. (1894). *Diseases of the skin: An outline of the principles and practice of dermatology.* Cassell.

Norton, S. A. (2007). What caused the Athenian itch in Hippocrates' on epidemics? *Journal of the American Academy of Dermatology, 57*(6), 1093–1094.

Osborne, E. D., & Walker, H. L. (1938). Contact and environmental allergens as a cause of eczema in infants and in children. *Archives of Dermatology and Syphilology, 38*(4), 511–525.

Rayer, P. F. O. (1845). *A theoretical and practical treatise on the diseases of the skin.* Carey and Hart.

Ring, J. (1985). 1st description of an "atopic family anamnesis" in the Julio-Claudian imperial house: Augustus, Claudius. Britannicus.

Rudikoff, D. (2014). The history of eczema and atopic dermatitis. In: *Atopic dermatitis and eczematous disorders* (pp. 11–24). CRC Press.

Scurlock, J. A., & Andersen, B. (2010). *Diagnoses in Assyrian and Babylonian medicine: Ancient sources, translations, and modern medical analyses.* University of Illinois Press.

Stelwagon, H. W. (1916). *A treatise on diseases of the skin: For advanced students and practitioners.* W.B. Saunders Company.

Stelwagon, L. (1891). Prurigo infantum; psoriasis-eczema; primary pigmented sarcoma of the skin; xeroderma pigmentosum; dermatitis herpetiformis. On the nature and treatment of eczema. *American Journal of Medical Sciences, 101*(1), 95–96.

Sulzberger, M. B., Wise, F., & Wolf, J. (1935). A tentative classification of allergic dermatoses. *The Journal of the American Medical Association, 104*(17), 1489–1490.

Sutton, R. L. (1928). *Diseases of the skin* (7th ed). CV Mosby Company.

Tilles, G., Wallach, D., & Taïeb, A. (2007). Topical therapy of atopic dermatitis: Controversies from Hippocrates to topical immunomodulators. *Journal of the American Academy of Dermatology, 56*(2), 295–301.

Towle, H. P., & Talbot, F. B. (1912). Infantile eczema and indigestion: Preliminary clinical study with illustrative cases. *American Journal of Diseases of Children, 4*(4), 219–228.

Unna, P. G., & Walker, N. (1896). *The histopathology of the diseases of the skin.* W. F. Clay.

Van Harlingen, A. (1889). Diseases of the skin and syphilis. In C. E. Sajous (Ed.), *Annual of the universal medical sciences.* F. A. Davis.

von Hebra, F., & Kaposi, M. (1872). *Traité des maladies de la peau: Comprenant les exanthèmes aigus* (vol. 1). G. Masson.

von Hebra, F. R., Fagge, C. H., Pye-Smith, P. H., Kaposi, M., & Tay, W. (1866). On diseases of the skin, including the exanthemata. *New Sydenham Society, 1*: 40–41.

Von Pirquet, C. E. (1911). Allergy. *Archives of Internal Medicine, 7*(3), 383–436.

von Plenck, J. J. R. (1796). *Doctrina de morbis cutaneis.* J. F. Van Overbeke.

Walker, C. (1918). Causation of eczema, urticaria and angioneurotic edema: By proteins other than those derived from food: Study XVIII. *The Journal of the American Medical Association, 70*(13), 897–900.

Wigley, J. E. M. (1953). The everlasting eczema: A retrospect. *Australasian Journal of Dermatology, 2*(1), 5–10.

Williams, H. C., Burney, P. G., Pembroke, A. C., & Hay, R. J. (1994). The U.K. Working Party's diagnostic criteria for atopic dermatitis. III. Independent hospital validation. *The British Journal of Dermatology, 131*(3), 406–416. https://doi.org/10.1111/j.1365-2133.1994.tb08532.x.

Wilson, E. (1871). Lectures on dermatology. *British Medical Journal, 1*(535), 332.

Wise, F., & Sulzberger, M. B. (1933). *Year book of dermatology and syphilology* (pp. 38–39). Year Book Publishers.

Wise, F., & Wolf, J. (1938). Eczema and its practical management: Clinical lecture at San Francisco session. *The Journal of the American Medical Association, 111*(23), 2106–2113.

Zavaleta, A. T., & Mom, A. M. (1948). Prurigo of Hebra. *Archives of Dermatology and Syphilology, 57*(6), 998–1008.

2

Atopy Redefined

LAWRENCE S. CHAN

KEY POINTS

- Although the original term *atopy* provides a general framework of understanding about allergic clinical conditions, this big umbrella now includes a group of patients who have heterogeneous clinical and laboratory-defined characteristics. Similarly, *atopic dermatitis*, the skin atopy, characterizes a group of patients with heterogeneous clinical and laboratory-based findings.
- Since the immune milieu in children is a dynamic system, atopic dermatitis manifested in childhood may have a different pathomechanism than those occurring in adulthood.
- The intrinsic subtype of atopic dermatitis, with its absence of an elevation in serum immunoglobulin E (IgE), may differ from the extrinsic subset of atopic dermatitis in pathophysiology, as IgE is a direct product of the important Th2 cytokine interleukin-4 (IL4).
- The atopic dermatitis patients with filaggrin gene mutation may manifest skin disease differently than those patients with intact skin barrier proteins, since skin barrier defect favors easy entry of pathogens and allergens, leading to triggering of cutaneous inflammatory processes.
- The potential pathophysiologic differences of onset age, IgE, and skin barrier protein mutation, together with varied clinical responses to targeted immune modulators, point to the need for redefining atopic dermatitis or for defining specific subsets according to their verified pathomechanisms. Refining atopy will facilitate more accurate and personalized management of atopic dermatitis.

Introduction

In this chapter, we intend to discuss redefining the term *atopy*. Before we begin the process, however, we should first clearly delineate the meaning of the original term. Thus we first ask, What is atopy? and What defines atopy?

According to *Merriam-Webster Dictionary* online, atopy (2019) is "a genetic disposition to develop an allergic reaction (such as allergic rhinitis or asthma) and produce elevated levels of IgE upon exposure to an environmental antigen and especially one inhaled or digested."

Another definition of atopy provided by ScienceDirect (2019) is "a personal and/or familial tendency, usually in childhood or adolescence, to become sensitized and produce IgE antibodies in response to ordinary exposure to allergens, usually proteins."

The American Academy of Allergy, Asthma & Immunology (AAAAI, 2019), an educational and training organization of nearly 7000 members of allergists and immunologists and a trusted information source for patients, states atopy is "the genetic tendency to develop allergic diseases such as allergic rhinitis, asthma and atopic dermatitis (eczema). Atopy is typically associated with heightened immune responses to common allergens, especially inhaled allergens and food allergens".

Historically, atopy was first described by Coca and Cooke in their 1923 article on the classification of hypersensitive phenomena. The term as they introduced it is derived from the Greek words *a* and *topos*, meaning "without" and "place," respectively. They aimed to designate a terminology place for disorders such as hay fever and asthma (Cohen, Dworetzky, & Frick, 2003). While the abovementioned definitions provide a general framework of understanding atopy, detailed evidence, as delineated later in this chapter, points to a need to redefine or to subdivide this diverse group of patients who were currently categorized in the single and large disease entity of atopy. These challenging data include heterogeneous clinical manifestations, existence and nonexistence of skin barrier protein defect, presence and absence of elevated levels of serum IgE, different degrees of altered immune milieu, and favorable and unfavorable clinical responses to targeted immunomodulatory therapy. In this chapter we provide evidence to argue for such a need for redefinition or subdivision, with the focus on skin perspective.

Clear definition of atopic dermatitis

The current lack of uniform clinical definition and objective test that could unequivocally confirm the diagnosis of atopic dermatitis has led to significant differences in determination of disease prevalence, performance of prediction models, and risk factors (Nakamura et al., 2019). The diagnostic criteria proposed by Hanifin and Rajka (1980) was deemed too complicated, and other diagnostic criteria were used in different geographic locations (Bos, van Leent, & Sillevis Smitt, 1998; Williams et al., 1994). Since diagnostic criteria define disease entity, the effect of imperfect definition could result in misleading laboratory and clinical research data.

Childhood-onset versus adult-onset subsets

The immune system in childhood has many differences compared to that in adulthood (Adeli et al., 2015; Georgountzou & Papadopoulos, 2017; Kollmann, Kampmann, Mazmanian, Marchant, & Levy, 2017; Olin et al., 2018; Simon, Hollander, & McMichael, 2015; Valiathan, Ashman, & Asthana, 2016; Vallejo, 2007). First, some immune components are not fully mature during childhood. In particular, many changes occur during the first year of life (Torok et al., 2019). Another difference is that adulthood, compared to childhood, has encountered more immune challenges and developed a lot more immune memories to these challenges, whether they are pathogenic or allergic in nature. As a result, the proportion of antigen-encountered lymphocytes becomes expanded in adults compared to that in childhood, which has a larger percent of naïve lymphocytes (Simon et al., 2015). In addition, we must consider a naturally occurring immune cell "aging" process that renders immune cells more "permissive" later in adult life (Vallejo, 2007). Immunologic parameter studies also point to a dynamic immune milieu occurring in infancy and childhood (Torok et al., 2019). Some known differences between the childhood and adult immune milieu are depicted here. Newborns predominantly rely on maternal circulation-containing antibodies for their immune defense, but over the first few months of life their thymus pours out substantial amounts of T cells, which become various subsets over the next few years (Olin et al., 2018; Simon et al., 2015). The CD4+ and CD8+ T cells in the peripheral blood increase from childhood to adulthood with an interesting decrease of B cells (Valiathan et al., 2016). The reduction of peripheral B cells in adulthood may simply reflect a greater entry of those cells from peripheral blood into the solid lymphoid organs (Torok et al., 2019). On the contrary, monocytes, NK cells, and regulatory T cells are decreasing from early childhood to adulthood (Adeli et al., 2015; Georgountzou & Papadopoulos, 2017; Simon et al., 2015). The differences between childhood and adult immune milieu are manifested not only in cell number but also in cell function. The innate immunity in the early postnatal period, for example, is represented by NK cells predominantly in cytokine-producing mode rather than in cytotoxic activities (Georgountzou & Papadopoulos, 2017). Responses to toll-like receptor stimulation are lower early in life (Georgountzou & Papadopoulos, 2017; Kollmann et al., 2017). IL10, one of the Th2 cytokines important in atopic dermatitis development, is higher in early infancy. Interestingly, the IL10 level decreases to a level below the adult's during infancy but then increases again until it reaches adult level (Georgountzou & Papadopoulos, 2017). So in theory, immune-mediated diseases that have onset during childhood differ from those that have onset during adulthood in terms of the immune system's ability to handle certain challenges and how the immune system responds to challenges, at least from an immunologic perspective. Even if childhood atopic dermatitis persists into adulthood, the different adult immune milieu could still modify the disease to some extent. Therefore appropriate treatments for childhood-onset disease may need to tailor-suit the immature and dynamic nature of immune milieu in the childhood, and the same for the adult-onset disease.

Intrinsic versus extrinsic subsets

Although, historically, all patients affected by atopic dermatitis are considered uniformly extrinsic, with a common finding of elevated serum IgE level, subsequently the concept of intrinsic atopic dermatitis, which characterizes a subgroup of patients who do not have abnormally high total serum IgE level or antigen-specific IgE, emerges (Ott et al., 2009; Roguedas-Contios & Misery, 2011; Schnopp, Grosch, Ring, Ollert, & Mempel, 2008). The robustness of this intrinsic form of atopic dermatitis is unsettled. While some academicians have named this intrinsic form of disease "nonallergic atopic dermatitis" or "atopiform dermatitis," other academic physicians did not utilize the same criteria to define this subtype of dermatitis in their clinical investigations (Bos, 2002; Bos et al., 1998, 2010; Roguedas-Contios & Misery, 2011). Some academic physicians argued that this intrinsic form of skin inflammation may not necessarily be atopic at all and that the term *atopiform* dermatitis would be more appropriate since atopiform will not indicate the disease as atopic or atopy, per se (Bos, 2002; Bos et al., 2010).

Since the Th2 cytokine IL4 is a prerequisite for IgE production in humans and a high IgE level could point to an upregulation of IL4, patients with intrinsic atopic dermatitis and a normal level of IgE may not have a prominently altered immune system that manifests with IL4 upregulation (Kuhn, Rajewsky, & Muller, 1991). So in theory, the patients affected by intrinsic atopic dermatitis may have had no altered internal immune milieu or have an altered immune milieu other than IL4 upregulation. From the clinical data, the intrinsic patients are primarily female and are the significant majority in infant atopic dermatitis (Roguedas-Contios & Misery, 2011). On the genetic level, a higher percentage of patients with extrinsic atopic dermatitis have IL4/IL13 receptor polymorphism, whereas a higher percentage of patients with intrinsic counterpart have β_2-adrenergic receptor polymorphism, probably implicating weakened adrenergic responses in intrinsic patients (Novak et al., 2002; Roguedas et al., 2006). In a study completed in 2000, the phenotypes of epidermal dendritic cells between these atopic subtypes were found to have some differences. Specifically, the expression of Fc epsilon RI in

TABLE 2.1	Differential characteristics between intrinsic and extrinsic atopic dermatitis	
Characteristics	**Intrinsic atopic dermatitis**	**Extrinsic atopic dermatitis**
Onset	Mostly infant onset	Variable
Patient gender	Mostly females	Both males and females
Serum IgE level	Normal	Upregulated
Tissue eosinophilia	Less numerous than extrinsic	More numerous than intrinsic
IL4/IL13 receptor		
Polymorphism	Lower percentage than extrinsic	Higher percentage than intrinsic
β_2-Adrenergic receptor		
Polymorphism	Higher percentage than extrinsic	Lower percentage than intrinsic
FcεRI in CD1a+		
Dendritic cells	Lower upregulation than extrinsic	Higher upregulation than intrinsic
IL4 (skin)	Upregulated, equal to extrinsic	Upregulated, equal to intrinsic
IL10 (skin)	Upregulated, equal to extrinsic	Upregulated, equal to intrinsic
IL1β (skin)	Upregulated, lower than extrinsic	Upregulated, higher than intrinsic
IL5 (skin)	Upregulated, lower than extrinsic	Upregulated, higher than intrinsic
IL13 (skin)	Upregulated, lower than extrinsic	Upregulated, higher than intrinsic
Th17 immune		
Activation	Higher than extrinsic	Lower than intrinsic
Contact allergens	More frequent to nickel and cobalt than extrinsic	Less frequent to nickel and cobalt than intrinsic

CD1a+ dendritic cells of extrinsic atopic dermatitis is significantly higher than that of intrinsic counterpart (Oppel et al., 2000).

The study of in vivo cytokine mRNA expressions did indeed reveal some differences between the skin of patients with intrinsic atopic dermatitis, compared to that of patients with extrinsic atopic dermatitis. The number of dermal eosinophil infiltration and the cytokine levels of IL5, IL13, and IL1β were higher in the skin of extrinsic atopic dermatitis patients than that of intrinsic atopic dermatitis patients, although these cytokine levels from both groups of patients were higher than normal subjects without atopic dermatitis. Interestingly, IL4 and IL10, the two major Th2 cytokines involved in atopic dermatitis development, were equally elevated in the skin of both groups of atopic dermatitis patients compared to normal subjects without atopic dermatitis (Jeong et al., 2003). In addition, peripheral blood count of eosinophils, serum eosinophil cationic protein level, and IL5 were higher or more detectable in patients with extrinsic atopic dermatitis, compared to those with intrinsic atopic dermatitis, which further supports the eosinophil differential between these two subsets (Park et al., 2006).

Another study pointed out that intrinsic atopic dermatitis patients tend to have higher sweat concentrations of nickel and a correspondingly higher frequency of positive patch test to nickel, compared to the extrinsic atopic dermatitis patients. These intrinsic patients also have greater

frequency of having cobalt allergy by patch test (Yamaguchi et al., 2013). From the perspective of contact allergen reaction, it is probably not appropriate to name an intrinsic form of atopic dermatitis as nonallergic atopic dermatitis (Bos et al., 1998). A study completed in 2013 showed that the patients affected with the intrinsic form of atopic dermatitis exhibited higher Th17 immune activation compared to those with extrinsic counterpart, although the Th2 immune activation is similar between the subtypes (Suarez-Farinas et al., 2013). The presence of clinical and immunologic differences between these two subtypes of dermatitis suggests a somewhat different pathophysiology between them. However, to definitively sort out these differences, the academic community would need to reach consensus criteria on various subtypes to guide subsequent clinical and translational investigations that will lead to improved understanding of the disease. The differential characteristics between these two subsets are depicted in Table 2.1.

Filaggrin-defect versus filaggrin-intact subsets

The key genetic mutation in association with atopic dermatitis is the loss-of-function mutation of the key skin barrier protein filaggrin, a stratum corneum component (see Chapter 11). Although this is highly relevant, and it is highly prevalent in Europe, affecting nearly 50% of the atopic dermatitis patients, it is not so prevalent in Asia or Africa. Only 10% to 20% atopic dermatitis patients in Asia have one or more filaggrin mutations (Nomura et al., 2008; Park, Park, Seok, Li, & Seo, 2016). In patients of African descent, the picture is somewhat muddy. Although atopy is disproportionally affecting black children, the rate of filaggrin mutation is not clearly determined. Recent studies have provided scientific evidence that loss-of-function mutation in certain filaggrin gene regions uncommon in the white patient population may be responsible for this population, and a modified method may be superior in delineating the mutations in this population (Margolis et al., 2018; Mathyer et al., 2018). Thus far we do not have comprehensive information on genetic mutations of skin barrier proteins other than filaggrin occurring in atopic dermatitis patients who have intact filaggrin. Since filaggrin defect, with the resulting skin barrier compromise leading to easy penetration of pathogens and allergens into the skin, would play an important role in the pathogenesis of atopic dermatitis, in theory the atopic dermatitis occurring in patients with filaggrin mutation would have a different pathogenic mechanism than those occurring in patients with intact skin barrier functions, at least from the skin barrier perspective. In fact, there is evidence to suggest that filaggrin defect confers distinct disease risks. Furthermore, the frequency of R501X mutation of the filaggrin gene in white subjects was three times higher in patients with atopic dermatitis and history of eczema herpeticum (25%) than in patients with atopic dermatitis and no history of eczema herpeticum (9%; Gao et al., 2009), suggesting that a difference in gene location of filaggrin mutation could confer a different disease phenotype. In addition, atopic dermatitis patients with filaggrin mutation tend to have more severe skin disease, earlier onset of disease, poorer skin hydration condition, recurrent bacterial infections, and increased risk of sustained molluscum contagiosum skin infection (Cai et al., 2012; Manti et al. 2017; Park et al., 2016).

Nonuniform clinical responses to immune modulatory therapeutics

One possible way to analyze pathogenic mechanism is through observation of clinical responsiveness to targeted immunomodulation therapies, such as biologics and small molecule inhibitors. In many prior reports on clinical trials for atopic dermatitis, subsets of patients can respond favorably or negatively to immunologic therapeutics. In one study, not all atopic dermatitis patients treated with interferon-gamma (IFN-γ), a prototypic Th1 cytokine that counters Th2 immune milieu, had experienced significant improvement, with percent improvement as low as 27% (Boguniewicz et al., 1990). In another study in which atopic dermatitis patients received omalizumab, an antibody-type biologic medication targeting IgE, only a subset of patients

with intact filaggrin and higher serum levels of phosphatidylcholines had a good clinical response (Hotze et al., 2014). Efalizumab, a T-cell activation and migration inhibitor, has also been examined for its efficacy for treating atopic dermatitis. A 12-week pilot trial of this subcutaneously administered biologic for 10 patients resulted in 6 patients who had at least 50% improvement in Eczema Area and Severity Index (EASI) score, and 1 patient with EASI score worsening as a result of this treatment (Takiguchi et al., 2007). In a 13-week study of systemic pimecrolimus for moderate to severe atopic dermatitis, the average improvement of EASI score was a little over 60% when patients received the highest trial doses (30 mg twice daily; Wolff et al., 2005). More recently, atopic dermatitis patients who responded favorably to biologic treatment of dupilumab, a humanized antibody against IL4Rα, the cellular receptor for IL4 and IL13, have upregulation of IL4, IL13, or both (Beck et al., 2014). Even with dupilumab, not all patients with atopic dermatitis received the same degrees of improvement (Beck et al., 2014; de Wijs et al. 2019; Faiz et al., 2019; Uchida et al. 2019). Therefore distinct therapeutic responses to specifically targeted molecules could assist researchers in defining the clinical subsets. Additional target therapies are discussed in a later chapter.

Future directions

How should we then approach this singly grouped disease with apparently heterogeneous clinical characteristics? Several suggestions are provided here, including a clear definition of clinical subsets, consensus on diagnostic criteria on subset determination, characterization of clinical trial findings according to patient subsets, and utilization of artificial intelligence and Big Data (omics) analytics to facilitate the disease subset determination process (Ghosh, Bernstein, Khurana Hershey, Rothenberg, & Mersha, 2018; Tartarisco et al., 2017). One academic group pointed out that there are overlapping genes and candidate genes derived from multiple omics data, including filaggrin, SPINK5, S100A8, and SERPINB3 in relationship to atopic dermatitis pathogenesis, and that there are overlapping immune pathways involving atopic dermatitis by Th2, NFκB, macrophage, fibroblast, and endothelial cell. These medical researchers have advocated that by integrating omics layers that often have complementary and synergistic effects, such as genome, epigenome, transcriptome, proteome, metabolome, lipidome, exposome, and microbiome data, we may be able to fully capture the information flow underlying atopic dermatitis manifestation (Ghosh et al., 2018). Exposome is defined as the sum of external factors that a person is exposed to during a lifetime (Stefanovic, Carsten, & Irvine, 2020). Ultimately, clinical researchers who devote their efforts in this disease and physicians who care for this group of patients would also need to come to a consensus on how to redefine the disease entity or to define subsets for this group of diseases. Without a consensus to follow there will be a continuous variation in the diagnosis and treatment for these patients that will not serve our patients well. Variation on definition of atopic dermatitis that has resulted in a substantial difference in disease prevalence estimation, prediction models' performance, and associated risk factor determination would need to be corrected (Nakamura et al., 2019). Once atopy is redefined and its subsets are delineated, clinicians will have a better understanding of the disease and will be able to provide the most suitable treatments accordingly. A recently published study, which was conducted on more than 30,000 participants evaluated from birth into midlife, identified 4 clinical subtypes of AD with regard to disease activity that continue into adulthood: high probability (2-3%), increasing (2-6%), decreasing (4%), and low probability (88-91%). These findings will open new opportunity for further defining AD subtypes that will help better management of the disease (Abuabara et al., 2021).

Summary

As the medical and scientific communities examine this group of patients categorized under the big umbrella of atopy, the data we gathered point to a need to redefine or to determine distinct subsets within this umbrella. Several aspects of the disease considered as the basis for subset determination include childhood onset versus adult onset, intrinsic versus extrinsic, filaggrin defect versus filaggrin intact, and excellent clinical response versus poor response to targeted immunomodulation therapy. In this new era of precision medicine (i.e., to deliver the right health care to the right person), a one-size-fits-all approach to atopic dermatitis management may no longer be the best practice. A personalized medicine strategy should be in our consideration as we proceed to provide the best care for patients affected by atopic dermatitis in this century and beyond (Cabanillas, Brehler, & Novak, 2017; Chan, 2019).

Further readings

Chan, L. S. (2019). Precision. In L. S. Chan & W. C. Tang (Eds.), *Engineering-medicine: Principles and applications of engineering in medicine*. CRC Press.

Coca, A. F., & Cooke, R. A. (1923). On the classification of the phenomena of hypersensitiveness. *Journal of Immunology, 8*(3), 163–182.

Czarnowicki, T., He, H., Krueger, J. G., & Guttman-Yassky, E. (2019). Atopic dermatitis endotypes and implications for targeted therapeutics. *The Journal of Allergy and Clinical Immunology, 143*, 1–11. https://doi.org/10.1016.j.jaci.2018.10.032.

Grammer, L. G., & Greenberger, P. A. (2018). *Patterson's allergic diseases* (8th ed.). Wolters Kluwer.

Katayama, I., Murota, H., & Satoh, T. (Eds.), (2017). *Evolution of atopic dermatitis in the 21st century*. Springer Nature.

Solomon, I., Llie, M. A., Draghici, C., Voiculescu, V. M., Caruntu, C., Boda, D., & Zurac, S. (2019). The impact of lifestyle factors on evolution of atopic dermatitis: An alternative approach. *Experimental and Therapeutic Medicine, 172*(2), 1078–1084. https://doi.org/10.3892/etm.2018.6980.

Sullivan, M., & Silverberg, N. B. (2017). Current and emerging concepts in atopic dermatitis pathogenesis. *Clinical Dermatology, 35*(4), 349–353. https://doi.org/10.1016/j.clindermatol.2017.03.006.

Tartarisco, G., Tonacci, A., Minciullo, P. L., Billeci, L., Pioggia, G., Incorvaia, C., & Gangemi, S. (2017). The soft computing-based approach to investigate allergic diseases: A systematic review. *Clinical and Molecular Allergy, 15*, 10. https://doi.org/10.1186/s12948-017-0066-3.

References

Abuabara K., Ye, M., Margolis, D. J., McCulloch, C. E., Malick, A. R., Silverwood R. J., et al. (2021). Patterns of atopic eczema disease activity from birth through midlife in 2 British birth cohorts. *JAMA Dermatol, 157*(10), 1191–1199. https://doi.org/10.1001/jamadermatol.2021.2489.

American Academy of Allergy Asthma & Immunology (2019). *Atopy definition.* https://www.aaaai.org/conditions-and-treatments/conditions-dictionary/atopy. Accessed 17.06.19.

Adeli K., Raizman, J.E., Chen Y., Higgins V., Nieuwesteeg M., Abdelhaleem M., et al. (2015). Complex biological profile of hematologic markers across pediatric, adult, and geriatric ages: Establishment of robust pediatric and adult reference intervals on the basis of the Canadian health measures survey. *Clinical Chemistry, 61*(8), 1075–1086. https://doi.org/10.1373/clinchem.2015.240531.

Atopy. (2019). *Merriam-Webster dictionary online.* https://www.merriam-webster.com/dictionary/atopy. Accessed 17.06.19.

Beck L. A., Thaçi, D., Hamilton, J.D., Graham, N.M., Bieber T., Rocklin R. Dupilumab treatment in adults with moderate-to-severe atopic dermatitis. *The New England Journal of Medicine, 371*(2), 130–139. https://doi.org/10.1058/NEJMoa1314768.

Boguniewicz, M., Jaffe, H. S., Izu, A., Sullivan, M. J., York, D., Geha, R. S., & Leung, D. Y. M. Recombinant gamma interferon in treatment of patients with atopic dermatitis and elevated IgE levels. *The American Journal of Medicine, 88*(4), 365–370. https://doi.org/10.1016/0002-9343(90)90490-5.

Bos. J. D. (2002). Atopiform dermatitis. *The British Journal of Dermatology, 147*(3), 426–429. https://doi.org/10.1046/j.1365-2133.2002.05010.x.

Bos, J. D., Brenninkmeijer, E. A., Schram, M. E., Middelkamp-Hup, M. A., Spuls, P. I., & Smitt, J. H. (2010). Atopic eczema or atopiform dermatitis. *Experimental Dermatology, 19*(4), 325–331. https://doi.org/10.1111/j.1600-0625.2009.01024.x.

Bos, J. D., van Leent, E. J., & Sillevis Smitt, J. H. (1998). The millennium criteria for the diagnosis of AD. *Experimental Dermatology, 7*(4), 132–138. https://doi.org/10.1111/j.1600-0625.1998.tb00313.x.

Cabanillas, B., Brehler, A-C, & Novak, N. (2017). Atopic dermatitis phenotypes and the need for personalized medicine. *Current Opinion In Allergy and Clinical Immunology, 174*(4), 309–315. https://doi.org/10.1097/ACI.0000000000000376.

Cai, S. C., Chen, H., Koh, W. P., Common, J. E., van Bever, H. P., McLean, W. H., et al. Filaggrin mutations are associated with recurrent skin infection in Singaporean Chinese patients with atopic dermatitis. *British Journal of Dermatology, 166*(1), 200–203. https://doi.org/10.1111/j.1365-2133.2011.10541.x.

Chan, L. S. (2019). Precision. In L. S. Chan & W. C. Tang (Eds.), *Engineering-medicine: Principles and applications of engineering in medicine*. CRC Press.

Coca, A. F., & Cooke, R. A. (1923). On the classification of the phenomena of hypersensitiveness. *Journal of Immunology, 8*(3), 163–182.

Cohen, S., Dworetzky, M., & Frick, O. L. (2003). The allergy archives: Pioneers and milestones. Coca and Cooke on the classification of hypersensitiveness. *The Journal of Allergy and Clinical Immunology, 111*(1), 205–210.

de Wijs, L. E. M., Bosma, A. L., Erler, N. S., Hollestein, L. M., Gerbens, L. A. A., Middelkamp-Hup, M. A., et al. (2019). Effectiveness of dupilumab treatment in 95 patients with atopic dermatitis: Daily practice data. *The British Journal of Dermatology.* https://doi.org/10.1111/bjd.18179.

Faiz, S., Jonathan G., Celine P., Marie J., Jean-David B., Ziad R., Audrey N., et al. (2019). Effectiveness and safety of dupilumab for the treatment of atopic dermatitis in a real-life French multicenter adult cohort. *The Journal of the American Academy of Dermatology, 81*(1):143–151. https://doi.org/10.1016/j.jaad.2019.02.053.

Gao, P-S. S., Nicholas, M. R., Hand, T., Murray, T., Boguniewicz, M., Hata, T. Filaggrin mutations that confer risk of atopic dermatitis confer greater risk for eczema herpeticum. *The Journal of Allergy and Clinical Immunology, 124*(3), 507–513. https://doi.org/10.1016/j.jaci.2009.07.034.

Georgountzou, A., & Papadopoulos, N. G. (2017). Postnatal innate immune development: from birth to adulthood. *Frontiers in Immunology, 8,* 957. https://doi.org/10.3389/fimmu.2017.00957.

Ghosh, D., Bernstein, J. A., Khurana Hershey, G. K., Rothenberg, M. E., & Mersha, T. B. (2018). Leveraging multilayered "omics" data for atopic dermatitis: A road map to precision medicine. *Frontiers in Immunology, 9,* 2727. https://doi.org/10.10.3389/fimmu.2018.02727.

Hanifin, J. M., & Rajka, G. (1980). Diagnostic features of atopic dermatitis. *Acta Dermato-Venereologica Supplementum, 92,* 44–47.

Hotze, M., Baurecht, H., Rodriguez, E., Chapman-Rothe, N., Ollert, M., Folster-Holst, R., et al. (2014). Increased efficacy of omalizumab in atopic dermatitis patients with wild-type filaggrin status and higher serum levels of phosphatidylcholines. *Allergy, 69*(1), 132–135. https://doi.org/10.1111/all.12234.

Jeong, C. W., An, K. S., Rho, N. K., Park, Y. D., Lee, D. Y., Lee, J. H., et al. (2003). Differential in vivo cytokine mRNA expression in lesion skin of intrinsic vs. extrinsic atopic dermatitis patients using semi quantitative RT-PCR. *Clinical and Experimental Allergy, 33*(12), 1717–1724. https://doi.org/10.1111/j.1365-2222.2003.01782.x.

Kollmann, T. R., Kampmann, B., Mazmanian, S. K., Marchant, A., & Levy, O. (2017). Protecting the newborn and young infant from infectious diseases: Lessons from immune ontogeny. *Immunity, 46*(3), 350–363. https://doi.org/10.1016/j.immuni.2017.03.009.

Kuhn, R., Rajewsky, K., & Muller, W. (1991). Generation and analysis of interleukin-4 deficient mice. *Science, 254*(5032), 707–710.

Manti, S., Amorini, M., Cuppari, C., Salpietro, A., Porcino, F., Leonardi, S., et al. (2017). Filaggrin mutations and Molluscum contagiosum skin infection in patients with atopic dermatitis. *Annals of Allergy, Asthma and Immunology, 119*(5), 446–451. https://doi.org/10.1016/j.anai.2017.07.019.

Margolis, D. J., Mitra, N., Gochnauer, H., Wubbenhorst, B., D'Andrea, K., Kraya, A., et al. (2018). Uncommon filaggrin variants are associated with persistent atopic dermatitis in African Americans. *The Journal of Investigative Dermatology, 138*(7), 1501–1506. https://doi.org/10.1016/j.jid.2018.01.029.

Mathyer, M. E., Ashley, M. Q., Colin, X. F. W. C., Denil, S. L. I. J., Kumar, M. G., Ciliberto, H. M., et al. (2018). Tiled array-based sequencing identifies enrichment of loss-of-function variants in the highly homologous filaggrin gene in African American children with severe atopic dermatitis. *Experimental Dermatology, 27*(9), 989–992. https://doi.org/10.1111/exd.13691.

Nakamura, T., Haider, S., Haider, S., Colicino, S., Murray, C. S., Holloway, J., et al., (2019). Different definition of atopic dermatitis: Impact on prevalence estimates and associated risk factors. *British Journal of Dermatology, 181*(6), 1272–1279. https://doi.org/10.1111/bjd.17853.

Nomura, T., Akiyama, M., Sandilands, A., Nemoto-Hasebe, I., Sakai, K., Nagasaki, A., et al. (2008). Specific filaggrin mutations cause ichthyosis vulgaris and are significantly associated with atopic dermatitis in Japan. *The Journal of Investigative Dermatology, 128*(6), 1436–1441. https://doi.org/10.1038.sj.jid.5701205.

Novak, N., Kruse, S., Kraft, S., Geiger, E., Kluken, H., Fimmers, R., et al. (2002). Dichotomic nature of atopic dermatitis reflected by combined analysis of monocyte immuophenotyping and single nucleotide polymorphisms of the interleukin-4/interleukin-13 receptor gene: The dichotomy of extrinsic and intrinsic atopic dermatitis. *The Journal of Investigative Dermatology, 119*(4), 870–875. https://doi.org/10.1046/j.1523-1747.2002.00191.x.

Olin, A., Henckel, E., Chen, Y., Lakshmikanth, T., Pou, C., Mikes, J., et al. (2018). Stereotypic immune system development in newborn children. *Cell, 174*(5), 1277–1292. https://doi.org/10.1016/j.cell.2018.06.045.

Oppel, T., Schuller, E., Gunther, S., Moderer, M., Haberstok, J., Bieber, T., & Wollenberg, A. (2000). Phenotyping of epidermal dendritic cells allows the differentiation between extrinsic and intrinsic forms of atopic dermatitis. *The British Journal of Dermatology, 143*(6), 1193–1198. https://doi.org/10.1046/j.1365-2133.2000.03887.x.

Ott, H., Stanzel, S., Ocklenburg, C., Merk, H.-F., Baron, J. M., & Lehmann, S. (2009). Total serum IgE as a parameter to differentiate between intrinsic and extrinsic atopic dermatitis. *Acta Dermato-Venereologica, 89*(3), 257–261. http://doi.org/10.2340/00015555-0527.

Park, J. H., Choi, Y. L., Namkung, J. H., Kim, W. S., Lee, J. H., Park, H. J., et al. (2006). Characteristics of extrinsic vs. intrinsic atopic dermatitis in infancy: Correlations with laboratory variables. *The British Journal of Dermatology, 155*(4), 778–783. https://doi.org/10.1111/j.1365-2133.2006.07394.x.

Park, K. Y., Park, M. K., Seok, J., Li, K., & Seo, S. J. (2016). Clinical characteristics of Korean patients with filaggrin-related atopic dermatitis. *Clinical and Experimental Dermatology, 41*(6), 595–600. https://doi.org/10.1111/ced.12854.

Roguedas, A.-M., Andrezet, M.-P., Scotet, V., Dupre-Goetghebeur, D., Ferec, C., & Misery, L. (2006). Intrinsic atopic dermatitis is associated with a beta-2 adrenergic receptor polymorphism. *Acta Dermato-Venereologica, 86*(5), 447–448. https://doi.org/10.2340/00015555-0134.

Roguedas-Contios, A.-M., & Misery, L. (2011). What is intrinsic atopic dermatitis? *Clinical Reviews in Allergy & Immunology, 41,* 233–236. https://doi.org/10.1007/s12016-011-8276-9.

Schnopp, C., Grosch, J., Ring, J., Ollert, M., & Mempel, M. (2008). Microbial allergen-specific IgE is not suitable to identify the intrinsic form of atopic dermatitis in children. *The Journal of Allergy and Clinical Immunology, 121*(1), 267–268e1. https://doi.org/10.1016/j.jaci.2007.06.052.

ScienceDirect. (2019). *Atopy.* https://www.sciencedirect.com/topics/medicine-and-dentistry/atopy. Accessed 17.06.19.

Simon, A. K., Hollander, G. A., & McMichael, A. (2015). Evolution of the immune system in humans from infancy to old age. *Proceedings Biological Sciences/The Royal Society, 282*(1821), 20143085. https://doi.org/10.1098/rspb.2014.3085.

Stefanovic, N., Carsten, F., & Irvine, A. D. (2020). The exposome in atopic dermatitis. *Allergy, 75*(1), 63–74. https://doi.org/10.1111/all.13946.

Suarez-Farinas, M., Dhingra, N., Gittler, J., Shemer, A., Cardinale, I., de Guzman Strong, C., et al. (2013). Intrinsic atopic dermatitis (AD) shows similar Th2 and higher Th17 immune activation compared to extrinsic AD. *The Journal of Allergy and Clinical Immunology*, *132*(2), 361–370. https://doi.org/10.1016/j.jaci.2013.04.046.

Takiguchi, R., Tofte, S., Simpson, B., Harper, E., Blauvelt, A., Hanifin, J., & Simpson, E. (2007). Efalizumab for severe atopic dermatitis: A pilot study in adults. *Journal of the American Academy of Dermatology*, *56*(2), 222–227. https://doi.org/10.1016/j.jaad.2006.08.031.

Tartarisco, G., Tonacci, A., Minciullo, P. L., Billeci, L., Pioggia, G., Incorvaia, C., et al. (2017). The soft computing-based approach to investigate allergic diseases: a systematic review. *Clinical and Molecular Allergy*, *15*, 10. https://doi.org/10.1186/s12948-017-0066-3.

Torok, K. S., Li, S. C., Jacobe, H. M., Taber, S. T., Stevens, A. M., Zulian, F., et al. (2019). Immunopathogenesis of pediatric localized scleroderma. *Frontiers in Immunology*, *10*, 908. https://doi.org/10.3389/fimmu.2019.00908.

Uchida, H., Kamata, M., Mizukawa, I., Watanabe, A., Agematsu, A., Nagata, M. et al. (2019). Real-world effectiveness and safety of dupilumab for the treatment of atopic dermatitis in Japanese patients: A single-centre retrospective study. *The British Journal of Dermatology*. https://doi.org/10.1111/bjd.18163.

Valiathan, R., Ashman, M., & Asthana, D. (2016). Effects of ageing on the immune system: Infants to elderly. *Scandinavian Journal of Immunology*, *83*(4), 255–266. https://doi.org/10.1111/sji.12413.

Vallejo, A. N. (2007). Immune remodeling: Lessons from repertoire alterations during chronological aging and in immune mediated disease. *Trends in Molecular Medicine*, *13*(3), 94–102. https://doi.org/10.1016/j.molmed.2007.01.005.

Williams, H. C., Burney, P. G. J., Hay, R. J., Archer, C. B., Shipley, M. J., & Hunter., J. J. A. (1994). The U.K. working party's diagnostic criteria for atopic dermatitis. I. Derivation of a minimum set of discriminators for atopic dermatitis. *The British Journal of Dermatology*, *131*, 383–396.

Wolff, K., Fleming, C., Hanifin, J., Papp, K., Reitamo, S., Rustin, M., et al. (2005). Efficacy and tolerability of three different doses of oral pimecrolimus in the treatment of moderate to severe atopic dermatitis: A randomized controlled trial. *The British Journal of Dermatology*, *152*(6), 1296–1303. https://doi.org/10.1111/j.1365-2133.2005.06674.x.

Yamaguchi, H., Kabashima-Kudo, R., Bito, T., Sakabe, J.-I., Shimauchi, T., Taisuke, I., et al. (2013). High frequencies of positive nickel/cobalt patch tests and high sweat nickel concentration in patients with intrinsic atopic dermatitis. *Journal of Dermatological Science*, *72*(3), 240–245. https://doi.org/10.1016/j.jdermsci.2018.07.009.

3

Atopy of the Skin

LAWRENCE S. CHAN

KEY POINTS

- Atopy of the skin is manifested as atopic dermatitis (atopic eczema).
- Histologically, the atopy of the skin is characterized by epidermal and dermal infiltration predominantly by lymphocytic cells as well as eosinophils and mast cells. In some patients, the granular cell layer is diminished because of the absence of filaggrin protein.
- The skin surface of patients affected by skin atopy is commonly characterized by lack of proper hydration (xerosis), and some patients have a genetic mutation of a key skin barrier component, filaggrin. We frequently observe pathogenic *Staphylococcus* colonization, with a relative decrease in commensal bacteria and overall microbial diversity, a phenomenon known as dysbiosis.
- Physiologically, patients affected by skin atopy bear heavy burdens of itch and pain, which in turn affects patients' sleep, circadian rhythm, and overall health. Severe disease associates with cardiovascular and cerebrovascular comorbidities.
- On the immunologic aspect, patients affected by skin atopy typically have deviations of both innate and adaptive systems. The documented findings include deficiency in antimicrobial peptides and helper T-cell imbalance that favors Th2 with upregulation on the expressions of interleukin-4 (IL4), IL5, IL10, IL13, IL31, and serum immunoglobulin E (IgE).

Introduction

When atopy occurs in the skin, the medical term is *atopic dermatitis* or *atopic eczema*. In this chapter, a bird's-eye view on major aspects of atopic dermatitis will be discussed, including the histology of inflammatory skin lesion, the skin surface abnormalities, the physiologic abnormalities of atopic dermatitis, and the altered immune milieu. The chapters that follow will expand the overview of atopic dermatitis with detailed delineation. This chapter, in fact, is the miniature representation of this entire book on clinical and basic sciences of atopic dermatitis.

Atopy of the skin under the microscope: histopathology

Historically, one of the earliest attempts by the medical community to understand the pathomechanism of disease is through a microscopic examination of disease tissue (histopathology), as it is an identification of what the disease is and what damages the disease causes at the tissue level. The basic process involves getting the disease tissue, preserving the tissue with formaldehyde (formalin), dehydrating the tissue in graded alcohol, embedding and hardening the tissue in paraffin, sectioning and placing thin sections of tissue on glass slides, rehydrating the tissue, and staining the tissue sections with routine combination stain of hematoxylin (for cell nucleus) and eosin (for cellular cytoplasm). After mounting the stained tissues with a coverslip, the tissues on slides can then be examined microscopically. Although not particularly high-tech compared to newer diagnostic methods, histopathology provides very important information regarding a particular disease, including tissues and level affected, structures and/or cells damaged, invading pathogens detected, inflammatory cells involved, cancerous cell type identified, and boundary of the cancerous tissue delineated. When needed, special stains other than hematoxylin/eosin are used to detect other components with better visualization. Giemsa stain is used to identify mast cells, periodic acid–Schiff (PAS) stain detects fungal elements, Gram stain reveals bacteria, Warthin-Starry stain labels spirochetes bacteria, and acid-fast stain identifies mycobacteria (Suvarna, Layton, & Bancroft, 2012). Besides these special staining techniques that utilize chemical stains, immunohistochemistry staining methods use antibody to identify certain cellular components for visualization after the sectioned tissues undergo certain antigen retrieval steps. These retrieval steps are necessary since formalin fixation disguises the antigenic epitope, and the unmasking steps are required to make these antigenic epitopes available for the antibody binding (Suvarna et al., 2012). Tissues obtained for regular histopathology can also be specially preserved and processed for electron microscopic examination if indications for the more detailed examination arise (Suvarna et al., 2012). We can apply molecular diagnostic methods to the tissue

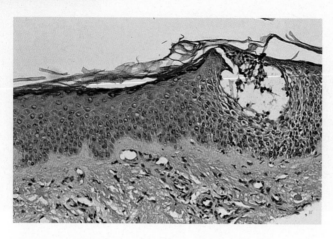

• **Fig. 3.1** Lesional skin of atopic dermatitis viewed under microscope. At the acute stage, atopic dermatitis histologically is characterized by intercellular edema of the epidermis (spongiosis), and dermal perivascular infiltration of mononuclear cells, with infrequent presence of eosinophils and mast cells.

sections processed through the routine formalin-fixed paraffinized tissues as well (Suvarna et al., 2012).

In the nonvesicular lesional skin of atopic dermatitis, one can commonly visualize a picture of inflammation with the following findings under the microscope (Fig. 3.1). In the acute inflammatory lesion, the epidermis shows psoriasiform hyperplasia and intercellular edema. Epidermal and dermal white blood cell infiltrations are composed primarily of lymphocytes with occasional monocytes/macrophages, neutrophils, eosinophils, and basophils. Mast cells and Langerhans cells are present. We can also observe some vascular changes, including endothelial cell hypertrophy, rare endothelial mitosis, and large activated nuclei, suggesting a process of angiogenesis. In chronically inflamed lesion, the epidermis is visibly different from the acute lesion, with the presence of hyperkeratosis and dyskeratosis besides psoriasiform hyperplasia. Varying degrees of intercellular edema and a few lymphocytes are present. In the dermis there are a moderate number of lymphocytes and monocytes/macrophages. The number of mast cells significantly increases (Mihm, Soter, Dvorak, & Frank Austen, 1976). The thickness of the granular layer of the epidermis in atopic dermatitis lesion can be similar to that of normal individuals, unless atopic dermatitis occurs in a person who has filaggrin gene mutation with a corresponding reduction of granular cell layer (Erickson & Kahn, 1970). More details of filaggrin mutation in atopic dermatitis are discussed in Chapters 5 and 11.

A bird's-eye view of the atopic skin surface

Skin barrier defect and hydration problem

The initial discovery of loss-of-function genetic mutation of filaggrin in nearly 50% of white patients affected by atopic dermatitis opens a new scientific window into the disease mechanism of atopic dermatitis and atopy in general

(Palmer et al., 2006). However, researchers subsequently determined that the filaggrin mutation occurred in much lower frequency in nonwhite atopic dermatitis patients (Nomura et al., 2008; Park, Park, Seok, Li, & Seo, 2016). Whether atopic dermatitis patients have other skin barrier protein defects aside from filaggrin is not known at the present time. Although some patients do not have a genetic mutation of skin barrier proteins, their barrier proteins can be deficient secondary to the Th2 cytokine upregulation. Experimentally, human epidermal keratinocytes, under the influence of IL4, or a combination of IL4/IL13, reduce their ability to synthesize various skin barrier proteins such as filaggrin, involucrin, and loricrin (Bao, Alexander, Zhang, Shen, & Chan, 2016; Bao et al., 2017; Di et al., 2016). Thus, in clinically observed inflammatory skin lesions, these skin barrier proteins may in fact be reduced secondary to inflammation without the corresponding gene mutation.

Intimately related to skin barrier function, skin hydration is reduced in patients affected by atopic dermatitis. Xerosis (dry skin) is a common finding in skin of atopic dermatitis patients and is a clinical diagnostic criterion for atopic dermatitis (Hanifin & Rajka, 1980). This improper hydration condition in atopic skin, predisposed to penetration of irritants and allergens, is documented by an increase of transepidermal water loss (Lee et al., 2006; Tupker, Pinnagoda, Coenraads, & Nater, 1990). More discussions on skin barrier defect in atopic dermatitis are available in Chapters 5, 11, 15, and 22.

Staphylococcus colonization and dysbiosis

Pathogenic *Staphylococcus aureus* species commonly colonize in 30% to 100% of atopic skin, and this abnormal colonization is associated with increased disease severity (Nakatsuji & Gallo, 2019). In addition, staphylococcal superantigen from pathogenic species can induce IL31, an itch-inducing cytokine, in skin and in peripheral blood mononuclear cells, leading to promotion of pruritus symptom (Kasraie, Niebuhr, & Werfel, 2010; Sonkoly et al., 2006). The upregulation of IL31 can then induce secretion of IL1 and IL6, which could then lead to cardiovascular comorbidities (discussed later) (Ivert et al., 2019; Kasraie et al., 2010; Kwa & Silverberg, 2017; Silverberg, 2019). When this invasive species takes root and expands its growth, it pushes out the skin commensal bacteria, leading to dysbiosis, a condition of alteration of resident commensal community with the disruption of symbiosis (Petersen & Round, 2014). The scientific community has now recognized that the microbiota (the microorganisms of a particular site) have an important role in immune development and maturation, and that alterations of microbiota have been observed in animal models and in human patients of several immune-mediated diseases, including inflammatory bowel diseases and diabetes (Petersen & Round, 2014). Since commensal bacteria serve a protective function for their hosts, their relative absence reduces one important defense against skin infection and inflammation. Together with reduction of skin barrier and skin-containing antimicrobial peptides, these deficiencies result in the clinical observation of frequent skin infection in patients affected by atopic dermatitis, including serious bacterial, fungal, and viral infections (Howell et al., 2006; Nakatsuji & Gallo, 2019; Sun & Ong, 2017). Although uncommon, systemic infections can occur and can be life threatening, and therefore should be recognized as a serious atopic dermatitis comorbidity (Wang, Boguniewicz, Boguniewicz, & Ong, 2020). In addition, the colonization of pathogenic *S. aureus* species creates substantial challenges for the diagnosis and treatment in patients of atopic dermatitis (Alexander et al., 2020). Greater details on the dysbiosis in atopic dermatitis are discussed in Chapter 6.

A bird's-eye view of the atopic physiology

The burdens of itch and pain

Itch and pain together generate substantial symptoms of atopic dermatitis. Recently, IL31, a cytokine upregulated in atopic dermatitis and a key component in causing pruritus, is identified as a link between activated T cells and itch in atopic skin inflammation. Pruritic symptom in atopic dermatitis links at least in part to the colonization of *S. aureus*, and superantigen (Staphylococcal enterotoxin B) that can induce IL31 in skin and in peripheral blood mononuclear cells (Fries & Varshney, 2013; Kasraie et al., 2010; Sonkoly et al., 2006). In a survey of 304 patients affected by atopic dermatitis, 91% of individuals reported that itch occurred at least once daily, and greater than 50% of patients reported pain and heat sensation in association with itch symptom (Dawn et al., 2009). As we will learn in the following section, these symptoms could lead to sleep disturbance and other psychologic and physiologic health hazards. More detailed discussions on pruritus and pain in atopic dermatitis are available in Chapters 16 and 25.

Sleep disturbance and the role of circadian rhythm and melatonin

One of the major health hazards that patients with atopic dermatitis face is sleep disturbance because of the chronic nature of itchiness and other disturbing sensations such as pain and heat (Dawn et al., 2009; Fishbein et al., 2015, 2018; Yu, Attarian, Zee, & Silverberg, 2016). Reduction of sleep quality has been reported in children affected by atopic dermatitis (Ramirez et al., 2019). How does sleep disturbance affect one's circadian rhythm and overall health?

According to information provided by the National Institute of General Medical Sciences (NIGMS, 2019), circadian rhythms are "physical, mental, and behavioral changes that follow a daily cycle." Living organisms, plants, animals, even bacteria have followed these rhythms. A related biologic phenomenon called biologic clock is defined as an organism's innate timing device composed of specific protein molecules that interact with different cells

in the body. The relationship between these two is that the biologic clock, the internal timing machine, generates the circadian rhythm and regulates it. In living organisms, there is a so-called master clock, which in humans and vertebrate animals is formed by a group of 20,000 neurons into a structure called suprachiasmatic nucleus (SCN) in the brain's hypothalamus. SCN receives input directly from the eyes, coordinates all the biologic clocks, and keeps the clocks in proper working order. Consequently, these rhythmic outputs affect human physiology and behavior. One example is sleep cycle. When there is less light coming from the eyes at late evening time, the stimulation of optic nerves is slower; that message is then related to SCN, which signals the brain to release more melatonin that induces drowsiness, leading to sleep (NIGMS, 2019) (Fig. 3.2).

Historically, the French astronomer and botanist Jean-Jacques de Mairan (1678–1771) was credited as being the first person to show that daily rhythms could be generated internally (i.e., endogenous rhythmicity). He observed that *Mimosa pudica*, a sensitive plant that folds its leaves when touched, folds up its leaves at nighttime and opens them again at daytime; however, the plant still folds its leaves at nighttime and opens them again at daytime when he placed the plant in total darkness (Refinetti, 2016). Augustin Pyramus de Candolle (1778–1841), a Swiss botanist, later showed that by placing the sensitive plant under continuous lighting, the plant still folds its leaves at nighttime and opens them at daytime; however, this occurred with a rhythm cycle duration shorter than 24 hours, effectively demonstrating the existence of an internal rhythmic clock (Refinetti, 2016). The first animal model that was used to illustrate the circadian rhythmicity was credited to Maynard Johnson, who published the findings in 1926 on circadian rhythm on mammals. While keeping deer mice *(Peromyscus leucopus)* in total darkness and constant temperature, he observed a circadian rhythm in the mice, with a cycle time slightly longer than 24 hours, further supporting an endogenously controlled rhythm (Johnson, 1926; Refinetti, 2016). Subsequently, many studies have been conducted in humans. Other key events of circadian rhythm research in the 2000s focused on SCN, molecular clock, and redox. Later, a majority of current research focused on the mechanism of biologic timing (Refinetti, 2016). The term designated to the study of circadian rhythm is *chronobiology* (NIGMS, 2019).

How does the disruption of normal sleep and circadian rhythm impact on human health? Both internal and external factors influence circadian rhythms. The principal factor for humans is daylight, which can turn on or off genes that control the molecular structure of biologic clocks, which then affects our energy, mood, emotion, and other physiologic functions. One does not need to go far to verify this: Simply recall an experience of jetlag that led to fatigue, lack of appetite, and emotional irritability. Studies conducted in the past decades have documented many diseases associated with disturbance of circadian cycle, including cardiovascular, gastrointestinal, neurologic, psychologic, neoplastic, endocrine,

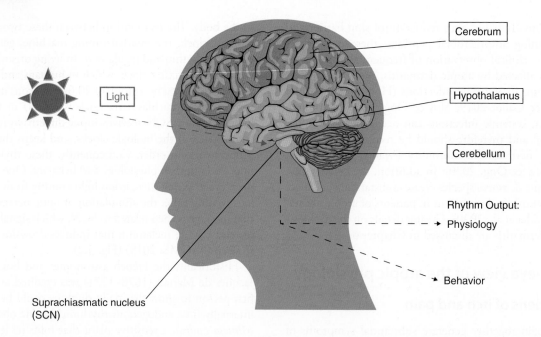

• **Fig. 3.2** Neurologic control of circadian rhythms. The brain structure suprachiasmatic nucleus, located in the area of hypothalamus, responds to input of light signal through the eyes. These neural signals would in turn affect human physiology and behavior by way of circadian rhythms. (Derived from NIGMS. [2019]. *Circadian rhythm.* <https://www.nigms.nih.gov/Education/Pages/Factsheet_CircadianRhythms.aspx>.)

and immunologic diseases (Colwell, 2015). Atopic dermatitis, being an immune-mediated disorder, is no exception (Chang & Chiang, 2016; Fishbein et al., 2015). Researchers reported that during an active phase of atopic dermatitis, both melatonin and β-endorphin levels in serum reduced (Munoz-Hoyos et al., 2007; Schwarz et al., 1988). Studies on the circadian rhythm in atopic dermatitis patients have focused on the central rather than the peripheral circadian rhythm, and a picture of misalignment of circadian rhythm has emerged with shifts in the peaks and troughs of cortisol secretion. In addition, some atopic dermatitis patients with suppressed levels of cortisol and adrenocorticotropic hormone may have reduction of natural secretion of melatonin. Many studies utilizing the techniques of actigraphy (monitor rest/activity cycles) and polysomnography (monitor brain waves, oxygen concentration, heart and respiratory rates, and movements) in recent years have documented the deficient sleep in children affected by atopic dermatitis. Sleep efficiency is defined by the ratio of the actual sleep time to the total record time in bed by polysomnography. In children, sleep disturbance because of atopic dermatitis has been associated with behavior problems, neurocognitive defect, lower IQ, attention-deficit hyperactivity, poorer performance of schoolwork, obesity, hypertension, and impaired linear growth (Fishbein et al., 2015).

The cardiovascular and cerebrovascular comorbidities

As an inflammatory skin disease, atopic dermatitis is characterized by increased serum levels of cytokines such as IL1 and IL6 (Greally, Hussain, Price, & Coleman, 1992; Toshitani, Ansel, Chan, Li, & Hanifin, 1993). It is therefore logical for one to speculate that these proinflammatory and proatherogenic cytokines (IL1 and IL6) could lead to increased cardiovascular and/or cerebrovascular comorbidity, as supported by findings of an in vitro study (Mohan, Zhang, Bao, Many, & Chan, 2017) and by evidence that such cytokine upregulation in another inflammatory skin disease (psoriasis) also linked to cardiovascular comorbidity (Garshick et al., 2019; Gelfand et al., 2006; Shiba et al., 2019). Other evidence supporting this link is that staphylococcal superantigen derived from *S. aureus* can induce IL31 from human monocytes/macrophages. Consequently, these induced IL31 cytokines can then enhance IL1 and IL6 secretions that might contribute to these vascular comorbidities (Kasraie et al., 2010). Recent clinical studies seem to point to evidence to support this link (Ivert et al., 2019; Kwa & Silverberg, 2017; Silverberg, 2019). Keep in mind, however, some studies reported no increase or minimum increase of cardiovascular risk in atopic dermatitis patients (Drucker & Harvey, 2019; Drucker, Qureshi, Dummer, Parker, & Li, 2017; Jachiet et al., 2019; Thyssen et al., 2018), and some academicians have questioned the adequacy of current epidemiologic tools utilized in the risk analysis (Thyssen et al., 2018). Nevertheless, the majority of evidence seems to settle in that the more severe the atopic dermatitis, the higher the risk of cardiovascular comorbidity (Ascott et al., 2019; Drucker & Flohr, 2018; Silverberg et al., 2018; Silverwood et al., 2018). This conclusion, similar to the reports from psoriasis studies (Garshick et al., 2019; Gelfand et al., 2006), seems to make sense from the immune mechanism perspective. The more severe disease would allow more proinflammatory and proatherogenic cytokines to be produced. Once these cytokines reach the blood vessels they could lead to cardiovascular or cerebrovascular comorbidities.

A bird's-eye view of the atopic immune deviation

The hygiene hypothesis

The hygiene hypothesis of allergy, first proposed by Strachan (1989), speculates that the arising of atopic dermatitis is due in major part to the modern family practice of keeping children in an excessively clean (hygienic) condition, so much so that the children grow up lacking exposure to certain pathogens (Flohr & Yeo, 2011; Okada, Kuhn, Feillet, & Bach, 2010). The absence of such common pathogens challenges children's immune systems, as the theory speculated, and can then lead to deviation from a balanced milieu toward to a Th2-dominant immune milieu. This theory is based, in part, on the epidemiologic findings that the substantial increase of atopic dermatitis prevalence is primarily observed in developed nations (which tend to have more stringent hygiene practices than developing nations) and that migrants moving from a low-incidence country to a high-incidence country tend to acquire the disease (Okada et al., 2010). One survey pointed out an inverse relationship between development of atopic dermatitis and exposures of endotoxin, early day care, farm animal and dog in early age, and helminth infections (Flohr & Yeo, 2011).

Innate immune deviation

The innate immune system is the first line of immune defense against invading pathogens, and it does not require prior training or memory to act effectively. Antimicrobial peptides are one of the major components that have a role in the skin immune defense (Howell et al., 2004). The altered immune milieu, particularly an increase of IL10 in atopic dermatitis, can suppress the expression of these antimicrobial peptides (Howell et al., 2005). Studies pointed to a deficiency of human skin-producing cathelicidin (LL37) and human β-defensin-2 in patients of atopic dermatitis, particularly on lesional skin (Hata et al., 2010; Ong et al., 2002). Such deficiencies have been linked to the serious bacterial, fungal, and viral infections (Hata et al., 2010; Howell et al., 2006; Nakatsuji & Gallo, 2019; Sun & Ong, 2017).

Adaptive immune deviation

Adaptive immune system requires a prior encounter of pathogens to develop a long-term cellular memory, such that a subsequent challenge by the same pathogens will lead to rapid generation and movement of immune armies, lymphocytes or antibodies, aiming to eliminate the invading enemies. Once the invading microorganisms are eliminated, the immune system will naturally shut down the inflammatory process. In chronic inflammatory disease atopic dermatitis, however, such an inflammatory process, once activated, will remain activated. Commonly, T-cell activation, IgE, Th2, Th17, and Th22 were upregulated, with predominant increase of IL4, IL5, IL6, IL10, IL13, and IL31 and variable increase in IL17 and IL22 (Bieber, 2019; Bos, Kapsenberg, & Sillevis Smitt, 1994; Brunner et al., 2019; Cooper, 1994; Moyle, Cevikbas, Harden, & Guttman-Yassky, 2019; Renert-Yuval & Guttman-Yassky, 2019; Roesner, Zeitvogel, & Heratizadeh, 2019). The continuous presence of these cytokines thus fuels the ongoing inflammation until external antiinflammatory medications stop it.

The early reports of total serum IgE level showed a substantial upregulation in patients with atopic dermatitis, and on the average the atopic dermatitis patients have 6793 ng/mL and 493 IU mL, compared to normal average levels of 160 ng/mL and 122 IU mL, respectively (Blaylock, 1976). More discussions of immune factors in atopic dermatitis are available in Chapters 13 and 14.

The skin-gut-lung link in atopic march

Literature accumulated over years of studies has pointed to a link between the skin, the intestine, and the lung in terms of the immune deviation and the resulting atopy manifestations, and it has been postulated that initial disruption of the skin epidermal barrier permits allergen sensitization and colonization by pathogens. As hypothesized, this initial skin disruption induces a Th2 inflammatory response and a thymic stromal lymphopoietin-mediated pathway that further promotes barrier breakdown at distant sites, including the intestinal and respiratory tract (Zhu, Zhu, Tran, Sivamani, & Shi, 2018). This may explain the atopic march phenomenon, defined as the initial clinical manifestation of skin atopy (i.e., atopic dermatitis) that will later expand to affect other organ systems, including the gastrointestinal and respiratory systems, resulting in food allergy, rhinitis, and asthma, as observed by clinicians (Han, Roan, & Ziegler, 2017; Oliveira & Torres, 2019). Additional discussions on the skin-gut-lung link are provided in Chapter 15.

Summary

In summary, atopic dermatitis is a chronic, itchy, inflammatory skin disease characterized by skin barrier defect, hydration deficiency, pathogenic bacterial colonization, chronic pruritus and skin inflammation, inefficient innate immune functions, and adaptive immune deviation. In addition, atopic dermatitis carries a heavy disease burden to the patient, as the itch and pain cause sleep disturbance and circadian rhythm alterations as well as cardiovascular and cerebrovascular comorbidities. Atopic dermatitis is not only a skin disease; it also has substantial systemic implications, as it can expand to affect the gastrointestinal and respiratory systems in the development of food allergy, rhinitis, and asthma. As detailed in Chapter 2, accumulative evidence gathered from clinical and laboratory investigations has pointed to a need to redefine this entity or to determine subsets within this big umbrella of atopic dermatitis. Overall, however, the general characteristics of atopic dermatitis described in this chapter, to a large extent, still hold true.

Further readings

Czarnowicki, T., He, H., Krueger, J. G., & Guttman-Yassky, E. (2019). Atopic dermatitis endotypes and implications for targeted therapeutics. *Journal of Allergy and Clinical Immunology, 143*(1), 1–11. https://doi.org/10.1016/j.jaci.2018.10.032.

Gause, W. C., & Artis, D. (Eds.), (2016). *The Th2 type immune response in health and diseases: From host defense and allergy to metabolic homeostasis and beyond.* Springer.

Medzhitov, R. (Ed.), *Innate immunity and inflammation (Cold Spring Harbor respectives in biology).* Cold Spring Harbor Laboratory Press.

Misery, L., & Stander, S. (Eds.), (2016). *Pruritus.* Springer.

Tham, E. H., & Leung, D. Y. M. (2019). Mechanisms by which atopic dermatitis predisposes to food allergy and the atopic march. *Allergy, Asthma & Immunology Research, 11*(1), 4–15. https://doi.org/10.4168/aair.2019.11.1.4.

Thyssen, J. P., & Maibach, H. I. (Eds.), (2014). *Filaggrin: Basic science, epidemiology, clinical aspects and management.* Springer.

References

Alexander, H., Paller, A. S., Traidl-Hoffmann, C., Beck, L. A., De Benedetto, A., Dhar, S., et al. (2020). The role of bacterial skin infections in atopic dermatitis: Expert statement and review from the international eczema council skin infection group. *The British Journal of Dermatology, 182*(6), 1331–1342. https://doi.org/10.1111/bjd.18643.

Ascott, A., Mulick, A., Yu, A. M., Prieto-Merino, D., Schmidt, M., Abuabara, K., et al. (2019). Atopic eczema and major cardiovascular outcomes: A systematic review and meta-analysis of population-based studies. *The Journal of Allergy and Clinical Immunology, 145*(5), 1821–1829. https://doi.org/10.1016/j.jaci.2018.11.030.

Bao, L., Alexander, J. B., Zhang, H., Shen, K., & Chan, L.S. (2016). Interleukin-4 downregulation of involucrin expression in human epidermal keratinocytes involves Stat6 sequestration of the coactivator CREB-binding protein. *Journal of Interferon and Cytokine Research, 36*(6), 374–381. https://doi.org/10.1089/jir.2015.0056.

Bao, L., Mohan, G. C., Alexander, J. B., Doo, C., Shen, K., Bao, J., & Chan, L. S. (2017). A molecular mechanism for IL-4 suppression of loricrin transcription in epidermal keratinocytes: Implication for atopic dermatitis pathogenesis. *Innate Immunity, 23*(8), 641–647. https://doi.org/10.1177/1753425917732823.

Bieber, T. (2019). Interleukin-13: Targeting an underestimated cytokine in atopic dermatitis. *Allergy.* https://doi.org/10.1111/all.13954.

Blaylock, W. K. (1976). Atopic dermatitis: Diagnosis and pathobiology. *The Journal of Allergy and Clinical Immunology, 57*(1), 62–79. https://doi.org/10.1016/0091-6749(76)90080-4.

Bos, J. D., Kapsenberg, M. L., & Sillevis Smitt, J. H. (1994). Pathogenesis of atopic eczema. *Lancet.* https://doi.org/10.1016/S0140-6736(94)92473-2.

Brunner, P. M., Pavel, A. B., Khattri, S., Leonard, A., Malik, K., Rose, S., et al. (2019). Baseline IL-22 expression in patients with atopic dermatitis stratifies tissue responses to fezakinumab. The *Journal of Allergy and Clinical Immunology, 143,* 1, 142–154.

Chang, Y.-S., & Chiang, B.-L. (2016). Mechanism of sleep disturbance in children with atopic dermatitis and the role of the circadian rhythm and melatonin. *International Journal of Molecular Sciences, 17*(4), 462. https://doi.org/10.3390/ijms.17040462.

Colwell. C. S. (2015). *Circadian Medicine.* Wiley.

Cooper, K. D. (1994). Atopic dermatitis: Recent trends in pathogenesis and therapy. *The Journal of Investigative Dermatology, 102*(1), 128–137. https://doi.org/10.1111/1523-1747.ep12371746.

Dawn, A., Papoiu, A. D. P., Chan, Y. H., Rapp, S. R., Rassette, N. & Yosipovitch, G. (2009). Itch characteristics in atopic dermatitis: Results of a web-based questionnaire. *The British Journal of Dermatology, 160*(3), 642–644. https://doi.org/10.1111/j.1365-2133.2008.08941.x.

Di, Z.-H., Ma, L., Qi, R.-Q., Sun, X.-D., Huo, W., Zhang, L., et al. (2016). T helper 1 and T help 2 cytokines differentially modulate expression of filaggrin and its processing proteases in human keratinocytes. *Chinese Medical Journal, 129*(3), 295–303. https://doi.org/10.4103/0366-6999.174489.

Drucker, A. M., Qureshi, A. A., Dummer, T. J. B., Parker, L., & Li, W. Q. (2017). Atopic dermatitis and risk of hypertension, type 2 diabetes, myocardial infarction and stroke in a cross-sectional analysis from the Canadian partnership for tomorrow project. *The British Journal of Dermatology, 177*(4), 1043–1051. https://doi.org/10.1111/bjd.15727.

Drucker, A. M., & Flohr, C. (2018). Revisiting atopic dermatitis and cardiovascular disease. *The British Journal of Dermatology, 179*(3), 801–802. https://doi.org/10.1111/bjd.16891.

Drucker, A. M., & Harvey, P. J. (2019). Atopic dermatitis and cardiovascular disease: What are the clinical implications? *The Journal of Allergy and Clinical Immunology, 143*(5), 1736–1738. https://doi.org/10.1136/j.jaci.2019.01.008.

Erickson, L., & Kahn, G. (1970). The granular layer thickness in atopy and ichthyosis vulgaris. *The Journal of Investigative Dermatology, 54*(1), 11–12. https://doi.org/10.1111/1523-1747.ep12551488.

Fishbein, A. B., Vitaterna, O., Haugh, I. M., Bavishi, A. A., Zee, P. C., Turek, F. W., et al. (2015). Nocturnal eczema: Review of sleep and circadian rhythms in children with atopic dermatitis and future research directions. *The Journal of Allergy and Clinical Immunology, 136*(5), 1170–1177. https://doi.org/10.1016/j.jaci.2015.08.028.

Fishbein, A. B., Mueller, K., Kruse, L., Boor, P., Sheldon, S., Zee, P., & Paller, A. S. (2018). Sleep disturbance in children with moderate/severe atopic dermatitis: A case-control study. *Journal of the American Academy of Dermatology, 78*(2), 336–341. doi:10.1016/j.jaad.2017.08.043.

Flohr, C., & Yeo, L. (2011). Atopic dermatitis and the hygiene hypothesis revisited. *Current Problems in Dermatology, 41,* 1–34. https://doi.org/10.1159/000323290.

Fries, B. C., & Varshney, A. K. (2013). Bacterial toxins-Staphylococcal enterotoxin B. *Microbiology Spectrum, 1*(2), 1–21. https://doi.org/10.1128/microbiolspec.AID-0002-2012.

Garshick, M. S., Barrett, T. J., Wechter, T., Azarchi, S., Scher, J. U., Neimann, A., et al.(2019). Inflammasome signaling and impaired vascular health in psoriasis. *Arteriosclerosis, Thrombosis, and Vascular Biology, 39*(4), 787–798. https://doi.org/10.1161/ATVBAHA.118.312246.

Gelfand, J. M., Neimann, A. L., Shin, D. B., Wang, X., Margolis, D. J., & Troxel, A. B. (2006). Risk of myocardial infarction in patients with psoriasis. *The Journal of the American Medical Association, 296*(14), 1735–1741. https://doi.org/10.1001/jama.296.14.1735.

Greally, P., Hussain, M. J., Price, J. F., & Coleman, R. (1992). Interleukin-1 alpha and soluble interleukin-2 receptor in atopic dermatitis. *Archives of Disease in Childhood, 67*(11), 1413. https://doi.org/10.1136/adc.67.11.1413.

Han, H., Roan, F., & Ziegler, S. F. (2017). The atopic march: Current insights into skin barrier dysfunction and epithelial cell-derived cytokines. *Immunological Reviews*, *278*(1), 116–130. https://doi.org/10.1111/imr.12546.

Hanifin, J. M., & Rajka, G. (1980). Diagnostic features of atopic dermatitis. *Acta Dermato-Venereologica*, *92*, 44–47.

Hata, T. R., Kotol, P., Boguniewicz, M., Taylor, P., Paik, A., Jackson, M., et al. (2010). History of eczema herpeticum is associated with the inability to induce human b-defensin (HBD)-2, HBD-3 and cathelicidin in the skin of patients with atopic dermatitis. *The British Journal of Dermatology*, *163*(3), 659–661. https://doi.org/10.1111/j.1365-2133.2010.09892.x.

Howell, M. D., Jones, J. F., Kisich, K. D., Streib, L. E., Gallo, R. L., & Leung, D. Y. M. (2004). Selective killing of vaccinia virus by LL-37: Implications for eczema vaccinatum. *Journal of Immunology*, *172*(3), 1763–1767. https://doi.org/10.4049/jimmunol.172.3.1763.

Howell, M. D., Novak, N., Bieber, T., Pastore, S., Girolomoni, G., Boguniewicz, M., et al. (2005). Interleukin-10 downregulates anti-microbial peptide expression in atopic dermatitis. *The Journal of Investigative Dermatology*, *125*(4), 738–745. https://doi.org/10.1111/j.0022-202X.2005.23776.x.

Howell, M. D., Gallo, R. L., Boguniewicz, M., Jones, J. F., Wong, C., Strieb, J. E., & Leung, D. Y. M. (2006). Cytokine milieu of atopic dermatitis skin subverts the innate immune response to vaccinia virus. *Immunity*, *24*(3), 341–348. https://doi.org/10.1016/j.immuni.2006.02.006.

Ivert, L. U., Emma, K. J., Dal, H., Lindelof, B., Wahlgren, C.-F., & Bradley, M. (2019). Association between atopic dermatitis and cardiovascular disease: A nationwide register-based case-control study from Sweden. *Acta Dermato-Venereologica*, *99*(10), 865-870. https://doi.org/10.2340/00015555-3235.

Jachiet, M., Nosbaum, A., Staumont-Salle, D., Seneschal, J., Viguier, M., Soria, A., et al. (2019). Low cardiovascular risk and poor quality of life associated with tobacco use and skin infections in adult atopic dermatitis: Result of a French multicenter study. *Journal of the European Academy of Dermatology and Venereology*, *33*(12), e451–e453. https://doi.org/10.1111/jdv.15774.

Johnson, M. S. (1926). Activity and distribution of certain wild mice in relation to biotic communities. *Journal of Mammalogy*, *7*, 245–277.

Kasraie, S., Niebuhr, M., & Werfel, T. (2010). Interleukin (IL)-31 induces pro-inflammatory cytokines in human monocytes and macrophages following stimulation with staphylococcal exotoxins. *Allergy*, *65*(6), 712–721. https://doi.org/10.1111/j.1398-9995.2009.02255.x.

Kwa, M. C., & Silverberg, J. I. (2017). Association between inflammatory skin disease and cardiovascular and cerebrovascular comorbidities in US adults: Analysis of nationwide inpatient sample data. *American Journal of Clinical Dermatology*, *18*(6), 813–823. https://doi.org/10.1007/s40257-017-0293-x.

Lee, C. H., Chuang, H. Y., Shih, C. C., Jong, S. B., Chang, C. H., & Yu, H. S. (2006). Transepidermal water loss, serum IgE and beta-endorphin as important and independent biological markers for development of itch intensity in atopic dermatitis. *The British Journal of Dermatology*, *154*(6), 1100–1107. https://doi.org/10.1111/j.1365-2133.2006.07191.x.

Mihm, M. C., Soter, N. A., Dvorak, H. F., & Austen K. F. (1976). The structure of normal skin and the morphology of atopic eczema. *The Journal of Investigative Dermatology*, *67*(3), 305–312. https://doi.org/10.1111/1523-1747.ep12514346.

Mohan, G. C., Zhang, H., Bao, L., Many, B., & Chan, L. S. (2017). Diacerein inhibits the pro-atherogenic & pro-inflammatory effects of IL-1 on human keratinocytes & endothelial cells. *PLoS One*, *12*(3), e1073981. https://doi.org/10.1371/journal.pone.0173981.

Moyle, M., Cevikbas, F., Harden, J. L., & Guttman-Yassky, E. (2019). Understanding the immune landscape in atopic dermatitis: The era of biologics and emerging therapeutic approaches. *Experimental Dermatology*, *28*(7), 756–768. https://doi.org/10.1111/exd.13911.

Munoz-Hoyos, A., Espin-Quirantes, C., Molina-Carballo, A., Uberos, J., Contreras-Chova, F., Narbona-Lopez, E., & Gutierrez-Salmeron, M. J. (2007). Neuroendocrine and circadian aspects (melatonin and beta-endorphin) of atopic dermatitis in the child. *Pediatric Allergy and Immunology*, *18*(8), 679–686. https://doi.org/10.1111/j.1399-3038.2007.00574.x.

Nakatsuji, T., & Gallo, R. L. (2019). The role of skin microbiome in atopic dermatitis. *Annals of Allergy, Asthma and Immunology*, *122*(3), 263–269. https://doi.org/10.1016/j.anai.2018.12.003.

National Institute of General Medical Sciences. (2019). Circadian rhythm. <https://www.nigms.nih.gov/Education/Pages/Factsheet_CircadianRhythms,aspx> Accessed 28.06.19.

Nomura, T., Akiyama, M., Sandilands, A., Nemoto-Hasebe, I., Sakai, K., Nagasaki, A., & Ota, M. (2008). Specific filaggrin mutations cause ichthyosis vulgaris and are significantly associated with atopic dermatitis in Japan. *The Journal of Investigative Dermatology*, *128*(6), 1436–1441. doi:10.1038/sj.jid.5701205.

Okada, H., Kuhn, C., Feillet, H., & Bach, J. F. (2010). The 'hygiene hypothesis' for autoimmune and allergic diseases: An update. *Clinical and Experimental Immunology*, *160*(1), 1–9. https://doi.org/10.1111/j.1365-2249.2010.04139.x.

Oliveira, C., & Torres, T. (2019). More than skin deep: The systemic nature of atopic dermatitis. *European Journal of Dermatology*, *29*(3), 250–258. https://doi.org/10.1684/ejd.2019.3557.

Ong, P. Y., Ohtake, T., Brandt, C., Strickland, I., Boguniewicz, M., Ganz, T., et al. (2002). Endogenous antimicrobial peptides and skin infections in atopic dermatitis. *The New England Journal of Medicine*, *347*(15), 1151–1160. https://doi.org/10.1056/NEJM/oa021481.

Palmer, C. N. A., Irvine, A. D., Terron-Kwiatkowski, A., Zhao, Y., Liao, H., Lee, S. P., et al. (2006). Common loss-of-function variants of the epidermal barrier protein filaggrin are a major predisposing factor for atopic dermatitis. *Nature Genetics*, *38*(4), 441–446. https://doi.org/10.1036/ng1767.

Park, K. Y., Park, M. K., Seok, J., Li, K., & Seo, S. J. (2016). Clinical characteristics of Korean patients with filaggrin-related atopic dermatitis. *Clinical and Experimental Dermatology*, *41*(6), 595–600. https://doi.org/10.1111/ced.12854.

Petersen, C., & Round, J. L. (2014). Defining dybiosis and its influence on host immunity and disease. *Cellular Microbiology*, *16*(7), 1024–1033. https://doi.org/10.1111/cmi.12308.

Ramirez, F. D., Chen, S., Langan, S. M., Prather, A. A., McCulloch, C. E., Kidd, S. A., et al. (2019). Association of atopic dermatitis with sleep quality in children. *JAMA Pediatrics*, *173*(5), e190025. doi:10.1001/jamapediatrics.2019.0025.

Refinetti, R. (2016). *Circadian physiology* (3rd Ed.). Boca Raton: CRC Press.

Renert-Yuval, Y., & Guttman-Yassky, E. (2019). What's new in atopic dermatitis. *Dermatologic Clinics*, *37*(2), 205–213. https://doi.org/10.1016/j.det.2018.12.007.

Roesner, L., Zeitvogel, J., & Heratizadeh, A. (2019). Common and different roles of IL-4 and IL-13 in skin allergy and clinical implications. *Current Opinion in Allergy and Clinical Immunology*, *19*(4), 319–327. https://doi.org/10.1097/ACI.0000000000000553.

Schwarz, W., Birau, N., Hornstein, O. P., Heubeck, B., Schonberger, A., Meyer, C., & Gottschalk, J. (1988). Alterations of melatonin secretion in atopic eczema. *Acta Dermato-Venereologica*, *68*(3), 224–229.

Shiba, M., Kato, T., Izumi, T., Miyamoto, S., Nakane, E., Haruna, T., & Inoko, M. (2019). Risk of myocardial infarction in patients with psoriasis: A cross-sectional patient-population study in a Japanese hospital. *Journal of Cardiology, 73*(4), 276–279. https://doi.org/10.1016/j.jjcc.2018.10.008.

Silverberg, J. I. (2019). Comorbidities and the impact of atopic dermatitis. *Annals of Allergy, Asthma and Immunology, 123*(2), P144–P151. https://doi.org/10.1016/j.anai.2019.04.020.

Silverberg, J. I., Gelfand, J. M., Margolis, D. J., Boguniewicz, M., Fonacier, L., Grayson, M. H., et al. (2018). Association of atopic dermatitis with allergic, autoimmune, and cardiovascular comorbidities in US adults. *Annals of Allergy, Asthma and Immunology, 121*(5), 604–612. https://doi.org/10.1016/j.anai.2018.07.042.

Silverwood, R. J., Forbes, H. J., Abuabara, K., Ascott, A., Schmidt, M., Schmidt, S. A. J., et al. (2018). Severe and predominantly active atopic eczema in adulthood and long term risk of cardiovascular disease: Population based cohort study. *British Medical Journal, 361*, k1786. doi:10.1136/bmj.k1786.

Sonkoly, E., Muller, A., Lauerma, A. I., Pivarcsi, A., Soto, H., Kemeny, L., et al. (2006). IL-31: A new link between T cells and pruritus in atopic skin inflammation. *Journal of Allergy and Clinical Immunology, 117*(2), 411–417. https://doi.org/10.1016/j.jaci.2005.10.033.

Strachan, D. P. (1989). Hay fever, hygiene, and household size. *British Medical Journal, 299*, 1259–1260.

Sun, Di, & Ong, P. Y. (2017). Infectious complications in atopic dermatitis. *Immunology and Allergy Clinics of North America, 37*(1), 75–93. https://doi.org/10.1016/j.iac.2016.08.015.

Suvarna, S. K., Layton, C., & Bancroft, J. D. (2012). *Bancroft's theory and practice of histological techniques* (7th ed). Livingston: Churchill.

Thyssen, J. P., Halling-Overgaard, A. S., Andersen, Y. M. F., Gislason, G., Skov, L., & Egeberg, A. (2018). The association with cardiovascular disease and type 2 diabetes in adults with atopic dermatitis: A systematic review and meta-analysis. *The British Journal of Dermatology, 178*(6), 1272–1279. https://doi.org/10.1111/bjd.16215.

Toshitani, A., Ansel, J. C., Chan, S. C., Li, S.-H., & Hanifin, J. M. (1993). Increased interleukin 6 production by T cells derived from patients with atopic dermatitis. *The Journal of Investigative Dermatology, 100*(3), 299–304. https://doi.org/10.1111/1523-1747.ep12469875.

Tupker, R. A., Pinnagoda, J., Coenraads, P. J., & Nater, J. P. (1990). Susceptibility to irritants: Role of barrier function, skin dryness and history of atopic dermatitis. *The British Journal of Dermatology, 123*(2), 199–205. doi:10.1111/j.1365-2133.1990.tb01847.x.

Wang, V., Boguniewicz, J., Boguniewicz, M., & Ong, P. Y. (2020). The infectious complications of atopic dermatitis. *Annals of Allergy, Asthma and Immunology, 126*(1), 3–12. https://doi.org/10.1016/j.anai.2020.08.002.

Yu, S. H., Attarian, H., Zee, P., & Silverberg, J. I. (2016). Burden of sleep and fatigue in US adults with atopic dermatitis. *Dermatitis: Contact, Atopic, Occupational, Drug: Official Journal of the American Contact Dermatitis Society, North American Contact Dermatitis Group, 27*(2), 50–58. https://doi.org/10.1097/DER.0000000000000161.

Zhu, T. H., Zhu, T. R., Tran, K. A., Sivamani, R. K., & Shi, V. Y. (2018). Epithelial barrier dysfunctions in atopic dermatitis: A skin-gut-lung model linking microbiome alteration and immune dysregulation. *The British Journal of Dermatology, 179*(3), 570–581. https://doi.org/10.1111/bjd.16734.

4

Epidemiology

JULIA ARZENO AND MARCIA HOGELING

KEY POINTS

- Atopic dermatitis is one of the most common inflammatory diseases of the skin, with both genetic and environmental etiologies.
- The prevalence of atopic dermatitis is increasing globally due to changes in climate, microbes, urbanization, among other factors.
- Atopic dermatitis can have broad effects on mental health, quality of life, development, and psychosocial function, which can affect patients and their families.
- The financial burden of atopic dermatitis is high with both primary and secondary costs.
- Access to dermatologists, especially pediatric dermatologists, is limited, and vulnerable patients are often disproportionately affected with limited access to specialist care.

Introduction

Atopic dermatitis is an inflammatory skin disorder. Descriptions of atopic dermatitis are found in Roman history dating back to 69 to 140 CE. The term *eczema*, meaning "boiling over," was first introduced in 543 CE to describe an "inward heat, which drives off the humors of the body from its surface like the seething of a boiling fluid" (Kramer, Strom, Ladizinski, & Lio, 2017). The term *atopic dermatitis* was introduced into the dermatology medical lexicon in 1933 by Fred Wise and Marion Sulzberger based on the term *atopy* to describe the association between asthma and allergic rhinitis (Kramer et al., 2017). This chapter delineates the epidemiology, which by definition deals with the incidence, prevalence, distribution, and sum of factors controlling the presence and absence of atopic dermatitis.

Prevalence, distribution, and generally recognized factors

Atopic dermatitis is now one of the most common inflammatory skin disorders both in the United States and worldwide. Prevalence estimates for atopic dermatitis range from 10% to 13% for children and 2% to 10 % for adults, as prevalence of atopic dermatitis decreases with age (McKenzie & Silverberg, 2019; Silverberg, 2017). The severity of atopic

dermatitis also tends to decrease with age. One pediatric study from 2017 evaluated the severity of atopic dermatitis in the United States. This study found that among pediatric patients with atopic dermatitis, 67% had mild disease, 26% had moderate disease, and 7% had severe disease, which correlates with 2.98 million children in the United States with moderate-to-severe disease (Drucker et al., 2017). The prevalence estimates vary both globally and within different settings in the United States. For example, prevalence estimates vary with urban versus rural living and within different socioeconomic populations. Globally, prevalence estimates are as low as 0.9% in India and as high as 11% to 24% in Japan, 24.6% in Colombia, and 30.48% in China (Guo et al., 2019; Silverberg, 2017; Sugiura et al., 1998). Prevalence estimates may be lower when using diagnostic criteria studies, such as the Hanifin and Rajka scales, than when studies are conducted with in-person dermatologists (Guo et al., 2019).

US prevalence estimates for atopic dermatitis also vary within different populations. Blacks and Hispanics have a higher prevalence of atopic dermatitis even after controlling for potential confounding factors, such as household incomes, health insurance, and parental education levels (Silverberg, 2017; Silverberg et al., 2018). Higher rates of more persistent, early-onset atopic dermatitis and higher rates of late-onset atopic dermatitis may contribute to the higher prevalence of atopic dermatitis seen in these populations (McKenzie & Silverberg, 2019). Increased severity of atopic dermatitis is associated with higher household incomes, the oldest child in the family, homes with a single mother, lower parental education levels, lower parental emotional health, and in areas with dilapidated housing and garbage on the streets (Silverberg & Simpson, 2014).

There are multiple names and clinical definitions for atopic dermatitis that contribute to differences in prevalence estimates (Nakamura et al., 2019). Overall, the prevalence of atopic dermatitis is increasing. This is a true increase in prevalence, not simply due to an increase in minor signs and symptoms or in the medical profession's use of the words *eczema* and *dermatitis* (Larsen, Diepgen, & Svensson, 1996). A study in Japan found that among Japanese children, the prevalence of atopic dermatitis has doubled in the past 20 years, and among 18-year-olds the prevalence is over five times greater than it was 20 years ago (Sugiura et al., 1998). In the United States, prevalence estimates have also shown an upward trend with a possible plateau around 2013 (Silverberg, 2017). This increase in prevalence has been attributed to changes in urbanization, pollution, microbes, climate, and diet.

With urbanization, the prevalence of atopic dermatitis in developing nations approaches that of developed nations; increasing trends toward urbanization may contribute to the overall increased prevalence of atopic dermatitis (Bonamonte et al., 2019). The leveling off of prevalence of atopic dermatitis with urbanization supports a role for environmental factors in the pathogenesis of atopic dermatitis (Bonamonte et al., 2019). Atopic dermatitis has a higher prevalence in cities than in the countryside. The hygiene hypothesis proposes that exposure to microbes early in life may induce immunologic tolerance and thereby decrease the risk of allergy development (Hesselmar et al., 2013). Urbanization may be associated with changes in hygiene, different microbial infections, increased use of antibiotics, and different exposures to diet and new allergens, which may contribute to the increased prevalence of atopic dermatitis in urban areas.

Urbanization may further be associated with an increased prevalence of atopic dermatitis secondary to the effects of pollution. Both indoor and outdoor pollution are known to exacerbate atopic dermatitis. Similarly, tobacco smoke exposure is associated with atopic dermatitis. Tobacco smoke increases levels of proinflammatory cytokines and reduces levels of antiinflammatory cytokines, contributing to oxidative damage, which decreases the skin barrier and has an irritant effect on the skin. Given that up to one-third of atopic dermatitis occurs within the first year of life, prenatal exposure to air pollution may play a role in the development of atopic dermatitis. One study showed that the prevalence of atopic dermatitis during the first year of life doubles with prenatal exposure to fine particulate matter and with postnatal exposure to tobacco smoke (Bonamonte et al., 2019).

Changes in microbes may contribute to differences in atopic dermatitis in urban areas compared to more rural areas. Exposure to bacterial endotoxins from dogs, farm animals, and commensal microbes may be protective against developing allergies (Bonamonte et al., 2019; Hesselmar et al., 2013). A 2013 study examined pacifier use in infants. Infants whose parents sucked the pacifier to clean it were less likely to develop asthma, eczema, and sensitization than infants whose parents did not clean the pacifier by sucking it, suggesting that the transfer of salivary microbiota may stimulate the immune system in infants and ultimately reduce the risk of allergy development (Hesselmar et al., 2013). Similarly, along the lines of the hygiene hypothesis, exposure to microbes on dishes may reduce the incidence of atopic dermatitis. A 2015 study found that allergic diseases were less common in children whose families hand-washed dishes compared to those who used a dishwashing machine, perhaps due to increased microbial exposure in

the less-efficient hand-washing technique (Hesselmar et al., 2013). The skin microbiome may contribute to differences in atopic dermatitis phenotypes. Antibiotic use is associated with an increased risk of atopic dermatitis, which may be related to changes in the microbiome. A recent study found increased levels of *Staphylococcus aureus* in atopic dermatitis patients compared to nonatopic controls. Furthermore, the study found a positive correlation between *S. aureus* levels and transepidermal water loss in patients with atopic dermatitis and food allergies but not in patients with atopic dermatitis alone or in nonatopic controls. These data suggest a potential link between the skin microbiome and atopic phenotypes (Leung et al., 2019). There has been no proven association between vaccinations and the prevalence of atopic dermatitis (Bonamonte et al., 2019).

In regard to climate, symptoms of atopic dermatitis worsen with increasing latitude and with decreasing outside temperature. This is thought to relate to the immunosuppressive effects of ultraviolet (UV) light. UV light aids in the conversion of *trans*-urocanic acid in filaggrin into *cis*-urocanic acid, which has an immunosuppressive effect. UV light has antiinflammatory effects by downregulating Langerhans cells and decreasing proinflammatory T-cell cytokines in the skin. Additionally, increased levels of vitamin D in response to sun exposure may improve atopic dermatitis. Vitamin D deficiency has been associated with more severe atopic dermatitis in photo-protected areas suggestive of a potential local protective effect from vitamin D (Bonamonte et al., 2019).

Atopic dermatitis is less common in developing countries, which may in part be related to diet. The traditional Western diet, consisting of refined cereals, red and preserved meats, and high in saturated and unsaturated fatty acids may be associated with an increased prevalence of atopic dermatitis (Bonamonte et al., 2019). More specifically, a high intake of fish during pregnancy has been shown to lower the risk of atopic dermatitis. There is a similar risk reduction in children who have a high intake of fish. This risk reduction is likely related to the high content of antiinflammatory n-3-polyunsaturated fatty acids. Similarly, some studies suggest a possible protective effect with an increased intake of fresh fruit and a negative effect with the intake of fast foods. However, despite these potential correlations, strict diet control has not shown to be effective in the management of atopic dermatitis. Nutrition and diet as a factor of atopic dermatitis are further discussed in Chapter 8.

Along the lines of increased inflammation worsening atopic dermatitis, increased screen time on electronic devices, which may contribute to obesity and inflammatory adipokines, has also been associated with increased atopic dermatitis (Bonamonte et al., 2019). Obesity has been shown to be associated with an increased incidence of bacterial and *Candida* skin infections as well as multiple inflammatory disorders, including psoriasis, rosacea, and hidradenitis suppurativa. A 2015 meta-analysis showed an association between increased weight and the prevalence of atopic dermatitis in North America and Asia, though a causal link has yet to be determined (Bonamonte et al., 2019; Hirt, Castillo, Yosipovitch, & Keri, 2019; Zhang & Silverberg, 2015). The data regarding breastfeeding for prevention of atopic dermatitis is controversial, with some studies suggesting that exclusive breastfeeding may actually increase the risk of atopic dermatitis due to decreased exposure to microbes early in life (Lien & Goldman, 2011). The data regarding the role of probiotics in reducing atopic dermatitis have also been mixed; however, maternal supplementation with probiotics during breastfeeding may play a role in reducing the incidence of atopic dermatitis by increasing antiinflammatory immunoregulatory factors in breast milk (Lien & Goldman, 2011). Furthermore, atopic dermatitis is a chronic inflammatory disorder, and like other chronic inflammatory conditions may increase the risk of malignancy, though evidence is contradictory, and there are many potential confounding factors (Hirt et al., 2019).

Some studies suggest that a decreased remission rate may also explain the increasing prevalence of atopic dermatitis. This decreased remission rate is attributed to an increase in the environmental factors previously described, social stressors, a fear of using topical corticosteroids, and more widespread use of home remedies, which often lack scientific evidence (Sugiura et al., 1998). Epidemiologic trends, potential contributors, and possible action items are summarized in Table 4.1.

Genetics as a controlling factor

Genetics plays a strong role in the pathogenesis of atopic dermatitis, with genetic alterations accounting for 90% of the susceptibility of early-onset atopic dermatitis (McAleer, O'Regan, & Irvine, 2018). The concordance rate for atopic dermatitis is significantly higher in monozygotic twins at 77% compared to only 15% in dizygotic twins (McAleer et al., 2018; Paller & Mancini, 2016). Furthermore, parental history of atopic dermatitis is a stronger predictor for developing atopic dermatitis than a personal history of either asthma or allergic rhinitis. For many years, atopic dermatitis was thought to result from immunologic defects resulting in a defective skin barrier, a theory known as the inside-outside hypothesis (Irvine, McLean, & Leung, 2011). It is now known that genetics do play a strong role in the development of atopic dermatitis, more likely through an outside-inside mechanism with defects affecting the skin barrier rather than immunology alone.

FLG encodes the protein filaggrin, or filament-aggregating protein. *FLG* is expressed throughout all layers of the epidermis, and filaggrin is an important structural component of the stratum corneum (Barker et al., 2007; Irvine et al., 2011; McAleer et al., 2018). Breakdown products of filaggrin play an important role in epidermal hydration, lipid processing, and barrier function (McAleer et al., 2018). Mutations in *FLG* are an important predisposing factor for childhood eczema. *FLG* mutations are present in 10% to 30% of atopic dermatitis patients, and genome-wide association studies suggest multiple other loci that may play a role in the development of atopic dermatitis (McAleer et al., 2018; Paller & Mancini, 2016).

FLG mutations are overexpressed in patients with atopic dermatitis compared to those without atopic dermatitis. In the atopic dermatitis cohort, there is a sixfold overrepresentation of null *FLG* alleles: 42% of patients in the atopic dermatitis cohort carry null mutations in *FLG*, whereas as only 8.8% of the general population carry null mutations in *FLG* (Barker et al., 2007). An estimated 20% to 50% of European and Asian children with moderate-to-severe atopic dermatitis have at least one *FLG* mutation (McAleer et al., 2018).

Patients with *FLG* mutations tend to have earlier-onset atopic dermatitis, greater disease severity, and are more likely to have disease persistence into adulthood. Carriers

TABLE 4.1	Factors affecting epidemiologic trends		
Epidemiologic trends	**Potential contributors**		**Possible actions items**
Blacks and Hispanics have higher prevalence	• Household income • Health insurance • Access to care • Difficulty in assessing erythema in skin of nonwhite patients, leading to delayed and underdiagnosis		• Increasing access to education • Revising assessment tools to better access atopic dermatitis severity in skin of nonwhite patients
Increasing prevalence in developing nations	• Environmental pollution association with urbanization • Decreased exposure to allergens early in life (hygiene hypothesis) • Climate change • Dietary changes • Obesity		• Environmental programs • Nutrition and education programs
Decreased remission rate	• Increasing prevalence • Social stressors • Fear of medications		• Patient and parent education • Drug development

of *FLG* mutations are also at increased risk for developing allergic and irritant contact dermatitis, asthma, hay fever, and food allergies (Irvine et al., 2011; McAleer et al., 2018). *FLG* is not expressed in the gastrointestinal or bronchial mucosa, so the increased risk for food allergies and asthma associated with filaggrin mutations supports the hypothesis that cutaneous sensitization and inflammation contribute to systemic development of atopy (McAleer et al., 2018).

Deficiencies in *SPINK5*, which encodes lymphoepithelial Kazal-type 5 (LETK1) may also play a role in the development of atopic dermatitis and Netherton syndrome. LETK1 is a serine protease inhibitor expressed in mucosal and epithelial surfaces. LETK1 normally inhibits kallikreins, which are important in regulating skin desquamation, inflammation, and maintaining the skin barrier (Kato et al., 2003). Increased serine protease results in proteolytic cleavage of the stratum corneum (Richard & Ringpfeil, 2018).

In addition to *FLG* and *SPINK5*, genome-wide association studies have found many genes that are associated with atopic dermatitis. Some of the proteins encoded by these genes include mattrin, which regulates lamellar body assembly and is encoded by *TMEM79*, zinc-dependent metalloproteinases encoded by *ADAMTS*, kinesin found in cilia encoded by *KIF3A*, and proteins involved in epithelial tissue and germ cell differentiation encoded by *OVOL1* (Esparza-Gordillo et al., 2009; Paternoster et al., 2011; Portelli, Hodge, & Sayers, 2015; Sun et al., 2011). A recent study examined different phenotypes of atopic dermatitis. Patients with atopic dermatitis and food allergies had increased amounts of keratin 5, 14, and 16 in the skin compared to patients with atopic dermatitis and no food allergies and compared to nonatopic controls. These data suggest that variation in protein expression may contribute to different atopic dermatitis phenotypes (Leung et al., 2019). There may also be differences in barrier components among atopic dermatitis phenotypes. Atopic dermatitis patients with food allergies may have lower levels of filaggrin and lower proportions of omega-hydroxy fatty acid sphingosine ceramide content compared to atopic dermatitis patients without food allergies and nonatopic controls (Leung et al., 2019). Genes, proteins and their respective functions, and mutational effects in atopic dermatitis are summarized in Table 4.2.

Socioeconomic burden perspectives

Atopic dermatitis can have severe implications on the socioeconomic status of affected patients and their families. Atopic dermatitis has the highest disability-adjusted life-years among skin disorders, reflecting both the high prevalence and significant patient burden (Silverberg, 2017). Multiple studies have shown that children with atopic dermatitis are more likely to have an increased number of sick days and poorer performance at school due to their symptoms from atopic dermatitis (Silverberg et al., 2018; Wan, Margolis, Mitra, Hoffstad, & Takeshita, 2019). Wan et al. (2019) conducted a survey looking at school absences in

TABLE 4.2	Important genes involved in skin barrier intnegrity	
Gene/protein	**Function(s)**	**Effect(s)**
FLG/filaggrin	Structural component of the stratum corneum	Reduced barrier function; associated with earlier-onset atopic dermatitis and increased disease severity
SPINK5/LETK1	Serine protease inhibitor; expressed in mucosal and epithelial surfaces; regulates skin desquamation, inflammation, and maintains skin barrier	Stratum corneum cleavage; defective barrier; mutation in Netherton syndrome
TMEM79/mattrin	Lamellar body assembly	Reduced barrier function
ADAMTS/zinc-dependent metalloproteinases	Tissue remodeling and inflammation	Reduced barrier function

children with atopic dermatitis. About 3% of children with atopic dermatitis miss 6 or more days of school over the course of 6 months due to their atopic dermatitis, which meets the definition for chronic school absenteeism in the United States. Children who are chronically absent from school are more likely to fall behind or drop out, which has potential negative long-term implications. Furthermore, black and Hispanic children were 1.5- to 3.4-fold more likely to miss at least 6 days of school because of atopic dermatitis compared to non-Hispanic white children, even after controlling for potential confounding factors, including sociodemographic factors, degree of atopic dermatitis control, health care visits, and other medical comorbidities (Wan et al., 2019). This discrepancy suggests that atopic dermatitis may have a greater negative impact on socioeconomics and quality of life in patients from ethnic minority groups (Wan et al., 2019).

The care associated with atopic dermatitis comes with increased health care utilization and an economic burden (Eckert et al., 2018). Patients with atopic dermatitis face both direct and indirect costs. Direct costs include office visit copays, hospitalizations, diagnostic and laboratory testing, over-the-counter medications and supplies, prescription medications, transportation, dietary and environmental changes, and special clothing (Mancini, Kaulback, & Chamlin, 2008). Indirect costs include those associated with pain and suffering, decreased performance and absences at work or school, and effects on ultimate career choice (Mancini et al., 2008). In 2012 emergency department visits for atopic dermatitis alone totaled over $265 million in the United States (Kwa & Silverberg, 2018). One study estimated that in the United States the total mean annual per-patient direct costs is over $10,000 more than direct patient costs for patients without atopic dermatitis (Eckert et al., 2018; Silverberg et al., 2018). Total national costs for atopic dermatitis range from $364 million (estimated cost in 1993) to $4.228 billion in 2004 (Bickers et al., 2006; Drucker et al., 2017; Mancini et al., 2008; Narla, Hsu, Thyssen, & Silverberg, 2017) with a breakdown of $1.009 billion for direct costs, $619 million for lost productivity, and $2.6 billion for decrements in quality of life (Bickers et al., 2006; Drucker et al., 2017). These costs were projected to reach $5.297 billion in 2015. With inflation and increased prevalence of atopic dermatitis, these costs are now likely significantly higher than reported in these studies.

Patients with atopic dermatitis also have an increased risk for hospitalization, which carries a high economic burden for the patient, patient's family, and health care system as a whole (Eckert et al., 2018; Hua & Silverberg, 2019). Patients with atopic dermatitis are more than twice as likely to have emergency room visits than nonatopic dermatitis controls and are more likely to be hospitalized (Eckert et al., 2018). Between 2002 and 2012 there were 6577 admissions for atopic dermatitis, which included 4330 adults and 2247 children (Narla et al., 2017). Inpatient costs associated with hospitalizations for atopic dermatitis range from $3 million per year for children to $8 million per year for adults, and actual costs are likely higher (Narla et al., 2017). Risk factors associated with hospitalization among patients with atopic dermatitis include black and other nonwhite races, having Medicaid or no insurance, outpatient physician interaction, an asthma attack in the past year, feeling depressed, attention-deficit hyperactivity disorder (ADHD), hay fever or respiratory allergy, digestive allergy, and infection (Hua & Silverberg, 2019). Overall, costs of atopic dermatitis continue to rise, particularly with the growing prevalence of atopic dermatitis (Mancini et al., 2008).

Atopic dermatitis causes further financial strain on families through indirect costs, such as when parents have to take time off work to care for their sick children. Studies estimate that parents of children with atopic dermatitis may spend 2 to 3 hours per day with eczema-related care (Lewis-Jones, 2006). Mothers of young children with atopic dermatitis report decreased employment, poor social support, and stress about parenting (Chamlin, 2006). In single-parent, low-income families, cost is rated as one of the most important negative factors associated with atopic dermatitis (Lewis-Jones, 2006).

Drug development also contributes to the overall cost of atopic dermatitis. Clinical trials are costly and once approved, medications can be formidably expensive. Dupilumab, which is US Food and Drug Administration (FDA) approved for atopic dermatitis, runs a price of $37,000 per year without insurance. Even if covered by insurance these medications

TABLE 4.3	Factors contributing to costs associated with atopic dermatitis care
Costs	**Contributors**
Costs to patient and family	*Direct costs:* office visit copays, hospitalizations, lab testing, medications, supplies, transportation, special diet/clothes *Indirect costs:* work/school absences, career choice, parental time off work
Costs to medical system	Emergency room visits, drug development, hospitalizations

increase costs for the health care system as a whole. Economic burdens of atopic dermatitis are summarized in Table 4.3.

The factor of barriers to care

In addition to costs, patients with atopic dermatitis face additional barriers to care. Access to specialist care is limited, and it can be difficult to schedule an appointment particularly during an acute flare. Among children with atopic dermatitis, the most common specialty pediatric patients see for their atopic dermatitis general pediatrics followed by dermatology, then other specialties suggesting a particular need for increased access to pediatric dermatologists (Singh & Silverberg, 2019). When looking at the type of visits, office visits for acute flares of atopic dermatitis were more likely to be seen by primary care physicians than by dermatologists. Conversely, follow-up visits for chronic atopic dermatitis are more likely to be seen by dermatologists, suggesting difficulty scheduling urgent visits with dermatologists for acute atopic dermatitis flares (Singh & Silverberg, 2019). Limited access to providers forces some patients to be seen in emergency department settings with providers who do not know their medical history and who do not regularly manage atopic dermatitis. One study found that 63% of medical visits for atopic dermatitis occurred in an emergency department, and that 60% of all emergency department visits occurred during normal working hours. These data suggest that patients resort to emergency department care due to lack of access to dermatology providers, not simply because flares occur outside normal working hours (Mancini et al., 2008). A 2018 study found that emergency department visits for atopic dermatitis compared to emergency department visits for other diagnoses were more likely to occur in patients with younger age, Medicaid or no insurance, and lower household incomes suggesting an increased need for access to pediatric dermatologists and a disproportionate effect of socioeconomics on emergency department use for patients with atopic dermatitis (Kwa & Silverberg. 2018).

Fears about medication use also contribute to barriers to care. In particular, fear about medication side effects contributes to lack of adherence to treatment regimens. Patients and parents may seek alternative therapies that can be costly and have little to no evidence of efficacy behind them (Chamlin, 2006). Over 17% of parents and adult patients cite concern about the potential side effects of medications as a reason for avoiding their use (Lewis-Jones, 2006). As such, education of patients with atopic dermatitis and all members of their care is essential to aid in adequate treatment and flare prevention (Lewis-Jones, 2006).

Psychosocial burden: physical health, mental health, and quality of life

Physical health and medical comorbidities

When compared to the general population, patients with eczema have a higher proportion of poor to fair overall health (Silverberg et al., 2018). Overall health is proportional to the severity of eczema: The more severe the eczema, the worse the overall health. Patients with eczema tend to have multiple comorbidities, including but not limited to the well-described atopic triad with allergic rhinitis and asthma (Simpson et al., 2016). In fact, eczema in infancy is one of the strongest risk factors for developing asthma and allergic rhinitis (von Kobyletzki et al., 2012). Children with eczema have over a twofold increase in odds of developing asthma and over a threefold increase in odds of developing rhinitis compared to children without eczema even after adjusting for potential confounding factors. The more severe the eczema and the earlier the onset of eczema, the higher the odds of developing asthma and rhinitis (von Kobyletzki et al., 2012). Patients with atopic dermatitis are also more likely to have hay fever, food allergies, mental health disturbances, and possible cardiometabolic comorbidities.

Quality of life

Multiple factors negatively impact the quality of life in patients with atopic dermatitis. Several reviews and studies have shown that the most burdensome symptom for patients with atopic dermatitis is pruritus followed by excessive dryness, scaling, inflammation, sleep disturbances, and increased skin pain (Avena-Woods, 2017). These symptoms interfere with normal lifestyle; patients report that they avoid social interactions because of their appearance and that their symptoms impact their daily activities, including the clothes they wear, owning pets, and sports participation (particularly swimming). Patients with atopic dermatitis also report that their symptoms interfere with developing personal relationships and with their performance at work and school (Simpson et al., 2016). In fact, nearly 23% of patients in one study reported that their skin prevented them from working or studying. Children also report feeling embarrassed about their skin condition and being teased by their peers, which can lead to social isolation (Lewis-Jones, 2006). In one study, nearly 32% of patients with severe atopic dermatitis reported being somewhat to very dissatisfied with life (Silverberg, 2017; Silverberg et al., 2018), and

another study of patients with atopic dermatitis reported an average Dermatology Life Quality Index (DLQI) score of 14.3, which correlates with having a very large impact on patient's lives. This is among the same level, if not greater than, other chronic medical conditions such as asthma and diabetes.

The most debilitating factor reported among patients with atopic dermatitis is pruritus (Silverberg, 2017; Silverberg et al., 2018; Vakharia et al., 2018). One study of pruritus in patients with atopic dermatitis found that itch intensity was rated as severe by 46.3% of patients, and 14.2% reported that their itch was unbearable (Simpson et al., 2016). Patients also report bleeding, oozing, cracking, flaking, and drying of the skin more than 5 days of the week (Simpson et al., 2016). Another study found that pruritus and soreness cause sleeplessness in over 60% of children with atopic dermatitis, and about 70% of patients reported that pruritus delayed their ability to fall asleep (Simpson et al., 2016; Lewis-Jones, 2006). Using a weighted average, sleep was disrupted on an average of 4.4 nights over a week among patients with atopic dermatitis (Simpson et al., 2016). More specifically, there is increased sleep latency and difficulty awakening in the morning (Lewis-Jones, 2006). This sleep deprivation can subsequently lead to daytime tiredness, mood changes, and impaired psychosocial functioning. Patients with atopic dermatitis are more likely to miss school due to both flares and fatigue, which may lead to further withdrawal and school avoidance (Lewis-Jones, 2006). Adequate sleep is important in developing children; sleep alterations have potential negative impacts on normal growth and development (e.g., altered sleep can alter growth hormone secretion) (Lewis-Jones, 2006). During atopic dermatitis flares, up to 89% of infants may have disturbed sleep. Sleep disturbances in children often affect the whole family. One study estimates that parents of children with atopic dermatitis lose 2.5 hours of sleep a night when their children are flaring, and up to 40% of siblings of affected children also experience sleep disturbances. To cope with sleep disturbances, parents of young children with atopic dermatitis may adopt cosleeping habits, which can further decrease parental sleep and can even perpetuate children's sleep disturbance beyond their flares (Chamlin, 2006).

Parents of children with atopic dermatitis also experience practical barriers, such as increased laundry, house cleaning, food preparation, and house dust mite regimens, that impact their day-to-day life (Lewis-Jones, 2006).

Mental health

A population-based, cross-sectional study looked at mental and physical health in several chronic medical conditions, including atopic dermatitis, anxiety or depression, autoimmune conditions, food allergy, asthma, heart disease, diabetes, high blood pressure, hay fever, and other serious chronic conditions. The mental health subscores for moderate atopic dermatitis were lower than almost all other disorders, and the mental health subscores for severe atopic dermatitis were drastically lower than all other disorders. Similarly, atopic dermatitis was associated with lower physical health and a lower quality of life. These differences persisted even when controlling for sociodemographic difference (Silverberg et al., 2018).

Sleep disturbances and the negative impact on quality of life contribute to behavioral symptoms seen in children with atopic dermatitis (Lewis-Jones, 2006). Sleep likely has a reciprocal relationship with mental health. Early life is a critical period for both physical and psychosocial health (Chamlin, 2006). Children learn and establish behavioral and sleep patterns early in life (Chamlin, 2006). Atopic dermatitis can interrupt the development of normal behavior and sleep patterns (Chamlin, 2006). One study estimates that nearly 25% of preschool-age children with severe atopic dermatitis have an increase in behavioral symptoms compared with only 5% of age-matched controls (Lewis-Jones, 2006). Behavioral effects occur in an age-dependent manner. Children with atopic dermatitis tend to have increased irritability, fussiness, and crying. Teenage years are an important time for the development of self-identity and self-esteem. Teenagers with atopic dermatitis report increased embarrassment, social isolation, and self-consciousness, which is similar to teenagers with acne. Symptoms are worse with increasing disease severity (Chamlin, 2006).

In children, disturbances in sleep increase daytime sleepiness and make waking up for school harder, which can contribute to the chronic school absenteeism previously described (Lewis-Jones, 2006). Daytime tiredness from loss of sleep also affects schoolwork, and children with atopic dermatitis are more likely to have impaired concentration, school avoidance, and school phobia. Social isolation, peer group rejection, teasing, and bullying can all lead to loss of confidence, mood changes, social withdrawal, and depression (Lewis-Jones, 2006). Some reports of children with eczema estimate up to double the rate of psychologic disturbances in school-age children compared to controls. Studies estimate that 43% to 50% of patients with atopic dermatitis suffer from anxiety, depression, or other mood disorders (Simpson

et al., 2016). A European study found that 15% of patients with atopic dermatitis reported suicidal ideation, and among patients with severe atopic disease this rose to 20% (Simpson et al., 2016). Additionally, atopic dermatitis is associated with a higher odds of hospitalization for all mental health disorders (Hsu, Smith, & Silverberg, 2019). Parents of children with atopic dermatitis also report emotional problems and report increased sadness, crying, guilt, and self-blame in addition to feelings of social isolation (Chamlin, 2006; Lewis-Jones, 2006). The physical and mental health burdens of atopic dermatitis are summarized in Table 4.4.

Summary

Overall, the prevalence of atopic dermatitis is increasing globally. Contributing factors include urbanization, genetics, and changes in microbes and climate. Atopic dermatitis results in significant burden for patients and their families with quality of life, socioeconomic, mental health, and development issues. There is limited access to pediatric dermatologists, and some of the most vulnerable patients often lack access to dermatologic care.

Further readings

Bonamonte, D., Filoni, A., Vestita, M., Romita, P., Foti, C., & Angelini, G. (2019). The role of the environmental risk factors in the pathogenesis and clinical outcome of atopic dermatitis. *BioMedical Research Internation*. https://doi.org/10.1155/2019/2450605.

Lewis-Jones. S. (2006). Quality of life and childhood atopic dermatitis: The misery of living with childhood eczema. *International Journal of Clinical Practice*, 60(8), 984–992. https://doi.org/10.1111/j.1742-1241.2006.01047.x.

Mancini, A. J., Kaulback, K., & Chamlin, S. L. (2008). The socioeconomic impact of atopic dermatitis in the United States: A systematic review. *Pediatric Dermatology*, 25(1), 1–6. https://doi.org/10.1111/j.1525-1470.2007.00572.x.

Silverberg. J. I. (2017). Public health burden and epidemiology of atopic dermatitis. *Dermatology Clinics*, 35(3), 283–289. https://doi.org/10.1016/j.det.2017.02.002.

Singh, P., & Silverberg, J. I. (2019). Outpatient utilization patterns for atopic dermatitis in the United States. *Journal of the American Academy of Dermatology*. https://doi.org/10.1016/j.jaad.2019.03.021.

References

Avena-Woods. C. (2017). Overview of atopic dermatitis. *The American Journal of Managed Care*, 23(8 Suppl), S115–S123.

Barker, J. N., Palmer, C. N., Zhao, Y., Liao, H., Hull, P. R., Lee, S. P., et al. (2007). Null mutations in the filaggrin gene (FLG) determine major susceptibility to early-onset atopic dermatitis that persists into adulthood. *Journal of Investigative Dermatology*, 127(3), 564–567. https://doi.org/10.1038/sj.jid.5700587.

Bickers, D. R., Lim, H. W., Margolis, D., Weinstock, M. A., Goodman, C., Faulkner, E., et al. (2006). The burden of skin diseases: 2004 a joint project of the American Academy of Dermatology Association and the Society for Investigative Dermatology. *Journal*

TABLE 4.4	Factors contributing to burdens associated with atopic dermatitis	
Burdens	**Contributors**
Physical health and medical comorbidities	Atopic triad: eczema, asthma, allergic rhinitis, food allergies, cardiometabolic comorbidities
Decreased quality of life	Pruritus, xerosis, scaling, inflammation, sleep disturbances, skin pain, which can lead to school absenteeism, peer teasing, social isolation
Mental health	Sleep disturbances during critical development periods, daytime sleepiness, social isolation, peer group rejection

of the American Academy of Dermatology, 55(3), 490–500. https://doi.org/10.1016/j.jaad.2006.05.048.

Bonamonte, D., Filoni, A., Vestita, M., Romita, P., Foti, C., & Angelini, G. (2019). The role of the environmental risk factors in the pathogenesis and clinical outcome of atopic dermatitis. *BioMed Research International, 2019*, 2450605. https://doi.org/10.1155/2019/2450605.

Chamlin. S. L. (2006). The psychosocial burden of childhood atopic dermatitis. *Dermatologic Therapy, 19*(2), 104–107. https://doi.org/10.1111/j.1529-8019.2006.00060.x.

Drucker, A. M., Wang, A. R., Li, W. Q., Sevetson, E., Block, J. K., & Qureshi, A. A. (2017). The burden of atopic dermatitis: summary of a report for the National Eczema Association. *Journal of Investigative Dermatology, 137*(1), 26–30. https://doi.org/10.1016/j.jid.2016.07.012.

Eckert, L., Gupta, S., Amand, C., Gadkari, A., Mahajan, P., & Gelfand, J. M. (2018). The burden of atopic dermatitis in US adults: Health care resource utilization data from the 2013 National Health and Wellness Survey. *Journal of the American Academy of Dermatology, 78*(1), 54–61.e1. https://doi.org/10.1016/j.jaad.2017.08.002.

Esparza-Gordillo, J., Weidinger, S., Folster-Holst, R., Bauerfeind, A., Ruschendorf, F., Patone, G., et al. (2009). A common variant on chromosome 11q13 is associated with atopic dermatitis. *Nature Genetics, 41*(5), 596–601. https://doi.org/10.1038/ng.347.

Guo, Y., Zhang, H., Liu, Q., Wei, F., Tang, J., Li, P., et al. (2019). Phenotypic analysis of atopic dermatitis in children aged 1-12 months: Elaboration of novel diagnostic criteria for infants in China and estimation of prevalence. *Journal of the European Academy of Dermatology and Venereology, 33*(8), 1569–1576. https://doi.org/10.1111/jdv.15618.

Hesselmar, B., Sjoberg, F., Saalman, R., Aberg, N., Adlerberth, I., & Wold, A. E. (2013). Pacifier cleaning practices and risk of allergy development. *Pediatrics, 131*(6), e1829–e1837. https://doi.org/10.1542/peds.2012-3345.

Hirt, P. A., Castillo, D. E., Yosipovitch, G., & Keri, J. E. (2019). Skin changes in the obese patient. *Journal of the American Academy of Dermatology, 81*(5), 1037–1057. https://doi.org/10.1016/j.jaad.2018.12.070. https://www.jaad.org/article/S0190-9622(19)30158-6/fulltext.

Hsu, D. Y., Smith, B., & Silverberg, J. I. (2019). Atopic dermatitis and hospitalization for mental health disorders in the United States. *Dermatitis, 30*(1), 54–61. https://doi.org/10.1097/der.0000000000000418.

Hua, T., & Silverberg, J. I. (2019). Atopic dermatitis is associated with increased hospitalization in US children. *Journal of the American Academy of Dermatology, 81*(3), 862–865. https://doi.org/10.1016/j.jaad.2019.05.019.

Irvine, A. D., McLean, W. H., & Leung, D. Y. (2011). Filaggrin mutations associated with skin and allergic diseases. *The New England Journal of Medicine, 365*(14), 1315–1327. https://doi.org/10.1056/NEJMra1011040.

Kato, A., Fukai, K., Oiso, N., Hosomi, N., Murakami, T., & Ishii, M. (2003). Association of SPINK5 gene polymorphisms with atopic dermatitis in the Japanese population. *British Journal of Dermatology, 148*(4), 665–669. https://doi.org/10.1046/j.1365-2133.2003.05243.x.

Kramer, O. N., Strom, M. A., Ladizinski, B., & Lio, P. A. (2017). The history of atopic dermatitis. *Clinics in Dermatology, 35*(4), 344–348. https://doi.org/10.1016/j.clindermatol.2017.03.005.

Kwa, L., & Silverberg, J. I. (2018). Financial burden of emergency department visits for atopic dermatitis in the United States. *Journal of the American Academy of Dermatology, 79*(3), 443–447. https://doi.org/10.1016/j.jaad.2018.05.025.

Larsen, F. S., Diepgen, T., & Svensson, A. (1996). The occurrence of atopic dermatitis in north Europe: An international questionnaire study. *Journal of the American Academy of Dermatology, 34*(5 Pt 1), 760–764. https://doi.org/10.1016/s0190-9622(96)90009-2.

Leung, D. Y. M., Calatroni, A., Zaramela, L. S., LeBeau, P. K., Dyjack, N., Brar, K., et al. (2019). The nonlesional skin surface distinguishes atopic dermatitis with food allergy as a unique endotype. *Science Translational Medicine, 11*(480), eaav2685. https://doi.org/10.1126/scitranslmed.aav2685. https://stm.sciencemag.org/content/scitransmed/11/480/eaav2685.full.pdf.

Lewis-Jones. S. (2006). Quality of life and childhood atopic dermatitis: The misery of living with childhood eczema. *International Journal of Clinical Practice, 60*(8), 984–992. https://doi.org/10.1111/j.1742-1241.2006.01047.x.

Lien, T. Y., & Goldman, R. D. (2011). Breastfeeding and maternal diet in atopic dermatitis. *Canadian Family Physician, 57*(12), 1403–1405.

Mancini, A. J., Kaulback, K., & Chamlin, S. L. (2008). The socioeconomic impact of atopic dermatitis in the United States: A systematic review. *Pediatric Dermatology, 25*(1), 1–6. https://doi.org/10.1111/j.1525-1470.2007.00572.x.

McAleer, M., O'Regan, G., & Irvine, A. (2018). Atopic dermatitis. In J. Schaffer, J. Bolognia, & L. Cerroni (Eds.), *Dermatology.* (4th ed.), (pp. 208–224). Philadelphia, PA: Elsevier.

McKenzie, C., & Silverberg, J. I. (2019). The prevalence and persistence of atopic dermatitis in urban United States children. *Annals of Allergy, Asthma & Immunology, 123*(2), 173–178.e1. https://doi.org/10.1016/j.anai.2019.05.014.

Nakamura, T., Haider, S., Colicino, S., Murray, C. S., Holloway, J., Simpson, A., et al. (2019). Different definitions of atopic dermatitis: Impact on prevalence estimates and associated risk factors. *British Journal of Dermatology, 181*(6), 1272–1279. https://doi.org/10.1111/bjd.17853.

Narla, S., Hsu, D. Y., Thyssen, J. P., & Silverberg, J. I. (2017). Inpatient financial burden of atopic dermatitis in the United States. *Journal of Investigative Dermatology, 137*(7), 1461–1467. https://doi.org/10.1016/j.jid.2017.02.975.

Paller, A. S., & Mancini, A. J. (2016). Eczematous eruptions in childhood: In *Hurwitz Clinical Pediatric Dermatology* (5th ed.), (pp. 38–72). Elsevier.

Paternoster, L., Standl, M., Chen, C. M., Ramasamy, A., Bonnelykke, K., Duijts, L., et al. (2011). Meta-analysis of genome-wide association studies identifies three new risk loci for atopic dermatitis. *Nature Genetics, 44*(2), 187–192. https://doi.org/10.1038/ng.1017.

Portelli, M. A., Hodge, E., & Sayers, I. (2015). Genetic risk factors for the development of allergic disease identified by genome-wide association. *Clinical & Experimental Allergy, 45*(1), 21–31. https://doi.org/10.1111/cea.12327.

Richard, G., & Ringpfeil, F. (2018). Ichthyoses, erythrokeratodermas, and related disorders. In J. Schaffer, J. Bolognia, & L. Cerroni (Eds.), *Dermatology.* Elsevier.

Silverberg. J. I. (2017). Public health burden and epidemiology of atopic dermatitis. *Dermatologic Clinics, 35*(3), 283–289. https://doi.org/10.1016/j.det.2017.02.002.

Silverberg, J. I., Gelfand, J. M., Margolis, D. J., Boguniewicz, M., Fonacier, L., Grayson, M. H., et al. (2018). Patient burden and quality of life in atopic dermatitis in US adults: A population-based cross-sectional study. *Annals of Allergy, Asthma & Immunology, 121*(3), 340–347. https://doi.org/10.1016/j.anai.2018.07.006.

Silverberg, J. I., & Simpson, E. L. (2014). Associations of childhood eczema severity: A US population-based study. *Dermatitis, 25*(3), 107–114. https://doi.org/10.1097/der.0000000000000034.

Simpson, E. L., Bieber, T., Eckert, L., Wu, R., Ardeleanu, M., Graham, N. M., et al. (2016). Patient burden of moderate to severe atopic dermatitis (AD): Insights from a phase 2b clinical trial of dupilumab in adults. *Journal of the American Academy of Dermatology*, *74*(3), 491–498. https://doi.org/10.1016/j.jaad.2015.10.043.

Singh, P., & Silverberg, J. I. (2019). Outpatient utilization patterns for atopic dermatitis in the United States. *Journal of the American Academy of Dermatology*. https://doi.org/10.1016/j.jaad.2019.03.021.

Sugiura, H., Umemoto, N., Deguchi, H., Murata, Y., Tanaka, K., Sawai, T., et al. (1998). Prevalence of childhood and adolescent atopic dermatitis in a Japanese population: Comparison with the disease frequency examined 20 years ago. *Acta Dermato-Venereologica*, *78*(4), 293–294.

Sun, L. D., Xiao, F. L., Li, Y., Zhou, W. M., Tang, H. Y., Tang, X. F., et al. (2011). Genome-wide association study identifies two new susceptibility loci for atopic dermatitis in the Chinese Han population. *Nature Genetics*, *43*(7), 690–694. https://doi.org/10.1038/ng.851.

Vakharia, P. P., Chopra, R., Sacotte, R., Patel, N., Immaneni, S., White, T., et al. (2018). Validation of patient-reported global severity of atopic dermatitis in adults. *Allergy*, *73*(2), 451–458. https://doi.org/10.1111/all.13309.

von Kobyletzki, L. B., Bornehag, C. G., Hasselgren, M., Larsson, M., Lindstrom, C. B., & Svensson, A. (2012). Eczema in early childhood is strongly associated with the development of asthma and rhinitis in a prospective cohort. *BMC Dermatology*, *12*, 11. https://doi.org/10.1186/1471-5945-12-11.

Wan, J., Margolis, D. J., Mitra, N., Hoffstad, O. J., & Takeshita, J. (2019). Racial and Ethnic differences in atopic dermatitis-related school absences among US children. *JAMA Dermatology*. https://doi.org/10.1001/jamadermatol.2019.0597.

Zhang, A., & Silverberg, J. I. (2015). Association of atopic dermatitis with being overweight and obese: A systematic review and meta-analysis. *Journal of the American Academy of Dermatology*, *72*(4), 606–16.e4. https://doi.org/10.1016/j.jaad.2014.12.013

5

Skin Barrier

HERA WU AND RAJA K. SIVAMANI

KEY POINTS

- The four layers of the epidermis—stratum corneum, stratum granulosum, stratum spinosum, and stratum basale—are composed of keratinocytes, which undergo differentiation and mature as they become more superficial until they are terminally differentiated at the stratum corneum.
- The dermis provides structure, houses epidermally derived appendages, and provides vascular supply to the skin.
- There are many factors that may contribute to the development of atopic dermatitis, including defects in the components of the physical barrier (notably the lipid matrix) and structural and adhesive proteins in the stratum corneum.
- Atopic dermatitis is characterized by immune dysregulation as part of a Th2-driven disease.
- Skin in atopic dermatitis has increased permeability to microbes, allergens, and irritants causing local and systemic inflammation.

Introduction

What constitutes the skin barrier? The skin is the largest barrier between the outside environment and the internal body, which is otherwise susceptible to dehydration, loss of nutrients, infection, DNA damage from light, and ultimately loss of form and function. The skin is composed of both cellular and extracellular components that create specialized structures that make up the physical and immunologic interfaces to the outside world. This chapter focuses on physical structures and functions of this barrier and the consequences of the defective barrier in atopic dermatitis.

Physical composition and function of the skin

The two major layers of the skin include the epidermis and the deeper dermis. Deeper still is the subcutaneous fat and fascia, which together are also often referred to as the hypodermis, though this is not part of the integument unlike the epidermis and dermis. A drawing of a three-dimensional (3D) model depicts various major components at different levels of the skin (Fig. 5.1).

In a 3D cross section of skin, various components and appendages are housed with the three major layers of the skin known as the epidermis, dermis, and hypodermis. The most superficial layer of skin, the epidermis, is anchored to the deeper layer, the dermis, at the dermal-epidermal junction (DEJ) by intercalating dermal papillae and ridges. The dermis consists of extracellular matrix (ECM) that houses various functional components such as blood vessels, lymphatics, nerves, glands, and skin appendages. The deepest layer of skin that is sometimes included as a skin layer though it is not part of the integument is the hypodermis. This layer is made of subcutaneous fat and fascia.

The epidermis is largely composed of stratified squamous keratinized cells called keratinocytes that populate each of the sublayers birthed at the deepest cell layer against the basement membrane and become more differentiated as the cells become more superficial. Within the epidermis there are four sublayers (strata): From most superficial to deepest they are stratum corneum, stratum granulosum, stratum spinosum, and stratum basale. An additional dense layer called stratum lucidum consists of enucleated flat keratinocytes between stratum granulosum and stratum corneum and exists in thick skin such as in palms and soles. The histologic features, main functions, and specialized cells of each strata are described in Table 5.1. Basal stem cells are bound to the basement membrane by hemidesmosomes, and keratinocytes are bound to adjacent cells by desmosomes and other intercellular proteins contributing to the permeability barrier created from epidermal layers. As cells travel superficially, they undergo differentiation called keratinization (also known as cornification) and enhance the amount and types of keratin filaments while they flatten, dehydrate, and eventually dispose of their nucleus and organelles at their terminal stage in the stratum corneum. At the surface, cells are surrounded by a keratinized envelope composed of transglutaminase cross-linked proteins and lipids, notably loricrin and involucrin (Agrawal & Woodfolk, 2014; Marks & Miller, 2013; Mescher, 2018) (Fig. 5.2).

The epidermis consists of four major sublayers or strata composed of keratinocytes. As cells migrate from the deepest to the most superficial strata, they undergo differentiation

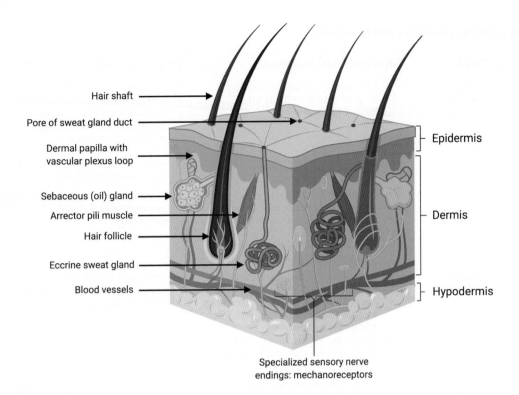

• **Fig. 5.1** Structural components of skin.

in a process called keratinization. The most superficial of the strata is the stratum corneum, which possesses terminally differentiated, enucleated, and dead keratinocytes that are flattened, dehydrated, and surrounded by a dense envelop of protein and lipids that serves as a water-resistant seal. Beneath it is the stratum granulosum named for its prominent keratinohyaline granules and Golgi-derived lamellar granules containing lipids that contribute to the water barrier. Deeper yet, the stratum spinosum is the thickest of the strata and is characterized by the intercellular bridges created by desmosomes, which anchor adjacent cells to one another. The stratum basale is the deepest of the strata and is a single layer of columnar cells attached to the basement membrane by hemidesmosomes. This is where the basal stem cells produce the new keratinocytes through mitosis. An additional dense layer called stratum lucidum (not pictured in Fig. 5.2) consists of enucleated flat keratinocytes just deep to the stratum corneum and exists in thick skin such as in palms and soles.

The DEJ is where the basement membrane lies and has a specialized 3D structure that anchors the epidermis to the dermis. Epidermal papillae and ridges show a wavy appearance in a superficial-to-deep cross section or a Swiss cheese model in a cross-sectional plane taken parallel to the skin surface at the DEJ.

The dermis consists of largely ECM made up of different protein fibers that provide the structural component of the skin. The dermal papillae consisting of the looser areolar connective tissue and its own vascular and lymphatic plexuses sit atop the reticular layer of the dermis, which contains more acellular irregular dense connective tissue. Fibroblasts are the main cells of the dermis producing ECM. Collagen is the predominant component of matrix responsible for the biomechanical properties associated with the strength of the dermal matrix by forming dense bundles of fibers. Other fibrillar proteins such as elastin, fibronectin, laminin, and fibrillins arrange around collagen to create a loose network that allows for the elasticity and flexibility of skin. Filling the spaces between fibers are the extrafibrillar matrix consisting of liquid binding glycosoaminoglycans (e.g., hyaluronan), proteoglycans, and glycoproteins that create a fluid medium for the movement of water, molecules, and immune cells. Additional cells in the dermal layer include macrophages, mast cells, adipocytes, Schwann cells, and stem cells.

Within the dermis there are several types of epidermally derived skin appendages, including sebaceous glands, sweat glands, and hair follicles. Blood vessels, lymphatics, and nerves also reside in the dermal and subcutaneous layers. Table 5.1 details the function of these structures (Krieg & Aumailley, 2011; Prost-Squarcioni, Fraitag, Heller, & Boehm, 2008; Ryan, Mortimer, & Jones, 1986). To sum up, the skin provides several protective barriers to the outside world, most notably the physical barrier provided by the many layers of skin, thermoinsulation from fat, water barrier created by keratinization and lipid-rich layer in epidermal stratum granulosum, and immunologic barrier created by various antigen-presenting cells and players in innate and adaptive immunity (Langerhans cells in the stratum spinosum, dendritic cells, macrophages, mast cells, and even recently discovered skin-resident T cells in the dermis and epidermis) (Clark, 2010). A properly functioning immunologic barrier is crucial in maintaining healthy skin, and these

TABLE 5.1 Skin layers: key features and functions

Skin layer	Strata	Key histologic feature(s)	Major function(s)
Epidermis	Stratum corneum	• Most superficial layer consisting of dead enucleate flattened keratinocytes and debris	• Keratinized dead skin cells provide water barrier and some physical barrier to environmental assaults such as penetration by foreign objects, organisms, toxic substances, friction, and extreme temperature • This layer along with the other most superficial layers of epidermis where most of the skin microbiome is located
	Stratum granulosum	• A few layers of flattened keratinocytes • Where keratinization is achieved • Prominent basophilic keratinohyaline granules • Golgi-derived lamellar granules containing various lipids	• Keratinization and lipid-containing lamellar granules provide a water barrier, preventing dehydration
	Stratum spinosum	• Intercellular bridges created between cells by desmosomes • Active synthesis of keratin filaments and assembly of tonofilaments that anchor to desmosomes • Usually the thickest layer of the epidermis especially in the epidermal ridges	• Contains Langerhans cells, the first major antigen-presenting cell in epidermis for immune response
	Stratum basale	• Single layer of columnar cells secured to dermal-epidermal junction (basement membrane) by hemidesmosomes • Mitotically active cells • Cells contain cytoskeletal keratins (intermediate filaments)	• Basal stem cells are the primary source of mitotic activity producing new keratinocytes • Contains melanocytes (pigment producing cells) involved in DNA protection from light • Contains Merkel cells (mechanoreceptors) involved in sensory response

Skin layer	Component	Major function(s)	
Dermis and skin appendages	Extracellular matrix	• Collagen is the major component of the dermis and responsible for strength • Fibrillar proteins contribute to elasticity and flexibility of skin • Extrafibrillar matrix binds liquid and allow nutrients, water, and immune cells to travel within dermis	
	Vascular plexuses	• Thermoregulation • Nutrient and waste processing • Allow circulatory immune cells to travel to and from skin	
	Lymphatic plexuses	• Clears proteins and fluid • Channel for macrophages and other immune cells to travel from the skin tissue	
	Sebaceous glands	• Produce sebum, a compound of lipids, cell debris, and keratin that nourishes and creates lubrication for skin preventing water loss	
	Apocrine glands	• Sweat glands usually associated with hair follicles that produce fatty liquid expulsed from gland tubules in response to stress • Thermoregulation by working together with eccrine glands through emulsification to create film of sweat to efficiently dissipate heat and discourage formation and loss of sweat drops • Liquid is broken to fatty acids by skin bacteria, which can cause characteristic odor	
	Eccrine glands	• Sweat glands that secrete watery sweat in response to emotional and thermal stress and sympathetic nervous system for role in thermoregulation by dissipating heat through water evaporation from skin surface	
	Hair follicles	• Extensions of the epidermal basal layer surround the base of these structures • Skin microbiome densely populates this area	
	Nerve endings	• Somatosensation. Sensory nerve endings, including free nerve endings (nocireceptors) and specialized tactile mechanoreceptors (Meissner corpuscles, Ruffini endings, Pacinian corpuscles, Merkel disks, and regionally specific Kraus end bulbs) that together provide detailed information on pain, temperature, light touch, deep pressure, low and high frequency vibrations, and skin stretch. Somatosensation allows protective feature of detecting damage to the skin or threatening contacts with the skin such as sharp objects or extreme temperatures that may damage tissue if not withdrawn	
Hypodermis	Subcutaneous fascia and fat	• Adipose tissue provides thermoinsulation, energy, and storage of nutrients; provides extra padding in places that experience more pressure such as buttocks, palms, and soles	

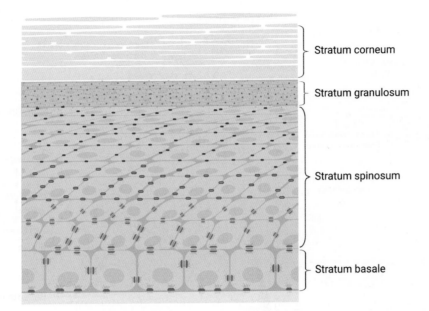

• **Fig. 5.2** Layers of the epidermis.

immune factors are discussed in greater detail in Chapters 7, 13, and 14. In addition to the native components of skin, the healthy skin microbiome is part of a functional barrier of skin, which is elucidated in Chapter 6.

The compromised skin barrier in atopic dermatitis

How is the skin barrier compromised in atopic dermatitis? This skin disease is caused by defective skin barrier proteins and a dysfunctional immune system. A component of atopic dermatitis can be genetic and as a result be a heritable disorder. Atopic dermatitis can also be part of other syndromes and diseases such as immunodeficiencies. In people who do not have primary immunodeficiencies, the disease is also associated with other allergic symptoms such as allergic rhinitis and asthma in the allergic triad, showing us that atopic dermatitis has a lot to do with the dysfunction of the immune system and is more than just simply a defect of the skin. There are many contributing factors in pathogenesis of atopic dermatitis and a variety of clinical presentations. In those who are diagnosed with the disease, changes to the environment or an acquired modification of the skin barrier and immune system can change its severity. In fact, some environmental factors can cause epigenetic changes that can cause atopic dermatitis. Fig. 5.3 depicts these barrier compromises in atopic dermatitis.

Loss of skin barrier function in atopic dermatitis is multifactorial. Measurable parameters of skin barrier loss include increased transepidermal water loss, increased stratum corneum pH, and decreased hydration. Histologic changes include spongiosis and hyperkeratosis of the epidermis and perivascular inflammation with prominent T-cell infiltration. Local immune dysregulation characterized by overexpression

of Th2 and Th22 cytokines change the expression or functions of various enzymes. Stratum corneum lipid matrix producing water barrier is abnormal in atopic dermatitis, where ceramides are decreased in amount or structures are shorter in length. Antimicrobial peptides are also inhibited by Th2 cytokines causing increased propensity for infections such as *Staphylococcus aureus*. Increase in kallikrein (KLK) activity and impaired tight junction proteins also decrease the function of proteins responsible for intercellular adhesion.

Mutations in filaggrin *(FLG)* gene seen in some individuals with atopic dermatitis cause abnormal filaggrin and downstream products such as natural moisturizing factors (NMFs). All of these factors can compromise the paracellular barrier in the epidermis, allowing water to escape the body and increase the permeability of skin to allergens, irritants, and haptans, which reinforce local inflammation when skin resident immune cells are activated. Local inflammation causes adaptive response with T-cell recruitment and activation and leads to systemic allergic responses with imbalance in Th1 and Th2 cytokines and overexpression of immunoglobulin E (IgE) antibodies. Additional external factors such as the scratch and itch cycle, *S. aureus* toxins, and dust mite proteases further compromise the skin barrier. The increase in skin pH, various alterations in intrinsic antimicrobial components, and immune dysfunction also result in shifts in the skin microbiome (dysbiosis). The multifactorial contributors to atopic dermatitis pathology create a self-reinforcing cycle of barrier and immune dysfunction.

Physical barrier disruption

There have been several skin-associated tissue factors identified that when altered produce problems in barrier function that contribute to atopic dermatitis. These barrier dysfunctions are listed in Table 5.2.

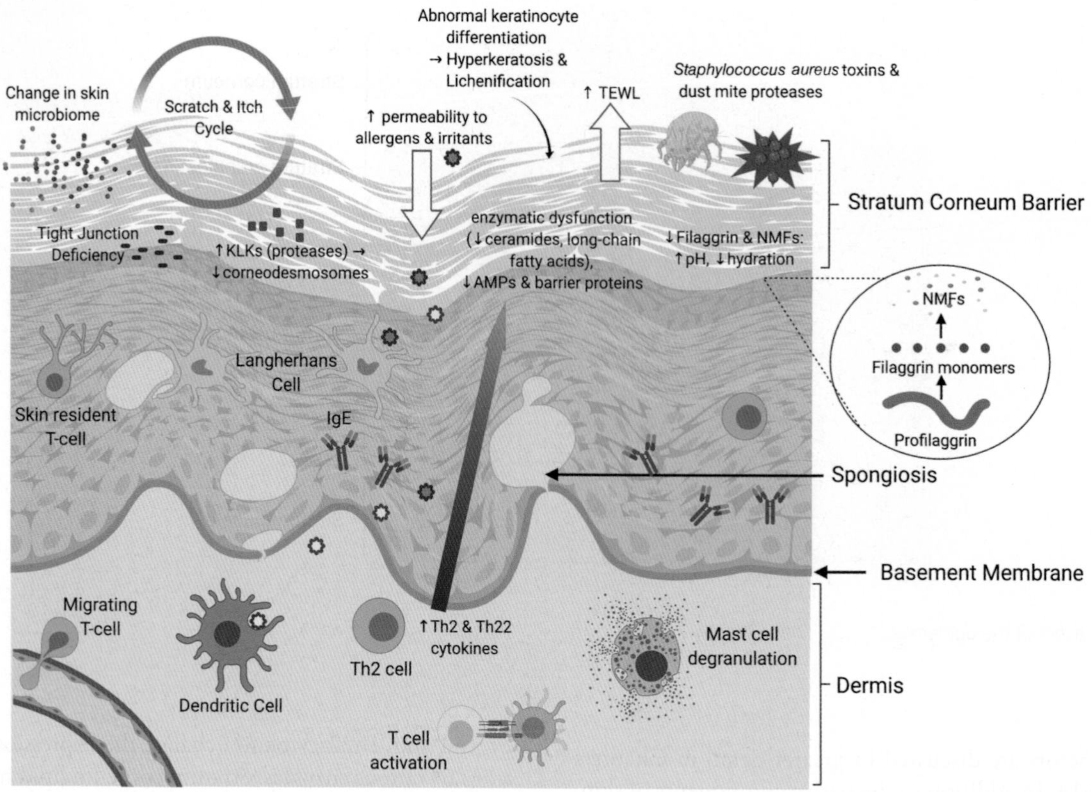

• **Fig. 5.3** Skin barrier dysfunction in atopic dermatitis. *AMP,* Antimicrobial peptides; *KLKs,* kallikreins; *NMFs,* natural moisturizing factors; *TEWL,* transepidermal water loss.

Characteristics of skin in atopic dermatitis associated with loss of barrier function include the following:
- Biophysical measures: increased transepidermal water loss, increased stratum corneum pH, and decreased hydration
- Histological: spongiosis of epidermis, hyperkeratosis of epidermis, perivascular inflammation with prominent T-cell infiltration
- Downstream effects of barrier dysfunction: increased allergen sensitization and resulting systemic allergic responses, including characteristic increased IgE levels
- Increased permeability to microbes, allergens, haptans, irritants, and water
- Local immune dysregulation: overexpression of Th2 and Th22 cytokines altering proteins and lipids in epidermis
- Markers of keratinocyte differentiation: proteins such as desmoglein-1, desmocolin-1, loricrin, and involucrin involved in barrier function are deficient in atopic dermatitis lesional skin (Agrawal & Woodfolk, 2014; Kim & Leung, 2018)

Filaggrin

FLG is a monomer subunit of a protein packed in keratinohyaline granules that are produced in terminally differentiated keratinocytes in the granular and cornified layers of the epidermis involved in maintaining the paracellular permeability barrier. *FLG* is a structural protein that binds keratinocyte filaments to increase the density of filament bundles, flattening keratinocytes to their terminal shape, which is crucial to the strength and integrity of the skin. Profilaggrin produced from *FLG* gene is broken down into monomeric filaggrin. Filaggrin is also broken down by proteases (e.g., cysteine peptidase and caspase-14) into free amino acids that function as NMFs to retain water and maintain skin pH. NMFs also strengthen stratum corneum and provide chemical, allergen, and microbial protection (Agrawal & Woodfolk, 2014).

When *FLG* gene is mutated to be nonfunctional (*FLG*-null) or has a lower number of intraexonic repeating units, this can cause a deficiency of *FLG* enough to cause a change in the morphology of keratinocytes and enhance skin inflammation. Compromised paracellular barrier causes leaky epithelium to allergens and haptens. *FLG* mutations can contribute to atopic dermatitis but is not sufficient to cause the disease in isolation, and individuals with null alleles often do not have the disease. About 25% to 50% of atopic dermatitis patients have a *FLG* mutation as a predisposing factor (Osawa, Akiyama, & Shimizu, 2011). Individuals with these mutations often are seen in persistent or early-onset atopic dermatitis. Methylation of the gene has also been correlated with risk for atopic dermatitis and points to epigenetic contributors to this disease development (Ziyab et al., 2013). Th2 predominant imbalance in atopic dermatitis has been implicated in the downregulation of *FLG* expression and is another contributor to barrier

TABLE 5.2 Skin barrier components, function, and disruption in atopic dermatitis (AD)

Skin barrier components	Derangements in AD skin	Downstream effects
Stratum corneum (SC) and epidermal barrier		
Lipid matrix	• Increase in lipid processing enzyme activity as a result of inflammation • Lamellar body and lipid processing impaired	• Decreased and shortened ceramides and long chain fatty acids • Increased stratum corneum permeability to water → increased transepidermal water loss (TEWL)
Filaggrin (FLG)	• Mutations in *FLG* gene (in some individuals with AD) or epigenetic modification cause deficiency	• Abnormal keratinocyte differentiation, shape, and resulting defects in paracellular barrier
Natural moisturizing factors (NMFs)	• NMFs, the free amino acids created by *FLG* breakdown, can be deficient in AD from *FLG* mutation or *FLG*-degrading enzyme (e.g., caspase-14) deficiency	• Increased pH of skin, resulting in microbiome dysbiosis • Decreased hydration (retention of water) of skin • Decreased protection of SC from chemical, allergen, and microbial protection
Kallikreins (KLKs)	• Abnormal expression and increased activity of protease KLKs	• Increased paracellular leakage as a result of desmosome degradation • Abnormal lipid processing, hyperkeratosis, increased risk for infection
Tight junctions (TJs)	• Impaired TJ subunits (claudins and occludins) as a result of exposure to allergens and bacteria	• Paracellular barrier compromised, increased TEWL
Terminal differentiation products	• Decreased desmoglein-1, desmocolin-1, loricrin, involucrin, along with other markers of terminal keratinocyte differentiation	• Impaired paracellular barrier, increased TEWL • Abnormal keratinocyte maturation and hyperkeratosis
Microbial barrier		
Skin microbiome	• Dysbiosis due to increased skin pH, altered lipid composition, and immune dysregulation	• Decreased induction of AMPs, increased risk for infection by virulent bacteria (particularly *Staphylococcus aureus*) and viral infections
Immune and antimicrobial barrier		
Antimicrobial peptides (AMPs)	• Overexpression of Th2 cytokines inhibits AMPs	• Increased risk for infection • Decreased regulation of inflammation • Impaired keratinocyte migration, proliferation, reepithelization, neovascularization, and wound healing
Th1:Th2 balance	• Th2 predominant imbalance and T-cell perivascular infiltration and local tissue inflammation	• Activation of proteases causing local tissue damage, enzymatic dysfunction in lipid processing, downregulation of AMPs, and terminal differentiation products of keratinocytes • Chronic inflammation from Th1, Th17, Th22 responses
Other barrier factors		
Sebaceous glands	• Gland hypoplasia, decreased sebocyte proliferation, decreased sebum	• Dry skin • Decreased delivery of antimicrobial lipids and antioxidants to skin surface
Histamine	• Exposure to allergens and irritants from compromised barrier causes increased allergic responses and mast cell degranulation → increased histamine	• Itch-and-scratch cycle causes damage to skin and increased introduction of allergens, irritants, and microbes
S. aureus colonization	• *S. aureus* is especially virulent in AD skin with combination of immune dysfunction, skin microbiome dysbiosis, and decreased skin protective factors	• Increased risk for infection • Infection and proteins can cause immune responses that decrease terminal differentiation factors in skin (including *FLG*, loricrin, keratin-1 and -10, and desmocollin-1)
Dust mite allergens	• Compromised skin allows increased penetration of dust mite allergens	• Enzymatic activity of dust mites break down extracellular matrix • Increased local and systemic allergic responses can predispose to development of AD

defect. Additionally, filaggrin-like proteins such as filaggrin-2 and hornerin have some evidence of increasing atopic dermatitis risk (Pellerin et al., 2013).

Tight Junctions (TJs)

TJs are proteins that are responsible for intercellular adhesion and thus contribute to the paracellular permeability barrier as well. Impaired TJ subunits, notably proteins called claudins and occludins, can contribute to atopic dermatitis skin defects. These subunit proteins are decreased by the exposure to certain allergens and bacteria (Ohnemus et al., 2008; Wan et al., 1999).

Stratum corneum lipid matrix

The stratum corneum lipid matrix is defective in atopic dermatitis skin due to a change in expression of enzymes that are involved in the synthesis and processing of free fatty acids and ceramides. Lipid-rich lamellar granules in the granular layer of the epidermis provide the hydrophobic seal in the most superficial epidermal layers. The extruded lipid matrix after processing by lipid processing enzymes becomes a mixture of ceramides, cholesterol, and free fatty acids. Ceramides in normal skin are the predominant lipid, but in cases of atopic dermatitis there is a decreased amount of ceramides, and those present are shorter in length (Janssens et al., 2012). This may be controlled by the increase in lipid processing enzyme activity or a result of inflammation (Sawada, Yoshida, Sugiura, & Imokawa, 2012).

Kallikreins

KLKs are a group of proteases responsible for desquamation by degrading intercellular proteins such as desmosomes of keratinocytes and are involved in regulating levels of lipid-processing enzymes and antimicrobial peptides (AMPs). In atopic dermatitis skin, there is abnormal expression and enhancing of activity of KLKs leading to abnormal lipid processing, hyperkeratosis, and increased risk for infection.

Null mutations of KLK inhibitors have been associated with severe variants of atopic dermatitis as part of the Netherton syndrome (Hvid et al., 2011; Komatsu et al., 2007).

Sebaceous glands

Sebaceous glands provide hormonally responsive lipid production that is extruded atop the stratum corneum to provide additional moisture retention as a hydrophobic barrier. Once extruded, the local skin microbiome atop the epidermis and those concentrated around glands break down lipids to free fatty acids and other byproducts. Additionally, sebum can also be responsible for delivering antimicrobial lipids and antioxidants. Decreased sebum, decreased sebocyte proliferation, and sebaceous gland hypoplasia are linked to lesional atopic dermatitis skin. Decreased sebum

production during childhood explains a correlation with the high prevalence for atopic dermatitis due to the decreased barrier protection afforded by sebum. Sebum gland development in the neonatal period and sebum composition (ratio of different lipids) can change in patients who develop atopic dermatitis. In fact, patients with hyperplastic or overactive sebaceous glands such as those found physiologically in pubescent teens or pathologically in acne vulgaris may be protective against eczematous skin conditions (Shi et al., 2015).

Immune barrier dysfunction and systemic dysregulation

Antimicrobial peptides

AMPs are part of the innate epithelial chemical barrier and as their name suggests have antibacterial properties and kill viruses and fungi. They also regulate inflammation. In healthy individuals, expression of AMPs is upregulated during states of inflammation and infection. This group of peptides include β-defensins and cathelicidin. For modulating inflammation these peptides can induce expression of interleukin-18 (IL18), IL6, IL10, macrophage inflammatory protein-3α, and RANTES. These also aid in normal skin cell functions by inducing keratinocyte migration, proliferation, reepithelization, neovascularization, and wound healing. In atopic dermatitis skin, overexpression of Th2 cytokines inhibits these peptides and can lead to an increased propensity for certain skin infections, notably *S. aureus* (Kim & Leung, 2018).

Imbalances in Th1 and Th2 cytokines and overexpression of IgE with system allergic responses is caused by a faulty barrier. Traditionally, atopic dermatitis is thought to be caused by Th2 predominant imbalance. T-cell perivascular infiltration and local tissue inflammation involve both Th1 and Th2 cytokines. Locally and systemically, the immune system is sensitized and goes into overdrive as a result of barrier dysfunction.

In rare cases, immune dysfunction can result from a single gene mutation such as in *CARD11*, a gene that produces a protein involved in pathway signaling in T cells (Dadi et al., 2018). Other primary immunodeficiencies can also include atopic dermatitis as part of their syndromes. Other common contributors to local and systemic immune dysfunction in atopic dermatitis are described in subsequent chapters.

Skin microbiome dysbiosis and superimposed infections

Atopic dermatitis skin is vulnerable to infection due to decreased AMPs and Th2 cytokine overexpression, particularly bacterial and viral infections. *S. aureus* infection is especially detrimental for atopic dermatitis skin by inhibiting the expression of late differentiation factors in keratinocytes (such as *FLG*, loricrin, keratin-1 and -10, and desmocollin-1), which may further compromise the paracellular barrier. Additionally, *S. aureus* bacterial components are associated with altered composition of intercellular lipids (Brauweiler, Hall, Goleva, & Leung, 2017; Son et al., 2014). Kaposi varicelliform eruption caused by herpes simplex, variola, or vaccinia virus can cause life-threatening infection. Dust mites can contain allergens that induce eczematous allergic responses as well as enzymes that break down cutaneous ECM components of skin and increase skin pH (Oida et al., 2017).

Healthy skin flora is necessary in maintaining a microbial barrier as certain bacteria in healthy skin suppress virulent bacteria and induce expression of AMPs, controlling inflammation. Skin pH helps determine skin microbial populations, and increased pH can increase susceptibility to infection. Healthy flora along with normal expression of skin proteins, enzymes, proteases, and inflammatory cytokine balance are crucial in maintaining normal acidic skin pH. In Chapter 6, the skin microbiome and its effects are described in detail (Ali & Yosipovitch, 2013).

Special populations: age and race matter

The predominant age group for atopic dermatitis is the pediatric population, which contributes to several factors in regard to an immature immune system and an immature skin barrier. In children there is a lack of Th1 response related to increase in IFN-gamma compared to adults, thus increasing the Th2 imbalance that can contribute to development or severity of atopic dermatitis. Pediatric populations have thinner skin and have larger surface area of skin leading to increased loss of fluids as evidenced by increased transepidermal water loss (TEWL). Increased prevalence of atopic dermatitis in the elderly population can be in part explained by age-related skin barrier dysfunction and the immune system's impaired ability to mount a Th1 response (Gupta et al., 2008; Leung, 2015).

In the United States, atopic dermatitis occurs in higher prevalence in the black population than whites; however, *FLG* mutations are more common in whites and Asians. Asians with atopic dermatitis have increased Th17 and Th22 responses than their white counterparts, with atopic dermatitis lesional morphology and histology more similar to psoriasis (Leung, 2015). TEWL in white atopic dermatitis patients is higher than in black patients. Black atopic dermatitis patients have the highest IgE serum levels among racial groups (Brunner & Guttman-Yassky, 2019). All of this can point to complex intrinsic differences in skin barrier function of specific racial groups and thus propensity to develop atopic dermatitis.

Challenges and complications in barrier healing and protection

Atopic dermatitis can be persistent and difficult to treat because of the cyclic nature of barrier compromise that develops due to many factors. Pruritus is often the dominant distressing symptom of atopic dermatitis created by histamine and inflammatory reactions in the skin and can be a driving force for damaging the skin through self-inflicted skin trauma. Scratching introduces barrier damage and microbes to the lesional skin, which exacerbates the disease and can lead to complications such as superimposed contact dermatitis and infections. The complex cascade of barrier dysfunction and introduction of components that cause allergic and immunologic response lead to chronic inflammation. Several external and internal factors can be addressed to disrupt this self-reinforcing cycle and ameliorate symptoms and prevent exacerbations.

When considering therapies for atopic dermatitis, addressing external factors that influence the skin barrier include control of triggers, including allergens, temperature, and modulating circadian changes in itch and inflammation. Moisturizing agents can aid in barrier repair. Immune dysfunction can be addressed through immunomodulating drugs and local suppressors of inflammationary response. Additional internal factors contributing to disease are hydration, gut health, hormones, nutrition, sleep quality, and psychosocial factors as a contributor to itch and perception of suffering from disease. Proper management requires a multifaceted approach to barrier protection, immune regulation, and disease prevention.

Summary

The skin is composed of epidermis and dermis that together create a physical and immune barrier between the environment and the internal body. In atopic dermatitis, the physical barrier is compromised due to an altered lipid matrix, impaired intercellular proteins, abnormal maturation and terminal differentiation products in keratinocytes, and other derangements leading to "leaky" skin with increased TEWL, decreased hydration, and increased permeability to microbes, allergens, and irritants. Atopic dermatitis is also caused by immune dysfunction with Th2 predominant cytokine imbalances, increased allergic responses, and increased local and systemic inflammation. Other alterations in microbiome, higher skin pH, and decreased antimicrobial skin factors such as AMPs create increased risk for serious infection. The contributing factors for development of atopic dermatitis are different between individuals with the disease, and there are challenges in addressing the complex processes at the skin and internally.

Further reading

Brunner, P. M., & Guttman-Yassky, E. (2019). Racial differences in atopic dermatitis. *Annals of Allergy, Asthma & Immunology, 122*(5), 449–455. https://doi.org/10.1016/j.anai.2018.11.015. https://www.ncbi.nlm.nih.gov/pubmed/30465859.

Chambers, E. S., & Vukmanovic-Stejic, M. (2019). Skin barrier immunity and ageing. *Immunology, 160*(2),116-125. https://doi.org/10.1111/imm.13152.

Drislane, C., & Irvine, A. D. (2020). The role of filaggrin in atopic dermatitis and allergic disease. *Annals of Allergy, Asthma & Immunology*, *124*(1), 36–43. https://doi.org/10.1016/j.anai.2019.10.008.

References

Agrawal, R., & Woodfolk, J. A. (2014). Skin barrier defects in atopic dermatitis. *Current Allergy and Asthma Reports, 14*(5), 433. https://doi.org/10.1007/s11882-014-0433-9. https://www.ncbi.nlm.nih.gov/pubmed/24633617.

Ali, S. M., & Yosipovitch, G. (2013). Skin pH: From basic science to basic skin care. *Acta Dermato-Venereologica, 93*(3), 261–267. https://doi.org/10.2340/00015555-1531. https://www.ncbi.nlm.nih.gov/pubmed/23322028.

Brauweiler, A. M., Hall, C. F., Goleva, E., & Leung, D. Y. M. (2017). *Staphylococcus aureus* lipoteichoic acid inhibits keratinocyte differentiation through a p63-Mediated Pathway. *Journal of Investigative Dermatology, 137*(9), 2030–2033. https://doi.org/10.1016/j.jid.2017.05.003. https://www.ncbi.nlm.nih.gov/pubmed/28528912.

Brunner, P. M., & Guttman-Yassky, E. (2019). Racial differences in atopic dermatitis. *Ann Allergy Asthma Immunol, 122*(5), 449–455. https://doi.org/10.1016/j.anai.2018.11.015. https://www.ncbi.nlm.nih.gov/pubmed/30465859.

Clark. R. A. (2010). Skin-resident T cells: the ups and downs of on site immunity. *Journal of Investigative Dermatology, 130*(2), 362–370. https://doi.org/10.1038/jid.2009.247. https://www.ncbi.nlm.nih.gov/pubmed/19675575.

Dadi, H., Jones, T. A., Merico, D., Sharfe, N., Ovadia, A., Schejter, Y., et al. (2018). Combined immunodeficiency and atopy caused by a dominant negative mutation in caspase activation and recruitment domain family member 11 (CARD11). *Journal of Allergy and Clinical Immunology, 141*(5), 1818–1830.e2. https://doi.org/10.1016/j.jaci.2017.06.047. https://www.ncbi.nlm.nih.gov/pubmed/28826773.

Gupta, J., Grube, E., Ericksen, M. B., Stevenson, M. D., Lucky, A. W., Sheth, A. P., et al. (2008). Intrinsically defective skin barrier function in children with atopic dermatitis correlates with disease severity. *Journal of Allergy and Clinical Immunology, 121*(3), 725–730.e2. https://doi.org/10.1016/j.jaci.2007.12.1161. https://www.ncbi.nlm.nih.gov/pubmed/18249438.

Hvid, M., Johansen, C., Deleuran, B., Kemp, K., Deleuran, M., & Vestergaard, C. (2011). Regulation of caspase 14 expression in keratinocytes by inflammatory cytokines–a possible link between reduced skin barrier function and inflammation? *Experimental Dermatology, 20*(8), 633–636. https://doi.org/10.1111/j.1600-0625.2011.01280.x. https://www.ncbi.nlm.nih.gov/pubmed/ 21539619.

Janssens, M., van Smeden, J., Gooris, G. S., Bras, W., Portale, G., Caspers, P. J., et al. (2012). Increase in short-chain ceramides correlates with an altered lipid organization and decreased barrier function in atopic eczema patients. *Journal of Lipid Research, 53*(12), 2755–2766. https://doi.org/10.1194/jlr.P030338. https://www.ncbi.nlm.nih.gov/pubmed/23024286.

Kim, B. E., & Leung, D. Y. M. (2018). Significance of skin barrier dysfunction in atopic dermatitis. *Allergy, Asthma and Immunology Research, 10*(3), 207–215. https://doi.org/10.4168/aair.2018.10.3.207. https://www.ncbi.nlm.nih.gov/pubmed/29676067.

Komatsu, N., Saijoh, K., Kuk, C., Liu, A. C., Khan, S., Shirasaki, F., et al. (2007). Human tissue kallikrein expression in the stratum corneum and serum of atopic dermatitis patients. *Experimental Dermatology, 16*(6), 513–519. https://doi.org/10.1111/j.1600-0625.2007.00562.x. https://www.ncbi.nlm.nih.gov/pubmed/17518992.

Krieg, T., & Aumailley, M. (2011). The extracellular matrix of the dermis: Flexible structures with dynamic functions. *Experimental Dermatology, 20*(8), 689–695. https://doi.org/10.1111/j.1600-0625.2011.01313.x. https://www.ncbi.nlm.nih.gov/pubmed/21615511.

Leung. D. Y. (2015). Atopic dermatitis: Age and race do matter!. *Journal of Allergy and Clinical Immunology, 136*(5), 1265–1267. https://doi.org/10.1016/j.jaci.2015.09.011. https://www.ncbi.nlm.nih.gov/pubmed/26549637.

Marks, J. G., & Miller, J. J. (2013). *Lookingbill & Marks' Principles of Dermatology* (5th ed.). Philadelphia: Elsevier.

Mescher. A. L. (2018). *Junqueira's Basic Histology: Text and Atlas* (15th ed.). New York, NY: McGraw-Hill. http://accessmedicine.mhmedical.com/content.aspx?bookid=2430&sectionid=190220001.

Ohnemus, U., Kohrmeyer, K., Houdek, P., Rohde, H., Wladykowski, E., Vidal, S., et al. (2008). Regulation of epidermal tight-junctions (TJ) during infection with exfoliative toxin-negative *Staphylococcus* strains. *Journal of Investigative Dermatology, 128*(4), 906–916. https://doi.org/10.1038/sj.jid.5701070. https://www.ncbi.nlm.nih.gov/pubmed/17914452.

Oida, K., Einhorn, L., Herrmann, I., Panakova, L., Resch, Y., Vrtala, S., et al. (2017). Innate function of house dust mite allergens: Robust enzymatic degradation of extracellular matrix at elevated pH. *World Allergy Organization Journal, 10*(1), 23. https://doi.org/10.1186/s40413-017-0154-3. https://www.ncbi.nlm.nih.gov/pubmed/28702111.

Osawa, R., Akiyama, M., & Shimizu, H. (2011). Filaggrin gene defects and the risk of developing allergic disorders. *Allergology International, 60*(1), 1–9. https://doi.org/10.2332/allergolint.10-RAI-0270. https://www.ncbi.nlm.nih.gov/pubmed/21173567.

Pellerin, L., Henry, J., Hsu, C. Y., Balica, S., Jean-Decoster, C., Mechin, M. C., et al. (2013). Defects of filaggrin-like proteins in both lesional and nonlesional atopic skin. *Journal of Allergy and Clinical Immunology, 131*(4), 1094–1102. https://doi.org/10.1016/j.jaci.2012.12.1566. https://www.ncbi.nlm.nih.gov/pubmed/23403047.

Prost-Squarcioni, C., Fraitag, S., Heller, M., & Boehm, N. (2008). [Functional histology of dermis]. *Annales De Dermatologie et de Venereologie, 135*(1 Pt 3), 5–20. https://doi.org/10.1016/S0151-9638(08)70206-0. https://www.ncbi.nlm.nih.gov/pubmed/18442658.

Ryan, T. J., Mortimer, P. S., & Jones, R. L. (1986). Lymphatics of the skin. Neglected but important. *International Journal of Dermatology, 25*(7), 411–419. https://doi.org/10.1111/j.1365-4362.1986.tb03443.x. https://www.ncbi.nlm.nih.gov/pubmed/3533796.

Sawada, E., Yoshida, N., Sugiura, A., & Imokawa, G. (2012). Th1 cytokines accentuate but Th2 cytokines attenuate ceramide production in the stratum corneum of human epidermal equivalents: An implication for the disrupted barrier mechanism in atopic dermatitis. *Journal of Dermatological Science, 68*(1), 25–35. https://doi.org/10.1016/j.jdermsci.2012.07.004. https://www.ncbi.nlm.nih.gov/pubmed/22884781.

Shi, V. Y., Leo, M., Hassoun, L., Chahal, D. S., Maibach, H. I., & Sivamani, R. K. (2015). Role of sebaceous glands in inflammatory dermatoses. *Journal of the American Academy of Dermatology, 73*(5), 856–863. https://doi.org/10.1016/j.jaad.2015.08.015. https://www.ncbi.nlm.nih.gov/pubmed/26386632.

Son, E. D., Kim, H. J., Park, T., Shin, K., Bae, I. H., Lim, K. M., et al. (2014). *Staphylococcus aureus* inhibits terminal differentiation of normal human keratinocytes by stimulating interleukin-6 secretion. *Journal of Dermatological Science, 74*(1), 64–71. https://doi.org/10.1016/j.jdermsci.2013.12.004. https://www.ncbi.nlm.nih.gov/pubmed/24398033.

Wan, H., Winton, H. L., Soeller, C., Tovey, E. R., Gruenert, D. C., Thompson, P. J., et al. (1999). Der p 1 facilitates transepithelial allergen delivery by disruption of tight junctions. *The Journal of Clinical Investigation, 104*(1), 123–133. https://doi.org/10.1172/JCI5844. https://www.ncbi.nlm.nih.gov/pubmed/10393706.

Ziyab, A. H., Karmaus, W., Holloway, J. W., Zhang, H., Ewart, S., & Arshad, S. H. (2013). DNA methylation of the filaggrin gene adds to the risk of eczema associated with loss-of-function variants. *Journal of the European Academy of Dermatology and Venereology, 27*(3), e420–e423. https://doi.org/10.1111/jdv.12000. https://www.ncbi.nlm.nih.gov/pubmed/23003573.

6

Skin and Gut Microbiome

PAUL BLACKCLOUD AND JENNIFER HSIAO

KEY POINTS

- The human microbiome consists of a wide variety of micro-organisms that assist in key physiologic processes.
- The majority of microbial diversity is found on the skin and in the gut; and microbial composition is influenced by multiple host factors.
- Disruption in microbiome homeostasis is termed dysbiosis and is associated with disease states such as atopic dermatitis.
- Flares of atopic dermatitis are associated with changes in the cutaneous microbiome, most notably increases in *Staphylococcus aureus* and loss of microbial diversity.
- The gut microbiome is influenced by multiple factors and evolves over time, with differences observed in patients with atopic dermatitis compared to controls.

Introduction

Interest in the human microbiome and its role in both normal human physiology and in disease has grown dramatically in recent years. Our understanding of the composition and abundance of organisms in the human body has increased as more precise techniques have been developed. No longer viewed as bystanders, commensal organisms are now understood to play vital physiologic roles, including nutrient metabolism, vitamin synthesis, barrier protection, and immune system development. Dysbiosis, a term used to describe imbalance in the healthy microbiome, can lead to increased inflammation and is associated with disease states. This chapter will explore the composition of the healthy microbiome and the changes that occur in dysbiosis and its impact on atopic dermatitis.

Microbiome

The human microbiome refers to the genetic material (collection of all genomes) of the community of organisms, including bacteria, fungi, and viruses, that inhabit the body both inside and out. This adds significant genetic information to the human body, as the amount of nonhuman cells is estimated to be in the trillions and accounts for at least as many human cells, and potentially even 10-fold more (Savage, 1977; Sender, Fuchs, & Milo, 2016). The majority of microbes reside in the intestinal tract, followed next by the skin (Sander, Sander, Isaac-Renton, & Croxen, 2019).

Use of sequencing techniques has led to a better understanding of the composition of the microbiome. These sequencing techniques can either be directed toward a specific genetic target or the genome as a whole (Byrd, Belkaid, & Segre, 2018). For bacteria, 16 S ribosomal RNA (rRNA) sequencing targets a conserved and yet highly variable region of bacterial genomes, allowing for increased detection of microbes compared to traditional culture techniques (Hiergeist, Gläsner, Reischl, & Gessner, 2015). For fungi, sequencing of ribosomal internal transcribed spacer (ITS) allows for identification to the species level (Schoch et al., 2012).

Whole genome (shotgun) sequencing, a technique used to analyze all genomic material in a given sample, has helped to further classify skin microbes. Compared to 16 S rRNA and ITS sequencing, this technique confers the additional benefits of identifying viral genes, classifying bacterial species to the strain level, and quantifying relative abundances at the kingdom level (Byrd et al., 2018). Using these techniques, the overall composition of the skin demonstrates highest abundance of bacteria, followed by viruses and lastly fungi (~4%), though site-specific compositional differences exist (Oh et al., 2014). Nineteen different phyla of bacteria have been identified on the skin, with the four predominant phyla among these being Actinobacteria, Firmicutes, Proteobacteria, and Bacteroidetes, with the most abundant genera being *Corynebacteria*, *Propionibacteria*, and *Staphylococci* (Grice et al., 2009). The most abundant viruses are bacteriophages (viruses that target bacteria), and the predominant fungal genus is *Malassezia* (Findley et al., 2013; Hannigan et al., 2015).

The predominant species found on human skin evolves over time, dependent upon various environmental and physiologic factors. As infants, the microbiome is first influenced by delivery method. Vaginal delivery results in colonization by common vaginal bacteria (*Lactobacillus, Prevotella, Sneathia*), while delivery through cesarean section leads to colonization with common skin bacteria (*Staphylococcus, Corynebacterium, Propionibacterium*) (Dominguez-Bello et al., 2010). Regardless of delivery method, this colonization is temporary, with diversification by body site occurring by 6 weeks of age (Chu et al., 2017). In prepubescence, the microbiome shifts to an abundance of Firmicutes (including *Streptococcaceae*), Bacteroidetes, and Proteobacteria, while changes in hormone levels at puberty result in increased sebum production and subsequent expansion of *Propionibacterium, Cornyebacterium*, and *Malassezia* (Byrd et al., 2018; Jo et al., 2016; Oh, Conlan, Polley, Segre, & Kong, 2012).

Beyond these age-related changes, multiple additional environmental factors have been shown to influence the skin microbiome, including pH, gender, ethnicity, geography, and ultraviolet (UV) exposure (Table 6.1). Healthy skin exhibits a lower skin pH (in the acidic range of 4–6), allowing for the growth of select bacteria (coagulase-negative *Staphylococcus, Corynebacteria*), while inhibiting pathogenic strains (*Staphylococcus aureus* and *Streptococcus pyogenes*) (Ali & Yosipovitch, 2013; Grice & Segre, 2011). Gender differences also influence the skin microbiome, likely due to inherent differences in hormone, sebum, and sweat production as well as differences in skin surface pH (Giacomoni, Mammone, & Teri, 2009; Grice & Segre, 2011). Numerous studies have also shown variations in the skin microbiome of patients with different ethnic and geographic backgrounds, which likely result from differences in diet and lifestyle among studied populations (Gupta, Paul, & Dutta, 2017). For example, *Propionibacteriaceae, Staphylococcaceae*, and *Streptococceacea* are more abundant on adult hands in the United States, while *Rhodobacteraceae* and *Nocardioidaceae*, bacteria commonly found in soil and aquatic environments, are more abundant on adults' hands in Tanzania (Hospodsky et al., 2014). UV light has an immunomodulatory influence on skin and can decrease skin *S. aureus* levels (Dotterud, Wilsgaard, Vorland, & Falk, 2008; Silva et al., 2006). Though influenced by many factors, once established, an individual's skin microbiome remains stable over time (Oh et al., 2016). Factors that influence skin microbiome are listed in Table 6.1.

Skin microbial communities also vary based on body location, which can be categorized by areas that are moist, dry, or sebaceous. Moist areas include the axillae, nostrils, antecubital and popliteal fossae, interdigital web spaces, inguinal creases, plantar heels, and umbilicus (skin creases). These areas tend to have greater abundance of *Corynebacterium* and *Staphylococcus*—microorganisms

TABLE 6.1	Factors influencing skin microbiome
Method of birth delivery	
Age	
Skin pH	
Gender	
Ethnicity	
Geography	
Ultraviolet exposure	

that thrive in environments with higher temperature and humidity. Dry areas include the forearms, palms, and buttocks. These areas tend to have more mixed populations, with an abundance of β-Proteobacteria and Flavobacteriales. Sebaceous areas include the glabella, alar crease, inside and behind the ear, occiput, upper chest, and back; these areas have the lowest amount of diversity, attributed to the anoxic and lipid-rich environment. Sebaceous areas are dominated by *Propionibacteria*, though *Staphylococci* are also present (Costello et al., 2009; Grice & Segre, 2011; Grice et al., 2009). Like bacteria, viruses tend to be less diverse at sebaceous sites (Hannigan et al., 2015). While *Malassezia* is the predominant fungus on the majority of skin surfaces, increased fungal diversity is seen on parts of the foot (Findley et al., 2013).

In its normal state, the skin microbiome is in a healthy homeostasis and consists primarily of commensal organisms, or those conferring benefit without causing harm, and transient microbes (Findley & Grice, 2014). This homeostasis is maintained by a combination of protective mechanisms inherent to the skin, as well as contributions from a diverse resident bacterial population. Keratinocytes produce numerous antimicrobial peptides (AMPs), including cathelicidin and β-defensin, that protect the skin barrier through multiple mechanisms, including direct attack on microbes and eliciting a host response (Schauber & Gallo, 2008).

Similar to innate host defense, commensal bacteria (*Staphylococcus epidermidis* being the most widely studied) also contribute to this balance through multiple mechanisms. Directly, *S. epidermidis* can produce peptides that inhibit growth of pathogenic organisms such as *S. aureus*, without disrupting other commensals (Cogen et al., 2010). Indirectly, *S. epidermidis* is capable of eliciting an immune response targeting pathogens through activation of toll-like receptors (Lai et al., 2009; Wanke et al., 2011). *S. epidermidis* has also been shown to inhibit the formation of *S. aureus* biofilms (Iwase et al., 2010).

Regulatory T cells (Tregs), a subset of CD4+ T cells, play an important role in immune regulation and maintaining homeostasis through promotion of tolerance to self-antigens. A greater number of regulatory T cells are present in infancy (Paller et al., 2019), and exposure to commensal bacteria on the skin early on in life plays a significant role in establishing this tolerance (Naik et al., 2012). Specifically, in the skin, the early presence of *S. epidermidis* is detected by antigen-presenting cells, presented to T cells that express the matching antigen receptor, which results in the expansion of a population of regulatory T cells that allows for tolerance to the organism (Scharschmidt, 2017; Scharschmidt et al., 2015). As a result, subsequent detection of *S. epidermidis* does not trigger inflammation (immune tolerance), but instead results in the induction of cytokine interleukin 1a (IL1a), which in turn acts as host defense, an example of immune-commensal crosstalk (Byrd et al., 2018; Naik et al., 2012, 2015). Early exposure is necessary for this commensal tolerance to occur (Scharschmidt et al., 2015). Since regulatory T cells play a key role in self-tolerance, dysfunctional or decreased number of Tregs are seen with autoimmune conditions (Dominguez-Villar & Hafler, 2018).

Skin dysbiosis

Dysbiosis refers to a disruption of the microbiome and a shift away from homeostasis, and is seen in disease states such as atopic dermatitis. A study published in 1989 highlighted epidemiologic data that correlated increases in the incidence of atopic dermatitis with improved personal cleanliness and smaller family sizes (with subsequent decreases in sibling contact), suggesting that a disruption in microbial exposure may contribute to atopic dermatitis (Strachan, 1989). This idea became known as the hygiene hypothesis. In support of this hypothesis were subsequent data that showed that exposure of children to microbial products (endotoxin) through their environment was protective against the development of atopic disease (Braun-Fahrländer et al., 2002).

Risk factors of skin dysbiosis

Patients with atopic dermatitis are at increased risk for dysbiosis through skin barrier dysfunction (Table 6.2). Extrinsically, as flares drive itch, scratching physically breeches the barrier. Intrinsic factors include the higher skin pH seen in these patients, which results in altered synthesis of protective lipids that creates an environment conducive to pathogen growth, including *Staphylococcus and Candida* (Ali & Yosipovitch, 2013). Loss-of-function mutations in filaggrin, a protein with multiple roles important to skin barrier function, including pH regulation and maintaining hydration, is a major risk

TABLE 6.2	Characteristics of skin dysbiosis in atopic dermatitis
Barrier Dysfunction	
Defective lipid matrix	
Decreased expression of tight junction proteins	
Increased production of proteases	
Scratching	
Filaggrin mutation	
Increased water loss	
Decreased hydration	
Increased pH	
Microbiome	
Decreased diversity	
Increased *Staphylococcus aureus*	
Immune Dysregulation	
Increased inflammation	
Increased Th2 response	
Allergic sensitization	
Decreased antimicrobial peptides	
Impaired innate and adaptive immune response	

Adapted from Weidinger, S., & Novak, N. (2016). Atopic dermatitis. *Lancet, 387*(10023), 1109–1122. doi:10.1016/S0140–6736(15)00149-X.

factor for the development of atopic dermatitis and is present in nearly half of patients (Palmer et al., 2006; Sandilands, Sutherland, Irvine, & McLean, 2009).

Patients with atopic dermatitis also produce fewer antimicrobial peptides, such as cathelicidin and β-defensins, predisposing individuals to increased *S. aureus* colonization (Nakatsuji et al., 2017). Antibiotics, commonly used as part of the treatment for atopic dermatitis, may be an additional contributor to dysbiosis through nonselective elimination of both beneficial and pathogenic bacteria (Nakatsuji & Gallo, 2019). Together, these factors contribute to a state of dysbiosis by altering the skin's natural defenses and allowing allergens and microbes to enter the skin (a state also known as leaky skin), ultimately resulting in inflammation (Hulshof, Van't Land, Sprikkelman, & Garssen, 2017).

Bacterial composition

In a healthy state, coagulase-negative staphylococci (CoNS) species such as *S. epidermidis, Staphylococcus lugdunensis,* and *Staphylococcus caprae* limit *S. aureus* colonization and pathogenicity (Paharik et al., 2017). In addition to CoNS, additional microbes beneficial to maintaining homeostasis have been identified. *Propionibacterium* and *Corynebacterium* may also limit growth of *S. aureus* through their ability to release porphyrins (Shi et al., 2016). *Streptococcus pneumoniae* is capable of killing *S. aureus* through release of hydrogen peroxide (Regev-Yochay, Trzcinski, Thompson, Malley, & Lipsitch, 2006). *Roseomonas mucosa*, a gram-negative bacterium, has also been shown to limit *S. aureus* growth and influence innate immune activation (Myles et al., 2016).

A shift to dysbiosis is marked by low bacterial diversity in general, though with higher levels of staphylococcal species (*S. aureus* and *S. epidermidis*), and a greater diversity of non-*Malassezia* fungi (Bjerre, Bandier, Skov, Engstrand, & Johansen, 2017). Since the 1970s, *S. aureus* has been known to colonize the skin in 30% to 100% of atopic dermatitis patients, in contrast to approximately 20% of those unaffected, and to contribute to atopic dermatitis flares (Leyden, Marples, & Kligman, 1974; Paller et al., 2019). Atopic dermatitis patients are particularly at risk for this colonization and subsequent dysbiosis due to reduced levels of antimicrobial peptides, a consequence of both suppression from increased Th2 cytokines and decreased coagulase-negative staphylococcal species (Nakatsuji & Gallo, 2019).

Importance of *Staphylococcus aureus*

Virulence of *S. aureus* starts with its ability to adhere to and penetrate atopic dermatitis skin (Baker, 2006) and is achieved through the expression of multiple proteins. The toxins produced by *S. aureus* can be categorized into three general groups based on function: toxins that damage cell membrane (which includes α- and δ-toxins), toxins that interfere with receptor function (which includes the superantigen enterotoxin), and secreted enzymes (proteases that alter host pathways) (Otto, 2014). Atopic dermatitis patients often exhibit reduced or impaired filaggrin expression, making these patients more susceptible to *S. aureus* toxins. Reduced filaggrin expression leads to reduced sphingomyelinase secretion, an enzyme that hydrolyzes sphingomyelin into ceramides, and which has been shown to protect keratinocytes specifically from α-toxin and cell death (Brauweiler et al., 2013). δ-Toxin has also been shown to cause mast cell degranulation, promote IL4 production, and lead to skin inflammation, as seen in atopic dermatitis (Nakamura et al., 2013). Numerous other proteins produced by *S. aureus* may contribute to atopic dermatitis, including those that allow adhesion to skin (clumping factor B, fibronectin-binding proteins), proinflammatory proteins (protein A, lipoproteins, phenol-soluble modulins), and those that inactivate AMPs (staphopain, aureolysin) (Geoghegan, Irvine, & Foster, 2018). The ability to form biofilms also helps protect *S. aureus* from host immune response and antibacterial treatment (Blicharz, Rudnicka, & Samochocki, 2019).

S. aureus density is increased in lesional skin of atopic dermatitis patients and correlates with its disease severity. During a disease flare, and even preceding the flare, higher levels of *S. aureus* and an overall decrease in microbial diversity are observed. As the flare resolves, levels of *S. aureus* fall, and microbial diversity is restored (Kong et al., 2012) (Fig. 6.1). It has also been observed that atopic dermatitis patients experiencing severe flares are colonized not only with *S. aureus*, but also with other strains that have great capability of inducing an inflammatory response, while those with less severe atopic dermatitis have a predominance of *S. epidermidis* (Byrd et al., 2017). Following treatment of flares, the microbiome shifts, with a decrease of *Staphylococcus* species and increases in *Streptococcus, Corynebacterium*, and *Propionibacterium* species (Kong et al., 2012).

Other factors

Although *S. aureus* is the most widely implicated and studied microbial contributor to dysbiosis in atopic dermatitis, other microbes such as *Propionibacterium, Streptococcus, Acinetobacter*, and *Malassezia* are also believed to play a role (Bjerre et al., 2017). Among other observations, lesion-prone

skin of atopic dermatitis patients is higher in *Streptococcus* and *Gemella* species but lower in *Dermacoccus*, a genus of bacteria capable of producing antiinflammatory and antimicrobial metabolites (Chng et al., 2016). Although *Malassezia* is considered part of the normal skin flora, as many as 80% of patients with atopic dermatitis are sensitized to and produce immunoglobulin E (IgE) against *Malassezia*, a response that drives inflammation (Glatz, Bosshard, Hoetzenecker, & Schmid-Grendelmeier, 2015). It has also been shown that a specific fungal protein from *Malassezia* (MGL_1304 from *Malassezia globosa*) is found in human sweat and causes histamine release from basophils, with increased levels of IgE against this protein seen in atopic dermatitis patients during flares and correlating with severity (Hiragun et al., 2013, 2014). Shifts in predominant *Malassezia* species (specifically *Malassezia restricta* and *M. globosa*) also occur, based on severity of disease. Though marked by a lower bacterial diversity, patients with atopic dermatitis have a higher diversity of fungi—specifically non-*Malassezia* fungi—when compared to controls, including the presence of *Candida* and *Cryptococcus* species (Zhang et al., 2011).

Additional factors found to support a diverse microbiome include emollient use (Glatz et al., 2018) and treatment of atopic dermatitis (Kong et al., 2012). However, treatments with antibacterial agents alone, aimed specifically toward reduction of *S. aureus*, do not seem to improve atopic dermatitis flares in the absence of clinical infection (Bath-Hextall, Birnie, Ravenscroft, & Williams, 2010). For example, though used widely in clinical practice as a means of decreasing *S. aureus* burden, current evidence suggests that bleach baths are too diluted to be bactericidal (Sawada et al., 2019) and that their use may confer no additional benefit over water bath alone (Chopra, Vakharia, Sacotte, & Silverberg, 2017). Together, these findings suggest a greater interplay among many factors in the connection between dysbiosis and atopic dermatitis.

Gut dysbiosis

The gut microbiome is composed of trillions of microbes and is postulated to assist crucial physiologic functions

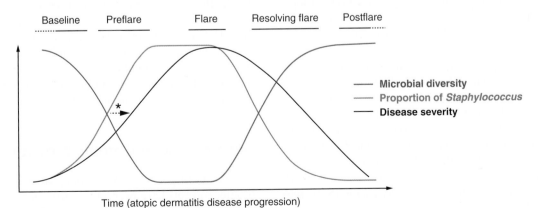

• **Fig. 6.1** Temporal association of atopic dermatitis severity and cutaneous microbiome. "(*) Proposed relationship among shifts in skin microbial diversity, the proportion of *Staphylococcus*, and disease severity." (Adapted with permission from Kong et al., 2012.)

such as nutrient and protein metabolism, vitamin synthesis, drug metabolism, and protection of the gut epithelial barrier (Jandhyala et al., 2015). It also plays a key role in the development of the early immune system. Though the womb was once considered sterile, colonization of the gut is now believed to begin in utero, with maternal bacteria identified in umbilical cord blood, amniotic fluid, meconium, and the placenta (Thum et al., 2012). Similar to the evolution seen on the skin, the gut microbiome also changes over time. The gut of neonates is briefly dominated by an abundance of *Enterobacteriaceae* and *Staphylococcus* before then evolving to a *Bifidobacterium*-predominant environment while breastfeeding. Once started on solid foods, the gut microbiome shifts to a predominance of Bacteroidetes and Firmicutes (Tanaka & Nakayama, 2017).

Establishment of the gut microbiome

Factors influencing the initial establishment and composition of the gut microbiome in infancy include timing of birth, delivery method, feeding method, and antibiotic use (Table 6.3). Preterm infants have decreased levels of *Bifidobacterium* and are at risk for further alterations in gut flora due to subsequent parenteral nutrition and antibiotic use (Lee et al., 2017). Vaginal delivery is associated with increased *Bifidobacterium* and *Bacteroides* species, while delivery by cesarean section is associated with higher numbers of *Streptococcus, Staphylococcus*, and *Clostridium difficile* (Kim & Kim, 2019; Penders et al., 2006). This influence of delivery method on the gut microbiome may even carry into adulthood (Goedert, Hua, Yu, & Shi, 2014). Infants born by cesarean section are at increased risk of development of atopic dermatitis compared to those born via vaginal delivery (Cuppari et al., 2015). Infants that are exclusively breastfed show increases in the class Actinobacteria (includes genus *Bifidobacteria*), while formula-fed infants have higher levels of Proteobacteria (which includes the genus *Escherichia*) (O'Sullivan, Farver, & Smilowitz, 2015). Though results are mixed, many studies have shown that breastfed infants are also at a decreased risk of developing atopic dermatitis, particularly those with a family history of atopy, with the American Academy of Allergy, Asthma, and Immunology recommending exclusive breastfeeding for 4 to 6 months to reduce this incidence (Fleischer, Spergel, Assa'ad, & Pongracic, 2013; Kim, 2017).

In addition to providing nutrition, breastmilk contains protective factors such as IgA, immune-modulating cytokines, bacteria (including *Bifidobacterium, Lactobacillus, Enterococcus*, and *Staphylococcus*), and human milk oligosaccharides (HMOs)—sugar molecules that support growth of beneficial bacteria (Le Doare, Holder, Bassett, & Pannaraj, 2018). Breastfed infants exhibit lower stool pH and increased amounts of acetate and lactate in their stool, metabolic byproducts of *Bifidobacteria* (Wopereis et al., 2018).

Exposure to antibiotics, whether through maternal delivery or directly, has also been shown to influence the early gut microbiome. For example, neonates exposed to maternal intrapartum antibiotics exhibit decreased levels of *Bacteroides* and *Bifidobacterium* and increased levels of *Enterobacteriaceae* (Tapiainen et al., 2019). Neonates receiving antibiotic therapy directly have increases in *Enterobacteriaceae* and decreases in *Bifidobacteria, Lactobacilli*, and *Bacteroides*, in addition to a greater loss of microbial diversity overall (Fjalstad, Esaiassen, Juvet, van den Anker, & Klingenberg, 2018; Penders et al., 2006). Exposure to antibiotics early in life is associated with an increased risk of the development of atopic dermatitis, as well as other allergic conditions (Ahmadizar et al., 2018).

Additional maternal factors that influence the microbiome of the infant include maternal weight changes, obesity, bacterial exposure, and genetics. Increases in maternal weight and obesity are associated with higher levels of *Bacteroides-Prevotella* and lower levels of *Clostridium histolyticum* in the infant (Collado, Isolauri, Laitinen, & Salminen, 2010). Maternal exposure to microbes may lead to epigenetic changes in gene expression in the mother. These changes may then be passed along to her offspring, influencing the development of an immune system tolerant to commensal bacteria in neonates (Abrahamsson, Wu, & Jenmalm, 2015). Genetics also influence gut microbiome, as supported by twin and family studies showing that microbiotas are more similar within monozygotic twins than dizygotic twins, and more similar among related compared to unrelated individuals (Goodrich et al., 2014).

Gut and the immune system

Early colonization of the gut influences the immune system by helping the body build immune tolerance to allow for maintenance of commensal organisms. Through toll-like receptors, the innate immune system first recognizes gut bacterial antigens, eliciting a signal cascade that leads to inhibition of an inflammatory response, tolerance of those founding organisms, and the start of differentiating commensal from pathogenic organisms (Lazar et al., 2018). Cytokines released then trigger an adaptive immune response, priming naïve T cells and inducing regulatory T cells that suppress both inflammation and induction of naïve T cells to other Th types and establishing a balance of Th1, Th2, and Th17 cells (Francino, 2014). Gut anaerobes also produce acetate, propionate, and butyrate, which are short chain fatty acids (SCFAs) known to decrease inflammation and contribute to immune cell development, while potentially conferring additional health benefits (Louis & Flint, 2017).

Gut dysbiosis and atopic dermatitis

Differences in gut bacteria in atopic patients compared to healthy controls have been observed in numerous studies. Though not consistent among studies, the gut microbiome of atopic dermatitis patients is generally associated with higher levels of *C. difficile, Enterococcus, Escherichia coli*, and

TABLE 6.3	Factors influencing infant microbiome		
Timing of Birth			
Preterm	↑	Clostridium difficile	(Penders et al., 2006)
	↑	Proteobacteria	(Dahl et al., 2018)
	↑	Enterococcus	(Dahl et al., 2018)
Delivery Method			
Cesarean section	↑	C. difficile	(Penders et al., 2006)
	↑	Klebsiella	(Liu et al., 2019)
	↑	Veillonella	(Liu et al., 2019)
	↑	Streptococcus	(Kim & Kim, 2019)
	↑	Staphylococcus	(Dominguez-Bello et al., 2010; Kim & Kim, 2019)
	↑	Cornyebacterium	(Dominguez-Bello et al., 2010)
	↑	Propionibacterium	(Dominguez-Bello et al., 2010)
	↓	Bifidobacterium	(Liu et al., 2019; Penders et al., 2006)
	↓	Bacteroides	(Penders et al., 2006)
	↓	Lactobacillus	(Dahl et al., 2018)
Vaginal delivery	↑	Bifidobacterium	(Liu et al., 2019)
	↑	Lactobacillus	(Dominguez-Bello et al., 2010)
	↑	Prevotella	(Dominguez-Bello et al., 2010)
	↑	Sneathia	(Dominguez-Bello et al., 2010)
Feeding Method			
Formula	↑	C. difficile	(Penders et al., 2006)
	↑	Proteobacteria	(O'Sullivan et al., 2015)
Breastfeeding	↑	Bifidobacterium	(Penders et al., 2006)
	↑	Actinobacteria	(O'Sullivan et al., 2015)
	↓	Escherichia coli	(Penders et al., 2006)
	↓	C. difficile	(Penders et al., 2006)
	↓	Bacteroides fragilis	(Penders et al., 2006)
Infant Antibiotic Exposure			
Direct	↑	Enterobacteriaceae	(Fjalstad et al., 2018)
	↓	Bifidobacterium	(Fjalstad et al., 2018; Penders et al., 2006)
	↓	Bacteroides	(Fjalstad et al., 2018; Penders et al., 2006)
	↓	Lactobacillus	(Fjalstad et al., 2018)
	↓	Lachnoclostridium	(Liu et al., 2019)
Maternal (peripartum)	↑	Enterobacteriaceae	(Tapiainen et al., 2019)
	↓	Bacteroides	(Tapiainen et al., 2019)
	↓	Bifidobacteria	(Tapiainen et al., 2019)
Maternal Weight			
Maternal obesity	↑	Clostridium histolyticum	(Collado et al., 2010)
	↓	Bacteroides-Prevotella	(Collado et al., 2010)

S. aureus and lower levels of Bifidobacteria, Bacteroides, and Lactobacillus, as well as decreased gut diversity in general (Dou et al., 2019; Oh et al., 2017; Zimmermann, Messina, Mohn, Finlay, & Curtis, 2019).

The implications of this imbalance relate to further immune dysregulation. Increases in pathogenic bacteria, such as C. difficile and E. coli, may decrease levels of beneficial bacteria while also producing toxins that increase intestinal permeability and lead to sensitization and development of atopy (Penders et al., 2007). As gut dysbiosis can disrupt barrier integrity and increase permeability, it has also been theorized that a subsequent release of lipopolysaccharide (LPS), a component of the outer membrane of gram-negative bacterial cell walls and well-described trigger of inflammation, leads to a "metabolic endotoxemia" that drives low-level inflammation (Cani, Osto, Geurts, & Everard, 2012). Though primarily studied in obesity and metabolic disorders, induction of low-level inflammation through this mechanism may also play a role in atopic dermatitis.

As commensal species play a protective role, particularly those within the genera of *Bifidobacterium* and *Bacteroides*, a decrease or other change in their composition can further drive inflammation (Kim & Kim, 2019). For example, *Faecalibacterium prausnitzii* is an anaerobe abundant in the gut and believed to confer antiinflammatory benefits in healthy individuals. Decreases of the organism are seen in intestinal conditions such as Crohn disease (Martín et al., 2017). However, nonintuitively, its presence has also been shown to be more abundant in patients with atopic dermatitis (Song, Yoo, Hwang, Na, & Kim, 2016). Authors of the study propose that in atopic dermatitis, it is a change in the subspecies of *F. prausnitzii* that occurs, shifting to strains that produce less SCFAs (butyrate and propionate). This strain shift and subsequent decrease in SCFAs then leads to increased gut permeability and skin inflammation (Song et al., 2016). Severity of disease has also been inversely correlated with the butyrate producer *Coprococcus eutactus*, with patients with severe atopic disease exhibiting lower levels of the bacteria compared to those with mild disease (Nylund, Satokari, Salminen, & de Vos, 2014).

Leaky gut

In the well-functioning intestinal lumen, many factors contribute to barrier protection, including a physical mucous layer, IgA antibodies, antimicrobial peptides, commensal organisms, and cellular junctions (tight junctions, adherens junctions) (Vancamelbeke & Vermeire, 2017). However, changes in the gut microbiome can contribute to intestinal barrier disruption (i.e., leaky gut). Atopic dermatitis patients have decreased levels of protective IgA and commensal bacteria, which can allow for passage of antigens (from pathogens, allergens, irritants) through the gut epithelium, triggering of inflammation, and ultimately an adaptive immune response, specifically the Th2 pathway (Zhu, Zhu, Tran, Sivamani, & Shi, 2018).

It is unknown whether initial alterations in the gut microbiome (leaky gut) or in the skin microbiome (leaky skin) is the driver of dysbiosis, though both likely contribute (Fig. 6.2). The inside-out theory attributes the start of the process with first imbalance in the gut. Gut dysbiosis leads to inflammation, a Th2 response, and the production of bacterial byproducts that may enter circulation, ultimately

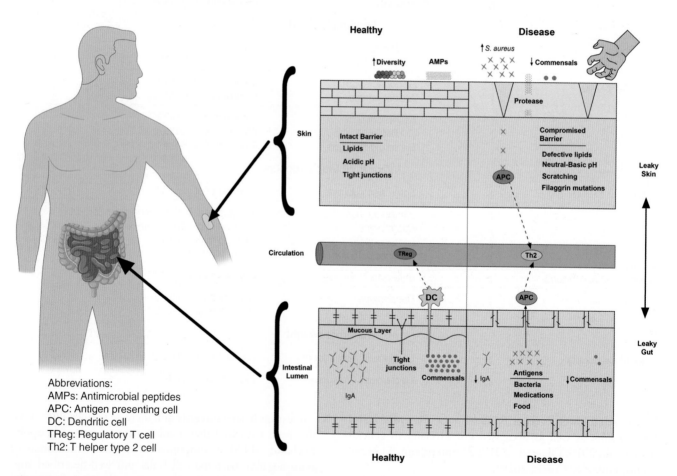

Abbreviations:
AMPs: Antimicrobial peptides
APC: Antigen presenting cell
DC: Dendritic cell
TReg: Regulatory T cell
Th2: T helper type 2 cell

• **Fig. 6.2**   The link between microbiome, dysbiosis, and intestinal and skin barrier defects. In the healthy state, the skin and gut exhibit a diverse microbiome with abundant commensals. Conversely, a state of dysbiosis is marked by a decrease in commensal organisms in both skin and gut, with an increase of *S. aureus* in the skin and increase in multiple antigens in the gut. Barrier protection is key to maintaining the healthy state, with the compromised barrier allowing pathogenic bacteria and environmental allergens to penetrate, leading to inflammation. This process of sensitization is referred to as "leaky skin." Alternatively, the gut also has multiple layers of protection, including tight junctions, a mucus layer, commensal bacteria and IgA, while the disease state is marked by decreases in IgA and commensals and compromise of the lumen, allowing antigens to penetrate with subsequent inflammatory response. This is referred to as "leaky gut." AMPs: Antimicrobial peptides; APC: Antigen presenting cell; DC: Dendritic cell; TReg: Regulatory T cell; Th2: T helper type 2 cell.

leading to skin dysbiosis and disease as a consequence (O'Neill, Monteleone, McLaughlin, & Paus, 2016; Slattery, MacFabe, & Frye, 2016). Alternatively, with the outside-in theory, cutaneous barrier disruption via a filaggrin mutation or skin dysbiosis leads to entry of toxins and allergens, with subsequent Th2 response and immune dysregulation (Silverberg & Silverberg, 2015). More research is needed to further investigate the relationship between the gut and skin microbiome and atopic dermatitis. Fig. 6.2 illustrates the link between the microbiome, dysbiosis, and intestinal and skin barrier defects.

Summary

Advances in microbial detection and quantification have allowed for a broader understanding of the composition of organisms that make up the human microbiome. Through this work, specific protective mechanisms provided by commensal organisms and their contributions toward a healthy state have also been elucidated. Disruption of this healthy state, or dysbiosis, can subsequently drive inflammation, and thus may be a key player in the development and exacerbation of conditions such as atopic dermatitis. Further understanding of the microbiome, dysbiosis, and the many factors that influence them may lead to novel therapeutic targets for both the prevention and treatment of disease.

Further readings

Abrahamsson, T. R., Wu, R. Y., & Jenmalm, M. C. (2015). Gut microbiota and allergy: The importance of the pregnancy period. *Pediatric Research*, *77*(1), 214–219. https://doi.org/10.1038/pr2014.165.

Bjerre, R. D., Bandier, J., Skov, L., Engstrand, L., & Johansen, J. D. (2017). The role of the skin microbiome in atopic dermatitis: A systematic review. *British Journal of Dermatology*, *177*(5), 1272–1278. https://doi.org/10.1111/bjd.15390.

Byrd, A. L., Belkaid, Y., & Segre, J. A. (2018). The human skin microbiome. *Nature Reviews Microbiology*, *16*(3), 143–155. https://doi.org/10.1038/nrmicro.2017.157.

Geoghegan, J. A., Irvine, A. D., & Foster, T. J. (2018). *Staphylococcus aureus* and atopic dermatitis: A complex and evolving relationship. *Trends in Microbiology*, *26*(6), 484–497. https://doi.org/10.1016/j.tim.2017.11.008.

Kong, H. H., Oh, J., Deming, C., Conlan, S., Grice, E. A., Beatson, M. A., et al. (2012). Temporal shifts in the skin microbiome associated with disease flares and treatment in children with atopic dermatitis. *Genome Research*, *22*(5), 850–859. https://doi.org/10.1101/gr.131029.111.

Paller, A. S., Kong, H. H., Seed, P., Naik, S., Scharschmidt, T. C., Gallo, R. L., et al. (2019). The microbiome in patients with atopic dermatitis. *Journal of Allergy and Clinical Immunology*, *143*(1), 26–35. https://doi.org/10.1016/j.jaci.2018.11.015.

Penders, J., Thijs, C., van den Brandt, P. A., Kummeling, I., Snijders, B., Stelma, F., et al. (2007). Gut microbiota composition and development of atopic manifestations in infancy: The KOALA birth cohort study. *Gut*, *56*(5), 661–667. https://doi.org/10.1136/gut.2006.100164.

Zimmermann, P., Messina, N., Mohn, W. W., Finlay, B. B., & Curtis, N. (2019). Association between the intestinal microbiota and allergic sensitization, eczema, and asthma: A systematic review.
Journal of Allergy and Clinical Immunology, *143*(2), 467–485. https://doi.org/10.1016/j.jaci.2018.09.025.

References

Abrahamsson, T. R., Wu, R. Y., & Jenmalm, M. C. (2015). Gut microbiota and allergy: The importance of the pregnancy period. *Pediatric Research*, *77*(1), 214–219. https://doi.org/10.1038/pr2014.165.

Ahmadizar, F., Vijverberg, S. J. H., Arets, H. G. M., Boer, A., Lang, J. E., Garssen, J., et al. (2018). Early-life antibiotic exposure increases the risk of developing allergic symptoms later in life: A meta-analysis. *Allergy*, *73*(5), 971–986. https://doi.org/10.1111/all.13332.

Ali, S. M., & Yosipovitch, G. (2013). Skin pH: From basic science to basic skin care. *Acta Dermato-Venereologica*, *93*(3), 261–267. https://doi.org/10.2340/00015555-1531.

Baker, B. S. (2006). The role of microorganisms in atopic dermatitis. *Clinical and Experimental Immunology*, *144*(1), 1–9. https://doi.org/10.1111/j.1365-2249.2005.02980.x.

Bath-Hextall, F. J., Birnie, A. J., Ravenscroft, J. C., & Williams, H. C. (2010). Interventions to reduce *Staphylococcus aureus* in the management of atopic eczema: An updated Cochrane review. *The British Journal of Dermatology*, *163*(1), 12–26. https://doi.org/10.1111/j.1365-2133.2010.09743.x.

Bjerre, R. D., Bandier, J., Skov, L., Engstrand, L., & Johansen, J. D. (2017). The role of the skin microbiome in atopic dermatitis: A systematic review. *The British Journal of Dermatology*, *177*(5), 1272–1278. https://doi.org/10.1111/bjd.15390.

Blicharz, L., Rudnicka, L., & Samochocki, Z. (2019). *Staphylococcus aureus*: An underestimated factor in the pathogenesis of atopic dermatitis? *Postepy Dermatol Alergol*, *36*(1), 11–17. https://doi.org/10.5114/ada.2019.82821.

Braun-Fahrländer, C., Riedler, J., Herz, U., Eder, W., Waser, M., Grize, L., et al. (2002). Environmental exposure to endotoxin and its relation to asthma in school-age children. *The New England Journal of Medicine*, *347*(12), 869–877. https://doi.org/10.1056/NEJMoa020057.

Brauweiler, A. M., Bin, L., Kim, B. E., Oyoshi, M. K., Geha, R. S., Goleva, E., & Leung, D. Y. (2013). Filaggrin-dependent secretion of sphingomyelinase protects against staphylococcal alpha-toxin-induced keratinocyte death. *The Journal of Allergy and Clinical Immunology*, *131*(2). https://doi.org/10.1016/j.jaci.2012.10.030. 421–7.e1-2.

Byrd, A. L., Belkaid, Y., & Segre, J. A. (2018). The human skin microbiome. *Nature Reviews Microbiology*, *16*(3), 143–155. https://doi.org/10.1038/nrmicro.2017.157.

Byrd, A. L., Deming, C., Cassidy, S. K. B., Harrison, O. J., Ng, W. I., Conlan, S., et al. (2017). *Staphylococcus aureus* and *Staphylococcus epidermidis* strain diversity underlying pediatric atopic dermatitis. *Science Translational Medicine*, *9*(397). https://doi.org/10.1126/scitranslmed.aal4651.

Cani, P. D., Osto, M., Geurts, L., & Everard, A. (2012). Involvement of gut microbiota in the development of low-grade inflammation and type 2 diabetes associated with obesity. *Gut Microbes*, *3*(4), 279–288. https://doi.org/10.4161/gmic.19625.

Chng, K. R., Tay, A. S., Li, C., Ng, A. H., Wang, J., Suri, B. K., et al. (2016). Whole metagenome profiling reveals skin microbiome-dependent susceptibility to atopic dermatitis flare. *Nature Microbiology*, *1*(9), 16106. https://doi.org/10.1038/nmicrobiol.2016.106.

Chopra, R., Vakharia, P. P., Sacotte, R., & Silverberg, J. I. (2017). Efficacy of bleach baths in reducing severity of atopic dermatitis: A systematic review and meta-analysis. *Annals of Allergy, Asthma and Immunology, 119*(5), 435–440. https://doi.org/10.1016/j.anai.2017.08.289.

Chu, D. M., Ma, J., Prince, A. L., Antony, K. M., Seferovic, M. D., & Aagaard, K. M. (2017). Maturation of the infant microbiome community structure and function across multiple body sites and in relation to mode of delivery. *Nature Medicine, 23*(3), 314–326. https://doi.org/10.1038/nm.4272.

Cogen, A. L., Yamasaki, K., Sanchez, K. M., Dorschner, R. A., Lai, Y., MacLeod, D. T., et al. (2010). Selective antimicrobial action is provided by phenol-soluble modulins derived from *Staphylococcus epidermidis*, a normal resident of the skin. *The Journal of Investigative Dermatology, 130*(1), 192–200. https://doi.org/10.1038/jid.2009.243.

Collado, M. C., Isolauri, E., Laitinen, K., & Salminen, S. (2010). Effect of mother's weight on infant's microbiota acquisition, composition, and activity during early infancy a prospective follow-up study initiated in early pregnancy. *American Journal of Clinical Nutrition, 92*(5), 1023–1030. https://doi.org/10.3945/ajcn.2010.29877.

Costello, E. K., Lauber, C. L., Hamady, M., Fierer, N., Gordon, J. I., & Knight, R. (2009). Bacterial community variation in human body habitats across space and time. *Science, 326*(5960), 1694–1697. https://doi.org/10.1126/science.1177486.

Cuppari, C., Manti, S., Salpietro, A., Alterio, T., Arrigo, T., Leonardi, S., & Salpietro, C. (2015). Mode of delivery and risk for development of atopic diseases in children. *Allergy and Asthma Proceedings, 36*(5), 344–351. https://doi.org/10.2500/aap.2015.36.3870.

Dahl, C., Stigum, H., Valeur, J., Iszatt, N., Lenters, V., Peddada, S., et al. (2018). Preterm infants have distinct microbiomes not explained by mode of delivery, breastfeeding duration or antibiotic exposure. *International Journal of Epidemiology, 47*(5), 1658–1669. https://doi.org/10.1093/ije/dyy064.

Dominguez-Bello, M. G., Costello, E. K., Contreras, M., Magris, M., Hidalgo, G., Fierer, N., & Knight, R. (2010). Delivery mode shapes the acquisition and structure of the initial microbiota across multiple body habitats in newborns. *Proceedings of the National Academy of Sciences of the United States of America, 107*(26), 11971–11975. https://doi.org/10.1073/pnas.1002601107.

Dominguez-Villar, M., & Hafler, D. A. (2018). Regulatory T cells in autoimmune disease. *Nature Immunology, 19*(7), 665–673. https://doi.org/10.1038/s41590-018-0120-4.

Dotterud, L. K., Wilsgaard, T., Vorland, L. H., & Falk, E. S. (2008). The effect of UVB radiation on skin microbiota in patients with atopic dermatitis and healthy controls. *International Journal of Circumpolar Health, 67*(2-3), 254–260. https://doi.org/10.3402/ijch.v67i2-3.18282.

Dou, J. H., Zeng, J. R., Wu, K., Tan, W. B., Gao, L. H., & Lu, J. Y. (2019). Microbiosis in pathogenesis and intervention of atopic dermatitis. *International Immunopharmacology, 69*, 263–269. https://doi.org/10.1016/j.intimp.2019.01.030.

Findley, K., & Grice, E. A. (2014). The skin microbiome: A focus on pathogens and their association with skin disease. *PLoS Pathogens, 10*(1), e1004436. https://doi.org/10.1371/journal.ppat.1004436.

Findley, K., Oh, J., Yang, J., Conlan, S., Deming, C., Meyer, J. A., et al. (2013). Topographic diversity of fungal and bacterial communities in human skin. *Nature, 498*(7454), 367–370. https://doi.org/10.1038/nature12171.

Fjalstad, J. W., Esaiassen, E., Juvet, L. K., van den Anker, J. N., & Klingenberg, C. (2018). Antibiotic therapy in neonates and impact on gut microbiota and antibiotic resistance development: A systematic review. *The Journal of Antimicrobial Chemotherapy, 73*(3), 569–580. https://doi.org/10.1093/jac/dkx426.

Fleischer, D. M., Spergel, J. M., Assa'ad, A. H., & Pongracic, J. A. (2013). Primary prevention of allergic disease through nutritional interventions. *Journal of Allergy and Clinical Immunology, 1*(1), 29–36. https://doi.org/10.1016/j.jaip.2012.09.003.

Francino. M. P. (2014). Early development of the gut microbiota and immune health. *Pathogens, 3*(3), 769–790. https://doi.org/10.3390/pathogens3030769.

Geoghegan, J. A., Irvine, A. D., & Foster, T. J. (2018). *Staphylococcus aureus* and atopic dermatitis: A complex and evolving relationship. *Trends in Microbiology, 26*(6), 484–497. https://doi.org/10.1016/j.tim.2017.11.008.

Giacomoni, P. U., Mammone, T., & Teri, M. (2009). Gender-linked differences in human skin. *Journal of Dermatological Science, 55*(3), 144–149. https://doi.org/10.1016/j.jdermsci.2009.06.001.

Glatz, M., Bosshard, P. P., Hoetzenecker, W., & Schmid-Grendelmeier, P. (2015). The role of *Malassezia* spp. in atopic dermatitis. *Journal of Clinical Medicine, 4*(6), 1217–1228. https://doi.org/10.3390/jcm4061217.

Glatz, M., Jo, J. H., Kennedy, E. A., Polley, E. C., Segre, J. A., Simpson, E. L., & Kong, H. H. (2018). Emollient use alters skin barrier and microbes in infants at risk for developing atopic dermatitis. *PLoS One, 13*(2), e0192443. https://doi.org/10.1371/journal.pone.0192443.

Goedert, J. J., Hua, X., Yu, G., & Shi, J. (2014). Diversity and composition of the adult fecal microbiome associated with history of cesarean birth or appendectomy: Analysis of the American Gut Project. *EBioMedicine, 1*(2-3), 167–172. https://doi.org/10.1016/j.ebiom.2014.11.004.

Goodrich, J. K., Waters, J. L., Poole, A. C., Sutter, J. L., Koren, O., Blekhman, R., et al. (2014). Human genetics shape the gut microbiome. *Cell, 159*(4), 789–799. https://doi.org/10.1016/j.cell.2014.09.053.

Grice, E. A., Kong, H. H., Conlan, S., Deming, C. B., Davis, J., Young, A. C., et al. (2009). Topographical and temporal diversity of the human skin microbiome. *Science, 324*(5931), 1190–1192. https://doi.org/10.1126/science.1171700.

Grice, E. A., & Segre, J. A. (2011). The skin microbiome. *Nature Reviews Microbiology, 9*(4), 244–253. https://doi.org/10.1038/nrmicro2537.

Gupta, V. K., Paul, S., & Dutta, C. (2017). Geography, ethnicity or subsistence-specific variations in human microbiome composition and diversity. *Frontiers in Microbiology, 8*, 1162. https://doi.org/10.3389/fmicb.2017.01162.

Hannigan, G. D., Meisel, J. S., Tyldsley, A. S., Zheng, Q., Hodkinson, B. P., SanMiguel, A. J., et al. (2015). The human skin double-stranded DNA virome: Topographical and temporal diversity, genetic enrichment, and dynamic associations with the host microbiome. *mBio, 6*(5): e01578-15. https://doi.org/10.1128/mBio.01578-15.

Hiergeist, A., Gläsner, J., Reischl, U., & Gessner, A. (2015). Analyses of intestinal microbiota: Culture versus sequencing. *ILAR Journal / National Research Council, Institute of Laboratory Animal Resources, 56*(2), 228–240. https://doi.org/10.1093/ilar/ilv017.

Hiragun, M., Hiragun, T., Ishii, K., Suzuki, H., Tanaka, A., Yanase, Y., et al. (2014). Elevated serum IgE against MGL_1304 in patients with atopic dermatitis and cholinergic urticaria. *Allergology International: Official Journal of the Japanese Society of Allergology, 63*(1), 83–93. https://doi.org/10.2332/allergolint.13-OA-0611.

Hiragun, T., Ishii, K., Hiragun, M., Suzuki, H., Kan, T., Mihara, S., et al. (2013). Fungal protein MGL_1304 in sweat is an allergen for atopic dermatitis patients. *The Journal of Allergy and Clinical Immunology, 132*(3), 608–615. https://doi.org/10.1016/j.jaci.2013.03.047.e4.

Hospodsky, D., Pickering, A. J., Julian, T. R., Miller, D., Gorthala, S., Boehm, A. B., & Peccia, J. (2014). Hand bacterial communities vary across two different human populations. *Microbiology*, *160*(Pt 6), 1144–1152. https://doi.org/10.1099/mic.0.075390-0.

Hulshof, L., Van't Land, B., Sprikkelman, A. B., & Garssen, J. (2017). Role of microbial modulation in management of atopic dermatitis in children. *Nutrients*, *9*(8), 854. https://doi.org/10.3390/nu9080854.

Iwase, T., Uehara, Y., Shinji, H., Tajima, A., Seo, H., Takada, K., et al. (2010). *Staphylococcus epidermidis* Esp inhibits *Staphylococcus aureus* biofilm formation and nasal colonization. *Nature*, *465*(7296), 346–349. https://doi.org/10.1038/nature09074.

Jandhyala, S. M., Talukdar, R., Subramanyam, C., Vuyyuru, H., Sasikala, M., & Reddy, D. N. (2015). Role of the normal gut microbiota. *World Journal of Gastroenterology*, *21*(29), 8787–8803. https://doi.org/10.3748/wjg.v21.i29.8787.

Jo, J. H., Deming, C., Kennedy, E. A., Conlan, S., Polley, E. C., Ng, W. I., et al. (2016). Diverse *Human Skin Fungal Communities in Children Converge in Adulthood. The Journal of Investigative Dermatology*, *136*(12), 2356–2363. https://doi.org/10.1016/j.jid.2016.05.130.

Kim, J. E., & Kim, H. S. (2019). Microbiome of the skin and gut in atopic dermatitis (AD): Understanding the pathophysiology and finding novel management strategies. *Journal of Clinical Medicine*, *8*(4), 444. https://doi.org/10.3390/jcm8040444.

Kim. J. H. (2017). Role of Breast-feeding in the development of atopic dermatitis in early childhood. *Allergy, Asthma & Immunology Research*, *9*(4), 285–287. https://doi.org/10.4168/aair.2017.9.4.285.

Kong, H. H., Oh, J., Deming, C., Conlan, S., Grice, E. A., Beatson, M. A., et al. (2012). Temporal shifts in the skin microbiome associated with disease flares and treatment in children with atopic dermatitis. *Genome Research*, *22*(5), 850–859. https://doi.org/10.1101/gr.131029.111.

Lai, Y., Di Nardo, A., Nakatsuji, T., Leichtle, A., Yang, Y., Cogen, A. L., et al. (2009). Commensal bacteria regulate toll-like receptor 3-dependent inflammation after skin injury. *Nature Medicine*, *15*(12), 1377–1382. https://doi.org/10.1038/nm.2062.

Lazar, V., Ditu, L. M., Pircalabioru, G. G., Gheorghe, I., Curutiu, C., Holban, A. M., et al. (2018). Aspects of gut microbiota and immune system interactions in infectious diseases, immunopathology, and cancer. *Frontiers in Immunology*, *9*, 1830. https://doi.org/10.3389/fimmu.2018.01830.

Le Doare, K., Holder, B., Bassett, A., & Pannaraj, P. S. (2018). Mother's milk: A purposeful contribution to the development of the infant microbiota and immunity. *Frontiers in Immunology*, *9*, 361. https://doi.org/10.3389/fimmu.2018.00361.

Lee, Y. Y., Hassan, S. A., Ismail, I. H., Chong, S. Y., Raja Ali, R. A., Amin Nordin, S., et al. (2017). Gut microbiota in early life and its influence on health and disease: A position paper by the Malaysian Working Group on Gastrointestinal Health. *Journal of Paediatrics and Child Health*, *53*(12), 1152–1158. https://doi.org/10.1111/jpc.13640.

Leyden, J. J., Marples, R. R., & Kligman, A. M. (1974). *Staphylococcus aureus* in the lesions of atopic dermatitis. *The British Journal of Dermatology*, *90*(5), 525–530. https://doi.org/10.1111/j.1365-2133.1974.tb06447.x.

Liu, Y., Qin, S., Song, Y., Feng, Y., Lv, N., Xue, Y., et al. (2019). The perturbation of infant gut microbiota caused by cesarean delivery is partially restored by exclusive breastfeeding. *Frontiers in Microbiology*, *10*, 598. https://doi.org/10.3389/fmicb.2019.00598.

Louis, P., & Flint, H. J. (2017). Formation of propionate and butyrate by the human colonic microbiota. *Environmental Microbiology*, *19*(1), 29–41. https://doi.org/10.1111/1462-2920.13589.

Martín, R., Miquel, S., Benevides, L., Bridonneau, C., Robert, V., Hudault, S., et al. (2017). Functional characterization of novel *faecalibacterium prausnitzii* strains isolated from healthy volunteers: A step forward in the use of *F. prausnitzii* as a next-generation probiotic. *Frontiers in Microbiology*, *8*, 1226. https://doi.org/10.3389/fmicb.2017.01226.

Myles, I. A., Williams, K. W., Reckhow, J. D., Jammeh, M. L., Pincus, N. B., Sastalla, I., et al. (2016). Transplantation of human skin microbiota in models of atopic dermatitis. *JCI Insight*, *1*(10): e86955. https://doi.org/10.1172/jci.insight.86955.

Naik, S., Bouladoux, N., Linehan, J. L., Han, S. J., Harrison, O. J., Wilhelm, C., et al. (2015). Commensal-dendritic-cell interaction specifies a unique protective skin immune signature. *Nature*, *520*(7545), 104–108. https://doi.org/10.1038/nature14052.

Naik, S., Bouladoux, N., Wilhelm, C., Molloy, M. J., Salcedo, R., Kastenmuller, W., et al. (2012). Compartmentalized control of skin immunity by resident commensals. *Science*, *337*(6098), 1115–1119. https://doi.org/10.1126/science.1225152.

Nakamura, Y., Oscherwitz, J., Cease, K. B., Chan, S. M., Muñoz-Planillo, R., Hasegawa, M., et al. (2013). Staphylococcus delta-toxin induces allergic skin disease by activating mast cells. *Nature*, *503*(7476), 397–401. https://doi.org/10.1038/nature12655.

Nakatsuji, T., Chen, T. H., Narala, S., Chun, K. A., Two, A. M., Yun, T., et al. (2017). Antimicrobials from human skin commensal bacteria protect against *Staphylococcus aureus* and are deficient in atopic dermatitis. *Science Translational Medicine*, *9*(378). https://doi.org/10.1126/scitranslmed.aah4680.

Nakatsuji, T., & Gallo, R. L. (2019). The role of the skin microbiome in atopic dermatitis. *Annals of Allergy, Asthma and Immunology*, *122*(3), 263–269. https://doi.org/10.1016/j.anai.2018.12.003.

Nylund, L., Satokari, R., Salminen, S., & de Vos, W. M. (2014). Intestinal microbiota during early life - impact on health and disease. *The Proceedings of the Nutrition Society*, *73*(4), 457–469. https://doi.org/10.1017/S0029665114000627.

O'Neill, C. A., Monteleone, G., McLaughlin, J. T., & Paus, R. (2016). The gut-skin axis in health and disease: A paradigm with therapeutic implications. *BioEssays*, *38*(11), 1167–1176. https://doi.org/10.1002/bies.201600008.

O'Sullivan, A., Farver, M., & Smilowitz, J. T. (2015). The influence of early infant-feeding practices on the intestinal microbiome and body composition in infants. *Nutrition and Metabolic Insights*, *8*(Suppl 1), 1–9. https://doi.org/10.4137/NMI.S29530.

Oh, J., Byrd, A. L., Deming, C., Conlan, S., Nisc Comparative Sequencing Program, Kong, H. H., & Segre, J. A. (2014). Biogeography and individuality shape function in the human skin metagenome. *Nature*, *514*(7520), 59–64. https://doi.org/10.1038/nature13786.

Oh, J., Byrd, A. L., Park, M., Nisc Comparative Sequencing Program, Kong, H. H., & Segre, J. A. (2016). Temporal stability of the human skin microbiome. *Cell*, *165*(4), 854–866. https://doi.org/10.1016/j.cell.2016.04.008.

Oh, J., Byrd, A. L., Deming, C., Conlan, S., Nisc Comparative Sequencing Program, Kong, H. H., & Segre, J. A. (2014). Biogeography and individuality shape function in the human skin metagenome. *Nature*, *514*(7520), 59–64.

Oh, J., Conlan, S., Polley, E. C., Segre, J. A., & Kong, H. H. (2012). Shifts in human skin and nares microbiota of healthy children and adults. *Genome Medicine*, *4*(10), 77. https://doi.org/10.1186/gm378.

Oh, S., Yap, G. C., Hong, P. Y., Huang, C. H., Aw, M. M., Shek, L. P. C., et al. (2017). Immune-modulatory genomic properties differentiate gut microbiota of infants with and without eczema. *PLoS One*, *12*(10): e0184955. https://doi.org/10.1371/journal. pone.0184955.

Otto, M. (2014). *Staphylococcus aureus* toxins. *Current Opinion in Microbiology*, *17*, 32–37. https://doi.org/10.1016/j.mib.2013. 11.004.

Paharik, A. E., Parlet, C. P., Chung, N., Todd, D. A., Rodriguez, E. I., Van Dyke, M. J., et al. (2017). Coagulase-negative staphylococcal strain prevents *Staphylococcus aureus* colonization and skin infection by blocking quorum sensing. *Cell host & microbe*, *22*(6), 746–756.e5. https://doi.org/10.1016/j.chom.2017.11.001.

Paller, A. S., Kong, H. H., Seed, P., Naik, S., Scharschmidt, T. C., Gallo, R. L., et al. (2019). The microbiome in patients with atopic dermatitis. *The Journal of Allergy and Clinical Immunology*, *143*(1), 26–35. https://doi.org/10.1016/j.jaci.2018.11.015.

Palmer, C. N., Irvine, A. D., Terron-Kwiatkowski, A., Zhao, Y., Liao, H., Lee, S. P., et al. (2006). Common loss-of-function variants of the epidermal barrier protein filaggrin are a major predisposing factor for atopic dermatitis. *Nature Genetics*, *38*(4), 441–446. https://doi.org/10.1038/ng1767.

Penders, J., Thijs, C., van den Brandt, P. A., Kummeling, I., Snijders, B., Stelma, F., et al. (2007). Gut microbiota composition and development of atopic manifestations in infancy: The KOALA Birth Cohort Study. *Gut*, *56*(5), 661–667. https://doi. org/10.1136/gut.2006.100164.

Penders, J., Thijs, C., Vink, C., Stelma, F. F., Snijders, B., Kummeling, I., et al. (2006). Factors influencing the composition of the intestinal microbiota in early infancy. *Pediatrics*, *118*(2), 511–521. https://doi.org/10.1542/peds.2005-2824.

Regev-Yochay, G., Trzcinski, K., Thompson, C. M., Malley, R., & Lipsitch, M. (2006). Interference between *Streptococcus pneumoniae* and *Staphylococcus aureus*: In vitro hydrogen peroxide-mediated killing by *Streptococcus pneumoniae*. *Journal of Bacteriology*, *188*(13), 4996–5001. https://doi.org/10.1128/JB.00317-06.

Sander, M. A., Sander, M. S., Isaac-Renton, J. L., & Croxen, M. A. (2019). The cutaneous microbiome: Implications for dermatology practice. *Journal of Cutaneous Medicine and Surgery*, *23*(4), 436–441. https://doi.org/10.1177/1203475419839939.

Sandilands, A., Sutherland, C., Irvine, A. D., & McLean, W. H. (2009). Filaggrin in the frontline: Role in skin barrier function and disease. *Journal of Cell Science*, *122*(Pt 9), 1285–1294. https:// doi.org/10.1242/jcs.033969.

Savage, D. C. (1977). Microbial ecology of the gastrointestinal tract. *Annual Review of Microbiology*, *31*, 107–133. https://doi. org/10.1146/annurev.mi.31.100177.000543.

Sawada, Y., Tong, Y., Barangi, M., Hata, T., Williams, M. R., Nakatsuji, T., & Gallo, R. L. (2019). Dilute bleach baths used for treatment of atopic dermatitis are not antimicrobial in vitro. *The Journal of Allergy and Clinical Immunology*, *143*(5), 1946–1948. https://doi.org/10.1016/j.jaci.2019.01.009.

Scharschmidt, T. C. (2017). Establishing tolerance to commensal skin bacteria: Timing is everything. *Dermatologic Clinics*, *35*(1), 1–9. https://doi.org/10.1016/j.det.2016.07.007.

Scharschmidt, T. C., Vasquez, K. S., Truong, H. A., Gearty, S. V., Pauli, M. L., Nosbaum, A., et al. (2015). A wave of regulatory T cells into neonatal skin mediates tolerance to commensal microbes. *Immunity*, *43*(5), 1011–1021. https://doi.org/10.1016/j. immuni.2015.10.016.

Schauber, J., & Gallo, R. L. (2008). Antimicrobial peptides and the skin immune defense system. *The Journal of Allergy and Clinical Immunology*, *122*(2), 261–266. https://doi.org/10.1016/j.jaci. 2008.03.027.

Schoch, C. L., Seifert, K. A., Huhndorf, S., Robert, V., Spouge, J. L., Levesque, C. A., et al. Wen Chen, & Fungal Barcoding Consortium. (2012). Nuclear ribosomal internal transcribed spacer (ITS) region as a universal DNA barcode marker for fungi. *Proceedings of the National Academy of Sciences of the United States of America*, *109*(16), 6241–6246. https://doi.org/10.1073/pnas.1117018109.

Sender, R., Fuchs, S., & Milo, R. (2016). Revised Estimates for the Number of Human and Bacteria Cells in the Body. *PLoS Biology*, *14*(8), e1002533. https://doi.org/10.1371/journal.pbio.1002533.

Shi, B., Bangayan, N. J., Curd, E., Taylor, P. A., Gallo, R. L., Leung, D. Y. M., & Li, H. (2016). The skin microbiome is different in pediatric versus adult atopic dermatitis. *The Journal of Allergy and Clinical Immunology*, *138*(4), 1233–1236. https://doi. org/10.1016/j.jaci.2016.04.053.

Silva, S. H., Guedes, A. C., Gontijo, B., Ramos, A. M., Carmo, L. S., Farias, L. M., & Nicoli, J. R. (2006). Influence of narrowband UVB phototherapy on cutaneous microbiota of children with atopic dermatitis. *Journal of the European Academy of Dermatology and Venereology*, *20*(9), 1114–1120. https://doi. org/10.1111/j.1468-3083.2006.01748.x.

Silverberg, N. B., & Silverberg, J. I. (2015). Inside out or outside in: does atopic dermatitis disrupt barrier function or does disruption of barrier function trigger atopic dermatitis? *Cutis*, *96*(6), 359–361.

Slattery, J., MacFabe, D. F., & Frye, R. E. (2016). The significance of the enteric microbiome on the development of childhood disease: A review of prebiotic and probiotic therapies in disorders of childhood. *Clinical Medicine Insights: Pediatrics*, *10*, 91–107. https:// doi.org/10.4137/CMPed.S38338.

Song, H., Yoo, Y., Hwang, J., Na, Y. C., & Kim, H. S. (2016). *Faecalibacterium prausnitzii* subspecies-level dysbiosis in the human gut microbiome underlying atopic dermatitis. *The Journal of Allergy and Clinical Immunology*, *137*(3), 852–860. https://doi. org/10.1016/j.jaci.2015.08.021.

Strachan, D. P. (1989). Hay fever, hygiene, and household size. *British Medical Journal*, *299*(6710), 1259–1260. https://doi.org/10.1136/ bmj.299.6710.1259.

Tanaka, M., & Nakayama, J. (2017). Development of the gut microbiota in infancy and its impact on health in later life. *Allergology International: Official Journal of the Japanese Society of Allergology*, *66*(4), 515–522. https://doi.org/10.1016/j.alit.2017.07.010.

Tapiainen, T., Koivusaari, P., Brinkac, L., Lorenzi, H. A., Salo, J., Renko, M., et al. (2019). Impact of intrapartum and postnatal antibiotics on the gut microbiome and emergence of antimicrobial resistance in infants. *Scientific Reports*, *9*(1), 10635. https://doi. org/10.1038/s41598-019-46964-5.

Thum, C., Cookson, A. L., Otter, D. E., McNabb, W. C., Hodgkinson, A. J., Dyer, J., & Roy, N. C. (2012). Can nutritional modulation of maternal intestinal microbiota influence the development of the infant gastrointestinal tract? *The Journal of Nutrition*, *142*(11), 1921–1928. https://doi.org/10.3945/jn.112.166231.

Vancamelbeke, M., & Vermeire, S. (2017). The intestinal barrier: A fundamental role in health and disease. *Expert Review of Gastroenterology & Hepatology*, *11*(9), 821–834. https://doi.org/1 0.1080/17474124.2017.1343143.

Wanke, I., Steffen, H., Christ, C., Krismer, B., Götz, F., Peschel, A., et al. (2011). Skin commensals amplify the innate immune response to pathogens by activation of distinct signaling pathways. *The Journal of Investigative Dermatology*, *131*(2), 382–390. https:// doi.org/10.1038/jid.2010.328.

Weidinger, S., & Novak, N. (2016). Atopic dermatitis. *Lancet*, *387*(10023), 1109–1122. https://doi.org/10.1016/S0140-6736(15)00149-X.

Wopereis, H., Sim, K., Shaw, A., Warner, J. O., Knol, J., & Kroll, J. S. (2018). Intestinal microbiota in infants at high risk for allergy: Effects of prebiotics and role in eczema development. *The Journal of Allergy and Clinical Immunology*, *141*(4), 1334–1342.e5. https://doi.org/10.1016/j.jaci.2017.05.054.

Zhang, E., Tanaka, T., Tajima, M., Tsuboi, R., Nishikawa, A., & Sugita, T. (2011). Characterization of the skin fungal microbiota in patients with atopic dermatitis and in healthy subjects. *Microbiology and Immunology*, *55*(9), 625–632. https://doi.org/10.1111/j.1348-0421.2011.00364.x.

Zhu, T. H., Zhu, T. R., Tran, K. A., Sivamani, R. K., & Shi, V. Y. (2018). Epithelial barrier dysfunctions in atopic dermatitis: A skin-gut-lung model linking microbiome alteration and immune dysregulation. *The British Journal of Dermatology*, *179*(3), 570–581. https://doi.org/10.1111/bjd.16734.

Zimmermann, P., Messina, N., Mohn, W. W., Finlay, B. B., & Curtis, N. (2019). Association between the intestinal microbiota and allergic sensitization, eczema, and asthma: A systematic review. *The Journal of Allergy and Clinical Immunology*, *143*(2), 467–485. https://doi.org/10.1016/j.jaci.2018.09.025.

7

Immunogens

VICTOR HUANG AND PEGGY A. WU

KEY POINTS

- Patients with atopic dermatitis are more susceptible to developing irritant contact dermatitis (ICD) and allergic contact dermatitis (ACD).
- ICD can present with phenotypic subtypes such as asteatotic ICD, airborne ICD, acneiform ICD, chronic ICD, and acute ICD with characteristic body sites involved, predominant morphologic features, time courses, and irritant sources.
- ACD is a type IV delayed hypersensitivity reaction and is preceded by prior sensitization to a hapten/allergen in contrast to ICD.
- Allergens that can cause ACD may have different pathologic and molecular signatures.
- The gold standard for diagnosing ACD is through patch testing.
- Treatments for atopic dermatitis can affect the reliability of patch testing results.

Introduction

Immunogens are external stimuli that perturb and penetrate the skin barrier resulting in the elicitation of inflammation. This chapter will review the relationship between atopic dermatitis (AD) and two conditions that predispose patients to immunogens: irritant contact dermatitis (ICD) and allergic contact dermatitis (ACD). Special considerations with regard to diagnosis and management of ICD and ACD in the context of AD are discussed.

Immunogens, outside in and inside out

The relationship between immunogens, the skin barrier, and the immune response is intertwined with outside-in versus inside-out factors in AD pathogenesis. The outside-in hypothesis of AD pathogenesis postulates that defects in the skin barrier allow greater penetration of irritants and immunogens eliciting the atopic march; this concept includes the idea that AD predisposes infants and children to other atopic diseases such as allergic rhinitis, allergic asthma, food allergy, and allergic keratoconjunctivitis. In contrast, the inside-out hypothesis suggests that innate immunologic factors predispose toward an atopic diathesis that results in skin barrier defects.

The inside-out hypothesis argues that a predisposition toward a polarized immune response gives rise to a defective skin barrier and that innate immune abnormalities lead to an aberrantly primed immune response. Support for this hypothesis comes from the observation that AD patients have an increased Th2 response, even in nonlesional skin. Tape stripping and using acetone to create skin barrier dysfunction in mice models leads to activation of innate immunity and increased Langerhans cell (LC) access to antigens along with upregulation of Th2 cytokines (Gittler et al., 2012). In mice, overexpression of Th2 cytokines leads the skin to spontaneously develop AD and skin barrier defects (Leung & Guttman-Yassky, 2014).

The outside-in hypothesis of AD pathogenesis is based on the observation that a percentage of AD patients have genetic defects in the stratum corneum and/or tight junctions located within the stratum granulosum, both of which are important barrier structures protecting the skin from the environment. Additional evidence for skin barrier defects initiating AD is provided by measures of epidermal dysfunction such as transepidermal water loss (TEWL) in AD. TEWL is increased in populations susceptible to AD such as neonates. Increased TEWL has been demonstrated in atopic versus normal skin, and studies have shown that even unaffected skin in patients with AD displays increased TEWL (Davidson et al., 2019). One of the best characterized genetic abnormalities associated with increased risk of AD is decreased expression of the epidermal differentiation protein filaggrin. The filaggrin *(FLG)* gene encodes the FLG protein, which is important for maintaining the skin barrier and preventing TEWL. Aside from structural deficiencies, decreased filaggrin can lead to increased Th2 cytokine production and production of endogenous proteases, increased interleukin-1 (IL1), and thymic stromal lymphopoietin (TSLP). These alterations in the immune milieu further erode the stratum corneum and skin barrier leaving it more penetrable to microbes and other immunogens. Nonetheless, filaggrin deficiency alone is not enough to account for most cases of AD. Although up to 40% of patients with severe AD have filaggrin mutations, only about 10% of European patients with AD are carriers.

Filaggrin mutations are rare in Asian populations and are not typically found in AD patients of African descent. While patients with filaggrin mutations often have dry skin, AD, and associated atopic diseases, most patients with AD do not have an *FLG* mutation (Leung & Guttman-Yassky, 2014). Other variants of genes encoding proteins in the epidermis associated with AD include filaggrin 2, hornerin, the cornified envelope precursor SPRR3, serine protease inhibitors, involucrin, loricrin as well as tight junction proteins such as the claudins (Leung & Guttman-Yassky, 2014). In this chapter we focus on immunogens as triggering factors for dermatitis primarily from the outside-in perspective.

Particularly, we focus on two types of immunogens: those related to irritant contact dermatitis (ICD) and to allergic contact dermatitis (ACD).

Irritant contact dermatitis–related immunogens

Irritants cause physical or chemical damage to the integument leading to a disruption of skin barrier integrity and the induction of inflammation. This inflammation results in ICD. No prior sensitization is necessary. ICD is a cytotoxic and inflammatory response to irritant stimuli resulting in several different clinical manifestations. Various clinical phenotypes of ICD have also been described based on the time course, predominant morphologic features, and irritant source. Examples include acute ICD, irritant reaction/chronic ICD, subjective irritation, frictional dermatitis, acneiform ICD, and airborne ICD. The prototypical ICD is acute ICD, typically due to a strong irritant, which can present with erythema, edema, vesicles, exudates with a sharp demarcation, and symptoms of burning, stinging, pain, and pruritus (Fig. 7.1). In contrast, chronic ICD and irritant reactions occur to mild irritants such as water, soap, and detergents; clinically, they appear as redness, scaling, and/or erosions (Fig. 7.2). Frictional dermatitis presents symptomatically with erythema, hyperkeratosis, scaling, and fissures in areas of friction. Asteatotic ICD is characterized by xerosis and superficial fissuring, and it commonly occurs on the lower extremities. Airborne ICD can occur to irritants in the air such as fibers, dust, fumes, and vapors.

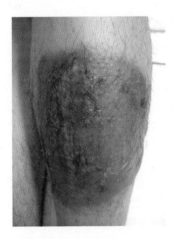

• **Fig. 7.1** Acute irritant contact dermatitis to garlic under occlusion. (From Xu, S., Heller, M., Wu, P. A., & Nambudiri V. E. [2014]. Chemical burn caused by topical application of garlic under occlusion. *Dermatology Online Journal, 20*[1], 21261.)

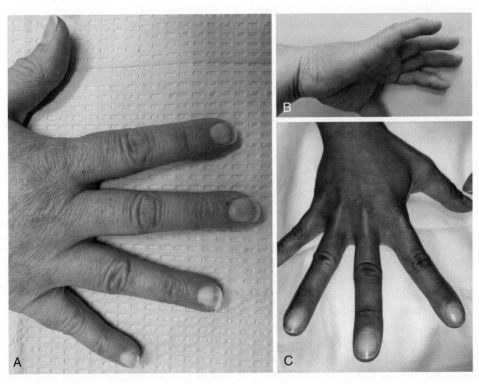

• **Fig. 7.2** Chronic irritant contact dermatitis of the hands. A, C. Erythematous patches with scale on the dorsal hands. B. Pink patches on the ulnar surface of the hand.

This dermatitis is predominant in exposed areas but can also affect covered areas by contaminating clothing. Finally acneiform ICD (due to metals, tars, metalworking fluids, chlorinated agents) can present as open and closed comedones, cysts, pustules, and nodules in a lateral distribution on the face and neck (Ale & Maibach, 2014).

Several mechanisms are involved to create the clinical presentation of ICD, including skin barrier disruption, keratinocyte damage, and release of proinflammatory mediators. While pure irritants do not directly induce an adaptive immune response, they can be a potent adjuvant for immune induction (Jacobs, Lehe, Hasegawa, Elliott, & Das, 2006). ICD triggers the innate immune system via similar pathways as those used by pathogens, and stimulates toll-like receptors (TLR) and cytosolic NOD-like receptors (NLR) present on both hematopoietic and non-hematopoietic cells to detect danger signals and activate inflammation. The activation of the innate immune system via TLR, reactive oxygen species, and NLRP3 inflammasomes can induce dendritic cells and in turn trigger the adaptive immune system. Indeed, a close connection between the two immune responses is increasingly recognized. Keratinocytes damaged with disruption of the skin barrier also release cytokines, upregulate major histocompatibility complex antigens, and release $IL1\alpha$, $IL1\beta$, and tumor necrosis factor (TNF).

ICD in patients with AD

The incidence of ICD is increased in patients with AD likely by several different mechanisms. Several epidemiologic studies document an increased rate of irritant reactions in patients with atopy, particularly in the occupational setting (Dickel, Bruckner, Schmidt, & Diepgen, 2003; Gittler, Krueger, & Guttman-Yassky, 2013; Landeck et al., 2012; Visser et al., 2013). Interestingly the most commonly used definition for AD in clinical trials, the Hanifin and Rajka criteria (Table 7.1) for AD, includes some features of ICD such as "tendency toward non specific hand or foot dermatitis" and "intolerance to wool and lipid solvents."

Pathogenesis of ICD in AD

The defects in the skin barrier associated with AD allow for increased penetration of irritants predisposing to ICD. Rates of occupational hand dermatitis are increased in patients with AD (Chew & Maibach, 2003). This may be due to deficiencies in the skin barrier. The interaction between filaggrin mutations and AD in patients with occupational dermatitis was studied in Germany and found that *FLG* mutations are present in 15.9% versus 8.3% of ICD patients and controls, respectively (Ale & Maibach, 2014). The odds ratio (OR) was 2.9 (95% confidence interval [CI], 1.33–3.28) for the combined *FLG*-deficient and AD phenotype. After adjusting for AD, the OR of 1.62 (95% CI, 1.01–2.58) continued to indicate an increased association. In the setting of occupational ICD, of 459 patients with

TABLE 7.1	Hanifin and Rajka criteria for atopic dermatitis, adapted from 1986 publication
Major criteria	
Chronic or chronically relapsing dermatitis	
Pruritus	
Typical morphology and distribution: Flexural lichenification or linearity, facial and extensor involvement in infants and children	
Personal and/or family history of atopy, asthma, allergic rhinitis, atopic dermatitis	
Minor criteria	
Immediate (type I) skin test reactivity	
Elevated serum immunoglobulin E	
Early age onset	
Tendency toward nonspecific hand or foot dermatitis	
Tendency toward cutaneous infections (i.e., *Staphylococcus aureus* and/or herpes simplex)/impaired cell-mediated immunity	
Xerosis	
Ichthyosis/palmar plantar hyper linearity/keratosis pilaris	
Recurrent conjunctivitis	
Dennie-Morgan infraorbital folds	
Keratoconus	
Anterior subcapsular cataracts	
Orbital darkening	
Facial pallor/facial erythema	
Pityriasis alba	
Chelitis	
Anterior neck folds	
Nipple eczema	
Perifollicular accentuation	
Itch when sweating	
Intolerance to wool or lipid solvents	
Food intolerance	
Disease course influenced by environmental/emotional factors	
White dermatographism/delayed blanch response	

From Andersen, R. M., Thyssen, J. P., & Maibach, H. I. (2016). Qualitative vs. quantitative atopic dermatitis criteria—in historical and present perspectives. *Journal of the European Academy of Dermatology and Venereology, 30*(4), 604–618. https://doi.org/10.1111/jdv.13442.

FLG mutations, 327 (71.2%) were atopic and 132 nonatopic. The *FLG*-deficient mutations in the setting of AD led to a more resistant clinical course of ICD with lower rates of recovery and higher use of topical corticosteroids (Landeck et al., 2012).

In addition to mutations in the skin barrier, patients with AD have inside-out genetic alterations in the cytokines involved in skin inflammation. One well-characterized factor is TNFα-308A. This polymorphism has been associated with susceptibility to ICD and ACD (Dittmar & Schuttelaar, 2017). TNFα-308A carriers have increased production of TNFα and a lower threshold to irritants such as sodium lauryl sulfate (SLS). In a case control study of 478 patients with occupational ICD, carriers of the TNFα-308A variant were more prone to developing ICD of the hands (Visser et al., 2013). TNFα is also released by keratinocytes when there is disruption of the skin barrier, which further induces inflammatory reactions and the cytokine cascade (Gittler et al., 2013). With the observation of the role for TNFα in ICD, TNFα may also be a target for treatment. It has been noted that injection of anti-TNFα antibodies may block some irritant reactions in animal models (Ale & Maibach, 2014; Piguet, Grau, Hauser, & Vassalli, 1991).

An objective demonstration of the increased risk of ICD in AD patients is demonstrated by a decreased threshold for susceptibility to SLS-induced irritant damage to the epidermis in patients with AD (Bandier, Carlsen, Rasmussen, Petersen, & Johansen, 2015). It is also known that ICD can predispose patients to ACD. When skin is pretreated with the irritant sodium dodecyl sulfate (SDS), the threshold for nickel concentration necessary to induce nickel allergic contact dermatitis is lowered (Allenby & Basketter, 1993).

Risk factors

Clinical risk factors for ICD in addition to AD include dry ambient conditions, cold temperatures, low humidity, and exposure to common irritants (e.g., detergents, friction, metalworking fluids, solvents, water, wet work, decreasing agents, disinfectants, antiseptics, acids, alkalis). Physical irritants include wood, fiberglass, plants, wool, paper, and chemical/cement/stone dust. Commonly affected areas include the hands and feet, particularly the dorsal aspect (vs. ventral due to thinner skin), face, and groin (Bains, Nash, & Fonacier, 2019).

Diagnosis

Diagnosis of ICD can only be made by adequate history, compatible clinical presentation, and negative patch test findings. In the clinical setting, skin biopsy is not reliable in distinguishing between AD, ICD, and ACD. One study examined 35 specimens from 28 patients with ICD, ACD, or AD and examined different histologic features such as presence of eosinophils, necrotic keratinocytes, parakeratosis, hypergranulosis, edema, neutrophils, crust, dermal infiltrates, erythrocyte extravasation, dermal fibrosis, and quantity of CD3, CD4, CD8, S100 staining and found a significant overlap of these findings in all three diagnoses (Frings, Böer-Auer, & Breuer, 2018). Only presence of eosinophils in the dermal infiltrate was significantly increased in the diagnosis of AD. The authors concluded that histopathology would not be able to dependably distinguish between ACD, ICD, and AD, but it could have a role in eliminating other papulosquamous diagnoses such as psoriasis in the differential diagnosis.

Management

Management of ICD focuses on identifying the irritants and prevention. If avoidance of known irritants is not possible, patients should protect the skin barrier with emollients as well as chemical or physical barriers such as gloves or clothing to cover at-risk areas. Barrier creams and skin conditioning products can be helpful as well as mild soap-free skin cleansers for washing, after which an emollient should be used. Washing and "wet-dry" cycles should be minimized as water itself can be a mild irritant. Irritation can also occur from sweat entrapment and friction of gloves. It is important to remove gloves to reduce perspiration and sweating and/or use a liner.

Because exposure to irritants can often occur in the occupational setting, educational measures should be implemented as secondary or tertiary prevention and motivation.

For any underlying inflammation, topical corticosteroids may be of help, although benefits would need to be balanced with potential compromise of the skin barrier function. The literature regarding steroid-sparing topical immunomodulators has been mixed with tacrolimus trending toward worsening SLS-irritated skin, whereas pimecrolimus was found to be effective. Psoralen and ultraviolet A (UVA) phototherapy may also be considered for their positive effects treating ICD and ACD (Ale & Maibach, 2014).

Allergic contact dermatitis–related immunogens

ACD can present in a myriad of ways. Erythema, scaling, edema, vesicles (especially in the acute phase), and hyperpigmentation can all be features (Fig. 7.3). Distinguishing characteristics include a linear or geometric configuration. In the patient with AD, ACD can present in areas not previously affected (such as the face) or as treatment-resistant areas.

Several key differences exist to distinguish ICD and ACD (Table 7.2). Key clinical differences are that ACD requires sensitization to a particular allergen and can be diagnosed with patch testing.

Several systematic reviews and meta-analyses have presented heterogenous findings estimating the incidence and risk of ACD in patients with and without AD. One systematic review found that although a third of children with AD who were patch tested were found to have at least one contact allergy, there was an increased rate of ACD in kids without AD versus those with AD (46.6% vs. 41.7%, $P < 0.001$) (Simonsen, Johansen, Deleuran, Mortz, & Sommerlund, 2017). Another systematic review and meta-analysis found adults and children with AD had a greater prevalence of contact sensitization when compared to the general population (OR, 1.5; 95% CI, 1.23–1.93) (Hamann et al., 2017). However, within the patch test population, patients with AD were less likely to be diagnosed with ACD (OR, 0.753; 95% CI, 0.632–0.90) (Hamann et al., 2017). Overall, pooled analysis showed no significant difference in contact sensitization between AD and controls (OR, 0.891; 95% CI, 0.771–1.03). One possible explanation was that patients with AD referred for patch testing are more likely to have severe and active disease with a higher elicitation threshold for contact sensitization (Owen, Vakharia, & Silverberg, 2018). Previous studies have found an inverse association between severe AD, asthma, and ACD with lower prevalence of contact sensitization when compared with controls (Thyssen, Johansen, Linneberg, Menné, & Engkilde, 2012).

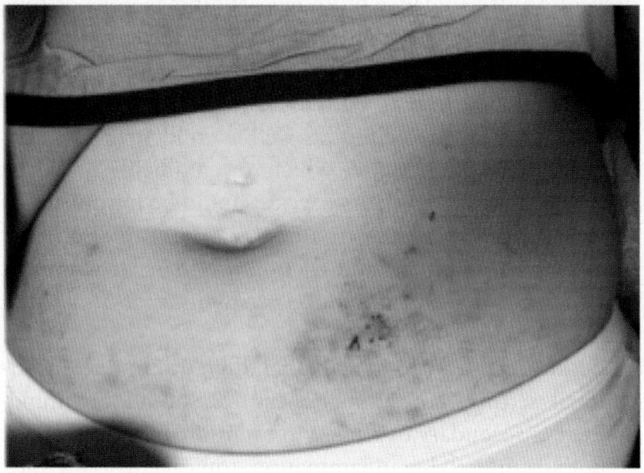

• **Fig. 7.3** Allergic contact dermatitis on the abdomen presenting as small erythematous, edematous papules coalescing into plaques on the abdomen.

TABLE 7.2 ACD versus ICD

Features	Allergic contact dermatitis	Irritant contact dermatitis
Causative agents	Low molecular weight haptens, lipid soluble	Acids, alkalis, surfactants, solvents, oxidants, enzymes
Genetic predisposition	More important	Less important
Sensitization and lag period	Necessary	Not necessary
Trigger	Interaction of antigen with primed T cells	Damage to keratinocytes
Cytokine release	Large	Moderate
T-cell activation	Early	Late
Mast cell activation	Some	Some
Langerhans cells	Increased	Decreased

Adapted from Marks, J. G., Anderson, B. E., & DeLeo, V. A. (2016). *Contact and occupational dermatology* (4th ed.). Jaypee Brothers Medical Publishers Pvt Ltd.

ACD pathogenesis

ACD is defined as a cell-mediated, type IV delayed hypersensitivity reaction to a specific immunogen (hapten). Haptens that penetrate the epidermis need to be low molecular weight, usually less than 500 Da, and lipid soluble. ACD takes place over two phases: the initial sensitization phase and an elicitation response (Mowad et al., 2016).

The sensitization phase starts when the hapten penetrates the epidermis, causing keratinocyte damage and cytokine release. That hapten interacts with host proteins, and is taken up and processed by an antigen presenting cell, most often Langerhans cells (LCs). The hapten becomes an immunogen after it is conjugated with endogenous proteins. The LC becomes activated by cytokines released from keratinocytes as it migrates to the lymph node. In the lymph node, the LC presents the antigen on its surface as an HLA-DR antigen complex to a naïve T cell. That T cell is trained to specifically recognize this antigen and create memory as well as effector T cells; it then expresses IL2 to stimulate T-cell proliferation of antigen-specific (usually CD8+) cells, which return to the site of the initial exposure. There the T cells release mediators such as TNFβ and γ-interferon to cause further inflammation and manifestation of rash. The process of sensitization takes place over 1 to 2 weeks (Fig. 7.4).

In the elicitation phase, reexposure to a recognized antigen occurs when the hapten penetrates the epidermis, is taken up and processed by LC, and is again presented as an antigen. Recognition of the antigen on the LC by a trained T cell leads to activation and expansion of that specific effector T-cell population within the skin. The activated T-cell release of γ-interferon stimulates nearby keratinocytes to express ICAM-1 and HLA-DR. The cycle of cytotoxic T-cell and keratinocyte activation also leads to mobilization of mast cells, macrophages, infiltrating leukocytes, and histamine release and results in inflammation, cellular destruction, and the clinical picture of a rash. The elicitation phase is more rapid and generally takes place over 3 to 5 days. This is the mechanism relied upon to identity culprit allergens in patch testing.

ACD in patients with AD

The exact association between ACD reactions to external immunogens and the relationship between ACD and AD is still debated. ACD had been understood to be a primarily Th1-mediated hypersensitivity reaction, but it is now known that the particular allergen of interest may dictate

Sensitization   **Elicitation**

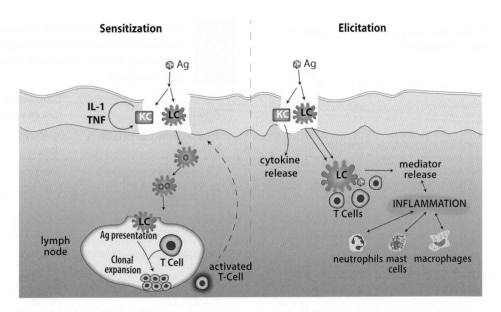

• **Fig. 7.4** The immune reactions of two phases of allergic contact dermatitis: sensitization phase *(left panel)*, elicitation phase *(right panel)*. (From Bolognia, J., Jorizzo, J., & Schaffer, J. (2012). *Dermatology* [3rd ed.]. Edinburgh: Saunders.)

whether Th2, Th17, and/or Th22 mediators also have a role. On the other hand, AD is primarily a Th2 response in the acute and chronic phases, with a Th1 contribution in the chronic phase (Owen et al., 2018). Within the context of AD, the pathogenesis of ACD is primarily Th2 rather than Th1 polarized (Dhingra, Gulati, & Guttman-Yassky, 2013). In the past, the increased Th2 response associated with AD was shown to decrease sensitization to allergens, primarily dinitrochlorobenzene (DCNB) in animal models (Correa da Rosa et al., 2015; Owen et al., 2018). More recently, with the use of gene expression and immunohisto-chemistry assays, one group found decreased expression of Th1 subset and Th2 subset genes with increased Th17/IL23 skewing for nickel-related responses in AD patients when compared with patients without AD. Rubber and fragrance allergens showed a similar trend leading to overall attenu-ated pattern of contact sensitization to those allergens in AD patients. The projected risk of ACD in AD patients from these translational studies conflicts with several epi-demiologic reports that have shown similar to higher ACD rates in patients with AD. In children, the rate of ACD in AD may be even higher than in adults (Simonsen et al., 2017). Several theories have been proposed to explain this finding. It is known that AD is associated with skin barrier disruption, which can lead to increased penetration of immunogens (Bandier et al., 2015; Leung & Guttman-Yassky, 2014). Patients with AD can have a twofold increase in skin absorption of irritants and contact allergens (Owen et al., 2018). As previously mentioned, skin irritants can lead to increased absorption of allergens and a decreased threshold necessary to stimulate ACD. Moreover, patients with AD, over the course of the lifetime, are more likely to use and be exposed to various skin products, emol-lients, and medications that may contain haptens causative of ACD.

Identifying the need to patch test patients with AD

Given the overlap between ACD and AD clinically, the two entities possibly coexisting within an individual patient, and the difference in treatment approach depending on that diagnosis, it is important to consider patch testing to make the diagnosis of ACD if suspected. ACD should be suspected if an existing dermatitis changes distribution, worsens, or occurs in a configuration more consistent with contact dermatitis such as with regional predominance of the head and neck, hand and foot, eyelids, or cheilitis, and if the dermatitis fails to improve with therapy or rebounds fol-lowing discontinuation of topical therapy. A recent expert consensus provided some recommendations when to con-sider patch testing in individuals with AD (Table 7.3).

Patch testing is not likely to be helpful in the setting of stable, controlled AD; patients on broad, systemic immu-nosuppression; patients undergoing phototherapy; and patients who are actively flaring. For patients who are flar-ing, efforts should be made to control the active dermatitis prior to patch testing, otherwise the risk of experiencing an angry back/excited skin syndrome during patch test-ing with uninterpretable results is increased (Cockayne & Gawkrodger, 2000). Guidelines for management of patients actively flared under consideration for patch test therapy are based on expert opinion. Expert consensus suggests that TNF inhibitors, methotrexate, and ustekinumab are less likely to affect patch testing results. Conversely, doses of prednisone greater than 10 mg a day, injection of intra-muscular triamcinolone less than 4 weeks prior to testing, topical corticosteroids or calcineurin inhibitors on patch test application sites within 1 week of patch testing, photo-therapy or sunburns less than 1 week prior to patch testing, azathioprine, cyclosporine, mycophenolate mofetil, and

TABLE 7.3	When to consider patch testing in patients with atopic dermatitis

If a previously controlled dermatitis worsens or changes in distribution, fails to improve with usual management
If dermatitis immediately rebounds upon discontinuation of topical treatments
If the dermatitis manifests in an atypical atopic dermatitis distribution or in a pattern that is suggestive of contact dermatitis such as eyelid predominance, perioral predominance, genital predominance, head and neck predominance, hand and foot predominance
If a dermatitis is severe or extensive or cannot be managed with topical therapy or moisturizers and one is considering systemic therapy
New-onset adult or adolescent atopic dermatitis without a childhood history of eczema

Adapted from Chen, J. K., Jacob, S. E., Nedorost, S. T., Hanifin, J. M., Simpson, E. L., Boguniewicz, M., et al. (2016). A pragmatic approach to patch testing atopic dermatitis patients: Clinical recommendations based on expert consensus opinion. *Dermatitis: Contact, Atopic, Occupational, Drug, 27*(4), 186–192. https://doi.org/10.1097/DER.0000000000000208.

TABLE 7.4	Results of poll of North American Contact Dermatitis Group (NACDG) members regarding effects of various agents on patch test reactions

Agent	Consensus recommendation
Topical corticosteroids on test site	Avoid between 3 and 7 days
Ultraviolet light exposure at test site (including phototherapy, sunburns)	Avoid for 1 week
Maximum dose of oral prednisone	≤10 mg, best if able to discontinue
Ideal oral prednisone washout time	3–5 days
Injection of intramuscular triamcinolone	Wait until 4 weeks after injection
Methotrexate	Little to no effect
Tumor necrosis factor inhibitors	Little to no effect
Ustekinumab	Little to no effect
Azathioprine	Dose-dependent inhibition of response
Cyclosporine	Dose-dependent inhibition of response
Mycophenolate mofetil	Dose-dependent inhibition of response
Systemic tacrolimus	Dose-dependent inhibition of response

Adapted from Fowler, J. F., Maibach, H. I., Zirwas, M., Taylor, J. S., Dekoven, J. G., Sasseville, D., et al. (2012). Effects of immunomodulatory agents on patch testing: Expert opinion 2012. *Dermatitis: Contact, Atopic, Occupational, Drug, 23*(6), 301–303. https://doi.org/10.1097/DER.0b013e318275969f.

tacrolimus are high risk for affecting patch test results (Table 7.4) (Fowler et al., 2012).

Patch testing patients with AD

Common contact allergens identified in children and adults with AD include bacitracin, carba mix, chromium, cinnamic aldehyde, cobalt, cocamidopropyl betaine, colophony, compositae mix, disperse blue, epoxy resin, formaldehyde, fragrance, benzisothiazolinones, lanolin, mercaptobenzothiazole, balsam of Peru, neomycin, nickel, p-tert butylphenol formaldehyde resin, p-phenylenediamine, potassium dichromate, quaternium 15, rubber or rubber mixes, sesquiterpene lactone, and topical antiseptics (Jacob et al., 2017). Within that list, various allergens have been highlighted depending on the published study. Lanolin and fragrances have been significantly associated in pediatric patients with AD, and in a retrospective analysis of 26,479 patients tested by the North American Contact Dermatitis Group (NACDG), lanolin allergy was more likely to be found in patients with AD (Owen et al., 2018). Other studies of ACD in AD patients have highlighted greater sensitization to potassium dichromate, phenylmercuric acetate, nickel, and cobalt (Landeck, Schalock, Baden, & González, 2011; Malajian & Belsito, 2013). As the list of possible allergens in AD patients is broad, it behooves the patch test practitioner to test comprehensively. When possible, patients should also be tested to their own products, as culprit agents are often found in the patient's own personal care products, including so-called hypoallergenic ones.

During patch testing, patients with AD are more likely to have irritant reactions, mild reactions, and borderline positive reactions (Owen et al., 2018). Further increasing the difficulty of deciphering patch test reactions in patients with AD is that they are less likely to display a crescendo pattern associated with ACD. This pattern of reactivity over the preliminary to final patch test reading at 72 hours or more can help distinguish ICD from ACD reactions. Whereas ICD reactions often have a decrescendo pattern where the reaction is stronger at the preliminary reading than at the final reading, ACD is more likely to have a crescendo pattern with the intensity of the reaction increasing over time.

Active AD or any preexisting dermatitis prior to patch testing is also a risk factor for angry back reaction, also known as excited skin syndrome. The angry back syndrome, which occurs when a generalized dermatitis affects patch testing areas, leading to false-positive and false-negative reactions, often yields indecipherable patch test results, which are not reproducible on subsequent patch test applications (Bruynzeel, van Ketel, von Blomberg-van der Flier, & Scheper, 1983; Cockayne & Gawkrodger, 2000).

Management of ACD in patients with AD

The mainstay of ACD management is avoiding the culprit allergen(s). Considering the underlying mechanisms of ACD within patients with AD, therapy for contact sensitization extends beyond avoiding the known trigger to addressing immune polarization as well as barrier deficiencies. Because skin barrier deficiency, and ICD, can predispose and/or lower thresholds to ACD, it is important to protect the skin barrier with emollients and physical barriers such as gloves.

One tool that has been very successful in helping in the management of ACD is the Contact Allergen Management Program (CAMP). This program specifically allows health care providers to filter out personal care products that contain a patient's patch test–positive allergens. Use of this tool has been significantly associated with decreased counseling time as well as increased success in managing ACD (Kist, el-Azhary, Hentz, & Yiannias, 2004).

Aside from avoidance, the management of ACD is similar to that of any dermatitis, with the therapeutic ladder ranging from emollients, topical medications, to systemic medications. Topical management with corticosteroids is frequently used. For longer term management, steroid sparing immunomodulatory agents such as tacrolimus, pimecrolimus, or crisaborole can be used. Skin directed phototherapy with ultraviolet (UV) B or UVA is another treatment option.

Most systemic medications that have the ability to affect patch testing results (doses of systemic corticosteroids ≥10 mg; antimetabolite such as methotrexate, azathioprine, or mycophenolate mofetil; γ-interferon antagonists such as cyclosporine and apremilast) can be used to manage severe ACD. Interestingly, although TNFα plays a critical role in development of ACD in the sensitization and elicitation phase, the TNF inhibitors such as infliximab, etanercept, and adalimumab have very little evidence in the form of case reports supporting their use in ACD (Sung, McGowan, Machler, & Jacob, 2019).

Dupilumab, a humanized monoclonal antibody that blocks IL4 and intralesional-13, key drivers of Th2 mediated disease, was Food and Drug Admininstration approved in 2017 and has emerged as a therapeutic treatment option for AD. Recent case reports of patients have noted its effect on ACD as well, although the effect on patch testing and ACD is more nuanced. Some patients who are unable to avoid their allergens experience relief from their ACD and AD while on dupilumab, including in cases of systemic contact dermatitis (Chipalkatti et al., 2018; Goldminz & Scheinman, 2018; Jacob, Sung, & Machler, 2019; Joshi & Khan 2018; Machler, Sung, Darwin, & Jacob, 2019). Positive reactions to allergens and patch testing while on dupilumab have been noted (Hoot, Desiree Douglas, & Falo, 2018). Although dupilumab does not appear to exert a dampening effect on

most patch test results, about 10.4% (13 of 125) of patch test reactions were lost in one series of patients on dupilumab (Raffi, Suresh, Botto, & Murase, 2019). In several of those cases (5 of 13), the patient also had a documented immunodeficiency. Another report noted a patient with prior positive reactions to nickel, composite mix, hydroperoxides of linalool (component of many fragrances) as well as bronopol and methylisothiazolinone (MI) experienced no reactions to nickel, composite today, and linalool upon repeat patch testing after 2 months of dupilumab (Raffi & Botto, 2019). When reaction patterns are compared with those prior to starting dupilumab therapy, a reduction in or absence of reactions (including loss of reaction to nickel; methylchoroisothiazolinone/methylisothiazolinone (MCI/MI) cinnamal, balsam of Peru) has been noted (Raffi & Botto, 2019; Stout & Silverberg, 2019). On the other hand, in one case dupilumab therapy for AD prompted a recall dermatitis to a positive reaction to colophony (Collantes-Rodríguez, Jiménez-Gallo, Ossorio-García, Villegas-Romero, & Linares-Barrios, 2019). The authors postulated that the dampened Th2 response led to increased Th1 reaction at the previous patch test site. The full effect of IL4 and IL13 blockade in ACD and AD are yet to be fully characterized.

Since the diagnoses of ACD and AD are often comorbid, another series illustrated the importance of performing an expanded series patch test in patients with facial dermatitis on dupilumab therapy, as ACD should be considered part of the differential diagnosis for residual disease (Suresh & Murase, 2018).

In theory, the biologics (e.g., dupilumab, JAK inhibitors) that are currently being used for AD may have some benefit in the management of ACD. This has yet to be explored, although there have been some promising case reports of dupilumab benefiting patients with both ACD and AD (Chipalkatti et al., 2019; Machler et al., 2019). There is some preliminary reports from the laboratory of JAK inhibitors being of potential use in treating ACD. No human studies on JAK inhibitors for ACD have been published to date (Fukuyama, Ehling, Cook, & Bäumer, 2015).

Immediate hypersensitivity reactions

Patients may misperceive ACD and the underlying delayed type hypersensitivity reaction with immediate hypersensitivity reactions. Immediate hypersensitivity reactions are immunoglobulin E (IgE) mediated, and they usually occur within 20 to 30 minutes of stimulus with mast cells as the main effector cell propagating the response. There is an intimate relationship between immediate hypersensitivity reactions and AD. Interwoven within the accepted clinical criteria for AD are the clinical criteria that AD patients have elevated IgE as well as increased skin hypersensitivity tests (Andersen, Thyssen, & Maibach, 2016). The 1980 Hanifin and Rajka criteria include "immediate (type I) skin test reactivity" as one of the minor features of AD. Common immediate hypersensitivity immunogens include dust mite and tree pollen, and positive reactions to those entities were considered part of the AD millennial diagnostic criteria (Andersen et al., 2016).

Approach to the patient with AD and ICD or ACD

In the clinical setting, both the outside-in and inside-out components of AD pathogenesis are important as they relate to the effects of immunogens on the skin of AD patients as well as the management approach. From the outside in, several studies have shown that early, daily emollient use to protect the skin barrier in high-risk infants leads to 50% reduction in AD by 6 months of age (Davidson et al., 2019; Leung & Guttman-Yassky, 2014). Conversely, use of broad and specific immunosuppressants and immunomodulators topically and systemically can resolve innate immunologic polarizations of AD as well as the associated epidermal defects. These options to prevent and treat AD are likely to also have an effect on ACD and ICD, two immunogen-modulated disorders that are over-represented in patients with AD.

Summary

AD, ICD, and ACD interact and contribute to altered host interactions with immunogens and increase risk for immunogen-mediated inflammation. Patients with AD are more likely to be susceptible to ICD due to deficiencies in the skin barrier. ICD occurs when irritants cause physical or chemical damage to the skin barrier and lead to induction of inflammation. ICD can present in different forms depending on the location of the body, strength of the irritant, and timing. It differs from ACD in that it does not require prior sensitization. Management is predominantly prevention and protection of the skin barrier with chemical or physical barriers. ACD is a manifestation of a delayed hypersensitivity reaction to a specific hapten or allergen. It requires prior sensitization, and our understanding of the mechanisms of ACD to various allergens is evolving. To make the diagnosis of ACD, patch testing needs to be performed. Even in a patient with a prior diagnosis of AD, patch testing can reveal new allergens. Management is predominantly avoidance of culprit allergens and protection of the skin barrier. There are various tools (e.g., CAMP) that can aid with avoidance. For ACD that cannot be managed with topical therapy, systemic therapy is an option. Newer biologics such as dupilumab may eventually play a role in the management of ACD.

Further readings

Mowad, C. M., Anderson, B., Scheinman, P., Pootongkam, S., Nedorost, S., & Brod, B. (2016) Allergic contact dermatitis: Patient management and education. *Journal of the American Academy of Dermatology, 74*(6),1043–1054.

Dermatologic Clinics: Allergic Contact Dermatitis. https://www.sciencedirect.com/journal/dermatologic-clinics/vol/38/issue/3.

References

Ale, I. S., & Maibach, H. I. (2014). Irritant contact dermatitis. *Reviews on Environmental Health, 29*(3), 195–206. https://doi.org/10.1515/reveh-2014-0060.

Allenby, C. F., & Basketter, D. A. (1993). An arm immersion model of compromised skin (II). Influence on minimal eliciting patch test concentrations of nickel. *Contact Dermatitis, 28*(3), 129–133. https://doi.org/10.1111/j.1600-0536.1993.tb03371.x.

Andersen, R. M., Thyssen, J. P., & Maibach, H. I. (2016). Qualitative vs. quantitative atopic dermatitis criteria—in historical and present perspectives. *Journal of the European Academy of Dermatology and Venereology, 30*(4), 604–618. https://doi.org/10.1111/jdv.13442.

Bains, Sonia N., Nash, Pembroke, & Fonacier, Luz (2019). Irritant contact dermatitis. *Clinical Reviews in Allergy & Immunology, 56*(1), 99–109. https://doi.org/10.1007/s12016-018-8713-0.

Bandier, J., Carlsen, B. C., Rasmussen, M. A., Petersen, L. J., & Johansen, J. D. (2015). Skin reaction and regeneration after single sodium lauryl sulfate exposure stratified by filaggrin genotype and atopic dermatitis phenotype. *The British Journal of Dermatology, 172*(6), 1519–1529. https://doi.org/10.1111/bjd.13651.

Bruynzeel, D. P., van Ketel, W. G., von Blomberg-van der Flier, B. M., & Scheper, R. J. (1983). Angry back or the excited skin syndrome. A prospective study. *Journal of the American Academy of Dermatology, 8*(3), 392–397. https://doi.org/10.1016/s0190-9622(83)70044-7.

Chew, Ai-Lean, & Maibach, Howard I. (2003). Occupational issues of irritant contact dermatitis. *International Archives of Occupational and Environmental Health, 76*(5), 339–346. https://doi.org/10.1007/s00420-002-0419-0.

Chipalkatti, Naina, Lee, Nicole, Zancanaro, Pedro, Dumont, Nicole, Donovan, Courtney, & Rosmarin, David (2018). Dupilumab as a treatment for allergic contact dermatitis. *Dermatitis, 29*(6), 347. https://doi.org/10.1097/DER.0000000000000414.

Chipalkatti, N., Lee, N., Zancanaro, P., Dumont, N., Kachuk, C., & Rosmarin, D. (2019). A retrospective review of dupilumab for atopic dermatitis patients with allergic contact dermatitis. *Journal of the American Academy of Dermatology, 80*(4), 1166–1167. https://doi.org/10.1016/j.jaad.2018.12.048.

Cockayne, S. E., & Gawkrodger, D. J. (2000). Angry back syndrome is often due to marginal irritants: A study of 17 cases seen over 4 years. *Contact Dermatitis, 43*(5), 280–282. https://doi.org/10.1034/j.1600-0536.2000.043005280.x.

Collantes-Rodríguez, Cristina, Jiménez-Gallo, David, Ossorio-García, Lidia, Villegas-Romero, Isabel, & Linares-Barrios, Mario (2019). Recall dermatitis at patch test sites in an atopic dermatitis patient treated with dupilumab. *Contact Dermatitis, 80*(1), 69–70. https://doi.org/10.1111/cod.13134.

Correa da Rosa, Joel, Malajian, Dana, Shemer, Avner, Rozenblit, Mariya, Dhingra, Nikhil, Czarnowicki, Tali, Khattri, Saakshi, et al. (2015). Patients with atopic dermatitis have attenuated and distinct contact hypersensitivity responses to common allergens in skin. *The Journal of Allergy and Clinical Immunology, 135*(3), 712–720. https://doi.org/10.1016/j.jaci.2014.11.017.

Davidson, Wendy F., Donald, Y. M. Leung, Beck, Lisa A., Berin, Cecilia M., Boguniewicz, Mark, Busse, William W., et al. (2019). Report from the National Institute of Allergy and Infectious Diseases Workshop on 'atopic dermatitis and the atopic march: Mechanisms and interventions.' *The Journal of Allergy and Clinical Immunology, 143*(3), 894–913. https://doi.org/10.1016/j.jaci.2019.01.003.

Dhingra, Nikhil, Gulati, Nicholas, & Guttman-Yassky, Emma (2013). Mechanisms of contact sensitization offer insights into the role of barrier defects vs. intrinsic immune abnormalities as drivers of atopic dermatitis. *The Journal of Investigative Dermatology*, *133*(10), 2311–2314. https://doi.org/10.1038/jid.2013.239.

Dickel, Heinrich, Bruckner, Thomas M., Schmidt, Anne, & Diepgen, Thomas L. (2003). Impact of atopic skin diathesis on occupational skin disease incidence in a working population. *The Journal of Investigative Dermatology*, *121*(1), 37–40. https://doi.org/10.1046/j.1523-1747.2003.12323.x.

Dittmar, Daan, & Schuttelaar, Marie L. (2017). Immunology and genetics of tumour necrosis factor in allergic contact dermatitis. *Contact Dermatitis*, *76*(5), 257–271. https://doi.org/10.1111/cod.12769.

Fowler, Joseph F., Maibach, Howard I., Zirwas, Matthew, Taylor, James S., Dekoven, Joel G., Sasseville, Denis, et al. (2012). Effects of immunomodulatory agents on patch testing: expert opinion 2012. *Dermatitis: Contact, Atopic, Occupational, Drug*, *23*(6), 301–303. https://doi.org/10.1097/DER.0b013e318275969f.

Frings, Verena G., Böer-Auer, Almut, & Breuer, Kristine (2018). Histomorphology and immunophenotype of eczematous skin lesions revisited-skin biopsies are not reliable in differentiating allergic contact dermatitis, irritant contact dermatitis, and atopic dermatitis. *The American Journal of Dermatopathology*, *40*(1), 7–16. https://doi.org/10.1097/DAD.0000000000000842.

Fukuyama, Tomoki, Ehling, Sarah, Cook, Elizabeth, & Bäumer, Wolfgang (2015). Topically administered janus-kinase inhibitors tofacitinib and oclacitinib display impressive antipruritic and anti-inflammatory responses in a model of allergic dermatitis. *The Journal of Pharmacology and Experimental Therapeutics*, *354*(3), 394–405. https://doi.org/10.1124/jpet.115.223784.

Gittler, Julia K., Krueger, James G., & Guttman-Yassky, Emma (2013). Atopic dermatitis results in intrinsic barrier and immune abnormalities: Implications for contact dermatitis. *The Journal of Allergy and Clinical Immunology*, *131*(2), 300–313. https://doi.org/10.1016/j.jaci.2012.06.048.

Gittler, Julia K., Shemer, Avner, Suárez-Fariñas, Mayte, Fuentes-Duculan, Judilyn, Gulewicz, Kara J., Wang, Claire Q. F., et al. (2012). Progressive activation of TH2/TH22 cytokines and selective epidermal proteins characterizes acute and chronic atopic dermatitis. *Journal of Allergy and Clinical Immunology*, *130*(6), 1344–1354. https://doi.org/10.1016/j.jaci.2012.07.012.

Goldminz, Ari M., & Scheinman, Pamela L. (2018). A case series of dupilumab-treated allergic contact dermatitis patients. *Dermatologic Therapy*, *31*(6), e12701. https://doi.org/10.1111/dth.12701.

Hamann, Carsten R., Hamann, Dathan, Egeberg, Alexander, Johansen, Jeanne D., Silverberg, Jonathan, & Thyssen, Jacob P. (2017). Association between atopic dermatitis and contact sensitization: A systematic review and meta-analysis. *Journal of the American Academy of Dermatology*, *77*(1), 70–78. https://doi.org/10.1016/j.jaad.2017.02.001.

Hoot, Joyce W., Desiree Douglas, J., & Falo, Louis D. (2018). Patch testing in a patient on dupilumab. *Dermatitis: Contact, Atopic, Occupational, Drug*, *29*(3), 164. https://doi.org/10.1097/DER.0000000000000357.

Jacobs, John, Lehe, Cynthia, Hasegawa, Hitoshi, Elliott, Graham, & Das, Pranab (2006). Both skin irritants and contact sensitizers induce Langerhans cell migration and maturation. *Experimental dermatology*, *15*(6), 432–440. https://doi.org/10.1111/j.0906-6705.2006.00420.x.

Jacob, Sharon E., McGowan, Maria, Silverberg, Nanette B., Pelletier, Janice L., Fonacier, Luz, Mousdicas, Nico, et al. (2017). Pediatric Contact Dermatitis Registry data on contact allergy in children with atopic dermatitis. *JAMA Dermatology*, *153*(8), 765–770. https://doi.org/10.1001/jamadermatol.2016.6136.

Jacob, Sharon E., Sung, Calvin T., & Machler, Brian C. (2019). Dupilumab for systemic allergy syndrome with dermatitis. *Dermatitis: Contact, Atopic, Occupational, Drug*, *30*(2), 164–167. https://doi.org/10.1097/DER.0000000000000446.

Joshi, Shyam R., & Khan, David A. (2018). Effective use of dupilumab in managing systemic allergic contact dermatitis. *Dermatitis: Contact, Atopic, Occupational, Drug*, *29*(5), 282–284. https://doi.org/10.1097/DER.0000000000000409.

Kist, Joseph M., el-Azhary, Rokea A., Hentz, Joseph G., & Yiannias, James A. (2004). The contact allergen replacement database and treatment of allergic contact dermatitis. *Archives of Dermatology*, *140*(12), 1448–1450. https://doi.org/10.1001/archderm.140.12.1448.

Landeck, Lilla, Schalock, Peter, Baden, Lynn, & González, Ernesto (2011). Contact sensitization pattern in 172 atopic subjects. *International Journal of Dermatology*, *50*(7), 806–810. https://doi.org/10.1111/j.1365-4632.2010.04754.x.

Landeck, L., Visser, M., Skudlik, C., Brans, R., Kezic, S., & John, S. M. (2012). Clinical course of occupational irritant contact dermatitis of the hands in relation to filaggrin genotype status and atopy. *The British Journal of Dermatology*, *167*(6), 1302–1309. https://doi.org/10.1111/bjd.12035.

Leung, Donald Y. M., & Guttman-Yassky, Emma (2014). Deciphering the complexities of atopic dermatitis: shifting paradigms in treatment approaches. *The Journal of Allergy and Clinical Immunology*, *134*(4), 769–779. https://doi.org/10.1016/j.jaci.2014.08.008.

Machler, Brian C., Sung, Calvin T., Darwin, Evan, & Jacob, Sharon E. (2019). Dupilumab use in allergic contact dermatitis. *Journal of the American Academy of Dermatology*, *80*(1), 281–281.e1. https://doi.org/10.1016/j.jaad.2018.07.043.

Malajian, Dana, & Belsito, Donald V. (2013). Cutaneous delayed-type hypersensitivity in patients with atopic dermatitis. *Journal of the American Academy of Dermatology*, *69*(2), 232–237. https://doi.org/10.1016/j.jaad.2013.03.012.

Mowad, Christen M., Anderson, Bryan, Scheinman, Pamela, Pootongkam, Suwimon, Nedorost, Susan, & Brod, Bruce (2016). Allergic contact dermatitis: Patient diagnosis and evaluation. *Journal of the American Academy of Dermatology*, *74*(6), 1029–1040. https://doi.org/10.1016/j.jaad.2015.02.1139.

Owen, Joshua L., Vakharia, Paras P., & Silverberg, Jonathan I. (2018). The role and diagnosis of allergic contact dermatitis in patients with atopic dermatitis. *American Journal of Clinical Dermatology*, *19*(3), 293–302. https://doi.org/10.1007/s40257-017-0340-7.

Piguet, P. F., Grau, G. E., Hauser, C., & Vassalli, P. (1991). Tumor necrosis factor is a critical mediator in hapten induced irritant and contact hypersensitivity reactions. *The Journal of Experimental Medicine*, *173*(3), 673–679. https://doi.org/10.1084/jem.173.3.673.

Raffi, Jodie, & Botto, Nina (2019). Patch testing and allergen-specific inhibition in a patient taking dupilumab. *JAMA Dermatology*, *155*(1), 120–121. https://doi.org/10.1001/jamadermatol.2018.4098.

Raffi, Jodie, Suresh, Raagini, Botto, Nina, & Murase, Jenny E. (2019). The impact of dupilumab on patch testing and the prevalence of co-morbid ACD in recalcitrant atopic dermatitis: A retrospective chart review. *Journal of the American Academy of Dermatology*. https://doi.org/10.1016/j.jaad.2019.09.028.

Simonsen, A. B., Johansen, J. D., Deleuran, M., Mortz, C. G., & Sommerlund, M. (2017). Contact allergy in children with atopic dermatitis: A systematic review. *The British Journal of Dermatology*, *177*(2), 395–405. https://doi.org/10.1111/bjd.15628.

Stout, Molly, & Silverberg, Jonathan I. (2019). Variable impact of dupilumab on patch testing results and allergic contact dermatitis in adults with atopic dermatitis. *Journal of the American Academy of Dermatology*, *81*(1), 157–162. https://doi.org/10.1016/j.jaad.2019.03.020.

Sung, Calvin T., McGowan, Maria A., Machler, Brian C., & Jacob, Sharon E. (2019). Systemic treatments for allergic contact dermatitis. *Dermatitis: Contact, Atopic, Occupational, Drug*, *30*(1), 46–53. https://doi.org/10.1097/DER.0000000000000435.

Suresh, Raagini, & Murase, Jenny E. (2018). The role of expanded series patch testing in identifying causality of residual facial dermatitis

following initiation of dupilumab therapy. *JAAD Case Reports*, *4*(9), 899–904. https://doi.org/10.1016/j.jdcr.2018.08.027.

Thyssen, J. P., Johansen, J. D., Linneberg, A., Menné, T., & Engkilde, K. (2012). The association between contact sensitization and atopic disease by linkage of a clinical database and a nationwide patient registry. *Allergy*, *67*(9), 1157–1164. https://doi.org/10.1111/j.1398-9995.2012.02863.x.

Visser, M. J., Landeck, L., Campbell, L. E., McLean, W. H. I., Weidinger, S., Calkoen, F., et al. (2013). Impact of atopic dermatitis and loss-of-function mutations in the filaggrin gene on the development of occupational irritant contact dermatitis. *The British Journal of Dermatology*, *168*(2), 326–332. https://doi.org/10.1111/bjd.12083.

8

Nutrition

JENNIFER M. FERNANDEZ AND COLLEEN COTTON

KEY POINTS

- Maternal supplementation of omega-3 polyunsaturated fatty acids may reduce risk of atopic dermatitis (AD).
- Fish intake during early childhood may decrease the risk of developing AD.
- Early oral introduction of potentially allergenic foods in combination with improved skin barrier function may decrease the risk of developing food allergies in patients with AD.
- Food allergy is common in patients with AD but usually does not exacerbate the condition directly.
- There is favorable evidence for vitamin D supplementation as an adjunctive treatment in AD.

Introduction

How does what we eat influence atopic dermatitis (AD)? Hundreds of studies of variable quality have attempted to answer this question. It is unclear whether the effects of diet on both AD risk and existing AD are mediated by pro- or antiinflammatory properties, skin barrier development, immune regulation, modulatory effects on the gut microbiome, or a combination of these. What is clear is that patients are gravitating toward more "natural" treatments or finding the "root cause" of AD, and dietary influences are one of the first places they may start.

The true relationship between nutrition and AD is difficult to tease out. One main reason is that high-quality dietary studies are difficult to perform, often resulting in inconclusive or inconsistent data. Observational studies rely heavily on patients' reports of what foods they consumed and when, rather than direct observation of dietary intake. Depending on timing of retrospective studies, they may ask questions about food intake months prior to data collection, resulting in recall bias due to omissions or inaccurate recollections. These studies also rely on patients having sound knowledge of food ingredients and portion sizes, and they often assume that diets do not vary significantly during the study period. Questionnaires are limited by how specific the questions may be (e.g., "fatty fish" vs. the specific type of fish). Other interventional trials may exhibit bias or lack randomization. Even randomized controlled trials (RCTs)

can have difficulty with blinding participants, patient adherence to dietary recommendations, and other methodologic challenges.

Other difficulties stem from the distinct phenotypes seen in AD. Often the questions to diagnose a child with AD are very broad. For example, "Has your child ever been diagnosed with eczema?" and "Has your child ever had a dry, itchy skin rash?" likely include many patients without AD. Eczema is often used as a catch-all term for any dry, itchy skin or scaly rash among patients and health care professionals alike. Even among those who are accurately classified as AD patients, there is variation in timing of onset, severity, responsiveness to therapy, associated comorbidities, and persistence over time. It is nearly impossible to control for this variability in large-scale population-based or cohort studies, though some have identified distinct AD phenotypes (Hu et al., 2019).

Here we attempt to summarize the highest-quality evidence currently available regarding nutrition and AD. The chapter is divided in two sections: how diet may affect the risk of an individual developing AD, and how diet may affect patients who have already developed AD.

Diet and the risk of AD development

Intrapartum maternal diet

Western diets are typically high in proinflammatory omega-6 polyunsaturated fatty acid (PUFA) and low in antiinflammatory omega-3 PUFA. This may contribute to the higher incidence of AD in developed countries. One German study of over 2600 children found that maternal intake of margarine and vegetable oils (high in omega-6 PUFAs) in the last 4 weeks of pregnancy increased risk of eczema during the first 2 years of life, while high maternal fish intake (high in omega-3 PUFAs) decreased this risk (Sausenthaler et al., 2007). A systematic review examined eight observational studies and four RCTs evaluating maternal intake of omega-3 PUFAs and its relationship to eczema in offspring. Half of the observational studies and half of the RCTs showed a protective effect of high omega-3 PUFAs/ fish intake (Best, Gold, Kennedy, Martin, & Makrides, 2016). A meta-analysis of the RCTs examining patients with eczema and a positive skin prick test (SPT) of any type showed a statistically significant decreased relative risk of 0.53 with maternal omega-3 PUFA supplementation. This relationship disappeared when all cases of eczema were included (Best et al., 2016), suggesting this protection may only extend to specific AD phenotypes. A separate meta-analysis failed to show a relationship between omega-3 PUFA supplementation and AD (Garcia-Larsen et al., 2018). A pooled analysis of 10 studies examining maternal fish intake only (rather than omega-3 PUFAs) failed to show any relationship with AD risk (Zhang et al., 2017).

Maternal vitamin intake may also have some impact. Increased maternal β-carotene consumption may result in lower AD risk at 16 to 24 months (Miyake, Sasaki, Tanaka, & Hirota, 2010). One study found that higher maternal folate intake from vitamin supplements, but not dietary folate, was associated with increased AD risk. This was unrelated to maternal serum folate levels (Dunstan et al., 2012). Higher late pregnancy maternal nicotinamide levels were associated with decreased AD risk at 12 months of age, but not at 6 months (El-Heis et al., 2016). Though nicotinamide is derived from dietary intake of vitamin B_3 and tryptophan, it remains unclear what diet is appropriate to achieve higher maternal nicotinamide levels, as additional nutrients and chemicals are related to this metabolic pathway (El-Heis et al., 2016). There is no evidence that direct supplementation of vitamin B_3 or tryptophan in pregnancy decreases AD risk. A systematic review and meta-analysis showed inconclusive evidence for any effect of other maternal vitamins or zinc intake on infant AD risk (Beckhaus et al., 2015).

The effect of varying types of carbohydrate consumption remains unclear. The United Kingdom (UK)–based Avon Longitudinal Study of Parents and Children showed no relationship between eczema and maternal free/added sugar intake (Bédard, Northstone, Henderson, & Shaheen, 2017). A multivariable analysis of over 600 mother-infant pairs demonstrated increased rates of AD in high-risk infants (first-degree family member with allergic disease) at 12 months of age in those whose mothers consumed higher levels of resistant starch and fiber from green vegetables in late pregnancy (Pretorius, Bodinier, Prescott, & Palmer, 2019). Finally, while several studies have not shown any relationship to maternal fruit and vegetable intake and AD, one study showed decreased AD risk at 16 to 24 months with increasing maternal consumption of citrus fruits (Miyake et al., 2010).

Both, a systematic review of 11 interventional studies and a Cochrane review failed to show a benefit to maternal dietary restriction of common food allergens during pregnancy (Kramer & Kakuma, 2014; Netting, Middleton, & Makrides, 2014). Two separate studies showed no effect of maternal Mediterranean diet on preventing the development of AD in offspring (Castro-Rodriguez et al., 2016; Chatzi et al., 2013). One Japanese study of maternal intake of natto, a fermented soybean food, showed that AD risk at 6 months of age decreased with daily consumption (Ozawa et al., 2014).

Breastfeeding and infant formula

The early infant diet is made up exclusively of human breast milk and/or an infant formula, with introduction of solid foods at around 4 to 6 months of age. Breast milk has beneficial effects on a child's overall development and immune system, and may modulate risk of atopy later in life (Ballard & Morrow, 2013). The effect of breastfeeding on AD remains controversial. One meta-analysis of 42 studies showed some low-quality evidence of decreased AD risk under 2 years of age with exclusive breastfeeding for 3 to 4 months (Lodge et al., 2015). A more recent meta-analysis of 27 prospective cohort studies showed no definitive relationship between either exclusive breastfeeding or total breastfeeding (any amount, whether combined or exclusive) and AD risk (Lin, Dai, Lu, Fan, & Yu, 2019). Family history of atopy appeared to influence the effect of exclusive breastfeeding, with decreased AD risk in those with a family history of atopy, and increased risk in those without (Lin et al., 2019). Yet another study in a UK cohort of over 14,000 children showed that breastfeeding for 1 to 6 weeks or more than 6 months actually increased AD risk at 5 years of age (Taylor-Robinson, Williams, Pearce, Law, & Hope, 2016). Given conflicting reports and significant study heterogeneity, no recommendation can be made regarding breastfeeding as a preventive measure for AD at this time. A Cochrane review showed no benefit to maternal restriction of common food allergens while breastfeeding in reducing AD risk. The authors additionally point out that mothers on restricted diets gain less weight and may actually be putting themselves and their infants at risk of poor nutrition (Kramer & Kakuma, 2014).

Standard infant formula is cow's milk based. Hydrolyzed formulas are composed of cow's milk proteins casein and whey broken down to varying degrees. The German Infant Nutritional Intervention (GINI) study compared intervention and nonintervention arms (GINIplus) for high-risk infants. It showed significantly less AD up to 6 and possibly 10 years of age when using hydrolyzed formula in the first 4 to 6 months of life (both with and instead of breast milk) compared to cow's milk formula (von Berg et al., 2017). Another study of high-risk nonexclusively breastfed infants in Singapore demonstrated decreased AD with partially hydrolyzed formulas (Botteman et al., 2018).

However, a Cochrane review found no evidence for hydrolyzed formulas preventing AD, either in comparison to exclusive breastfeeding or cow's milk formulas (Osborn, Sinn, & Jones, 2018). A more recent birth cohort from France showed increased AD in high-risk infants who received partially hydrolyzed formula instead of nonhydrolyzed formula (Davisse-Paturet et al., 2019). Based on these more recent studies, the recommendation to give hydrolyzed formula to high-risk infants if exclusive breastfeeding is not possible may need to be reconsidered.

Other types of formulas include amino acid–based (also known as elemental formula) and soy formulas. Amino acid–based formulas are not recommended for patients with AD in the absence of a documented cow's milk protein allergy. Based on a Cochrane review, using soy formula instead of cow's milk formula is not recommended to prevent food allergy or AD in at-risk infants (Osborn & Sinn, 2006).

Dietary risk factors

There is concern that the Western diet (i.e., high in refined carbohydrates, saturated fat, and red meat, and low in fruits and vegetables) may increase AD risk (Flohr & Mann, 2014). Consumption of fast food three or more times per week was associated with an increased risk of severe eczema, whereas consumption of fresh fruits (once or twice per week for adolescents and three or more times per week for children) was protective against AD in an international study (Ellwood et al., 2013). AD is less prevalent in areas with higher consumption of fish, vegetables, and cereal- and nut-based protein (Ellwood et al., 2013). Rice, kimchi, and coffee decreased AD risk in Korean adults in another survey study of 17,497 participants, whereas AD risk increased with consumption of meats and processed foods such as instant noodles (Park, Choi, & Bae, 2016).

Incorporating fish into the diet with the introduction of solid food may decrease AD risk. Eating fish at least once weekly decreased the odds of developing eczema by 28% by the age of 6 years in a questionnaire-based study of 4264 mother-infant pairs (Øien, Schjelvaag, Storrø, Johnsen, & Simpson, 2019). A meta-analysis also showed decreased AD risk with fish intake during the first 12 months of life (Zhang et al., 2017).

Though dairy has been reported as a trigger food for AD (Nosrati et al., 2017), some evidence indicates that dairy products such as milk may actually be protective against AD. Consumption of milk and butter, as well as fresh fruit, pulses (beans, lentils, and peas), and rice three or more times per week decreased AD risk among 3209 children 6 to 7 years of age (Cepeda et al., 2015). In a cross-sectional survey of 6- and 7-year-olds in Spain, milk, butter, and nuts were associated with a decreased AD risk when consumed three or more times per week (Suárez-Varela et al., 2010).

Avoidance of gluten is a commonly employed dietary tactic to minimize AD risk that is lacking in evidence. Several dietary associations have been drawn regarding AD from food frequency questionnaires. As part of the Nurses' Health Study II (NHS-II), a prospective cohort study of women 25 to 42 years of age, 63,443 responses were analyzed for AD risk factors. Neither gluten intake nor a proinflammatory diet increased AD risk (Bridgman et al., 2019; Drucker, Qureshi, Thompson, Li, & Cho, 2019).

Diet and existing AD

Skin barrier and food sensitization

There is an intimate relationship between AD and food allergy. While food allergies are more common in patients with AD, a common misconception is that food allergy frequently causes or exacerbates AD. In fact, the so-called atopic march starts with eczema, with an estimated 30% of patients subsequently developing food allergies, and only rarely do food allergies exacerbate AD (Celakovská & Bukač, 2014). There has been a recent international shift in dietary recommendations for avoidance of food allergy. Previously, parents were advised to consider withholding highly allergenic foods (e.g., peanuts, eggs) during early life to prevent allergy in high-risk children. However, the Learning Early About Peanut Allergy (LEAP) study, which showed that early introduction of peanuts decreased incidence of peanut allergy, has shifted the focus toward early introduction of allergenic foods to promote tolerance in both high- and low-risk infants (Toit et al., 2015).

Mouse models were the first to show that removal of the stratum corneum followed by antigen exposure induces a Th2 inflammatory response and migration of sensitized Langerhans cell (Strid, Hourihane, Kimber, Callard, & Strobel, 2004). Additionally, in vitro human keratinocytes have shown increased epidermal permeability, decreased filaggrin expression, and improved integrity of the stratum corneum in the presence of histamine. These immune responses are important parts of the dual-allergen exposure hypothesis, which speculates that low-dose environmental exposure of a disrupted skin barrier to food allergens can lead to allergy (also known as transcutaneous sensitization), while high-dose exposure orally to those same allergens can induce tolerance (Lack, 2008). If the stratum corneum is damaged by trauma, such as with scratching induced by active AD, histamine can increase the risk of transcutaneous sensitization (Gutowska-Owsiak et al., 2014). Early-life environmental peanut exposure also has a higher risk of peanut allergy in patients with filaggrin mutations than those without, independent of AD (Brough et al., 2014).

The relative balance of cutaneous versus oral exposure may ultimately be what determines food allergy development. This hypothesis could explain why eczema developed before 6 months of age (when oral solid food intake may be more restricted) is associated with higher risk of food allergy than eczema developed after 6 months of age (Hill et al., 2008), and why patients with more severe AD and/or who apply peanut-containing topical products are more likely to develop peanut allergy (Lack, Fox, Northstone, Golding, & Avon Longitudinal Study of Parents and Children Study Team, 2003). The dual-allergen exposure hypothesis is changing the way that physicians approach food allergy, encouraging early oral exposure of potential culprit foods to promote tolerance. The way we approach AD treatment is also changing. Early and aggressive management of infantile AD with topical steroids and emollients to restore the skin barrier may have a lasting effect on patients and their ultimate development of food allergies.

Food allergy and sensitivity

Patients with AD are more likely to show sensitization to multiple foods (Giannetti et al., 2019). Both patients and physicians commonly perceive that diet affects severity of AD as well as frequency of flares. The study of food-triggered AD has produced a vast array of literature, and it remains a somewhat controversial topic. Note that just because a patient has both AD and food allergy does not mean that exposure to their allergen will impact their AD. The two conditions can and frequently do coexist independently.

Immediate allergic reactions are what patients generally consider as food allergies and are mediated by food-specific immunoglobulin E (IgE). These reactions typically occur within minutes to a few hours of food ingestion and may cause urticaria, gastrointestinal (GI) symptoms, wheezing, and, at their most severe, anaphylaxis. AD can be indirectly aggravated by these immediate reactions with pruritus and subsequent scratching. However, direct exacerbation of AD is likely the result of a delayed eczematous reaction. This is an eczema flare due to a delayed hypersensitivity mediated by T cells rather than IgE. These occur 6 to 48 hours after exposure. Patients may not have immediate reactions to the same food, making a history of food-specific exacerbation unreliable.

Systemic allergic contact dermatitis is a type of delayed hypersensitivity to specific allergens found in a variety of foods, rather than specific foods themselves. This can be difficult to diagnose, as it may be mistaken for or superimposed on AD. Common culprits include nickel (beans, lentils, whole wheat bread, canned products, shellfish) and balsam of Peru (citrus fruits, tomatoes, chocolate, colas, cinnamon, and vanilla) (Fabbro & Zirwas, 2014).

Food allergy testing

Food allergy testing in AD has unique challenges and high false-positive rates. The skin of AD patients is more reactive, and overall serum IgE levels can be elevated. For this reason antigen-specific IgE (sIgE) testing is preferred over radioallergosorbent testing (RAST) or SPT for diagnosing immediate allergic reactions, though all have relatively low positive predictive values in AD patients. SPT and sIgE are most helpful if they are negative, as these tests have a high negative predictive value in patients with AD and effectively exclude a food allergy (Sampson, 2003). In contrast, late reactions may be missed with IgE-specific testing alone, and even if this testing is positive, it has a low specificity for these types of reactions (Breuer, Heratizadeh et al., 2004). A meta-analysis examining atopy patch testing (APT) in the detection of food allergy in patients with AD found a pooled sensitivity of 53.6% and specificity of 88.6% (Luo, Zhang, & Li, 2019). Double-blind, placebo-controlled food challenges are considered the gold standard, but these are often expensive, time consuming, and may require medical intervention for the patient in the event of a severe reaction.

Egg

Hen's egg allergy accounts for up to 70% of food allergies in AD patients, and up to 40% of patients with egg allergy will have AD (Niggemann, Sielaff, Beyer, Binder, & Wahn, 1999; Samady et al., 2019). The two proteins typically responsible

for egg allergy are ovomucoid protein (most common, heat stable) and ovalbumin (heat labile), with the majority of egg allergens found in egg whites (Caubet & Wang, 2011). Approximately 85% of patients will have developed complete tolerance by preschool age (Doğruel, Bingöl, Yılmaz, & Altıntaş, 2016). The rate of reduction in egg white sIgE may predict which patients will achieve tolerance (Kim et al., 2019). Egg-sensitive children have more allergic disease, including higher rates of severe and persistent AD, as well as concomitant asthma and rhinoconjunctivitis (Ricci et al., 2006). In infants with a suspected egg allergy and positive egg sIgE, there is some evidence supporting an egg-free diet to improve AD (Bath-Hextall, Delamere, & Williams, 2008). Though commonly practiced, there is little evidence to support egg exclusion in AD patients without suspected or documented egg allergy.

Peanut

Peanut allergy is found in 6.6% of all patients with infantile AD (Spergel et al., 2015). Persistence of AD correlates with presence of peanut allergy, and though tolerance with age has been reported, it is uncommon and does not occur in patients with severe food allergy symptoms at onset (Gray, Levin, & Du Toit, 2019; Horwitz, Hossain, & Yousef, 2009). Introducing peanuts early to children with AD and/or egg allergy decreases development of peanut allergy (Toit et al., 2015). US guidelines recommend introduction of peanuts at 6 months of age for patients with mild to moderate AD, and consideration of preexposure testing in addition to early introduction for those with severe AD (Greenhawt, 2017). Since refined peanut oils remove and/or denature the allergenic proteins, they are generally safe for use in patients allergic to peanuts (Paller et al., 2003).

Cow's milk

Cow's milk allergy is common in children with AD and may account for up to half of food allergies in this population (Niggemann et al., 1999). Allergy to cow's milk can cause both early and late skin reactions and may affect the skin alone without involvement of the GI tract (Breuer, Heratizadeh et al., 2004; Niggemann et al., 1999). Reactions in children with AD allergic to cow's milk are more likely to involve urticaria than those without (Giannetti et al., 2019). Cow's milk allergy is often outgrown by late childhood, and presence or absence of AD does not impact timing or likelihood of achieving tolerance (Giannetti et al., 2019). There is very little evidence regarding other nonhuman sources of milk in cow's milk–allergic children with AD.

Wheat and gluten

Wheat allergy usually develops in infancy and can be associated with gluten as well as other various allergenic proteins. Wheat can cause both immediate and delayed reactions in AD patients (Breuer, Heratizadeh et al., 2004; Niggemann et al., 1999). Both types of reactions often occur without other systemic symptoms such as vomiting, diarrhea, rhinitis, or stridor (Niggemann et al., 1999) and are considered a separate entity from celiac disease or nonceliac gluten sensitivity (Elli et al., 2015). Children with wheat allergy often become tolerant by 3 to 5 years of age. A study of AD patients 14 years of age or older showed that AD was exacerbated by wheat in about 5% of patients and improves with an elimination diet (Celakovská, Ettlerová, Ettler, Vanecková, & Bukac, 2011). In wheat-allergic AD patients, IgE antibodies to gliadin are typically seen in SPTs, RAST, and immunoblotting (Varjonen, Vainio, & Kalimo., 2000), though as mentioned previously these are not the tests of choice for diagnosing food allergy in patients with AD.

Soy

Soy protein, derived from soybeans, is a popular nonmeat protein substitute found in many processed foods. Soy allergy in children with AD usually causes late or eczematous reactions, although rarely immediate reactions can be seen (Breuer, Heratizadeh et al., 2004; Niggemann et al., 1999). About 27% of AD patients may be sensitized to soy without any clinical relevance (Celakovská, Ettlerová, Ettler, Vaněčková, & Bukač, 2014). Tolerance typically develops by adolescence. However, older patients can develop a "late" soy allergy that may be associated with birch pollen or peanut allergy (Savage, Kaeding, Matsui, & Wood, 2010).

Birch pollen–related foods

As part of the atopic march, allergic rhinoconjunctivitis often occurs in patients with AD. Allergy to birch pollen can result in oral allergy syndrome and late eczematous reactions due to cross-reactivity of birch pollen sIgE with proteins in a variety of fruits and vegetables, including celery, carrots, hazelnut, apples, and kiwi. This phenomenon plays an important role in areas where birch trees are native, including North America and Northern and Central Europe. Foods that were previously tolerated can suddenly lead to both immediate and late reactions in AD patients of all ages once sensitized to birch pollen (Breuer, Wulf et al., 2004; Wassmann-Otto, Heratizadeh, Wichmann, & Werfel, 2018).

Elimination diets and other dietary interventions

Several other types of diets have been explored in AD. Elemental diets with an amino acid–based formula for 6 weeks were not beneficial for children under 3 years of age (Leung et al., 2004). Elimination diets in which patients only consumed five to eight different foods in addition to whey or casein protein supplementation are not effective, and adherence to these strict diets is quite poor (Mabin, Sykes, & David., 1995).

In one survey of 169 adult AD patients, 87% had tried eliminating specific foods from their diet (Nosrati et al., 2017). Multiple foods were reported to improve or exacerbate AD, both by their intake and by their elimination (Nosrati et al., 2017) (Table 8.1). Evidence does not support elimination diets in the management of AD, and in fact, strict elimination diets may increase the risk for nutrient deficiencies and obtunded growth and development

TABLE 8.1	Patient-reported Exacerbating and alleviating foods in 169 patients with AD
Food	**%**
Exacerbating foods	
Dairy	24.8
Gluten	18.3
Alcohol	17.1
Sugar	16.5
Tomato	13.0
Citrus	10.0
Eggs	7.1
Meat, soda, spicy foods, processed foods, seafood	<5.0
Improved when removed	
White flour products	53.6
Gluten	51.4
Nightshades	51.4
Junk foods	51
Alcohol	50.8
Dairy	50.7
High fat foods	43.6
Tobacco	40.4
Shellfish	36.8
Caffeine	33.3
Pork	32.2
Red meat	24.1
Sodium/salt	23.2
Alleviating foods	
Dietary supplements[a]	25.4
Water	14.2
Vegetables	11.8
Oils[b]	9.5
Fruits	6.5
Fish	1.7
Improved when added	
Vegetables	47.6
Organic foods	39.5
Fish oil/omega-3	35.0
Fruits	34.6
Vitamin D	34.4
Probiotics	28.7

[a]Probiotics, vitamin D, vitamin C, zinc, or omega-3.
[b]Primrose, hempseed, cod liver, and coconut oils.
Adapted from Nosrati, A., Afifi, L., Danesh, M. J., Lee, K., Yan, D., Beroukhim, K., et al. (2017). Dietary modifications in atopic dermatitis: Patient-reported outcomes. *Journal of Dermatological Treatment*, 28(6), 523–538. https://doi.org/10.1080/09546634.2016.1278071.

(Finch, Munhutu, & Whitaker-Worth, 2010). Malnutrition can also retard skin barrier repair. Removal of specific foods based only on testing may also be harmful. In one study, 13% of those who eliminate foods they previously ate without reaction based on positive SPTs or sIgE levels subsequently developed intolerance and failed an oral food challenge (Eapen, Kloepfer, Leickly, Slaven, & Vitalpur, 2019). Intolerance developed as early as 3 months after food elimination (Eapen et al., 2019). When special diets are attempted, duration should be limited to 4 to 8 weeks to evaluate the effect of dietary interventions before resuming a normal diet (Finch et al., 2010).

Micronutrients

In addition to major food items, micronutrients may also play a role in AD. In the following paragraphs, the relationship between AD and several vitamins, minerals, and trace elements is discussed. Micronutrient studies have several unique challenges. Serum levels of micronutrients are often unreliable and may not accurately reflect nutrient intake. Micronutrients are rarely ingested in isolation, and micronutrient absorption can be influenced by other micronutrients (e.g., absorption of calcium is enhanced by vitamin D but inhibited by iron). Bioavailability of synthetic supplements can differ from naturally occurring nutrients found in food, and these different forms can have different impacts in the body. The combination of these effects makes it difficult to identify the effect of specific nutrients.

Vitamin C

Vitamin C is a water-soluble vitamin commonly found in fruits and vegetables with conflicting evidence in AD. It acts as an antioxidant by reducing toxic substances that can damage cells and is required for many biochemical reactions in the body, including synthesis of collagen (Gottschlich et al., n.d.). Oxidative stress plays an important role in the pathogenesis of AD (Ji & Li, 2016), and body tissue can succumb to oxidative stress with vitamin C deficiency (Mahan, Escott-Stump, Raymond, & Krause, 2012). One study showed higher dietary vitamin C intake correlated with increased AD risk (Laitinen, Kalliomäki, Poussa, Lagström, & Isolauri, 2005), while two other studies showed that AD patients had inadequate vitamin C intake (Kim, Sim, Park, Kim, & Choi, 2016; Yang, Kim, & Lee, 2016). Yet another study showed no relationship between AD and dietary or plasma vitamin C (Oh, Chung, Kim, Kwon, & Cho, 2010).

Vitamin D

Vitamin D is a fat-soluble vitamin involved in calcium homeostasis. It requires synthesis from cholecalciferol to the active form of calcitriol. Thought to play a role in modulating the immune system (Mutgi & Koo, 2013), vitamin D is commonly referred to as the "sunshine vitamin" because sun exposure triggers cholecalciferol production in the skin (Mahan et al., 2012). Dietary sources include cod liver oil, salmon, mackerel, tuna, fortified dairy products, and fortified orange juice (Mahan et al., 2012). Though optimal vitamin D levels are heavily debated, a 25-hydroxyvitamin D level of 40 to 60 ng/mL is recommended as it is associated with a 15% reduction in all-cause mortality (Grant, 2009). Levels up to 100 ng/mL can be considered safe (Holick, 2017). Toxicity is extremely rare and can only be induced by supplementation, not sun exposure (Holick, 2017).

Vitamin D deficiency is often seen in AD patients (Cheng et al., 2014; Yang et al., 2016). Low vitamin D is associated with increased AD severity in children (Wang et al., 2014). Additionally, low levels of vitamin D (<30 ng/mL) are correlated with increased risk of bacterial skin infections in AD (Samochocki et al., 2013). Several studies suggest that vitamin D supplementation may decrease severity and alleviate symptoms of AD. A recent meta-analysis of vitamin D supplementation trials concluded that supplementation with 1600 IU/day of cholecalciferol may lead to a clinically significant reduction in AD severity (Hattangdi-Haridas, Lanham-New, Wong, Ho, & Darling, 2019).

Vitamin E

Vitamin E is a fat-soluble vitamin with antioxidant properties commonly found in nuts and oils (Mahan et al., 2012). In one study of 65 patients, those who received vitamin E supplementation of 400 IU/day for 4 months had improved pruritus, lesion severity, and SCORAD index with no side effects (Jaffary, Faghihi, Mokhtarian, & Hosseini, 2015). Vitamin E supplementation has been associated with decreased IgE levels in AD patients (Tsoureli-Nikita, Hercogova, Lotti, & Menchini, 2002), and dietary intake of vitamin E may play a role in protecting against AD (Oh et al., 2010).

Zinc

Zinc, a mineral abundantly found in red meat and poultry, is an important component of many enzymatic reactions essential for nutrient metabolism (Mahan et al., 2012). In one study of 101 patients, zinc levels in AD were lower than controls, and 8 weeks of zinc supplementation led to improvement in eczema assessment severity index (EASI) scores, transepidermal water loss (TEWL), pruritus, and sleep (Kim, Yoo, Jeong, Ko, & Ro, 2014). The authors recommend 10 to 20 mg/day of zinc supplementation until normal levels are restored, followed by age-based maintenance dosing of 3 to 5 mg/day for ages 1 to 8 years, 8 mg/day for ages 9 to 14 years, and 9 to 10 mg/day for ages 15 years and older (Kim et al., 2014). Caution should be exercised with supplementation as zinc can impair copper absorption, causing copper deficiency. Copper should be supplemented with a zinc to copper ratio of 10:1 (Vaughn, Foolad, Maarouf, Tran, & Shi, 2019).

Other vitamins, minerals, and trace elements

Other micronutrients may play a role in AD. In a 12-month study of nicotinamide 500 mg twice daily compared to placebo, TEWL decreased by 6% to 7% (Chen, Martin, Dalziell, Halliday, & Damian, 2016). No direct studies have examined the relationship between nicotinamide and AD. Though iron plays a vital role in oxidation-reduction reactions, free radicals generated in iron metabolism can increase oxidative stress and cause tissue damage. A small study showed that those with AD had higher levels of iron in the dermis compared to controls but normal serum iron levels (Leveque et al., 2003). Another study with 162 participants found no difference in serum iron levels between AD patients and controls, and serum iron levels were not correlated with AD severity (Toyran et al., 2012).

Several studies have investigated the relationship between AD and selenium, a trace element with antioxidant properties. Similar levels of urinary selenium were seen in 27 children with AD when compared to 25 healthy controls (Omata et al., 2001). In a group of 60 adults with AD, supplementation with 600 mcg of selenium for 12 weeks did not improve AD severity (Fairris et al., 1989).

Summary

There is an intimate relationship between AD and nutrition. Both maternal and personal diet can influence the risk of developing AD. While no strong recommendations can be made, it appears that increased omega-3 PUFAs during pregnancy and fish during early life may decrease risk of AD. Fermented and fresh foods may protect against AD, while fast foods and processed foods may increase risk. Empirically avoiding highly allergenic foods, whether during pregnancy, breastfeeding, or infancy, does not reduce the risk of developing AD. Uncontrolled AD increases risk for developing food allergy, likely via the dual-allergen exposure hypothesis. Food allergies can in turn exacerbate AD through immediate or late reactions, though infrequently. Elimination diets can be dangerous to patients and do not improve AD. Vitamin D supplementation may improve AD in some patients. Summary tables of nutrition-related recommendations with associated levels of evidence from each section are described in Tables 8.2 and 8.3.

The relationship between AD and nutrition continues to have its controversies, including the role of breastfeeding, hydrolyzed formulas, and additional micronutrients. While

TABLE 8.2	Summary and level of evidence for nutrition recommendations in risk of atopic dermatitis (AD)	
Food type	Recommendations	Level of evidence
Omega-3 PUFAs/ fish oil	Increased maternal intake may protect against AD in offspring.	B
β-Carotene	Increased maternal intake may protect against AD in offspring.	B
Folate	Increased maternal intake of folate from vitamin supplements may increase risk of AD in offspring. No effect of dietary folate intake.	B
Zinc	No relationship between maternal intake and risk of AD in offspring.	B, C
Carbohydrates	Conflicting evidence regarding relationship between maternal intake and risk of AD in offspring, no recommendations can be made.	B
Breastfeeding	Conflicting evidence regarding relationship between maternal intake and risk of AD in offspring, no recommendations can be made.	B
Restrictive diets	No decreased risk of AD in offspring, maternal restrictive diets should be avoided.	B
Formula	Conflicting evidence regarding hydrolyzed formulas vs. breastfeeding vs. cow's milk formula and risk of AD. No recommendations can be made, unless a documented cow's milk allergy exists in which case avoidance of cow's milk formula is recommended. Soy formula does not decrease risk of AD.	B
Western diet	Increased consumption of refined carbohydrates, saturated fats, red meat, and other processed/fast foods may increase AD risk. Increased consumption of fresh or citrus fruits may protect against AD.	C
Fish	Increased fish consumption in early childhood at least once weekly may decrease AD risk.	B, C
Dairy	Increased dairy consumption in childhood may decrease AD risk.	C
Gluten	No relationship between dietary intake and risk of AD.	C

PUFAs, Polyunsaturated fatty acids.

| TABLE 8.3 | Summary and level of evidence for nutrition recommendations in existing atopic dermatitis (AD) |

Food type	Recommendations	Level of evidence
Solid foods	Recommend early oral exposure of potentially allergenic foods to promote tolerance. Early and aggressive management to repair skin barrier disruption in AD may decrease development of food allergy.	B, C
Egg	Elimination of egg in patients with suspected egg allergy and specific IgE to egg may improve AD.	B
Peanut	Early introduction of peanuts to patients with AD and/or egg allergy decreases development of peanut allergy.	A
Cow's milk	Cow's milk allergy may exacerbate AD in some patients.	B
Wheat/gluten	Wheat and gluten may exacerbate AD in about 5% of teenage AD patients.	B
Soy	Soy may cause delayed eczematous reactions in some AD patients.	B
Birch pollen–related foods	Patients with AD and allergic rhinoconjunctivitis to birch pollen may experience delayed eczematous reactions with consumption of foods related to birch pollen (e.g., carrots, celery, kiwi).	C
Elimination/restrictive diet	Elimination diets are not recommended in AD, as they may increase the risk of developing food intolerance and malnutrition.	B
Vitamin C	Conflicting evidence, no recommendations can be made.	B, C
Vitamin D	Supplementation with 1600 IU daily of cholecalciferol may decrease severity of AD.	A, B
Vitamin E	Vitamin E supplementation may decrease severity of AD.	A
Zinc	Zinc supplementation may decrease severity of AD.	B
Selenium	No effect of selenium supplementation on severity of AD.	A

well-designed studies are difficult to perform, there are numerous questions that require additional investigation.

Further readings

Bergmann, M. M., Caubet, J.-C., Boguniewicz, M., & Eigenmann, P. A. (2013). Evaluation of food allergy in patients with atopic dermatitis. *The Journal of Allergy and Clinical Immunology: In Practice, 1*(1), 22–28. https://doi.org/10.1016/j.jaip.2012.11.005.

Robison, R. G., & Singh, A. M. (2019). Controversies in allergy: Food testing and dietary avoidance in atopic dermatitis. *The Journal of Allergy and Clinical Immunology: In Practice, 7*(1), 35–39. https://doi.org/10.1016/j.jaip.2018.11.006.

Tham, E. H., Rajakulendran, M., Lee, B. W., & Van Bever, H. P. S. (2020). Epicutaneous sensitization to food allergens in atopic dermatitis: What do we know? *Pediatric Allergy and Immunology, 31*(1), 7–18. https://doi.org/10.1111/pai.13127.

Vaughn, A. R., Foolad, N., Maarouf, M., Tran, K. A., & Shi, V. Y. (2019). Micronutrients in atopic dermatitis: A systematic review. *The Journal of Alternative and Complementary Medicine, 25*(6), 567–577. https://doi.org/10.1089/acm.2018.0363.

References

Ballard, O., & Morrow, A. L. (2013). Human milk composition: Nutrients and bioactive factors. *Pediatric Clinics of North America, 60*(1), 49–74. https://doi.org/10.1016/j.pcl.2012.10.002.

Bath-Hextall, F. J., Delamere, F. M., & Williams, H. C. (2008). Dietary exclusions for established atopic eczema. *Cochrane Database of Systematic Reviews, 23*(1), CD005203. https://doi.org/10.1002/14651858.cd005203.pub2.

Beckhaus, A. A., Garcia-Marcos, L., Forno, E., Pacheco-Gonzalez, R. M., Celedón, J. C., & Castro-Rodriguez, J. A. (2015). Maternal nutrition during pregnancy and risk of asthma, wheeze, and atopic diseases during childhood: A systematic review and meta-analysis. *Allergy, 70*(12), 1588–1604. https://doi.org/10.1111/all.12729.

Bédard, A., Northstone, K., Henderson, A. J., & Shaheen, S. O. (2017). Maternal intake of sugar during pregnancy and childhood respiratory and atopic outcomes. *The European Respiratory Journal, 50*(1), 1700073. https://doi.org/10.1183/13993003.00073-2017.

von Berg, A., Filipiak-Pittroff, B., Krämer, U., Link, E., Heinrich, J., Koletzko, et al. (2017). The german infant nutritional intervention study (gini) for the preventive effect of hydrolyzed infant formulas in infants at high risk for allergic diseases. Design and selected results. *Allergologie Select, 1*(1), 28–38. https://doi.org/10.5414/ALX01462E.

Best, K. P., Gold, M., Kennedy, D., Martin, J., & Makrides, M. (2016). Omega-3 long-chain PUFA intake during pregnancy and allergic disease outcomes in the offspring: A systematic review and meta-analysis of observational studies and randomized controlled trials. *The American Journal of Clinical Nutrition, 103*(1), 128–143. https://doi.org/10.3945/ajcn.115.111104.

Botteman, M. F., Bhanegaonkar, A. J., Horodniceanu, E. G., Ji, X., Lee, B. W., Shek, L. P., et al. (2018). Economic value of using partially hydrolysed infant formula for risk reduction of atopic dermatitis in high-risk, not exclusively breastfed infants in singapore. *Singapore Medical Journal*, 59(8), 439–448. https://doi.org/10.11622/smedj.2017113.

Breuer, K., Heratizadeh, A., Wulf, A., Baumann, U., Constien, A., Tetau, D., et al. (2004). Late eczematous reactions to food in children with atopic dermatitis. *Clinical and Experimental Allergy: Journal of the British Society for Allergy and Clinical Immunology*, 34(5), 817–824. https://doi.org/10.1111/j.1365-2222.2004.1953.x.

Breuer, K., Wulf, A., Constien, A., Tetau, D., Kapp, A., & Werfel, T. (2004). Birch pollen-related food as a provocation factor of allergic symptoms in children with atopic eczema/dermatitis syndrome. *Allergy*, 59(9), 988–994. https://doi.org/10.1111/j.1398-9995.2004.00493.x.

Bridgman, A. C., Qureshi, A. A., Li, T., Tabung, F. K., Cho, E., & Drucker, A. M. (2019). Inflammatory dietary pattern and incident psoriasis, psoriatic arthritis, and atopic dermatitis in women: A cohort study. *Journal of the American Academy of Dermatology*, 80(6), 1682–1690. https://doi.org/10.1016/j.jaad.2019.02.038.

Brough, H. A., Simpson, A., Makinson, K., Hankinson, J., Brown, S., Douiri, A., et al. (2014). Peanut allergy: Effect of environmental peanut exposure in children with filaggrin loss-of-function mutations. *The Journal of Allergy and Clinical Immunology*, 134(4), 867–875.e1. https://doi.org/10.1016/j.jaci.2014.08.011

Castro-Rodriguez, J. A., Ramirez-Hernandez, M., Padilla, O., Pacheco-Gonzalez, R. M., Pérez-Fernández, V., & Garcia-Marcos, L. (2016). Effect of foods and mediterranean diet during pregnancy and first years of life on wheezing, rhinitis and dermatitis in preschoolers. *Allergologia Et Immunopathologia*, 44(5), 400–409. https://doi.org/10.1016/j.aller.2015.12.002.

Caubet, J. C., & Wang, J. (2011). Current understanding of egg allergy. *Pediatric Clinics of North America*, 58(2), 427–443, xi. https://doi.org/10.1016/j.pcl.2011.02.014.

Celakovská, J., & Bukač, J. (2014). Analysis of food allergy in atopic dermatitis patients - association with concomitant allergic diseases. *Indian Journal of Dermatology*, 59(5), 445–450. https://doi.org/10.4103/0019-5154.139867.

Celakovská, J., Ettlerová, K., Ettler, K., Vanecková, J., & Bukac, J. (2011). The effect of wheat allergy on the course of atopic eczema in patients over 14 years of age. *Acta Medica (Hradec Kralove)*, 54(4), 157–162.

Celakovská, J., Ettlerová, K., Ettler, K., Vaněčková, J., & Bukač, J. (2014). Food hypersensitivity in patients suffering from atopic dermatitis and sensitization to soy. *Indian Journal of Dermatology*, 59(1), 106. https://doi.org/10.4103/0019-5154.123545.

Cepeda, A. M., Del Giacco, S. R., Villalba, S., Tapias, E., Jaller, R., Segura, A. M., et al. (2015). Garcia-Larsen, A traditional diet is associated with a reduced risk of eczema and wheeze in Colombian children. *Nutrients*, 7(7), 5098–5110. https://doi.org/10.3390/nu7075098.

Chatzi, L., Garcia, R., Roumeliotaki, T., Basterrechea, M., Begiristain, H., Iñiguez, C., et al. (2013). Mediterranean diet adherence during pregnancy and risk of wheeze and eczema in the first year of life: INMA (Spain) and RHEA (Greece) mother-child cohort studies. *The British Journal of Nutrition*, 110(11), 2058–2068. https://doi.org/10.1017/S0007114513001426.

Chen, A. C., Martin, A. J., Dalziell, R. A., Halliday, G. M., & Damian, D. L. (2016). Oral nicotinamide reduces transepidermal water loss: A randomized controlled trial. *The British Journal of Dermatology*, 175(6), 1363–1365. https://doi.org/10.1111/bjd.14648.

Cheng, H. M., Kim, S., Park, G. H., Chang, S. E., Bang, S., Won, C. H., et al. (2014). Low vitamin D levels are associated with atopic dermatitis, but not allergic rhinitis, asthma, or IgE sensitization,

in the adult Korean population. *Journal of Allergy and Clinical Immunology*, 133(4), 1048–1055. https://doi.org/10.1016/j.jaci.2013.10.055.

Davisse-Paturet, C., Raherison, C., Adel-Patient, K., Divaret-Chauveau, A., Bois, C., Dufourg, M. N., et al. (2019). Use of partially hydrolysed formula in infancy and incidence of eczema, respiratory symptoms or food allergies in toddlers from the ELFE cohort. *Pediatric Allergy and Immunology*, 30(6), 614–623. https://doi.org/10.1111/pai.13094.

Doğruel, D., Bingöl, G. ülbin, Yılmaz, M., & Altıntaş, D. U. (2016). The ADAPAR birth cohort study: Food allergy results at five years and new insights. *International Archives of Allergy and Immunology*, 169(1), 57–61. https://doi.org/10.1159/000443831.

Drucker, A. M., Qureshi, A. A., Thompson, J. M., Li, T., & Cho, E. (2020). Gluten intake and risk of psoriasis, psoriatic arthritis and atopic dermatitis among US women. *Journal of the American Academy of Dermatology*, 82(3), 661–665. https://doi.org/10.1016/j.jaad.2019.08.007.

Dunstan, J. A., West, C., McCarthy, S., Metcalfe, J., Meldrum, S., Oddy, W. H., et al. (2012). The relationship between maternal folate status in pregnancy, cord blood folate levels, and allergic outcomes in early childhood. *Allergy*, 67(1), 50–57. https://doi.org/10.1111/j.1398-9995.2011.02714.x.

Eapen, A. A., Kloepfer, K. M., Leickly, F. E., Slaven, J. E., & Vitalpur, G. (2019). Oral food challenge failures among foods restricted because of atopic dermatitis. *Annals of Allergy, Asthma & Immunology*, 122(2), 193–197. https://doi.org/10.1016/j.anai.2018.10.012.

El-Heis, S., Crozier, S. R., Robinson, S. M., Harvey, N. C., Cooper, C., Inskip, H. M., & Godfrey, K. M. (2016). Higher maternal serum concentrations of nicotinamide and related metabolites in late pregnancy are associated with a lower risk of offspring atopic eczema at age 12 months. *Clinical and Experimental Allergy: Journal of the British Society for Allergy and Clinical Immunology*, 46(10), 1337–1343. https://doi.org/10.1111/cea.12782.

Elli, L., Branchi, F., Tomba, C., Villalta, D., Norsa, L., Ferretti, F., et al. (2015). Diagnosis of gluten related disorders: Celiac disease, wheat allergy and non-celiac gluten sensitivity. *World Journal of Gastroenterology*, 21(23), 7110–7119. https://doi.org/10.3748/wjg.v21.i23.7110.

Ellwood, P., Asher, M. I., García-Marcos, L., Williams, H., Keil, U., Robertson, C. et al. (2013). Do Fast Foods Cause Asthma, Rhinoconjunctivitis and Eczema? Global findings from the International Study of Asthma and Allergies in Childhood (ISAAC) Phase Three. *Thorax*, 68(4), 351–360. https://doi.org/10.1136/thoraxjnl-2012-202285.

Fabbro, S. K., & Zirwas, M. J. (2014). Systemic contact dermatitis to foods: Nickel, BOP, and more. *Current Allergy and Asthma Reports*, 14(10), 463. https://doi.org/10.1007/s11882-014-0463-3.

Fairris, G. M., Perkins, P. J., Lloyd, B., Hinks, L., & Clayton, B. E. (1989). The Effect on Atopic Dermatitis of Supplementation with Selenium and Vitamin E. *Acta Dermato-Venereologica*, 69(4), 359–362.

Finch, J., Munhutu, M. N., & Whitaker-Worth, D. L. (2010). Atopic dermatitis and nutrition. *Clinics in Dermatology*, 28(6), 605–614. https://doi.org/10.1016/j.clindermatol.2010.03.032.

Flohr, C., & Mann, J. (2014). New insights into the epidemiology of childhood atopic dermatitis. *Allergy*, 69(1), 3–16. https://doi.org/10.1111/all.12270.

Garcia-Larsen, V., Ierodiakonou, D., Jarrold, K., Cunha, S., Chivinge, J., Robinson, Z., et al. (2018). Diet during pregnancy and infancy and risk of allergic or autoimmune disease: A systematic review and meta-analysis. *PLoS Medicine*, 15(2). https://doi.org/10.1371/journal.pmed.1002507.

Giannetti, A., Cipriani, F., Indio, V., Gallucci, M., Caffarelli, C., & Ricci, G. (2019). Influence of atopic dermatitis on cow's milk allergy in children. *Medicina*, *55*(8), 460. https://doi.org/10.3390/medicina55080460.

Gottschlich, M. M., DeLegge, M. H., Mattox, T., Mueller, C., Worthington, P. and Guenter, P. n.d. "The A.S.P.E.N. NUTRITION SUPPORT CORE CURRICULUM," American Society for Parenteral and Enteral Nutrition, 848.

Grant, W. B. (2009). Critique of the U-shaped serum 25-hydroxyvitamin D level-disease response relation. *Dermato-Endocrinology*, *1*(6), 289–293. https://doi.org/10.4161/derm.1.6.11359.

Gray, C. L., Levin, M. E., & Du Toit, G. (2019). Acquisition of tolerance to egg and peanut in African food-allergic children with atopic dermatitis. *South African Medical Journal*, *109*(5), 323. https://doi.org/10.7196/SAMJ.2019.v109i5.13339.

Greenhawt, M. (2017). The national institutes of allergy and infectious diseases sponsored guidelines on preventing peanut allergy: A new paradigm in food allergy prevention. *Allergy and Asthma Proceedings*, *38*(2), 92–97. https://doi.org/10.2500/aap.2017.38.4037.

Gutowska-Owsiak, D., Salimi, M., Selvakumar, T. A., Wang, X., Taylor, S., & Ogg, G. S. (2014). Histamine exerts multiple effects on expression of genes associated with epidermal barrier function. *Journal of Investigational Allergology & Clinical Immunology*, *24*(4), 231–239.

Hattangdi-Haridas, S. R., Lanham-New, S. A., Wong, Wilfred H. S., Ho, Marco H. K., & Darling, A. L. (2019). Vitamin D deficiency and effects of vitamin D supplementation on disease severity in patients with atopic dermatitis: A systematic review and meta-analysis in adults and children. *Nutrients*, *11*(8), 1854. https://doi.org/10.3390/nu11081854.

Hill, D. J., Hosking, C. S., de Benedictis, F. M., Oranje, A. P., Diepgen, T. L., Bauchau, V., & EPAAC Study Group, (2008). Confirmation of the association between high levels of immunoglobulin E food sensitization and eczema in infancy: An international study. *Clinical and Experimental Allergy: Journal of the British Society for Allergy and Clinical Immunology*, *38*(1), 161–168. https://doi.org/10.1111/j.1365-2222.2007.02861.x.

Holick, M. F. (2017). The vitamin D deficiency pandemic: Approaches for diagnosis, treatment and prevention. *Reviews in Endocrine and Metabolic Disorders*, *18*(2), 153–165. https://doi.org/10.1007/s11154-017-9424-1.

Horwitz, A. A., Hossain, J., & Yousef, E. (2009). Correlates of outcome for atopic dermatitis. *Annals of Allergy, Asthma & Immunology: Official Publication of the American College of Allergy, Asthma, & Immunology*, *103*(2), 146–151. https://doi.org/10.1016/S1081-1206(10)60168-8.

Hu, C., Duijts, L., Erler, N. S., Elbert, N. J., Piketty, C., Bourdès, V., Blanchet-Réthoré, S., et al. (2019). Most associations of Early-life environmental exposures and genetic risk factors poorly differentiate between eczema phenotypes: The generation R study. *British Journal of Dermatology*, *181*(6), 1190–1197. https://doi.org/10.1111/bjd.17879.

Jaffary, F., Faghihi, G., Mokhtarian, A., & Hosseini, S. M. (2015). Effects of oral vitamin E on treatment of atopic dermatitis: A randomized controlled trial. *Journal of Research in Medical Sciences*, *20*(11), 1053. https://doi.org/10.4103/1735-1995.172815.

Ji, H., & Li, X. K. (2016). Oxidative stress in atopic dermatitis. *Oxidative Medicine and Cellular Longevity*, *2016*, 1–8. https://doi.org/10.1155/2016/2721469.

Kim, J. D., Kim, S. Y., Kwak, E. J., Sol, In. S., Kim, M. J., Kim, Y. H., et al. (2019). Reduction rate of specific IgE level as a predictor of persistent egg allergy in children. *Allergy, Asthma & Immunology Research*, *11*(4), 498–507. https://doi.org/10.4168/aair.2019.11.4.498.

Kim, So. Y., Sim, S., Park, B., Kim, J. H., & Choi, H. G. (2016). High-fat and low-carbohydrate diets are associated with allergic rhinitis but not asthma or atopic dermatitis in children. *PLoS One*, *11*(2). https://doi.org/10.1371/journal.pone.0150202.

Kim, J. E., Yoo, S. R., Jeong, M. G., Ko, J. Y., & Ro, Y. S. (2014). Hair zinc levels and the efficacy of oral zinc supplementation in patients with atopic dermatitis. *Acta Dermato-Venereologica*, *94*(5), 558–562. https://doi.org/10.2340/00015555-1772.

Kramer, M. S., & Kakuma, R. (2014). Maternal dietary antigen avoidance during pregnancy or lactation, or both, for preventing or treating atopic disease in the child: Maternal dietary antigen avoidance during pregnancy or lactation, or both, for preventing or treating atopic disease in the child. *Evidence-Based Child Health: A Cochrane Review Journal*, *9*(2), 447–483. https://doi.org/10.1002/ebch.1972.

Lack. G. (2008). Epidemiologic risks for food allergy. *The Journal of Allergy and Clinical Immunology*, *121*(6), 1331–1336. https://doi.org/10.1016/j.jaci.2008.04.032.

Lack, G., Fox, D., Northstone, K., Golding, J., & Avon longitudinal study of parents and children study team, (2003). Factors associated with the development of peanut allergy in childhood. *The New England Journal of Medicine*, *348*(11), 977–985. https://doi.org/10.1056/NEJMoa013536.

Laitinen, K., Kalliomäki, M., Poussa, T., Lagström, H., & Isolauri, E. (2005). Evaluation of diet and growth in children with and without atopic eczema: Follow-up study from birth to 4 years. *British Journal of Nutrition*, *94*(4), 565–574. https://doi.org/10.1079/BJN20051503.

Leung, T. F., Ma, K. C., Cheung, L. T. F., Lam, C. W. K., Wong, E., Wan, H., & Hon, E. K. L. (2004). A randomized, single-blind and crossover study of an amino acid-based milk formula in treating young children with atopic dermatitis. *Pediatric Allergy and Immunology*, *15*(6), 558–561. https://doi.org/10.1111/j.1399-3038.2004.00197.x.

Leveque, N., Robin, S., Muret, P., Mac-Mary, S., Makki, S., & Humber, P. (2003). High iron and low ascorbic acid concentrations in the dermis of atopic dermatitis patients. Dermatology (Basel, Switzerland) *207*(3): 261–264. https://doi.org/10.1159/000073087.

Lin, B., Dai, Ru, Lu, L., Fan, X., & Yu, Y. (2020). Breastfeeding and atopic dermatitis risk: A systematic review and meta-analysis of prospective cohort studies. *Dermatology (Basel, Switzerland)*, 236, 345–360. https://doi.org/10.1159/000503781.

Lodge, C. J., Tan, D. J., Lau, M. X. Z., Dai, X., Tham, R., Lowe, A. J., et al. (2015). Breastfeeding and asthma and allergies: A systematic review and meta-analysis. *Acta Paediatrica (Oslo, Norway: 1992)*, *104*(467), 38–53. https://doi.org/10.1111/apa.13132.

Luo, Y., Zhang, G. Q., & Li, Z. Y. (2019). The diagnostic value of APT for food allergy in children: A systematic review and meta-analysis. *Pediatric Allergy and Immunology: Official Publication of the European Society of Pediatric Allergy and Immunology*, *30*(4), 451–461. https://doi.org/10.1111/pai.13031.

Mabin, D. C., Sykes, A. E., & David, T. J. (1995). Controlled trial of a few foods diet in severe atopic dermatitis. *Archives of Disease in Childhood*, *73*(3), 202–207. https://doi.org/10.1136/adc.73.3.202.

Mahan, L. K., Escott-Stump, S., Raymond, J. L., & Krause, M. V. (2012). *Krause's Food & the Nutrition Care Process - E-Book* (13th ed.). St. Louis, MO: Saunders.

Miyake, Y., Sasaki, S., Tanaka, K., & Hirota, Y. (2010). Consumption of vegetables, fruit, and antioxidants during pregnancy and wheeze and eczema in infants. *Allergy*, *65*(6), 758–765. https://doi.org/10.1111/j.1398-9995.2009.02267.x.

Mutgi, K., & Koo, J. (2013). Update on the role of systemic vitamin D in atopic dermatitis: Atopic dermatitis and systemic vitamin D. *Pediatric Dermatology*, *30*(3), 303–307. https://doi.org/10.1111/j.1525-1470.2012.01850.x.

Netting, M. J., Middleton, Philippa F., & Makrides, Maria (2014). Does maternal diet during pregnancy and lactation affect outcomes in offspring? A systematic review of food-based approaches. *Nutrition (Burbank, Los Angeles County, Calif.)*, *30*(11–12), 1225–1241. https://doi.org/10.1016/j.nut.2014.02.015.

Niggemann, B., Sielaff, B., Beyer, K., Binder, C., & Wahn, U. (1999). Outcome of double-blind, placebo-controlled food challenge tests in 107 children with atopic dermatitis. *Clinical and Experimental Allergy: Journal of the British Society for Allergy and Clinical Immunology*, *29*(1), 91–96. https://doi.org/10.1046/j.1365-2222.1999.00454.x.

Nosrati, A., Afifi, L., Danesh, M. J., Lee, K., Yan, Di, Beroukhim, K., et al. (2017). Dietary modifications in atopic dermatitis: Patient-reported outcomes. *Journal of Dermatological Treatment*, *28*(6), 523–538. https://doi.org/10.1080/09546634.2016.1278071.

Oh, S.-Y., Chung, J., Kim, M.-K., Kwon, S. O., & Cho, B.-H. (2010). Antioxidant nutrient intakes and corresponding biomarkers associated with the risk of atopic dermatitis in young children. *European Journal of Clinical Nutrition*, *64*(3), 245–252. https://doi.org/10.1038/ejcn.2009.

Øien, T., Schjelvaag, A., Storrø, O., Johnsen, R., & Simpson, M. R. (2019). Fish consumption at one year of age reduces the risk of eczema, asthma and wheeze at six years of age. *Nutrients*, *11*(9), E1969. https://doi.org/10.3390/nu11091969.

Omata, N., Tsukahara, H., Ito, S., Ohshima, Y., Yasutomi, M., Yamada, A., Jiang, M., et al. (2001). Increased oxidative stress in childhood atopic dermatitis. *Life Sciences*, *69*(2), 223–228. https://doi.org/10.1016/s0024-3205(01)01124-9.

Osborn, D. A., & Sinn, J. K. H. (2006). Soy formula for prevention of allergy and food intolerance in infants. *The Cochrane Database of Systematic Reviews*, (4), CD003741. https://doi.org/10.1002/14651858.CD003741.pub4.

Osborn, D. A., Sinn, J. K. H., & Jones, L. J. (2018). Infant formulas containing hydrolysed protein for prevention of allergic disease. *The Cochrane Database of Systematic Reviews*, *2018*(10). https://doi.org/10.1002/14651858.CD003664.pub6.

Ozawa, N., Shimojo, N., Suzuki, Y., Ochiai, S., Nakano, T., Morita, Y., et al. (2014). Maternal intake of Natto, a Japan's traditional fermented soybean food, during pregnancy and the risk of eczema in Japanese babies. *Allergology International: Official Journal of the Japanese Society of Allergology*, *63*(2), 261–266. https://doi.org/10.2332/allergolint.13-OA-0613.

Paller, A. S., Nimmagadda, S., Schachner, L., Mallory, S. B., Kahn, T., Willis, I., & Eichenfield, L. F. (2003). Fluocinolone acetonide 0.01% In peanut oil: Therapy for childhood atopic dermatitis, even in patients who are peanut sensitive. *Journal of the American Academy of Dermatology*, *48*(4), 569–577. https://doi.org/10.1067/mjd.2003.174.

Park, S., Choi, H. S., & Bae, J. H. (2016). Instant noodles, processed food intake, and dietary pattern are associated with atopic dermatitis in an adult population (KNHANES 2009-2011). *Asia Pacific Journal of Clinical Nutrition*, *25*(3), 602–613. https://doi.org/10.6133/apjcn.092015.23.

Pretorius, R. A., Bodinier, M., Prescott, S. L., & Palmer, D. J. (2019). Maternal fiber dietary intakes during pregnancy and infant allergic disease. *Nutrients*, *11*(8), E1767. https://doi.org/10.3390/nu11081767.

Ricci, G., Patrizi, A., Baldi, E., Menna, G., Tabanelli, M., & Masi, M. (2006). Long-term follow-up of atopic dermatitis: Retrospective analysis of related risk factors and association with concomitant allergic diseases. *Journal of the American Academy of Dermatology*, *55*(5), 765–771. https://doi.org/10.1016/j.jaad.2006.04.064.

Samady, W., Warren, C., Kohli, S., Jain, R., Bilaver, L., Mancini, A. J., & Gupta, R. (2019). The prevalence of atopic dermatitis in children with food allergy. *Annals of Allergy, Asthma & Immunology: Official Publication of the American College of Allergy, Asthma, & Immunology*, *122*(6), 656–657.e1. https://doi.org/10.1016/j.anai.2019.03.019.

Samochocki, Z., Bogaczewicz, J., Jeziorkowska, R., Sysa-Jędrzejowska, A., Glińska, O., Karczmarewicz, E., et al. (2013). Vitamin D effects in atopic dermatitis. *Journal of the American Academy of Dermatology*, *69*(2), 238–244. https://doi.org/10.1016/j.jaad.2013.03.014.

Sampson, H. A. (2003). The evaluation and management of food allergy in atopic dermatitis. *Clinics in Dermatology*, *21*(3), 183–192. https://doi.org/10.1016/s0738-081x(02)00363-2.

Sausenthaler, S., Koletzko, S., Schaaf, B., Lehmann, I., Borte, M., Herbarth, O., et al., (2007). Maternal diet during pregnancy in relation to eczema and allergic sensitization in the offspring at 2 y of age. *The American Journal of Clinical Nutrition*, *85*(2), 530–537. https://doi.org/10.1093/ajcn/85.2.530.

Savage, J. H., Kaeding, A. J., Matsui, E. C., & Wood, R. A. (2010). The natural history of soy allergy. *The Journal of Allergy and Clinical Immunology*, *125*(3), 683–686. https://doi.org/10.1016/j.jaci.2009.12.994.

Spergel, J. M., Boguniewicz, M., Schneider, L., Hanifin, J. M., Paller, A. S., & Eichenfield, L. F. (2015). Food allergy in infants with atopic dermatitis: Limitations of food-specific IgE Measurements. *Pediatrics*, *136*(6), e1530–1538. https://doi.org/10.1542/peds.2015-1444.

Strid, J., Hourihane, J., Kimber, I., Callard, R., & Strobel, S. (2004). Disruption of the stratum corneum allows potent epicutaneous immunization with protein antigens resulting in a dominant systemic Th2 response. *European Journal of Immunology*, *34*(8), 2100–2109. https://doi.org/10.1002/eji.200425196.

Suárez-Varela, M. M., García-Marcos A. L., Kogan, M. D., Costa F. J., Martínez Gimeno, A., Aguinaga Ontoso, I., et al. (2010). Diet and prevalence of atopic eczema in 6 to 7-year-old schoolchildren in Spain: ISAAC phase III. *Journal of Investigational Allergology & Clinical Immunology*, *20*(6), 469–475.

Taylor-Robinson, D. C., Williams, H., Pearce, A., Law, C., & Hope, S. (2016). Do early-life exposures explain why more advantaged children get eczema? Findings from the U.K. Millennium Cohort Study. *The British Journal of Dermatology*, *174*(3), 569–578. https://doi.org/10.1111/bjd.14310.

Toit, G. Du, Roberts, G., Sayre, P. H., Bahnson, H. T., Radulovic, S., Santos, A. F., et al. (2015). Randomized trial of peanut consumption in infants at risk for peanut allergy. *The New England Journal of Medicine*, *372*(9), 803–813. https://doi.org/10.1056/NEJMoa1414850.

Toyran, M., Kaymak, M., Vezir, E., Harmancı, K., Kaya, A., Giniş, T., ... Kocabaş, C. N. (2012). Trace element levels in children with atopic dermatitis. *Journal of Investigational Allergology and Clinical Immunology*, *22*(5), 341–344.

Tsoureli-Nikita, E., Hercogova, J., Lotti, T., & Menchini, G. (2002). Evaluation of dietary intake of vitamin E in the treatment of atopic dermatitis: A study of the clinical course and evaluation of the immunoglobulin E serum levels. *International Journal of Dermatology*, *41*(3), 146–150.

Varjonen, E., Vainio, E., & Kalimo, K. (2000). Antigliadin IgE - indicator of wheat allergy in atopic dermatitis. *Allergy, 55*(4), 386–391. https://doi.org/10.1034/j.1398-9995.2000.00451.x.

Vaughn, A. R., Foolad, N., Maarouf, M., Tran, K. A., & Shi, V. Y. (2019). Micronutrients in atopic dermatitis: A systematic review. *The Journal of Alternative and Complementary Medicine, 25*(6), 567–577. https://doi.org/10.1089/acm.2018.0363.

Wang, S. S., Hon, K. L., Kong, A. P., Pong, H. N., Wong, G. W., & Leung, T. F. (2014). Vitamin D deficiency is associated with diagnosis and severity of childhood atopic dermatitis. *Pediatric Allergy and Immunology, 25*(1), 30–35. https://doi.org/10.1111/pai.12167.

Wassmann-Otto, A., Heratizadeh, A., Wichmann, K., & Werfel, T. (2018). Birch pollen-related foods can cause late eczematous reactions in patients with atopic dermatitis. *Allergy, 73*(10), 2046–2054. https://doi.org/10.1111/all.13454.

Yang, Ae-Ri, Kim, Y. N., & Lee, B. H. (2016). Dietary intakes and lifestyle patterns of Korean children and adolescents with atopic dermatitis: Using the fourth and fifth Korean National Health and Nutrition Examination Survey (KNHANES IV,V), 2007–11. *Ecology of Food and Nutrition, 55*(1), 50–64. https://doi.org/10.1080/03670244.2015.1072813.

Zhang, G. Q., Liu, B., Li, J., Luo, C.-Qi, Zhang, Q., Chen, J. L., et al. (2017). Fish intake during pregnancy or infancy and allergic outcomes in children: A systematic review and meta-analysis. *Pediatric Allergy and Immunology, 28*(2), 152–161. https://doi.org/10.1111/pai.12648.

9

Oxidative Stress, Environmental Factors, and Pollutants

ALEKSI J. HENDRICKS, ALYSSA M. THOMPSON, AND VIVIAN Y. SHI

KEY POINTS

- The worldwide prevalence of atopic dermatitis (AD) has risen over recent decades, paralleling industrial and urban growth.
- Airborne pollutants induce oxidative damage at the skin interface with the outside world, setting in motion a cycle of inflammation, skin barrier disruption, and repeated irritant entry in AD.
- Common forms of environmental pollution found to affect the skin barrier and AD include cigarette smoke, particulate matter, volatile organic compounds, and traffic-related air pollution.
- Strategies to mitigate pollution-induced barrier dysfunction include avoiding and blocking pollutant exposure, regular skin cleansing, and emollient application to repair and bolster the skin barrier.
- Future research should aim to more fully characterize the mechanisms by which pollutants impact AD in real-world settings and seek to identify effective topical formulations to protect the skin against airborne pollutants.

Introduction

When we consider the variety of external factors that may influence the development of atopic dermatitis (AD), it is logical that environmental pollution comes to the forefront, as it has been strongly associated with the development of other atopic diatheses, including asthma, allergic rhinitis, and food allergies.

Before we discuss the impact of pollution, however, it would be prudent that we first define the term *pollution*. According to the *Merriam-Webster Dictionary online*, pollution (2021) is "the action of polluting, especially by environmental contamination with man-made waste." (Merriam-Webster). Thus human activities, whether intentional or unintentional, produce waste and byproducts that can become triggering factors for the development of AD. Having defined pollution, let us now delineate its impact on AD by examining published data in the literature.

The prevalence of AD has been steadily rising in recent decades, particularly in certain regions. Despite a global increase in the number of children with AD, developed countries such as New Zealand and the United Kingdom that previously reported high rates of AD have experienced a plateau at around 10% to 15% (Asher et al., 2006; Nutten, 2015). However, AD prevalence is growing in lower income developing nations, with rates higher than 15% and up to 24.6% reported in countries of Southeast Asia, Africa, and Latin America (Asher et al., 2006; Nutten, 2015). The increased incidence of AD parallels expansion in urbanization and industrialization worldwide, and investigation of the role of airborne pollution in relation to AD has become increasingly relevant. One of the major areas of study centers on the role of pollution in skin barrier dysfunction.

General mechanism of pollution-induced barrier dysfunction

The general mechanisms of pollution-induced skin barrier dysfunction result from excess oxidative stress that in turn induces inflammation. Airborne pollution generates reactive oxygen species, which deplete the skin's antioxidant defenses. This pro- versus antioxidant imbalance, favoring prooxidants, results in oxidative damage to keratinocytes, decreased cell adhesion, and barrier dysfunction as indicated by increased transepidermal water loss (TEWL), decreased hydration, and increased pH (Jin et al., 2018; Kim, Han et al., 2016; Magnani et al., 2016). Compromised skin barrier integrity allows for easy entry of pathogens, irritants, and immunogens (Han et al., 2018; Kim, Han et al., 2016; Magnani et al., 2016), fueling inflammation and the itch-scratch cycle in AD (Han et al., 2016; Kim, Han et al., 2016). Signaling cascades involved in pollutant-induced skin barrier damage include the NFκB inflammatory pathway (Magnani et al., 2016) and aryl hydrocarbon receptor (AhR) (Mancebo & Wang, 2015; Schnass et al., 2018). Airborne pollutants have been found to increase NFκB signaling and promote expression of proinflammatory cytokines that lead to skin redness, swelling, itch, and pain. AhR acts as a chemical sensor in keratinocytes, leading to downstream activation of inflammation and itch mediators as well as epidermal antioxidant defense mechanisms (Furue et al., 2017).

Cigarette smoke

Cigarette smoke from burning tobacco contains antigenic and carcinogenic compounds such as nicotine, polycyclic aromatic hydrocarbons, and metal residues (Arnson, Shoenfeld, & Amital, 2010). Muizzuddin, Ken Marenus, and Maes (1997) evaluated TEWL as an indicator of barrier function in a cohort of 100 patients, including active heavy smokers, passive smokers, and nonsmokers. Average TEWL did not differ between active and passive smokers but was significantly lower in nonsmokers compared to both active and passive smoking groups (11 vs. $16 g/m^2/h$, $P < .001$) (Muizzuddin et al., 1997). These results suggest that both active and passive exposures to cigarette smoke are associated with reduced capacity of the epidermis to retain water.

Cigarette smoke has also been identified as an exacerbating factor in AD. Within a cohort of 7000 Korean schoolchildren, exposure to environmental tobacco smoke during the mother's pregnancy and children's infancy was associated with a twofold greater risk of AD development (Yi et al., 2012). In a large survey-based study of over 145,000 Korean adolescents, more than 10,000 respondents reported AD symptoms within the last 12 months. Among this subset of adolescents with AD symptoms, researchers found a significant association with both active and passive cigarette smoking, and the strongest association was observed in those who actively smoked more than 20 days per month (odds ratio [OR] = 1.18) (Kim, Sim, & Choi, 2017).

While increased TEWL and higher prevalence of AD symptoms have been demonstrated in association with smoking, further research is needed to better understand the relationship between cigarette pollution and AD exacerbation. Nevertheless, convincing evidence exists to support smoking cessation for skin as well as general health.

Particulate matter

Particulate matter (PM) describes liquid or solid particles in gas suspension and is classified according to its aerodynamic diameter (Mancebo & Wang, 2015). Ultrafine PM (<0.1 µm in diameter) is emitted from diesel engines. Fine PM (0.1–2.5 µm) is generated from open fires, power plants, and car exhaust. Coarse PM (2.5–10 µm) originates from soil, dust, and industrial emissions (Mancebo & Wang, 2015).

PM has been demonstrated to induce skin barrier dysfunction in vivo. In a study using live pigs, which have skin similar in structure and function to that of humans, dorsal skin treated with solubilized PM exhibited a twofold increase in TEWL compared to vehicle control, as well as loss of epidermal structural proteins (Pan et al., 2015).

PM stimulates keratinocyte production of matrix metalloproteinases, induces inflammatory cytokines, and activates the NFκB signaling pathway (Dajee et al., 2006; Jin et al., 2018; Kim, Bae et al., 2017; Magnani et al., 2016). Furthermore, PM has been shown to have dose- and time-dependent cytotoxic effects on cultured skin cells (Jin et al., 2018; Magnani et al., 2016).

PM has shown detrimental effects in both healthy and AD skin in animal models, with increased susceptibility to PM-induced damage in the barrier-disrupted state of AD. Jin et al. (2018) demonstrated the capacity of PM to penetrate barrier-disrupted skin and incite an inflammatory response in mice. PM was identified in the hair follicles of both intact and tape-stripped skin but was also present intercellularly in samples of barrier-disrupted epidermis. Repetitive topical application of PM followed by occlusive dressing led to neutrophil-predominant dermal inflammation in both intact and barrier-disrupted mouse skin (Jin et al., 2018). Han et al. (2018) used a rat model of capsaicin-induced AD to study the effects of vaporized glyoxal, a major source of PM production. Exposure to glyoxal vapor exacerbated pruritus and dermatitis in rats with existing AD but did not induce AD symptoms in healthy animals (Han et al., 2018), indicating that preexisting barrier disruption is required for PM to exacerbate AD. Increased skin *Staphylococcus aureus* colonization was observed in both AD and healthy animals following glyoxal exposure, demonstrating the potential of PM to contribute to cutaneous dysbiosis (imbalance of the microbiota), a major driving factor in AD pathogenesis (Han et al., 2018).

Studies in human populations have also identified correlations between PM and AD symptoms. A study of 21 Korean pediatric AD patients revealed a temporal association between elevated PM levels in urban areas and increase in reported AD symptoms (Oh et al., 2018). Fine PM (<2.5 µm in diameter) levels had a stronger positive correlation with AD symptoms compared to coarse PM (2.5–10 µm in diameter) with respective ORs of 1.399 and 1.215 per 10-µg/m³ increase in PM exposure (Oh et al., 2018). A population-based cross-sectional study of over 5000 Taiwanese adults identified a modest association between frequent fine PM exposure and development of AD (adjusted OR = 1.05) (Tang et al., 2017). Based on these findings, it appears that fine PM may be most detrimental, as it can penetrate the epidermal barrier of tape-stripped skin (Jin et al., 2018) and may inflict greater damage with high PM concentrations or prolonged exposure time.

Volatile organic compounds

Volatile organic compounds (VOCs) are carbon-based substances that readily vaporize at ambient air pressure and are important contributors to indoor air pollution. Common VOCs are organic solvents such as benzene, toluene, xylene, and formaldehyde, which are released from household items, including cleaning supplies, wallpaper, new furniture, plastics, and plywood (Kim, Kim, Lim, Lee, & Kim, 2016).

Airborne formaldehyde has been demonstrated to induce skin barrier dysfunction. Huss-Marp et al. (2006) evaluated 12 AD subjects and 12 healthy subjects exposed to dust mite allergen and subsequently to a mixture of 22 VOCs in a total body chamber. Compared to purified air control, a mean 34% increase in TEWL was observed at 48 hours post-VOC exposure in both healthy and AD subjects, without significant difference between the two groups (Huss-Marp et al., 2006). Furthermore, six of seven AD patients patch tested with house dust mite allergen exhibited an enhanced skin reaction following VOC exposure, demonstrating that VOCs can exacerbate the atopic response to allergens (Huss-Marp et al., 2006). Kim, Han et al. (2016) found that exposure to formaldehyde caused an increase in TEWL and skin pH in both healthy and AD subjects. The median increase in TEWL was 2.5 and $1.4 \, g/m^2/h$ in AD and healthy skin, respectively (Kim, Han et al., 2016). A more pronounced increase in skin pH was also observed in AD compared to healthy skin (0.11 vs. 0.04 pH units), indicating that individuals with existing AD are more susceptible to VOC-induced barrier damage. These findings are in agreement with animal studies conducted by Han et al. (2016), who found that formaldehyde fume exposure exacerbated pruritus and dermatitis in a rat model of AD.

Investigations of real-world VOC indoor pollution exposure have also demonstrated a negative impact on skin barrier function. In a cross-sectional study of over 4000 Korean schoolchildren, those living in homes that had been remodeled within the preceding 12 months had more than a threefold greater risk of AD compared to those who did not live in areas of remodeling (Lee et al., 2017). A combination of recent remodeling and food allergy synergistically increased the risk of AD in children by sevenfold (Lee et al., 2017). Kim, Kim et al. (2016) studied the effects of plant-based wallpaper compared to PVC (polyvinyl chloride)-based wallpaper, and reported that AD children who live in apartments with higher formaldehyde and VOC levels in indoor air had significantly higher SCORAD indexes. The authors found that ecofriendly wallpapering was associated with an increase in natural VOCs, also known as phytoncides, that are given off by trees and plants. Higher levels of natural VOCs correlated with improvement in AD symptoms, suggesting that plant-based VOCs may have positive effects on barrier integrity (Kim, Kim et al., 2016).

Traffic-related air pollution

Traffic-related air pollution (TRAP) includes both PM and VOC pollutants, which were described previously, in addition to gaseous components such as nitrogen oxides (NO, NO_2, N_2O), SO_2, CO, and O_3 generated from gasoline and diesel-powered engines (Mancebo & Wang, 2015). He et al. (2006) found that exposure of human skin to 0.8 ppm O_3 for 2 hours led to a nearly 50% reduction in colony-forming units of resident microflora compared to nonpolluted air exposure alone. This effect is of interest in relation to dysbiosis in AD, where alteration of resident skin flora and

predisposition to *S. aureus* colonization are widely observed (Kong et al., 2012), although a direct link between TRAP exposure and *S. aureus* colonization has not been established.

TRAP exposure is of particular relevance as many regions in the world become increasingly urbanized. To evaluate the health effects of this trend, a longitudinal study of the influence of air pollution in healthy German women was initiated in 1985. Follow-up during 2008–2009 identified a 7.9% incidence of AD symptoms after age 55. The investigators reported a significant positive association between incidence of AD symptoms and exposure to TRAP, with TRAP exposure determined by measuring levels of PM and nitrogen oxides in 2008–2009 and back-extrapolating to baseline levels (Schnass et al., 2018).

During the prenatal and infancy periods, TRAP exposure is associated with increased risk of AD. A prospective cohort of mother-child pairs in Osaka, Japan, was followed from mothers' pregnancy to 16 to 24 months of children's age and assessed for risk of asthma and AD development in relation to proximity of the child's residence to the nearest main road (Miyake et al., 2010). Within this cohort of 756 children, 8.9% developed physician-diagnosed AD by age 16 to 24 months. Compared to children living more than 200 m from the nearest main road, those living within 50 m had a significantly higher risk of doctor-diagnosed AD (adjusted OR = 2.26, P = .03) (Miyake et al., 2010). Although this study does not distinguish the effects of pre- versus postnatal TRAP exposure, the findings indicate a role of TRAP in childhood development of AD and its possible contribution to the rising prevalence of AD in industrialized and developing countries over recent decades. However, direct effects of TRAP on the skin barrier have not been investigated.

A summary of study findings regarding the effects of specific pollutants on skin barrier function and AD is presented in Table 9.1.

Solutions

As we anticipate continued urbanization and industrial growth in the coming years, preventive and protective strategies are crucial to combat the health effects of airborne pollution. In the context of AD, three main routes of intervention should be pursued: (1) dedicated avoidance of pollutant exposure and reducing harm to the skin barrier through choice of nonirritating materials; (2) thorough, regular cleansing to remove pollutants from the skin surface; and (3) protection of the skin barrier against pollutant entry. Patients should be encouraged to wash their skin daily, preferably at the end of the day after exposure to ambient pollution. Emollients should be applied immediately after cleansing for skin barrier repair and protection. Further research is needed to determine the ideal ingredients and formulations for barrier protection and repair, which may vary by pollutant. The potential role of topical antioxidants and antiinflammatory compounds as adjuvant therapy is an additional area of future investigation, as NFκB inhibitors (Dajee et al., 2006) and vitamin and trace

TABLE
9.1   **Effects of pollutants on skin barrier function and atopic dermatitis**

Author	Study design	Results
Cigarette smoke		
Muizzuddin et al. (1997)	Cohort of 100 subjects, including active smokers, passive smokers, nonsmokers	Increased TEWL in active and passive smokers compared to nonsmokers
Yi et al. (2012)	Survey-based study of 7000 Korean children	2-fold greater risk of AD in children exposed to cigarette smoke during mother's pregnancy or children's infancy
Kim et al. (2017) Kim, Kim et al. (2017)	Survey-based study of over 145,000 Korean adolescents	Significant association between both active and passive smoking and AD symptoms within the last 12 months, strongest in those who actively smoke >20 days/month
Particulate matter (PM)		
Pan et al. (2015)	Dorsal pig skin treated with solubilized PM	2-fold increase in TEWL in PM-treated skin compared to vehicle control. Loss of stratum corneum structural proteins cytokeratin, filaggrin, and epidermal tight junction protein E-cadherin
Jin et al. (2018)	Solubilized PM applied topically to intact and tape-stripped mouse skin	PM penetrates epidermal barrier of tape-stripped mouse skin and incites neutrophilic dermal inflammation in both intact and tape-stripped skin
Han et al. (2018)	Rat model of AD exposed to vaporized glyoxal	Exacerbation of pruritus and dermatitis in rats with existing AD. Increased *Staphylococcus aureus* colonization in both AD and healthy rats
Oh et al. (2018)	Study of 21 Korean children living in urban areas	Temporal association between elevated ambient PM levels and exacerbation of AD symptoms
Tang et al. (2017)	Population-based study of over 5000 Taiwanese adults	Modest association between frequent $PM_{2.5}$ exposure and development of AD
Volatile organic compounds (VOCs)		
Huss-Marp et al. (2006)	12 healthy and 12 AD subjects sensitized to house dust mite allergen and exposed to an aerosol mixture of 22 VOCs	34% increase in TEWL 48 h after VOC exposure in both AD and healthy skin. Enhanced reaction to house dust mite patch testing in AD patients exposed to aerosolized VOCs
Kim et al. (2016) Kim, Han et al. (2016)	AD and healthy subjects exposed to formaldehyde fumes	Increased TEWL and skin pH in both healthy and AD subjects, with more pronounced increase in AD skin
Han et al. (2016)	Rat model of AD exposed to formaldehyde fumes	Exacerbation of pruritus and dermatitis with increase in serum levels of IgE and Th1 cytokines
Lee et al. (2017)	Cross-sectional study of 4000 Korean schoolchildren	>3-fold higher risk of AD in children living in homes remodeled in the previous year compared to those living in nonremodeled residences. 7-fold greater risk of AD in children with food allergy living in recently remodeled homes
Kim et al. (2016) Kim, Kim et al. (2016)	Assessment of indoor VOC levels with PVC- vs. plant-based wallpaper and association with AD symptoms	Higher SCORAD indexes in children living in apartments with PVC-based wallpaper and elevated indoor levels of VOCs
Traffic-related air pollution (TRAP)		
He et al. (2006)	Human skin exposed to 0.8 ppm O_3 for 2 h	50% reduction in resident skin flora following exposure to ozone vs. air alone
Schnass et al. (2018)	Prospective cohort study of healthy German women over age 55	Positive correlation between TRAP exposure and development of AD after age 55
Miyake et al. (2010)	Prospective cohort study of Japanese mother-child pairs	>2-fold increased risk of AD in children living within 50 m of the nearest main road compared to those living >200 m away

AD, Atopic dermatitis; *PVC*, polyvinyl chloride; *SCORAD*, SCORing Atopic Dermatitis; *TEWL*, transepidermal water loss.

mineral formulations (Maarouf, Vaughn, & Shi, 2018) may augment cutaneous defense against oxidative damage and resulting inflammation.

While emollients and antioxidants may prove helpful in reducing and reversing pollutant-induced skin barrier dysfunction, larger-scale modifications to building and urban planning may yield greater results in minimizing or preventing barrier dysfunction. These adjustments will require the combined efforts of regulatory agencies, health care providers, public health researchers, urban planners, engineering industries, and the informed public to acknowledge the negative health impact of environmental pollution and encourage more thoughtful selection of materials used in buildings, factories, and vehicles in our increasingly urban society.

Summary

Environmental pollutants may contribute to the development and exacerbation of AD. While many of the exact mechanisms by which airborne pollution affects AD and skin barrier function remain incompletely understood, emerging evidence demonstrates negative effects of common pollutants on the skin in both animal- and population-based studies. Protective and preventive measures of cleansing, moisturizing, and wearing nonirritating barrier materials are practical approaches to minimize pollutant exposure during daily activities.

Further readings

Asante-Duah. K. (2018). *Public health risk assessment for human exposure to chemicals* (2nd ed.). Springer.

Brusseau, M. L., Pepper, I. L., & Gerba, C. P. (Eds.), (2019). *Environmental and pollution science* (3rd ed.). Academic Press.

Seigneur. C. (2019). *Air pollution: Concepts, theory, and application.* Cambridge University Press.

References

Arnson, Y., Shoenfeld, Y., & Amital, H. (2010). "Effects of tobacco smoke on immunity, inflammation and autoimmunity." *Journal of Autoimmunity, 34*(3), J258–J265. https://doi.org/10.1016/j.jaut.2009.12.003.

Asher, M. I., Montefort, S., Bjorksten, B., Lai, C. K., Strachan, D. P., Weiland, S. K., & Williams, H. (2006). "Worldwide time trends in the prevalence of symptoms of asthma, allergic rhinoconjunctivitis, and eczema in childhood: ISAAC Phases One and Three repeat multicountry cross-sectional surveys." *Lancet, 368*(9537), 733–743. https://doi.org/10.1016/s0140-6736(06)69283-0.

Dajee, M., Muchamuel, T., Schryver, B., Oo, A., Alleman-Sposeto, J., De Vry, C. G., et al. (2006). Blockade of experimental atopic dermatitis via topical NF-kappaB decoy oligonucleotide. *The Journal of Investigative Dermatology, 126*(8), 1792–1803. https://doi.org/10.1038/sj.jid.5700307.

Furue, M., Uchi, H., Mitoma, C., Hashimoto-Hachiya, A., Chiba, T., Ito, T., et al. (2017). "Antioxidants for healthy skin: The emerging role of aryl hydrocarbon receptors and nuclear factor-erythroid 2-related factor-2. *Nutrients, 9*(3), 223. https://doi.org/10.3390/nu9030223.

Han, R. T., Back, S. K., Lee, H., Lee, J., Kim, H. Y., Kim, H. J., & Na, H. S. (2016). "Formaldehyde-induced aggravation of pruritus and dermatitis is associated with the elevated expression of Th1 cytokines in a rat model of atopic dermatitis." *PLoS ONE, 11*(12), e0168466. https://doi.org/10.1371/journal.pone.0168466.

Han, R. T., Kim, H. Y., Ryu, H., Jang, W., Cha, S. H., Kim, H. Y., et al. (2018). "Glyoxal-induced exacerbation of pruritus and dermatitis is associated with staphylococcus aureus colonization in the skin of a rat model of atopic dermatitis." *Journal of Dermatological Science, 90*(3), 276–283. https://doi.org/10.1016/j.jdermsci.2018.02.012.

He, Q. C., Tavakkol, A., Wietecha, K., Begum-Gafur, R., Ansari, S. A., & Polefka, T. (2006). "Effects of environmentally realistic levels of ozone on stratum corneum function." *International Journal of Cosmetic Science, 28*(5), 349–357. https://doi.org/10.1111/j.1467-2494.2006.00347.x.

Huss-Marp, J., Eberlein-Konig, B., Breuer, K., Mair, S., Ansel, A., Darsow, U., et al. (2006). Influence of short-term exposure to airborne Der p 1 and volatile organic compounds on skin barrier function and dermal blood flow in patients with atopic eczema and healthy individuals. *Clinical and Experimental Allergy, 36*(3), 338–345. https://doi.org/10.1111/j.1365-2222.2006.02448.x.

Jin, S. P., Li, Z., Choi, E. K., Lee, S., Kim, Y. K., Seo, E. Y., et al. (2018). Urban particulate matter in air pollution penetrates into the barrier-disrupted skin and produces ROS-dependent cutaneous inflammatory response in vivo. *Journal of Dermatological Science, 91*(2), 175–183. https://doi.org/10.1016/j.jdermsci.2018.04.015.

Kim, H. J., Bae, I. H., Son, E. D., Park, J., Cha, N., Na, H. W., et al. (2017). Transcriptome analysis of airborne PM2.5-induced detrimental effects on human keratinocytes. *Toxicology Letters, 273*, 26–35. https://doi.org/10.1016/j.toxlet.2017.03.010.

Kim, J., Han, Y., Ahn, J. H., Kim, S. W., Lee, S. I., Lee, K. H., & Ahn, K. (2016). Airborne formaldehyde causes skin barrier dysfunction in atopic dermatitis. *The British Journal of Dermatology, 175*(2), 357–363. https://doi.org/10.1111/bjd.14357.

Kim, J., Kim, H., Lim, D., Lee, Y. K., & Kim, J. H. (2016). Effects of indoor air pollutants on atopic dermatitis. *International Journal of Environmental Research and Public Health, 13*(12), 1220. https://doi.org/10.3390/ijerph13121220.

Kim, S. Y., Sim, S., & Choi, H. G. (2017). Atopic dermatitis is associated with active and passive cigarette smoking in adolescents. *PLoS ONE, 12*(11), e0187453. https://doi.org/10.1371/journal.pone.0187453.

Kong, H. H., Oh, J., Deming, C., Conlan, S., Grice, E. A., Beatson, M. A., et al. (2012). Temporal shifts in the skin microbiome associated with disease flares and treatment in children with atopic dermatitis. *Genome Research, 22*(5), 850–859. https://doi.org/10.1101/gr.131029.111.

Lee, W. S., Lee, K. S., Lee, S., Sung, M., Lee, S. J., Jee, H. M., et al. (2017). Home remodeling and food allergy interact synergistically to increase the risk of atopic dermatitis. *BioMed Research International, 2017*, 3793679. https://doi.org/10.1155/2017/3793679.

Maarouf, M., Vaughn, A. R., & Shi, V. Y. (2018). Topical micronutrients in atopic dermatitis-An evidence-based review. *Dermatologic Therapy, 31*(5), e12659. https://doi.org/10.1111/dth.12659.

Magnani, N. D., Muresan, X. M., Belmonte, G., Cervellati, F., Sticozzi, C., Pecorelli, A., et al. (2016). Skin damage mechanisms related to airborne particulate matter exposure. *Toxicological Sciences, 149*(1), 227–236. https://doi.org/10.1093/toxsci.kfv230.

Mancebo, S. E., & Wang, S. Q. (2015). "Recognizing the impact of ambient air pollution on skin health." *Journal of the European Academy of Dermatology and Venereology, 29*(12), 2326–2332. https://doi.org/10.1111/jdv.13250.

Miyake, Y., Tanaka, K., Fujiwara, H., Mitani, Y., Ikemi, H., Sasaki, S., et al. (2010). Residential proximity to main roads during pregnancy and the risk of allergic disorders in Japanese infants: The Osaka Maternal and Child Health Study. *Pediatric Allergy and Immunology, 21*(1 Pt 1), 22–28. https://doi.org/10.1111/j.1399-3038.2009.00951.x.

Muizzuddin, N., Ken Marenus, P. V., & Maes, D. (1997). Effect of cigarette smoke on skin. *Journal of the Society of Cosmetic Chemists, 48*(5), 235–242.

Nutten. S. (2015). Atopic dermatitis: global epidemiology and risk factors. *Annals of Nutrition & Metabolism, 66*(Suppl 1), 8–16. https://doi.org/10.1159/000370220.

Oh, I., Lee, J., Ahn, K., Kim, J., Kim, Y. M., Sun Sim, C., & Kim, Y. (2018). "Association between particulate matter concentration and symptoms of atopic dermatitis in children living in an industrial urban area of South Korea." *Environmental Research, 160*, 462–468. https://doi.org/10.1016/j.envres.2017.10.030.

Pan, T. L., Wang, P. W., Aljuffali, I. A., Huang, C. T., Lee, C. W., & Fang, J. Y. (2015). "The impact of urban particulate pollution on skin barrier function and the subsequent drug absorption.". *Journal of Dermatological Science, 78*(1), 51–60. https://doi.org/10.1016/j.jdermsci.2015.01.011.

Pollution. (2021). *Merriam-Webster dictionary online* https://www.merriam-webster.com/dictionary/pollution?src=search-dict-box.

Schnass, W., Huls, A., Vierkotter, A., Kramer, U., Krutmann, J., & Schikowski, T. (2018). Traffic-related air pollution and eczema in the elderly: Findings from the SALIA cohort. *International Journal of Hygiene and Environmental Health* https://doi.org/10.1016/j.ijheh.2018.06.002.

Tang, K. T., Ku, K. C., Chen, D. Y., Lin, C. H., Tsuang, B. J., & Chen, Y. H. (2017). Adult atopic dermatitis and exposure to air pollutants—a nationwide population-based study. *Annals of Allergy, Asthma and Immunology, 118*(3), 351–355. https://doi.org/10.1016/j.anai.2016.12.005.

Yi, O., Kwon, H. J., Kim, H., Ha, M., Hong, S. J., Hong, Y. C., et al. (2012). Effect of environmental tobacco smoke on atopic dermatitis among children in Korea. *Environmental Research, 113*, 40–45. https://doi.org/10.1016/j.envres.2011.12.012.

10

Clinical Evidence: External Factors

LAWRENCE S. CHAN

KEY POINTS

- The fact that up to 50% of atopic dermatitis (AD) patients have loss-of-function genetic mutations of skin barrier protein filaggrin points to a cutaneous weakness that allows external factors to trigger skin inflammation in AD.
- Various studies documented that between 30% and 100% of patients with AD have pathogenic *Staphylococcus aureus* colonization on their skin, and this colonization worsens skin inflammation. Powerful evidences point to the colonization of *S. aureus*, paralleling a dysbiosis phenomenon with displacement of commensal bacteria and reduction of skin surface microbial diversity, as a contributing factor for AD development.
- Patients with AD are prone to have frequent skin infections.
- Patients with AD, particularly those with severe disease, tend to have heightened skin sensitivity to various contact allergens and are more likely to develop contact allergic reactions.
- Environmental pollutions are associated with the development of AD.

Introduction

When the loss-of-function filaggrin gene mutation was first revealed in the medical literature as a strong link to patients affected with atopic dermatitis (AD), the general sentiment of the medical community was that of an excitement for possessing a key to point to external factors as the cause of AD since the skin barrier defect would naturally open doors for invading actors to enter and trigger the inflammatory process manifested in AD (Palmer et al., 2006). Combining with the clinical evidences that AD patients commonly have pathogenic bacterial colonization in their skin and frequent skin infections with bacterial, fungal, and viral microorganisms, there are strong data to support external causes for the development of AD. The principal goal of this chapter is therefore to examine and analyze those relevant clinical data to delineate the degree these external factors are contributing to the disease development. In discussing the external factors as the contributors for AD development, we must at the same time reason if external factors alone will be sufficient to cause the disease to develop.

Although clinical data are generally not considered as robust as those collected through laboratory investigations, it nevertheless provides a supporting documentation from a different angle. In a way, clinical evidence provides a sense of reality or a sense of living proof. Any medical theory or purely laboratory-based research result unsupported by clinical evidence will be called into question of whether the theory is correct or that data are relevant for the actual disease.

First, we define what is clinical evidence. According to the online 2019 *Oxford Dictionary*, the term *clinical* relates "to the observation and treatment of actual patients rather than theoretical or laboratory studies." Oxford Living Dictionaries. (2019) Another dictionary defines *clinical* as "(of a disease or condition) causing observable and recognizable symptoms." *Merriam-Webster Dictionary* defines clinical (2019) this way: "of, relating to, or conducted in or as if in a clinic: such as a: involving direct observation of the patient or b: based on or characterized by observable and diagnosable symptoms." Clinical evidence therefore will be the collected data gathered from the clinical observations or studies.

Thus, to collect clinical evidence, we gather all the data relating to the symptoms and signs of what we can observe, obtain, measure about and from actual patient encounter, rather than by theoretic consideration, speculation, or purely laboratory investigation. However, laboratory data are also part of the supporting evaluation of clinical data and of documenting clinical evidence. One simple example is the clinical evaluation of early clinical failure of treatment of a gram-negative bacteria sepsis (bloodstream infection). To collect clinical evidence accurately and correctly, the clinical investigators first establish that all these patients indeed have bloodstream infection by gram-negative bacteria documented by results of blood culture, a laboratory method. Moreover, the clinical researchers have to measure many parameters to develop a set of criteria for determining the "predictors" for early clinical failure. These parameters would include some "purely clinical data" such as blood pressure, respiratory rate, altered mental status, but also include other "laboratory data" such as white blood cell count. Together, these collected data provide the valuable predictors for early clinical failure on treatment for gram-negative sepsis (Rac et al., 2019). Similarly, to collect clinical data and to document clinical evidence in relation to development of AD, some laboratory-generated information, such as bacterial culture determinations, skin histopathology findings, genetic mutation information in skin barrier protein, immunologic status, and other clinically supportive laboratory data, is also included. The following discussions delineate clinical findings to suggest that external factors play a significant role in AD development.

Staphylococcus aureus colonization

Pathogenic bacterial species colonized in the skin of AD patients is a well-documented finding. Pathogenic *Staphylococcus aureus* species colonize in about 30% to 100% of AD patients' skin. This kind of colonization displaced other commensal bacteria species beneficial to the human hosts, and this abnormal colonization is associated with increased disease severity (Geoghegan, Alan, & Foster, 2018; Nakatsuji & Gallo, 2019). Theoretically, several molecules expressed by *S. aureus* may contribute to the inflammation of AD:

- δ-toxin from these bacteria is capable of stimulating mast cells leading to inflammatory cytokine release.
- α-toxin from these bacteria can damage keratinocytes leading to damage-related inflammatory responses.
- Phenol-soluble modulins are stimulatory to keratinocytes for cytokine release.
- Protein A can trigger keratinocyte inflammatory responses and act as superantigens to generate B-lymphocyte immune activation (Geoghegan et al., 2018).
- Enterotoxin B from *S. aureus* is capable of triggering leukocyte expression of a pruritus-inducing cytokine interleukin 31 (IL31), and experimental overexpression of IL31 in mice actually triggers skin inflammation (Dillon et al., 2004; Sonkoly et al., 2006).

In one study, bacterial culture survey points out that a *S. aureus*–predominant colonization is associated with a severe disease phenotype, and a *Staphylococcus epidermidis*–predominant colonization is linked to a milder disease phenotype of AD (Byrd et al., 2017). But a mere association of *S. aureus* colonization does not prove a contributing role of these bacteria in triggering the disease development. One of the best studies that links *S. aureus* colonization to AD development is a Switzerland-conducted prospective birth cohort study. In this study of 149 white, fully term healthy infants, the researchers obtained bacterial culture at birth and at seven time points over their first 2 years of life. These infants were examined and followed by the physicians to monitor the development of skin disease at birth; at age day 1, 3, and 7; and at age 1, 3, 6, 12, and 24 months. At age 3 months, the investigators found that *S. aureus* colonization was significantly more prevalent in those patients who developed AD later on, compared to those infants who did not develop the skin disease. Furthermore, the prevalence of colonization increased 2 months before the onset of AD and at the time of disease onset. In addition, the patients who had

positive *S. aureus* colonization developed AD at a younger age than those patients without the bacterial colonization (Meylan et al., 2017). There were additional negative effects of *S. aureus* colonization. These colonized bacteria not only settled in the skin but also pushed away the commensal skin bacteria such as *S. epidermidis*, which normally provides their own antimicrobial peptides and enhances human-producing antimicrobial peptides for immune defenses of human skin (Gallo & Nakatsuji, 2011). A proposed mechanism of how *S. aureus* colonization would trigger AD development is depicted in Fig. 10.1. More discussions on the role of *S. aureus* in AD are detailed in Chapter 6.

Skin infection

With the discovery of skin barrier defect, a logical reasoning to follow might be to ask if such defect would lead to a tendency of frequent skin infection in patients affected by AD. Indeed, AD has been associated with the serious bacterial, fungal, and viral infections. Eczema herpeticum and eczema vaccinatum are two such well-documented examples. However, these infections are also linked to a deficiency of innate immune defense in patients with AD, therefore raising a question of the relative contribution between internal and external actors (Hata et al., 2010; Howell et al., 2006; Nakatsuji & Gallo, 2019; Sun & Ong, 2017). Having stated the fact that frequent skin infections do occur in patients with AD, how these infections would then contribute to the development of AD is not clear. Obviously these infection events could certainly exacerbate the existing skin inflammation, but whether these infections directly trigger the skin inflammation has not been well studied.

Allergic contact dermatitis

When skin barrier function is compromised, allergens exposed to the skin may have an easy entry into the epidermis to induce allergic contact dermatitis. Once contact dermatitis, an inflammatory process by itself, begins, the development of AD could then be triggered. So the two logical questions to ask include: Are patients with AD prone to have more frequent occurrence of allergic contact dermatitis? and Do these contact allergic events lead to the typical inflammatory skin disease AD? Although the data are conflicting, existing medical publications as a whole seem to support a notion that contact allergy is a common problem in children with AD (Jacob et al., 2017; Simonsen, Johansen, Deleuran, Mortz, & Sommerlund, 2017). In one study, the survey results suggested that AD developed in early childhood might associate with adolescent onset of contact allergy to fragrances. However, the results of this study did not point to allergen as a causative factor for AD development, only a simple association (Lagrelius et al., 2019). In another study, researchers have found that patients with AD were more likely to develop positive patch test reactions to ingredients in personal care products and topically applied antibiotics and corticosteroids (Rastogi, Patel, Singam, &

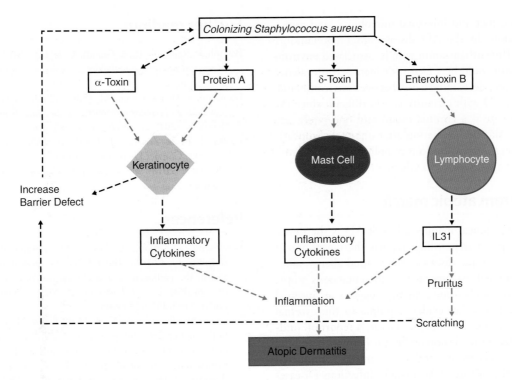

• **Fig. 10.1** Proposed mechanisms of atopic dermatitis development initiated by the external factor of colonizing pathogenic bacteria *Staphylococcus aureus*. *Black dash arrows* indicate releasing, resulting in, or leading to; *green dash arrows* indicate triggering, stimulating; *red dash arrow* indicates injury inducing.

Silverberg, 2018). A study focused on difficult-to-treat AD found that this subset of patients indeed had a high prevalence of concomitant allergic contact dermatitis and were commonly sensitized to multiple allergens (polysensitized) (Boonstra, Rustemeyer, & Middelkamp-Hup, 2018). In a Danish children study, investigators found that 30% of children with AD had at least one positive patch test reaction, and 17% of these patients had at least one contact allergic reaction relevant to their current skin symptoms, and that the risk of contact allergy significantly correlated with the AD severity. In addition, the fact that metal and skincare products were the most frequently identified allergens in this Danish study also pointed to the potential role of the external factors (Simonsen et al., 2018). In another study of Dutch patients, children with AD had significantly more frequent allergic reactions to lanolin alcohol and fragrances, although the overall sensitization prevalence between atopic and nonatopic children was similar (Lubbes, Rustemeyer, Sillevis Smitt, Schuttelaar, & Middelkamp-Hup, 2017). Whether these allergic contact dermatitis events directly trigger the development of AD is not well documented. An inflammatory event of allergic contact dermatitis could certainly exacerbate AD. In addition, the similar clinical morphology between AD and allergic contact dermatitis renders efforts to establish this explicit link very challenging. The association of AD with allergic contact dermatitis is also an immunologic puzzle since their disease mechanisms differ from an immune standpoint. Classically defined, AD is primarily a type 2-axis immune disease, and allergic contact dermatitis is a classic type 1 cell-mediated immune

phenomenon (Crepy, Audrey, & Lynda, 2019). Recent studies, however, pointed to possible common pathways, such as skin barrier defect, between allergic contact dermatitis and AD (Pootongkam & Nedorost, 2014). More details on the role of allergens in AD are discussed in Chapter 7.

Environmental pollution

The discovery of skin barrier defect in patients with AD also raises the question whether the environmental pollution, airborne or by other means, may affect the development of AD. It is reasonable to speculate that when skin barrier function is deficient, the environmental pollutants could enter the skin easier. Once they enter the skin, these pollutants could in effect become irritants/allergens from an immunologic standpoint, inducing skin inflammation that we observe as AD. There were some evidences pointed to this possible link. A study conducted in South Korea found associations between development of AD and road density in patients' home communities and between development of AD and road proximity to patients' homes, suggesting that traffic-related air pollution positively affected the development of AD (Yi et al., 2017). In another South Korean survey, smoking was associated with development of AD in patients age 12 to 18 years, suggesting a link between the fume of cigarette smoke and AD (Lee, Oh, Choi, & Rha, 2017). The fact that the incidence of AD in developing countries is slowly catching up with that of developed nations underlines the importance of environmental factors, such as hygiene practice, bacterial endotoxin exposure, animal contact, diet and intestinal microbiota, and atmospheric pollution, in the AD disease onset (Bonamonte et al., 2019). Thus urbanization with its associated environmental pollution could be a factor for increased prevalence of AD. To be sure, developing a link between environmental pollutions and AD with certainty is very difficult since the pollutant exposure is a chronic event, and one rarely sees the immediate skin inflammation after one such exposure. More details on the contributions of pollution in the development of AD are discussed in Chapter 9.

Evidence from atopic march

One interesting clinical manifestation of AD is the development of atopic march, which reports the development of noncutaneous atopic diseases such as food allergy, allergic rhinitis, and asthma preceded by the cutaneous atopic disease AD. Although some evidence suggests an internal immune deviation, other evidence points to the external exposure as an important influence factor. A report on findings from the recent workshop on "atopic dermatitis and the atopic march: mechanisms and interventions" conducted by the National Institute of Allergy and Infectious Diseases provides some insights. Exposure to family dogs at birth was inversely associated with development of AD and other allergy sensitization by age 1 year and recurrent wheezing by age 3 years. Moreover, a growing body of evidence has pointed to cutaneous exposure to environmental peanut allergen (through skin barrier defect) as a leader for food allergy development. In addition, patients with AD that progresses to food allergy, especially peanut allergy, has substantial increased risk of developing airway allergic disease. Accordingly, the recommendations from this workshop support investigations of the effectiveness of early prophylactic treatments of emollients or other skin barrier enhancers for the prevention of AD and atopic march (Davidson et al., 2019). Readers are encouraged to examine evidence pointing to internal immune dysregulation as a contributing factor for AD development in Chapter 18.

Summary

To summarize, there are many external factors identified in association with the development of AD or as potential contributing components for the development of AD. Among them are the colonization of pathogenic bacteria, other skin infections, allergens, and environmental pollutions. The big question is whether external factors alone are sufficient to induce AD or whether internal immune milieu alterations are also required to get the disease fired up. This question is germane since nearly all people are exposed to these external factors but only a fraction develop the AD disease. As of today, powerful evidences linking external factors to development of AD are limited to the colonization of the pathogenic species *S. aureus*. In Chapter 18 we will examine clinical evidences pointing to internal triggering factors that contribute to the development of AD.

Further readings

Bagnoli, F., Rappuoli, R., & Grandi, G. (Eds.), (2017). *Staphylococcus aureus: Microbiology, pathology, immunology, therapy and prophylaxis*. Springer.

Cavaillon, J.-M., & Singer, M. (Eds.), (2018). *Inflammation: From molecular and cellular mechanisms to the clinic*. Wiley-VCH.

de Nevers. N. (2017). *Air pollution control engineering*. Waveland Press.

Fowler, J. F., & Zirwas, M. J. (2019). *Fisher's contact dermatitis* (7th ed.). Contact Dermatitis Institute.

Ley, K. (Ed.), (2018). *Inflammation: Fundamental mechanisms*. World Scientific.

References

Bonamonte, D., Filoni, A., Vestita, M., Romita, P., Foti., C., & Angelini, G. (2019). The role of the environmental risk factors in the pathogenesis and clinical outcome of atopic dermatitis. *BioMed Research International*, *2019*, 2450605. https://doi.org/10.1155/2019/2450605.

Boonstra, M., Rustemeyer, T., & Middelkamp-Hup, M. A. (2018). Both children and adult patients with difficult-to-treat atopic dermatitis have high prevalences of concomitant allergic contact dermatitis and are frequently polysensitized. *Journal of the European Academy of Dermatology and Venereology*, *32*(9), 1554–1561. https://doi.org/10.1111/jdv.14973.

Byrd, A. L., Deming, C., Cassidy, S. K. B., Harrison, O. J., Ng, W. -I., Conlan, S., et al., (2017). *Staphylococcus aureus* and *Staphylococcus epidermidis* strain diversity underlying pediatric atopic dermatitis. *Science Translational Medicine*, *9*(397), eaal4651. https://doi.org/10.1126/scitranslmed.aal4651.

Clinical. (2019). Merriam-Webster online. https://merriam-webster.com/dictionary/clinical. Accessed 05.06.2019.

Crepy, M.-N., Nosbaum, A., & Bensefa-Colas, L. (2019). Blocking type 2 inflammation by dupilumab does not control classic (type 1-driven) allergic contact dermatitis in chronic hand eczema. *Contact Dermatitis*, *81*(2), 145–147. https://doi.org/10.1111/cod.13266.

Davidson, W. F., Leung, D. Y. M. , Beck, L. A., Berin, C. M., Boguniewicz, M., Busse, W. W., et al. (2019). Report from the National Institute of Allergy and Infectious Diseases workshop on 'atopic dermatitis and the atopic march: Mechanisms and interventions'. *The Journal of Allergy and Clinical Immunology*, *143*(3), 894–913. https://doi.org/10.1016/j.jaci.2019.01.003.

Dillon, S. R., Sprecher, C., Hammond, A., Bilsborough, J., Rosenfeld-Franklin, M., Presnell, et al. (2004). Interleukin 31, a cytokine produced by activated T cells, induces dermatitis in mice. *Nature Immunology*, *5*(7), 752–760. https://doi.org/10.1038/ni1084.

Gallo, R. L., & Nakatsuji, T. (2011). Microbial symbiosis with the innate immune defense system of the skin. *The Journal of Investigative Dermatology*, *131*(10), 1974–1980. https://doi.org/10.1038/jid.2011.182.

Geoghegan, J. A., Irvine, A. D., & Foster, T. J. (2018). *Staphylococcus aureus* and atopic dermatitis: A complex and evolving relationship. *Trends in Microbiology*, *26*(6), 484–497. https://doi.org/10.1016/j.tim.2017.11.008.

Hata, T. R., Kotol, P., Boguniewicz, M., Taylor, P., Paik, A., Jackson, M., Nguyen, M., et al. (2010). History of eczema herpeticum is associated with the inability to induce human b-defensin (HBD)-2, HBD-3 and cathelicidin in the skin of patients with atopic dermatitis. *British Journal of Dermatology*, *163*(3), 659–661. https://doi.org/10.1111/j.1365-2133.2010.09892x.

Howell, M. D., Wollenberg, A., Gallo, R. L., Flaig, M., Streib, J. E., Wong, C., Pavicic, T., et al. (2006). Cathelicidin deficiency predisposes to eczema herpeticum. *The Journal of Allergy and Clinical Immunology, 117*(4), 836–841.

Jacob, S. E., McGowan, M., Silverberg, N. B., Pelletier, J. L., Fonacier, L., Mousdicas, N. et al., (2017). Pediatric contact dermatitis registry data on contact allergy in children with atopic dermatitis. *JAMA Dermatology, 153*(8), 765–770. https://doi.org/10.1001/jamadermatol.2016.6136.

Lagrelius, M., Wahigren, C. F., Matura, M., Bergstrom, A., Kull, I., & Liden., C. (2019). Atopic dermatitis at preschool age and contact allergy in adolescence: A population-based cohort study. *The British Journal of Dermatology, 180*(4), 782–789. https://doi.org/10.1111/bjd.17449.

Lee, K. S., Oh, I. H., Choi, S. H., & Rha, Y. H. (2017). Analysis of epidemiology and risk factors of atopic dermatitis in Korean children and adolescents from the 2010 Korean national health and nutrition examination survey. *BioMed Research International, 2017*, 5142754. https://doi.org/10.1155/2017/5142754.

Lubbes, S., Rustemeyer, T., Sillevis Smitt, J. H., Schuttelaar, M.-L. A., & Middelkamp-Hup, M. A. (2017). Contact sensitization in Dutch children and adolescents with and without atopic dermatitis—a retrospective analysis. *Contact Dermatitis, 76*(3), 151–159. https://doi.org/10.1111/cod.12711.

Meylan, P., Lang, C., Mermound, S., Johannsen, A., Norrenberg, S., Hohl, D., et al. (2017). Skin colonization by *Staphylococcus aureus* precedes the clinical diagnosis of atopic dermatitis. *The Journal of Investigative Dermatology, 137*(12), 2497–2504. https://doi.org/10.1016/j.jid.2017.07.834.

Nakatsuji, T., & Gallo, R. L. (2019). The role of skin microbiome in atopic dermatitis. *Annals of Allergy, Asthma and Immunology, 122*(3), 263–269. https://doi.org/10.1016/j.anai.2018.12.003.

Oxford Living Dictionaries. 2019. Clinical. https://en.oxforddictionaries.com/definition/clinical. Accessed 05.06.2019.

Palmer, C. N. A., Irvine, A. D., Terron-Kwiatkowski, A., Zhao, Y., Liao, H., Lee, S. P., et al. (2006). Common loss-of-function variants of the epidermal barrier protein filaggrin are a major predisposing factor for atopic dermatitis. *Nature Genetics, 38*(4), 441–446. https://doi.org/10.1036/ng1767.

Pootongkam, S., & Nedorost, S. (2014). Allergic contact dermatitis in atopic dermatitis. *Current Treatment Option in Allergy, 1*, 329–336. https://doi.org/10.1007/s40521-014-0028-7.

Rac, H., Gould, A. P., Bookstaver, P. B., Justo, J. A., Kohn, J., & Al-Hasan, M. N. (2019). Evaluation of early clinical failure criteria for gram-negative bloodstream infections. *Clinical Microbiology and Infection, 26*(1), 73–77. https://doi.org/10.1016/j.cmi.2019.05.017.

Rastogi, S., Patel, K. R., Singam, V., & Silverberg, J. I. (2018). Allergic contact dermatitis to personal care products and topical medications in adults with atopic dermatitis. *Journal of the American Academy of Dermatology, 79*(6), 1028–1033, E6. https://doi.org/10.1016/j.jaad.2018.07.017.

Simonsen, A. B., Johansen, J. D., Deleuran, M., Mortz, C. G., & Sommerlund., M. (2017). Contact allergy in children with atopic dermatitis: A systematic review. *The British Journal of Dermatology, 177*(2), 395–405. https://doi.org/10.1111/bjd.15628.

Simonsen, A. B., Johansen, J. D., Deleuran, M., Mortz, C. G., Skov, L., & Sommerlund, M. (2018). Children with atopic dermatitis may have unacknowledged contact allergies contributing to their skin symptoms. *Journal of the European Academy of Dermatology and Venereology, 32*(3), 428–436. https://doi.org/10.1111/jdv.14737.

Sonkoly, E., Muller, A., Lauerma, A. I., Pivarcsi, A., Soto, H., Kemeny, L., et al. (2006). IL-31: A new link between T cells and pruritus in atopic skin inflammation. *The Journal of Allergy and Clinical Immunology, 117*(2), 411–417. https://doi.org/10.1016/j.jaci.2005.10.033.

Sun, D., & Ong, P. Y. (2017). Infectious complications in atopic dermatitis. *Immunology and Allergy Clinics of North America, 37*(1), 75–93. https://doi.org/10.1016/j.iac.2016.08.015.

Yi, S. J., Shon, C., Min, K. D., Kim, H. C., Leem, J. H., Kwon, H. J., et al. (2017). Association between exposure to traffic-related air pollution and prevalence of allergic diseases in children, Seoul, Korea. *BioMed Research International, 2017*, 4216107. https://doi.org/10.1155/2017/4216107.

11

Keratinocytes

LAWRENCE S. CHAN

KEY POINTS

- Epidermis is the outermost layer of skin surface that forms the first line of defense against invaders from the environment. Keratinocyte is the epidermis's principle cell type responsible for generating and maintaining the integrity of the epidermis.
- Besides being the structural foundation of the epidermis, keratinocytes also possess functions capable of interacting with their environment immunologically.
- Keratinocytes are capable of expressing neurologic factors that contribute to the itch sensation, which is a characteristic clinical finding in atopic dermatitis.
- Weakness of skin integrity at the epidermal level would allow easy entry of environmental pathogens or allergens into the skin, leading to chronic inflammatory processes as observed in atopic dermatitis.
- Internally altered immune milieu enhancing cytokines of helper T-cell subset 2 could trigger the release of proinflammatory components from epidermal keratinocytes, lessen keratinocyte's contribution to epidermal barrier, reduce keratinocyte's ability in wound healing, decrease keratinocyte's role in host defense, and thereby diminish the integrity of the skin and promote an inflammatory milieu of the skin and beyond.

Introduction

In this chapter, the roles of keratinocytes from an internal factor perspective are analyzed in relationship to the disease atopic dermatitis. Situated at the very surface of the human body, epidermis, the functional products of keratinocyte, is logically the first line of defense to ensure the body's safety against invading enemies, whatever they may be. Daily, the human body is being attacked by countless invaders: bacteria, fungi, viruses, parasites, chemicals, allergens, pollutants, and the like. For most of the invading incidences, the body manages them handily by physically blocking their entry inside, thanks to skin defense. From time to time, however, the first line of defense, the skin, is weakened or damaged either by internal defects or by external factors. These unwanted invaders enter the body through the skin

portal, causing harm and disease. Atopic dermatitis, manifested as itchy, chronic, inflammatory lesions primarily in exposed skin areas, is generally recognized to be due in part to the compromise of skin integrity, an internal factor. We have thoroughly discussed the external factors contributing to the disease when the skin barrier is weakened in the previous section of this book. In this section, we will examine what internal factors could contribute to the disease development. Since keratinocyte is the major cell type that forms the skeleton of the epidermis, it is therefore prudent to examine the role of keratinocyte in relationship to the development of atopic dermatitis. In this chapter, the structural and functional roles of keratinocyte in the skin integrity are first discussed, followed by examination of sensation, wound healing, and immunologic roles of keratinocyte in the skin, and then by delineation of the structural and immunologic effects on keratinocyte by three of the prominent atopic dermatitis-related cytokines, interleukin-10 (IL10), IL13, and particularly IL4. Studies have documented that these three cytokines are upregulated in the skin of patients affected by atopic dermatitis. In addition, IL4 is determined to be the sole initiating factor in an animal model of atopic dermatitis (Chan, Robinson, & Xu, 2001).

Keratinocyte: Roles in skin structure and integrity

It is best to demonstrate the structural and functional roles of keratinocyte when we view them from a histologic (tissue level) perspective (i.e., to see the location and the relative abundance of keratinocytes in the epidermis and the proximal relationship between keratinocytes and other cell types that are involved in the immune functions). Fig. 11.1 depicts this information visually. As illustrated, keratinocyte is the principle cell type of the epidermis. From findings of accumulative research studies, we now know that keratinocytes are responsible for the structural integrity of the epidermis and to some extent the entire skin. It is now clear that the basal (lowest) layer of the keratinocytes are the epidermal stem cells, which proliferate and give birth to keratinocytes that will differentiate and move to the upper layers of the epidermis. With proper calcium condition, the keratinocytes differentiate. As the differentiated keratinocytes move up toward the superficial portion of the skin, they form the suprabasal cell layer, then the granular layer, and die and convert into a keratin layer, the stratum corneum

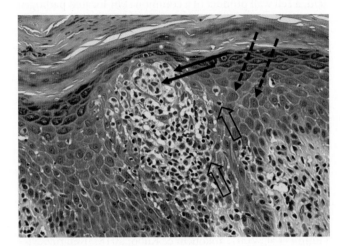

• **Fig. 11.1** Histology of inflamed human skin (atopic dermatitis) depicting the keratinocytes as the major epidermal cell type and the proximal relationship between keratinocytes *(dotted arrows)* and immune cells. Lymphocytes are abundantly observed in this histology at both the epidermis and the dermis as round, small cells with basophilic nuclei *(hollow arrows)*. Langerhans cells have larger cytoplasm and pale basophilic nuclei *(solid arrows)*.

of the skin. In Fig. 11.1, one can also observe two common immune cells present in the skin, the lymphocytes and the Langerhans cells.

Roles in epidermal structure

Looking at the epidermis from a brick-and-mortar model, the keratinocyte, being the major (90%) cellular component of the epidermis, has the right to be considered the bricks of the epidermis (see Fig. 11.1). What about the mortar aspect of the equation? Between adjacent cells, keratinocyte-produced intercellular proteins (desmogleins and desmocollins) and intracellular proteins (plakoglobin, desmoplakins, plakophilins, intermediate filaments, etc.) form intercellular structures called desmosomes and other adherence components that act as strong bonding to glue the epidermis together (Fig. 11.2). When one of these intercellular components (e.g., desmoglein) is weakened either by external factors such as bacterial toxin or by internal causes such as autoantibodies, the adherence and coherence of epidermis are lost, resulting in keratinocyte cell-cell separation (acantholysis), leading to intraepidermal blister formation and epidermal loss. An excellent clinical example in support of the epidermal coherence functions of keratinocyte is staphylococcal scalded skin syndrome, which occurs when the bacterial endotoxin breaks down desmoglein-1, leading to blister formation (Amagai, Matsuyoshi, Wang, Andi, & Stanley., 2000). Pemphigus vulgaris, a life-threatening form

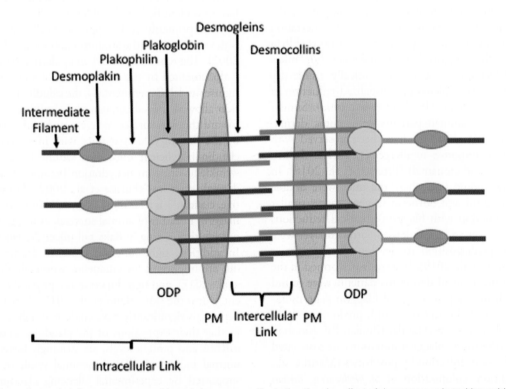

• **Fig. 11.2** A schematic presentation of a human epidermal desmosome, illustrating the glue effect of desmosomes in making epidermis a coherent tissue by their cell-cell connections. The intercellular linking is accomplished by desmogleins and desmocollins, whereas the intracellular linking is achieved by intermediate filaments, desmoplakin, plakophilin, plakoglobin, and the anchoring outer dense plaque *(ODP)*. *PM*, Plasma membrane of keratinocyte. (From Garrod, D., & Chidgey, M. (2007). Desmosome structure, composition and function. *Biochimica et Biophysica Acta, 1778*(3), 572–587; Najor, N. A. (2018). Desmosomes in human disease. *Annual Review of Pathology, 13*, 51–70.)

of intraepidermal blistering skin disease due to autoantibodies against desmogleins-1 and -3 and other nondesmoglein adhering proteins, provides another strong clinical evidence for the important role of keratinocyte in epidermal integrity (Chan, 2016; Spindler et al., 2018).

Roles in barrier proteins: Stratum corneum

To prevent undesirable substance or pathogens from entering the skin, keratinocytes produce proteins and form the corresponding protein-dominant physical barriers between the skin and the outside world in a form of keratin layer (i.e., the stratum corneum). Keratinocytes are the sole cell type that provides these proteins, which include filaggrin, involucrin, and loricrin (McLean, 2016; Smith et al., 2006). Filaggrin, a protein with an apparent molecular weight of 37 kD, is derived from a high-molecular-weight precursor profilaggrin (Fleckman, Beverly, & Karen, 1985). Filaggrin gene mutations have been documented in European patients with ichthyosis vulgaris and atopic dermatitis initially (Palmer et al., 2006; Smith et al., 2006) and have subsequently been identified in other populations in a worldwide distribution (Debinska, Danielewicz, Drabik-Chamerska, Kalita, & Boznanski, 2017; Enomoto et al., 2008; Margolis et al., 2018; Pigors et al., 2018). Clinical evidence supports their skin barrier functional roles. For example, filaggrin gene loss-of-function mutations, particularly the *R501X* mutation, has been significantly linked to allergen polysensitivity (defined as positivity to three or more allergic compounds) in patch testing, supporting the notion that a defect of filaggrin allows the easy penetration of allergen into the skin to trigger allergic reactions (Elhaji et al., 2019). In the filaggrin-deficient flaky tail (*ft/ft*) mice, skin barrier defect was evident from clinically visible dry skin and from electron microscopy-visualized reduction of stratum corneum contents (Presland et al., 2000). Similar to polysensitivity in human patients with atopic dermatitis, these flaky tail mice also have been observed with increased immune responses to allergens (nickel, 2, 4-dinitrofluorobenzene, and cinnamal) (Petersen et al., 2018). In an experimental mouse line where the mice were double deficient for filaggrin and hornerin (a gene shares similar structure and function with filaggrin), marked reductions of skin granular layer and a condensed cornified layer were observed, with predisposition to develop allergic contact dermatitis (Rahrig et al., 2019). In a study performed in the Indian subcontinent, hand dermatitis patients were found to have a much higher percentage of filaggrin gene mutation (33.7% vs. 3.5% in control group), predominantly in the S2889X polymorphism (Handa, Khullar, Pal, Kamboj, De, 2019). Furthermore, filaggrin mutations are associated with increased risk of infection by poxviruses (Manti et al., 2017). In addition, colonization of *Staphylococcus aureus* is significantly increased in atopic dermatitis patients with filaggrin mutations (Clausen et al., 2017). Elimination of filaggrin gene expression in keratinocytes (knocked down by lentivirus) not only led to loss of skin barrier protein

filaggrin production but also resulted in inhibition of keratinocyte cell adhesion, migration, and proliferation and in promotion of apoptosis and altered cell cycle progression (Dang, Ma, Meng, An, Pang, 2016).

Normal skin barrier functions could also be weakened by external substances. For example, exposure to lipoteichoic acid, a cell wall product of a common skin-located pathogen *S. aureus*, could lead to decreased expression of skin barrier proteins filaggrin and loricrin (Brauweiler, Goleva, & Leung, 2019).

Roles in barrier proteins: Epidermal tight junction

The second type of physical skin barrier structure, besides the stratum corneum mentioned already, is the tight junction—the intercellular junction sealing assembly between adjacent keratinocytes in the stratum granulosum, just below the stratum corneum (Basler et al., 2016; Brandner et al., 2002, 2015; Furuse et al., 2002; Kitajima, Eguchi, Ohno, Mori, & Yaoita, 1983; Pummi et al., 2001; Yokouchi & Kubo, 2018). Keratinocytes are the providers of these tight junction proteins. A schematic presentation of an epidermal tight junction is shown in Fig. 11.3. Several epidermal tight junction–associated mRNAs have been identified in human keratinocytes, including claudins-1, -4, -7, -8, -11, -12, -17, -23, ZO (zonula occludens), and occludin (De Benedetto, Rafaels et al., 2011; Furuse et al., 2002; Pummi et al., 2001). While claudin-1 protein has been identified in all epidermal cell layers, ZO-1 protein is found primarily in the uppermost cell layers, and occludin is detected only in the stratum granulosum (Brandner et al., 2002). The role of claudin-1 in epidermal barrier protection is documented by the construction of a claudin-1–deficient mouse model. Experimentally, the caludin-1–deficient mouse skin allowed the subcutaneously administered tracer diffuse toward the skin surface, whereas such diffusion was blocked by the skin of wild type mice with intact claudin-1. These claudin-1–deficient mice died within 1 day of birth with wrinkled skin from dehydration because of severe transepidermal water loss (Furuse et al., 2002). From this perspective, claudin-1 is a far more essential skin barrier protein than filaggrin in terms of animal survival, as filaggrin deficiency is not life threatening in flaky tail mice (Presland et al., 2000). In addition, tight junction proteins claudin-1 and occludin are important for cutaneous wound healing (Volksdorf et al., 2017), and tight junction is a physical blocker for viral entry into the skin (Rahn et al., 2017). Patients with atopic dermatitis significantly have epidermal tight junction defects in that their expressions of the claudin-1 and -23, in both mRNA and protein levels, are strikingly lower compared to normal individuals. The functional result of this defect is supported by experimental silencing claudin-1 expression in mice, which leads to diminishing tight junction function (De Benedetto, Rafaels et al., 2011; De Benedetto, Slifka et al., 2011; Duan et al., 2016; Furuse et al., 2002). The reduction of claudin-1 expressions occurs only in lesional skin

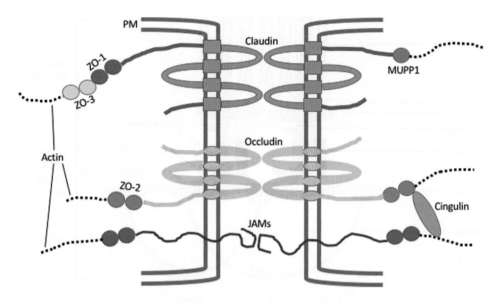

• **Fig. 11.3** Schematic presentation of a human epidermal tight junction, illustrating these structures and structural components that provide a second physical skin barrier function. *JAMs*, Junctional adhesion molecules; *MUPP1*, multi-PDZ protein-1; *PM*, plasma membranes of keratinocytes at the stratum granulosum level; *ZO*, zonula occludens. (From Basler, K., et al. (2016). The role of tight junctions in skin barrier function and dermal absorption. *Journal of Controlled Release, 242*, 105–118.)

(not in nonlesional skin) of atopic dermatitis patients, suggesting the reduction is related to the inflammatory process and not because of genetic mutation (Yuki, Toblishi, Kusaka-Kikushima, Ota, & Tokura, 2016). This inflammation-induced reduction of lesional skin claudin-1 in atopic dermatitis is supported by a study conducted in human epidermal equivalent, documenting the suppression of keratinocytes' claudin-1 by a trio of atopic dermatitis-related cytokines, IL4, IL13, and IL31 (Gruber et al., 2015). The tight junction protein expression, formation, and function are also influenced and regulated by a variety of proteins, enzymes, and cytokines, including IL1, CD44, somatostatin, kinase-directed phosphorylation, a Rho-family protein GTPases Rac, activation of toll-like receptor-2 (TLR2), epidermal growth factor receptor (EGFR), adenosine triphosphate (ATP)–powered calcium-pump protein 2C1, histamine, IL33, IL17, enolase-1, antimicrobial peptide LL37, keratin-76, integrin-linked kinase, activated protease-activated receptor-2, and receptor tyrosine kinase EphA2 (Akiyama et al., 2014; Aono, & Yohei, 2008; DiTommaso et al., 2014; Gschwandtner et al., 2013; Kirschner et al., 2011; Mertens, Rygiel, Olivo, van der Kammen, & Collard, 2005; Nadeau, Henehan, & De Benedetto, 2018; Perez White et al., 2017; Raiko et al., 2012; Roziomiy & Markov, 2010; Ryu et al., 2018; Sayedyahossein, Rudkouskaya, Leclerc, & Dagnino, 2016; Tohgasaki et al., 2018; Tran et al., 2012; Vockel, Breitenbach, Kreienkamp, & Brandner, 2010; Yuki et al., 2011, 2016).

Roles in epidermal-dermal adhesion

Keratinocytes are essential providers not only for structure and proteins needed for the integrity of the epidermis but also for the proteins that contribute to the adherence between the epidermis and dermis, the dermal-epidermal junction,

or skin basement membrane zone. This role is accomplished through the keratinocytes' synthesis of several important skin basement membrane anchoring proteins, α6β4-integrin (Vidal et al., 1995), type XVII collagen (or bullous pemphigoid antigen II) (Giudice, Daryl, & Luis, 1992), type VII collagen (Parente et al., 1991), and laminin 5/laminin 332 (Marinkovich, Lunstrum, & Burgeson, 1992), which are essential connecting components of the skin basement membrane at the junction between epidermis and dermis (Fig. 11.4) (Has, Nystrom, Hossein Saeidian, Bruckner-Tuderman, & Uitto, 2018). The functional importance of these keratinocyte-produced skin basement membrane components is vividly illustrated in both genetic skin diseases (epidermolysis bullosa group of diseases) and autoimmune skin diseases. When these keratinocyte-produced skin basement membrane components are weakened either by genetic defect (Aberdam et al., 1994; Christiano et al., 1993; Jonkman et al., 1995; Vidal et al., 1995) or by assault from autoantibodies in autoimmune diseases (Kirtschig, Peter Marinkovich, Burgeson, & Yancey, 1995; Ujiie et al., 2014; Woodley et al., 1988), the whole skin integrity is compromised, leading to dermal-epidermal separation, subepidermal blister formation, and even epidermis loss. In addition, keratinocytes synthesize another lower lamina lucida 105-kD protein that has yet to be fully characterized. When this 105-kD protein was targeted by autoantibodies from a patient, skin weakness occurred and subepidermal blisters developed, further supporting a role of keratinocytes in skin basement membrane stability (Chan et al., 1993, 1995).

Keratinocyte: Roles in cutaneous sensation

Recently, the traditional concept that intraepidermal nerve fibers are the sole transducers of neural signal has been

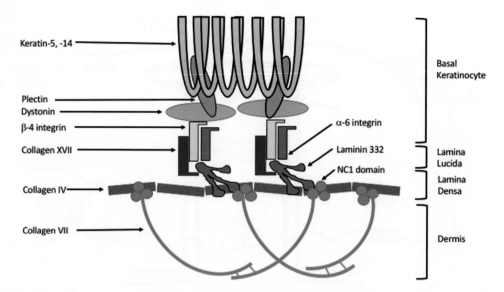

• **Fig. 11.4** Schematic presentation of a human skin basement membrane zone, illustrating the locations of various structural components and the relationship between basal keratinocytes and the basement membrane components. Importantly, the keratinocyte-producing proteins, α6β4-integrin, type XVII collagen, together with laminin 332, anchor the basal keratinocytes through the lamina lucida and onto the lamina densa. From there, type VII collagen, also a product of keratinocytes, helps anchor to the dermis. Collaboratively, these adhesion protein connections firmly link the basal cell to the basement membrane and the dermis. (From Shinkuma, S., McMillan, J. R., & Shimizu, H. (2011). Ultrastructure and molecular pathogenesis of epidermolysis bullosa. *Clinical Dermatology, 29*(4), 412–419.)

challenged, and the role of keratinocytes in neural signaling is proposed. The putative sensory role of keratinocyte was proposed based on the findings that keratinocytes express diverse sensory receptors that are present in sensory neurons such as transient receptor potential vallinoid-1 (TRPV1) and TRPV4 (Luo et al., 2018; Talagas & Misery, 2019). Since TRPV1 is a known transducer for pain, heat, and to a less extent itch, and TRPV4 is a heat transducer, keratinocytes' roles for cutaneous sensation cannot be neglected. Moreover, the findings that specific and selective activation of TRPV1 in keratinocytes can induce pain and that targeted stimulation of TRPV4 in keratinocytes can result in itch sensation leading to scratch behavior support a potential role of keratinocytes in skin sensation (Chen et al., 2016; Talagas & Misery, 2019). Moreover, lineage-specific deletion of keratinocyte TRPV4 reduced chronic itch in animal model (Luo et al., 2018). In addition, the findings that keratinocytes possess neuropeptide substance P and that keratinocytes express nerve growth factor, in response to neuropeptide activation of the ERK1/2 and JNK MAPK transcriptional pathways, also support their roles in cutaneous sensation (Shi, Wang, David Clark, & Kingery, 2013). The relevance of this keratinocyte's role in skin sensation in the disease of atopic dermatitis is that eczema is well characterized for its pruritic clinical presentation (Yosipovitch, Berger, & Fassett, 2020).

Keratinocyte: Role in wound healing

When skin is injured, the repair process will be initiated. The sequence of events in wound healing starts with hemostasis (to stop blood loss), inflammation (to stop invaders), angiogenesis

(to repair blood supply for nutrient and oxygen delivery), growth (to restore dermal structures), reepithelialization (to close epidermal gap and seal off external barrier), and remodeling (to fine-tune structure and function). On a cellular level, the wound healing process mobilizes a variety of cells and involves spatial and temporal synchronization of many cellular and molecular actions. The near last step of wound healing is the process of reepithelialization where keratinocytes play the most important role. In essence, this process will involve proliferation of epidermal stem cells at the basal layer of the epidermal wound edge and differentiation of hair follicle unipotent stem cells to keratinocytes. The subsequent formation of epithelial tongues (migration front), migration of these keratinocytes across the dermal wound bed, and differentiation of these keratinocytes into suprabasal, granular, and stratum corneum layers will accomplish the epidermal barrier repair (Rodrigues, Kosaric, Bonham, & Gurtner, 2019). IL4, the major cytokine that positively influences the development of atopic dermatitis, also seems to play a negative role in wound healing. In an animal model of atopic dermatitis triggered by an overexpression of IL4 in the basal epidermis, reepithelization and final wound healing were delayed compared to that of wild type mice; and such delay would likely have negative consequence for atopic dermatitis, as it will prolong the skin barrier defect that allows external invaders to enter the skin, thus flaming the ongoing inflammatory responses (Zhao, Bao, Chan, DiPietro, & Chen, 2016).

Keratinocyte: Roles in immune regulation

As depicted in Fig. 11.1, at the tissue level, keratinocytes are in physical contact with immune cells such as lymphocytes and

Langerhans cells. Since lymphocytes are the major immune cells in the adaptive immune system responsible for immune memory and the effector cells for defense against previously recognized pathogens, their proximal relationship to keratinocytes is worth noting. The importance of this keratinocyte-lymphocyte relationship is even more pronounced given the facts that there are nearly twice the amount of lymphocytes present in the skin than those present in the circulation and that most CLA+ memory effector T cells are located in the skin, as recently reported in the scientific literature (Clark et al., 2006). Langerhans cells are the professional antigen-presenting cells responsible for immune recognition and immune activation. Vaccination through epidermis-restricted microperforation can effectively activate keratinocytes and Langerhans cells, resulting in excellent antibody responses (Herve et al., 2019). In addition, Langerhans cells are also responsible for maintaining skin homeostasis by activating resident regulatory T cells (Seneschal, Clark, Gehad, Baecher-Allan, & Kupper, 2012). In the following paragraphs, the roles of keratinocytes in both innate and adaptive immune responses will be discussed.

Role in innate immune responses

Keratinocytes produce skin-localized antimicrobial substances, which can be a good and immediately available defense against invading microorganism, by mounting their innate immune responses.

Normal human keratinocytes regularly produce, usually in response to injury or infection challenge, many antimicrobial peptides (also described as host defense peptides) known for their innate immune defense functions. These peptides include two major families: human β-defensins and cathelicidins, and others (Niyonsaba, Kiatsurayanon, & Ogawa, 2016; Schauber & Gallo, 2008; Takahashi & Gallo 2017). Besides maintaining a homeostasis with commensal microorganisms in a symbiosis manner, these peptides function to defend against invading bacteria, viruses, fungi, and to a less extent parasites. They can also activate surrounding cells, keratinocytes or immune cells, to regulate many biologic functions, including angiogenesis, epithelialization, and immunity. Sometimes the roles of these peptides are also implicated in allergic disease, including atopic dermatitis (Niyonsaba et al., 2016). In atopic dermatitis patients, some of these peptides failed to be properly induced, thus allowing infection to set in (Takahashi & Gallo 2017). Although cathelicidins are also produced by neutrophils and other immune cells, besides keratinocytes, their strategic location at the front layer of the skin (therefore being the first to encounter pathogens) makes keratinocytes' roles in host defense particularly important. β-defensins are primarily located in epithelial surfaces, including the skin (Chieosilapathem, Ogawa, & Niyonsaba, 2017).

Keratinocytes, when encountering pathogens, can respond by releasing immune substances. In the presence of West Nile virus infection, human keratinocytes release type I and type III interferon inflammatory responses, including mRNAs of CXCL10 and interferon-induced proteins, as well other proinflammatory cytokines and chemokines, including tumor necrosis factor-α (TNF-α), IL6, CXCL1, CXCL2, CXCL8, and CCL20 (Garcia et al., 2018).

One of the common skin infections encountered by humans is from fungi. When exposed to dermatophytes in culture, human keratinocytes upregulate their mRNAs of many cytokines and chemokines, including IL1, IL2, IL4, IL6, IL8, IL10, IL13, IL15, IL16, IL17, and interferon-gamma (IFN-γ), and significantly increase secretion, compared to control, of many cytokines and chemokines, including eotaxin, eotaxin-2, G-CSF, GMCSF, ICAM-1, IFN-γ, IL1, IL2, IL3, IL4, IL6, IL7, IL8, IL13, IL15, IL16, IL17, IP10, and MCP-1 (Shiraki, Ishibashi, Hiruma, Nishikawa, & Ikeda, 2006).

Besides the cytokines and chemokines reported in human keratinocytes in responding to pathogen exposure, other cytokine present in keratinocyte includes IL20 (Blumberg et al., 2001). Furthermore, keratinocytes express many adhesion, activation, or cytokine receptors on their cell surfaces, including IL4R, IL20R, IL31R, CD95, IFN-γR1/CD119, IL2Rγ/CD132, ICAM-1, HLA-DR, and B7/BB1 (Blumberg et al., 2001; Cornelissen et al., 2012; El Darzi, Bazzi, Daoud, Echtay, Bahr, 2017; Junghans, 1996; Prens et al., 1996). Therefore, with a variety of immune receptors, keratinocytes can respond to immune signals, cytokines, and other stimulatory signals released by other cells. Their responses in turn would result in changing of immune milieu.

One of the most recent findings implicating keratinocyte's roles in atopic dermatitis is the acryl hydrocarbon receptor (AhR) on the surface of keratinocytes (Hidaka et al., 2017; Kim, Kim, Chung, Choi, & Park, 2014). The expression of this receptor, critical for the effects of major environmental pollutants on the human body, is highly upregulated in the skin of patients with atopic dermatitis (Kim et al., 2014). Consistent to this observation is the documentation that a transgenic mouse line constitutively expressing AhR in keratinocytes developed severe inflammatory skin lesions resembling atopic dermatitis in human patients (Tauchi et al., 2005). Experimentally, the link between AhR and atopic dermatitis is determined to be in the activation of AhR, leading to induced expression of artemin, alloknesis, epidermal hyperinnervation, severe pruritus, and the subsequent inflammatory process (Hidaka et al., 2017). Artemin is a member of the glial cell line–derived neurotrophic factor family with a variety of neuronal functions (Ikeda-Miyagawa et al., 2015). Alloknesis is a term describing abnormal itch sensation that can be induced by innocuous stimuli and by the absence of a keratinocyte-expressing and endogenous corticosteroid-activating enzyme 11β-hydroxysteroid dehydrogenase-1 (Matsumoto, Murota, Terao, & Katayama, 2018).

Role in adaptive immune responses

In addition to their innate immune functions, studies have pointed to a bigger role of keratinocytes in skin adaptive immunity. Keratinocytes can also orchestrate T-cell immunity in various adaptive immune responses (Klicznik, Szenes-Nagy, Campbell, & Gratz., 2018; Richmond et al., 2017). In a study aiming to examine the antigen-presenting abilities of keratinocyte, investigators generated a transgenic mouse model in which these epidermal cells exclusively present a myelin basic protein (MBP) peptide covalently linked to the major histocompatibility complex class II β-chain, under inflammatory conditions. These researchers found that inflammation induced by epicutaneous contact sensitization led to an expansion of MBP-specific CD4+ T cells in the skin. In addition, repeated applications of contact sensitizer to these mice preceding a systemic MBP immune administration, a classic method of immune desensitization, reduced the reactivity of these MBP-specific T cells and lessened the symptoms of the resulting experimental autoimmune encephalitis. Thus keratinocytes are shown that they can present antigen to T cells, and presenting neo-self antigen under the inflamed condition by keratinocyte can modulate CD4+ T cells' autoimmune aggressiveness at a distant organ (Meister et al., 2015). In another experimental study, coculture of epidermal professional antigen-presenting Langerhans cells with T cells in the presence of keratinocytes resulted in an enhanced acquired immunity compared to the condition in the absence of keratinocytes, suggesting a role of keratinocyte in augmenting antigen presentation (Sugita et al., 2007). The proximity of keratinocytes to Langerhans cells and lymphocytes in the epidermis also supports this role from a histologic perspective (see Fig. 11.1). In another experiment where human CD40 was transgenically expressed in mice under the control of keratin-14 promoter, which drives CD40 expression in basal keratinocytes exclusively, selective engagement of keratinocyte CD40 resulted in enhanced cell-mediated immune responses, supporting a notion that CD40 engagement by keratinocyte could amplify cutaneous and regional T-cell immune responses in vivo (Fuller, Nishmura, & Noelle, 2002). In an animal model of vitiligo using a conditional STAT-1–knockout mouse, investigators have discovered that the keratinocyte-generated IFN-γ signaling was essential for proper T-cell homing to the epidermis and for the disease progression, without the need of participation from professional immune cells, endogenous T cells, Langerhans cells, or γδ T cells (Richmond et al., 2017). A 2019 publication documented that the MHCII expressions in keratinocytes could be induced by association with commensal bacteria (*Staphylococcus epidermidis*), thus these friendly bugs could promote the antigen-presenting abilities of keratinocytes for the purpose of host defense (Tamoutounour et al., 2019).

Keratinocyte's barrier proteins: Impacts of IL4 and other Th2 cytokines

IL4, the most important cytokine in the helper T-cell subset 2 (Th2) family, has significant involvement in the development of atopic dermatitis (Beck et al., 2014; Chan et al.,

2001). In its absence, the IL4-knockout mice showed a substantial reduction of serum levels of immunoglobulin E (IgE), which is essential for allergic skin reaction and typically elevated in human patients affected by atopic dermatitis (Kuhn, Rajewsky, & Muller, 1991). In fact, the most significant way IL4 exhibits in relationship to atopic dermatitis is in a mouse model of atopic dermatitis, in which IL4 has been transgenically inserted and expressed in basal epidermis through a promoter of keratin-14, a basal keratinocyte-located keratin (Chan et al., 2001). The keratin-14/IL4 transgenic mice (but not the nontransgenic mice) spontaneously developed a very itchy and chronically inflammatory skin disease primarily affecting the hairless skin of mice (Fig. 11.5), with high total serum IgE, staphylococcal skin infection, and prominent skin infiltration of lymphocytes, mast cells, and eosinophils (Fig. 11.6) (Chan et al., 2001). Using clinical criteria for human atopic dermatitis, the manifestations of these diseased mice fulfill the diagnostic criteria for human atopic dermatitis (Hanifin & Rajka, 1980). From a different angle, a recently successful treatment of atopic dermatitis by the biologic medication dupilumab, a humanized antibody directly against IL4 receptor alpha, provides another strong support for the essential role of IL4 in atopic dermatitis development (Beck et al., 2014; Blauvelt et al., 2017). Therefore it is both academically interesting and theoretically important to examine what the results of interaction between IL4 and keratinocyte would show and how these results would affect the skin environment in a way that is contributing to the development or sustaining the disease atopic dermatitis. Toward that end, we seek to answer the question, How are epidermal keratinocytes impacted when the internally altered immune system produces and releases an excessive amount of IL4?

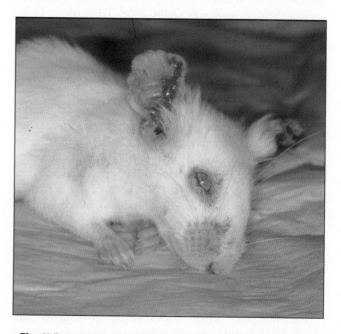

• **Fig. 11.5** Clinical photograph of a keratin-14/IL4 transgenic mouse, showing the acute inflammatory lesions located primarily in hairless skin surfaces.

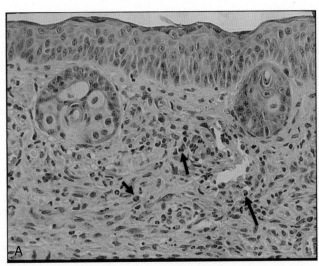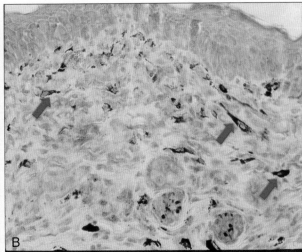

• **Fig. 11.6** Histopathology of a chronic skin lesion obtained from a keratin-14/IL4 transgenic mouse. Prominent mononuclear cell infiltration is visualized here, as well as some eosinophils *(arrows)* (A, hematoxylin & eosin stain). Numerous mast cells *(arrows)* are present in a chronic skin lesion (B, Giemsa stain). Some histologic changes in the epidermis, including acanthosis (thickening), and spongiosis are observed (A, B).

Th2 cytokines and keratinocyte's physical barrier proteins

Experimental data now clearly show that IL4 negatively impacts keratinocyte's abilities to produce the essential epidermal barrier protein production (Bao, Alexander, Zhang, Shen, & Chan, 2016a; Bao, Zhang, Mohan, Shen, & Chan, 2016b; Bao et al., 2017). In the following paragraphs the details of these impacts are depicted.

IL4 suppresses involucrin mRNA and protein production

Involucrin, one of the skin barrier proteins synthesized by keratinocyte, showed reduced expression in the lesional skin of atopic dermatitis patients, using ELISA on human skin extracts (Seguchi et al., 1996). In the nonlesional skin of the keratin-14/IL4 transgenic mice, we found that the mRNA and protein levels of involucrin are substantially reduced, compared to the wild type mice, suggesting that the involucrin reduction was likely due to the impact of IL4, not by an inflammatory process per se (Bao, Alexander et al., 2016a). To determine if IL4 could affect the expression of this protein, immortalized human keratinocyte HaCaT cells exposed to IL4 in different concentrations for 24 hours were extracted for examination of the mRNA expressions of involucrin by reverse transcription and then real-time polymerase chain reaction (PCR) in our laboratory. IL4 suppresses the involucrin expressions in a dose-dependent manner. This downregulation of involucrin in the protein level by IL4 was also confirmed by Western blot analysis (Fig. 11.7) (Bao, Alexander et al., 2016a). In addition, this IL4 suppression mechanism has been attributed to the Stat6 signaling pathway experimentally (Bao, Alexander et al., 2016a). This finding supports the notion that internal

immune dysregulation with IL4 upregulation can by itself lead to a reduction of skin barrier protein involucrin, thus impairing the skin barrier function.

IL4 downregulates loricrin mRNA and protein levels

Another skin barrier protein produced by keratinocyte is loricrin, which is also downregulated in the skin of atopic dermatitis patients (Kim, Leung, Boguniewicz, & Howell, 2008). To screen for the potential impact of IL4 on loricrin expressions, we examined nonlesional skin from the keratin-14/IL4 transgenic mice for the mRNA and protein levels by reverse transcription real-time PCR and Western blot analysis. After we determined that both mRNA and protein levels of loricrin were downregulated in the IL4 transgenic mice skin, we incubated IL4 with primary human keratinocyte in culture to examine its direct impact on loricrin expression. Just like the experimental results shown in the involucrin study, IL4 substantially downregulated the mRNA and protein levels of loricrin (Fig. 11.8) (Bao et al., 2017). Furthermore, we also determined that the IL4 regulatory mechanism on loricrin was through the Stat6 signaling channel, the same pathway involved in involucrin (Bao, Alexander et al., 2016a; Bao et al., 2017).

Combined IL4/IL13 reduces filaggrin expression

The expression of another important skin barrier protein, filaggrin, is similarly decreased in the lesional and nonlesional skin of patients affected by atopic dermatitis (Seguchi et al., 1996). In examination for the effects of Th2 cytokine on its expression, IL4, in combination with

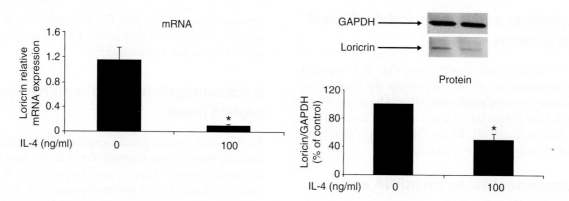

A   mRNA

B   Protein

Involucrin →

GAPDH →

IL-4 (ng/ml)   0   20   50   100   IL-4 (ng/ml)   0   20

• **Fig. 11.7** The mRNA and protein of involucrin, a skin barrier protein component, are downregulated by the presence of IL4 in a dose-dependent manner. HaCat cells, from a human keratinocyte cell line, were incubated with increasing concentrations of IL4 for 24 hours and their mRNA (panel A) and protein (panel B) levels were analyzed with real-time RT-PCR and Western blot methods, respectively. Human glyceraldehyde 3-phosphate dehydrogenase (GAPDH) was used as an internal control. (Reprint with author permission from Bao, L., Alexander, J. B., et al. (2016). Interleukin-4 downregulation of involucrin expression in human epidermal keratinocytes involves Stat6 sequestration of the coactivator CREB-binding protein. *Journal of Interferon & Cytokine Research, 36*, 374–381.)

mRNA

GAPDH ——

Loricrin ——

Protein

IL-4 (ng/ml)   0   100

IL-4 (ng/ml)   0   100

• **Fig. 11.8** The skin barrier protein component loricrin suppressed by IL4 in both mRNA and protein levels. Primary human keratinocytes were incubated with or without IL4 for 24 hours and their mRNA *(left panel)* and protein *(right panel)* were assayed by real-time RT-PCR and Western blot analyses, respectively. Human glyceraldehyde 3-phosphate dehydrogenase (GAPDH) was used as an internal control. "*" = "$p < 0.05$, compared to medium only (without IL-4)." (Reprint with author permission from Bao, L., et al. (2017). A molecular mechanism for IL-4 suppression of loricrin transcription in epidermal keratinocytes: Implication for atopic dermatitis pathogenesis. *Innate Immunity, 23*(8), 641–647.)

IL13, another Th2 cytokine upregulated in atopic dermatitis, significantly reduced the expression of filaggrin. Using real-time PCR performed on extracted mRNAs from normal and immortalized human keratinocyte in culture with or without cytokines, the combination of Th2 cytokines IL4/IL13 (50 mg/mL) significantly reduced the mRNAs of filaggrin (normalized with β-actin mRNAs), compared to media control, whereas the Th1 cytokine IFN-γ acted the opposite way. The mechanism of such filaggrin alternation by Th2 cytokines might be through upregulation of filaggrin proteinases kallikreins (KLK), KLK7, KLK5, matriptase, and channel-acting serine proteases-1 (CAP1) and through downregulation of caspase 14 (Di et al., 2016). Therefore dysregulation of internal immune milieu that results in upregulation of IL14 and IL13, such as documented in patients with atopic dermatitis, might cause the reduction of skin barrier protein filaggrin, leading to an immune-mediated, rather than a gene-based, skin barrier defect in those patients with no filaggrin gene mutation.

IL4 abrogates stratum corneum cohesion

Another experimental data supporting the disruptive role of IL4 on skin barrier function is revealed by a study that shows its effects of stratum corneum. Repeated injections of IL4 into hairless mice dermis, below the epidermis, resulted in compromised stratum corneum cohesion, possibly because of IL4's effect to reduce epidermal cell differentiation as it decreased the expression of desmoglein-1 (assayed by semiquantitative reverse transcription-polymerase chain reaction (RT-PCR)) and the amount of corneodesmosomes (revealed by electron microscopy) (Hatano et al., 2013). Corneodesmosome is a class of proteins that functions to hold together the corneocytes, terminally differentiated keratinocytes of stratum corneum. Degradation of corneosome would lead to desquamation (Pierard, Goffin, Hermanns-Le, & Pierard-Franchimont, 2000).

IL13 suppresses skin basement membrane proteins type IV collagen and integrin-α6

Interestingly, the atopic dermatitis–related cytokine, IL13, also exerts downregulatory effects on the in vitro synthesis of type IV collagen and integrin-α6 using a skin equivalent as study model. These effects correlate with the reduction of these two proteins in the skin of patients with atopic dermatitis (Shin et al., 2014). Thus these findings suggest that the IL13-induced basement membrane defect in atopic dermatitis may further add to the skin barrier malfunction in these patients.

IL4/IL13/IL31 trio cytokines reduce tight junction protein claudin-1

Utilizing a human epidermal equivalent model, investigators have shown that a combination of three cytokines (IL4, IL13, IL31), which are commonly upregulated in atopic dermatitis immune milieu, reduced claudin-1 protein expression in a semiquantitative manner. It is not clear how much a role IL4 plays relative to the other two cytokines (IL13, IL31). Although claudin-1 level was reduced in lesional skin of atopic dermatitis patients, its level in nonlesional skin of patients remained normal, suggesting that the claudin-1 reduction in atopic dermatitis was a result of an inflammatory process in a general sense (Gruber et al., 2015). In another study with skin equivalent model, IL17 (not IL4) reduced claudin-1 expression (Yuki et al., 2016).

Th2 cytokines and keratinocyte's immune barrier proteins

It has been well documented that patients affected by atopic dermatitis suffered frequent, recurrent, and at times severe infection events caused by bacteria and viruses (Howell, Boguniewicz, et al., 2006; Howell, Gallo, et al., 2006). Thus our understanding of the underlying mechanisms relating to this infection predisposition is essential for patient management. Besides the undesirable impacts on physical skin barrier proteins, IL4 and other Th2 cytokines also have a negative impact on antimicrobial proteins produced by keratinocyte. In one study using the human keratinocyte cell line HaCaT, the combination of IL4 and IL13 negatively affected the microbial protein β-defensin expressions induced by TNF-α and IFN-γ, through the STAT6 pathway of signaling (Albanesi et al., 2007). In a study investigating the immune milieu in atopic dermatitis skin regarding the response to vaccinia virus, researchers have identified the roles of negative impact by Th2 cytokines IL4 and IL13, through modulating the antimicrobial peptide cathelicidin LL37 leading to enhancement of vaccinia virus replication

(Howell et al., 2006a). In other study, the expressions of human β-defensin-3 stimulated by anti-CD3 antibodies in human HaCaT cells was substantially suppressed by atopic dermatitis–associated Th2 cytokines, IL10 alone, double combination of IL4 and IL13, or triple combination of IL4/IL10/IL13 (Howell et al., 2006b). Subsequently, a study showed that the combination of IL4 and IL13 suppressed the production of human keratinocyte's human β-defensin-3 by inhibiting the S100 calcium-binding protein A11 (S100/A11) (Howell et al., 2008). IL10, IL13, or a combination of IL10 and IL13, suppressed the anti-CD3–stimulated expressions of human β-defensin-2 and cathelicidin LL37 in HaCaT cells (Howell et al., 2005). Although IL17-producing T cells infiltrated the atopic dermatitis skin lesion, the IL17-dependent upregulation of human β-defensin-2 in human keratinocyte was suppressed partially by the combination effects of IL4 and IL13 (Eyerich et al., 2009). In another study, IL4, when incubated with an immortalized human keratinocyte cell line of HaCaT cells, downregulated the genes encoding for antimicrobial proteins or factors involved in antimicrobial peptide production, including IFN-κ, S100s, toll-like receptors, and several chemokines (Bao, Shi, & Chan, 2013).

IL4 and keratinocyte's inflammatory protein production

Experimental data also determine that IL4 has a significant and direct impact on keratinocyte's production of inflammatory-related proteins (Bao, Chau, Bao, Tsoukas, & Chan, 2018). In one study, IL4 added to the human HaCaT cell culture resulted in upregulation of multiple atopic dermatitis-related chemokines, including CCL3L1, CCL8, CCL24, CCL25, CCL26, CXCL6, and CXCL16. In the same study, IL4 also enhanced the expressions of other proinflammatory cytokines/factors, including IL1α, IL12Rβ2, IL19, IL20, IL25, IL31RA, OSMR, and nitric oxide synthase-2 (Bao et al., 2013). In another study, IL4 upregulated expression of IL19, a cytokine that stimulates Th2 cytokine production, in human keratinocyte through the Stat6 signaling pathway (Bao, Alexander, Shi, Mohan, & Chan, 2014). IL4 also enhanced keratinocyte expressions of CXCR3 chemokine, IP10 (IFN-induced protein of 10 kDa), Mig (monokine induced by IFN-γ), and I-TAC (IFN-induced alpha-chemoattractant). Since CXCR3 chemokine, acting on CXCR3 receptors, is a potent chemoattractant for T lymphocytes, it is therefore not surprising to visualize prominent T-cell infiltrates in the atopic dermatitis lesional skin (Albanesi et al., 2000). IL4, and the other atopic dermatitis–associated Th2 cytokine IL13, enhanced CCL26 (eotaxin-3) production by human keratinocyte HaCaT cells. Since CCL26 is a strong eosinophil chemoattractant, the finding of CXCR3 upregulation by IL4 is consistent with one of the skin pathologic characteristics of atopic dermatitis: prominent eosinophil infiltration (Kagami et al., 2005). The mechanism of IL4 upregulation

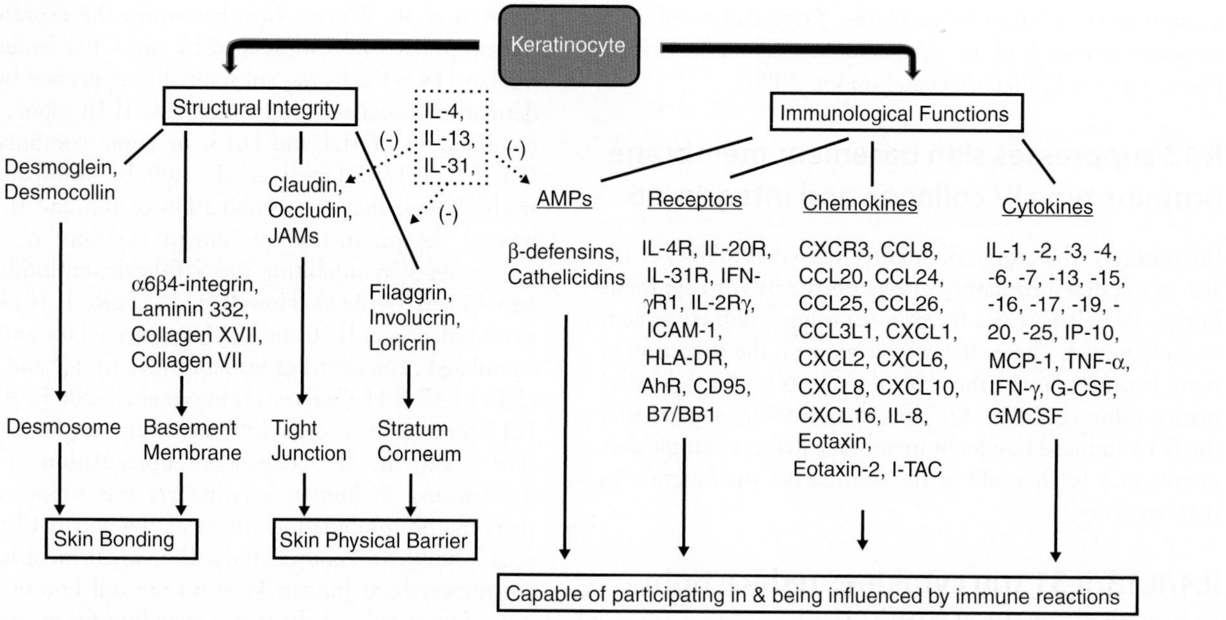

• **Fig. 11.9** Summary illustration of the roles of keratinocyte in the skin, regarding the skin structural integrity and the ability to take part in and be influenced by immune reactions, in relationship to the development of chronic, itchy, inflammatory disease atopic dermatitis. *AMPs*, Antimicrobial peptides; *JAMs*, junctional adhesion molecules.

of CCL26 is determined to be through the Stat6 signaling pathway (Bao, Shi, & Chan, 2012).

Summary

To analyze the roles of keratinocytes in atopic dermatitis from an internal factor's perspective, we discuss the structural and functional contributions of keratinocytes for the skin barrier integrity and what internal factors can influence keratinocytes in ways that favor an immune state of inflammation and easy infection. Fig. 11.9 summarizes the essential information described in this chapter. Keratinocytes, the major cell type in the epidermis, are not only the structural backbone of the epidermis; they are also participants of the immune functions. Structurally, keratinocytes are responsible for the production and renewal of the various layers of the epidermis. In addition, keratinocytes are responsible for production of various protein products essential for barrier functions and structural integrity of the epidermis and the entire skin. Thus, when the structures of keratinocytes and their products are weakened internally, the physical skin barrier and its integrity will be threatened and their protective and cohesive functions will be reduced, allowing pathogens and allergens to penetrate the skin. From the immunologic perspective, keratinocytes possess the machinery to synthesize various immunologic components that can affect the immune milieu of the skin and the body. Therefore, when the immune milieu is altered internally, keratinocytes can be affected in two ways. First, the altered immune milieu can trigger proinflammatory responses from keratinocytes, leading to a vicious cycle of inflammation. Second, the altered immune components could have significant impacts on keratinocytes, including alternation of keratinocytes' effectiveness to provide immune skin barrier and proper immune functions. Giving such important roles of keratinocytes for the epidermis and the skin, it is therefore essential to understand the roles keratinocytes play in the development and sustaining of the disease called atopic dermatitis, as this chapter attempts to convey.

Further readings

Agner, T. (Ed.), (2016). *Skin barrier function*. Karger: Basel, Switzerland.

Kabashima, K. (Ed.), (2016). *Immunology of the skin: Basic and clinical sciences in skin immune responses*. Springer: New York, NY USA.

Kudryashova, E., Seveau, S. M., & Kudryashov, D. S. (2017). Targeting and inactivation of bacterial toxins by human defensins. *Biological Chemistry*, 398(10), 1069–1085. https://doi.org/10.1515/hsz-2017-0106.

Harder, J., & Schroder, J.-M. (Eds.). (2017). *Antimicrobial peptides: Role in human health and disease*. Springer: New York, NY USA.

Megahed. M. (2004). *Histopathology of blistering diseases: With clinical, electron microscopic, immunological and molecular biological correlations*. Springer: New York, NY USA.

Montagna, W., & Parakkal, P. F. (1974). *The structure and function of skin* (3rd ed.). Academic Press: Cambridge, MA USA.

Tur, E. (Ed.), (2007). *Environmental factors in skin diseases*. Karger: Basel, Switzerland.

Wang, G. (Ed.), (2017). *Antimicrobial peptides: Discovery, design, and novel therapeutic strategies* (2nd ed.). CAB International: Oxfordshire, England.

References

Aberdam, D., Galliano, M. -F., Vailly, J., Pulkkinen, L., Bonifas, J., Christiano, A. M., et al. (1994). Herlitz's junctional epidermolysis bullosa is linked to mutations in the gene (LAMC2) for the γ2 subunit of nicein/kalinin (LAMININ-5). *Nature Genetics*, *6*(3), 299–304.

Akiyama, T., Niyonsaba, F., Kiatsurayanon, C., Nguyen, T. T., Ushio, H., Fujimura, T., et al. (2014). The human cathelicidin LL-37 host defense peptide upregulates tight junction-related proteins and increases human epidermal keratinocyte barrier function. *Journal of Innate Immunity*, *6*(6), 739–753. https://doi.org/10.1159/000362789.

Albanesi, C., Scarponi, C., Sebastiani, S., Cavani, A., Federici, M., De Pita, O., et al. (2000). IL-4 enhances keratinocyte expression of CXCR3 agonistic chemokines. *Journal of Immunology*, *165*(3), 1395–1402. https://doi.org/10.4049/jimmunol.165.3.1395.

Albanesi, C., Fairchild, H. R., Madonna, S., Scarponi, C., De Pita, O., Leung, D. Y. M., & Howell, M. D. (2007). IL-4 and IL-13 negatively regulate TNF-alpha- and IFN-gamma-induced beta-defensin expression through STAT-6, suppressor of cytokine signaling (SOCS)-1, and SOCS-3. *Journal of Immunology*, *179*(2), 984–992. https://doi.org/10.4049/jimmunol.179.2.984.

Amagai, M., Matsuyoshi, N., Wang, Z. H., Andi, C., & Stanley, J. R. (2000). Toxin in bullous impetigo and Staphylococcal scalded-skin syndrome targets desmoglein 1. *Nature Medicine*, *6*(11), 1275–1277.

Aono, S., & Hirai, Y. (2008). Phosphorylation of claudin-4 is required for tight junction formation in a human keratinocyte cell line. *Experimental Cell Research*, *314*(18), 3326–3339. https://doi.org/10.1016/j.yexcr.2008.08.012.

Bao, L., Alexander, J. B., Shi, V. Y., Mohan, G. C., & Chan, L. S. (2014). Interleukin-4 up-regulation of epidermal interleukin-19 expression in keratinocytes involves the binding of signal transducer and activator of transcription 6 (Stat6) to the imperfect Stat6 sites. *Immunology*, *143*(4), 601–608. https://doi.org/10.1111/imm.12339.

Bao, L., Alexander, J. B., Zhang, H., Shen, K., & Chan, L. S. (2016a). Interleukin-4 downregulation of involucrin expression in human epidermal keratinocytes involves Stat6 sequestration of the coactivator CREB-binding protein. *Journal of Interferon and Cytokine Research*, *36*(6), 374–381. https://doi.org/10.1089/jir.2015.0056.

Bao, L., Chau, C., Bao, J., Tsoukas, M. M., & Chan, L. S. (2018). IL-4 dysregulates microRNAs involved in inflammation, angiogenesis and apoptosis in epidermal keratinocytes. *Microbiology and Immunology*, *62*(11), 732–736. https://doi.org/10.1111/1348-0421.12650.

Bao, L., Mohan, G. C., Alexander, J. B., Doo, C., Shen, K., Bao, J., & Chan, L. S. (2017). A molecular mechanism for IL-4 suppression of loricrin transcription in epidermal keratinocytes: Implication for atopic dermatitis pathogenesis. *Innate Immunity*, *23*(8), 641–647. https://doi.org/10.1177/1753425917732823.

Bao, L., Shi, V. Y., & Chan, L. S. (2012). IL-4 regulates chemokine CCL26 in keratinocytes through the Jak1, 2/Stat6 signal transduction pathway: Implication for atopic dermatitis. *Molecular Immunology*, *50*(1-2), 91–97. https://doi.org/10.1016/j.molimm.2011.12.008.

Bao, L., Shi, V. Y., & Chan, L. S. (2013). IL-4 up-regulates epidermal chemotactic, angiogenic, and pro-inflammatory genes and down-regulates antimicrobial genes in vivo and in vitro: Relevant in the pathogenesis of atopic dermatitis. *Cytokine*, *61*(2), 419–425. https://doi.org/10.1016/j.cyto.2012.10.031.

Bao, L., Zhang, H., Mohan, G. C., Shen, K., & Chan, L. S. (2016b). Differential expression of inflammation-related genes in IL-4 transgenic mice before and after the onset of atopic dermatitis skin lesions. *Molecular and Cellular Probes*, *30*(1), 30–38. https://doi.org/10.1016/j.mcp.2015.11.001.

Basler, K., Bergmann, S., Heisig, M., Naegel, A., Zorn-Kruppa, M., & Brandner, J. M. (2016). The role of tight junctions in skin barrier function and dermal absorption. *Journal of Controlled Release*, *242*, 105–118. https://doi.org/10.1016/j.jconrel.2016.08.007.

Beck, L. A., Thaci, D., Hamilton, J. D., Graham, N. M., Bieber, T., Rocklin, R., et al. (2014). Dupilumab treatment in adults with moderate-to-severe atopic dermatitis. *The New England Journal of Medicine*, *371*(2), 130–139. https://doi.org/10.1056/NEJMoa1314768.

Blauvelt, A., de Bruin-Weller, M., Gooderham, M., Cather, J. C., Weisman, J., Pariser, D., et al. (2017). Long-term management of moderate-to-severe atopic dermatitis with dupilumab and concomitant topical corticosteroids (LIBERTY AD CHRONOS): A 1-year, randomised, double-blinded, placebo-controlled, phase 3 trial. *Lancet*, *389*(10086), 2287–2303. https://doi.org/10.1016/S0140-6736(17)31191-1.

Blumberg, H., Conklin, D., Xu, W., Grossmann, A., Brender, T., Carollo, S., et al. (2001). Interleukin 20: Discovery, receptor identification, and role in epidermal function. *Cell*, *104*(1), 9–19.

Brandner, J. M., Kief, S., Grund, C., Rendl, M., Houdek, P., Kuhn, C., et al. (2002). Organization and formation of the tight junction system in human epidermis and cultured keratinocytes. *European Journal of Cell Biology*, *81*(5), 253–263. https://doi.org/10.1078/0171-9335-00244.

Brandner, J. M., Zorn-Kruppa, M., Yoshida, T., Moll, I., Beck, L. A., & De Benedetto, A. (2015). Epidermal tight junctions in health and disease. *Tissue Barriers*, *3*(1-2), e974451. https://doi.org/10.4161/21688370.2014.974451.

Brauweiler, A. M., Goleva, E., & Leung, D. Y. M. (2019). *Staphylococcus aureus* lipoteichoic acid damages the skin barrier through an IL-1 mediated pathway. *Journal of Investigative Dermatology*, *139*(8), 1753–1761.E4. https://doi.org/10.1016/j.jid.2019.02.006.

Chan, L. S. (2016). *Pemphigus vulgaris: Scientific basis, clinical presentations, diagnostic methodology, and management strategies*. Hauppauge (NY): Nova Science Publisher.

Chan, L. S., Fine, J.-D., Briggaman, R. A., Woodley, D. T., Hammerber, C., Drugge, R. J., & Cooper, D. (1993). Identification and partial characterization of a novel 105-kDalton lower lamina lucida autoantigen associated with a novel immune-mediated subepidermal blistering disease. *The Journal of Investigative Dermatology*, *101*(3), 262–267.

Chan, L. S., Robinson, N., & Xu, L. (2001). Expression of interleukin-4 in the epidermis of transgenic mice results in a pruritic inflammatory skin disease: An experimental animal model to study atopic dermatitis. *The Journal of Investigative Dermatology*, *117*(4), 977–983.

Chan, L. S., Wang, X.-S., Lapiere, J. C., Marinkovich, M. P., Jones, J. C. R., & Woodley, D. T. (1995). A newly identified 105-kD lower lamina lucida autoantigen is an acidic protein distinct from the 105-KD gamma 2 chain of laminin-5. *The Journal of Investigative Dermatology*, *105*(1), 75–79.

Chen, Y., Fang, Q., Wang, Z., Zhang, J. Y., MacLeod, A. S., Hall, R. P., & Liedtke, W. B. (2016). Transient receptor potential vanilloid 4 ion channel functions as a pruriceptor in epidermal keratinocytes to evoke histaminergic itch. *The Journal of Biological Chemistry*, *291*(19), 10252–10262. https://doi.org/10.1074/jbc.M116.716464.

Chieosilapathem, P., Ogawa, H., & Niyonsaba, F. (2017). Current insight into the role of human β-defensins in atopic dermatitis. *Clinical and Experimental Immunology*, *190*(2), 156–166. https://doi.org/10.1111/cei.13013.

Christiano, A. M., Greenspan, D. S., Hoffman, G. G., Zhang, X., Tamai, Y., Lin, A. N., et al. (1993). A missense mutation in type

VII collagen in two affected siblings with recessive dystrophic epidermolysis bullosa. *Nature Genetics, 4*(1), 62–66.

Clark, R. A., Chong, B., Mirchandani, N., Brinster, N. K., Yamanaka, K. -I., Dowgiert, R. K., & Kupper, T. S. (2016). The vast majority of CLA+ T cells are resident in normal skin. *Journal of Immunology, 176*, 4431–4439.

Clausen, M. L., Edslev, S. M., Andersen, P. S., Clemensen, K., Krogfelt, K. A., & Agner, T. (2017). *Staphylococcus aureus* colonization in atopic eczema and its association with filaggrin gene mutations. *The British Journal of Dermatology, 177*(5), 1394–1400. https://doi.org/10.1111/bjd.15470.

Cornelissen, C., Marquardt, Y., Czaja, K., Wenzel, J., Frank, J., Luscher-Firzlaff, J., et al. (2012). IL-31 regulated differentiation and filaggrin expression in human organotypic skin models. *The Journal of Allergy and Clinical Immunology, 129*(2), 426–433. https://doi.org/10.1016/j.jaci.2011.10.042.

Dang, N., Ma, X., Meng, X., An, L., & Pang, S. (2016). Dysregulated function of normal human epidermal keratinocytes in the absence of filaggrin. *Molecular Medicine Reports, 14*(3), 2566–2572. https://doi.org/10.3892/mmr.2016.5539.

De Benedetto, A., Rafaels, N. M., McGirt, L. Y., Ivanov, A. I., Georas, S. N., Cheadle, C., et al. (2011a). Tight junction defects in patients with atopic dermatitis. *The Journal of Allergy and Clinical Immunology, 127*(3), 773–786. https://doi.org/10.1016/j.jaci.2010.10.018.

De Benedetto, A., Slifka, M. K., Rafaels, N. M., Kuo, I. -H., Georas, S. N., Boguniewicz, M., et al. (2011b). Reduction in claudin-1 may enhance susceptibility to HSV-1 infections in atopic dermatitis. *The Journal of Allergy and Clinical Immunology, 128*(1), 242–246.E5. https://doi.org/10.1016/j.jaci.2011.02.014.

Debinska, A., Danielewicz, H., Drabik-Chamerska, A., Kalita, D., & Boznanski, A. (2017). Filaggrin loss-of-function mutations as a predictor for atopic eczema, allergic sensitization and eczema-associated asthma in Polish children population. *Advances in Clinical and Experimental Medicine, 26*(6), 991–998. https://doi.org/10.17219/acem/61430.

Di, Z. -H., Ma, L., Qi, R. -Q., Sun, X. -D., Huo, W., Zhang, L., et al. (2016). T helper 1 and T help 2 cytokines differentially modulate expression of filaggrin and its processing proteases in human keratinocytes. *Chinese Medical Journal, 129*(3), 295–303. https://doi.org/10.4103/0366-6999.174489.

DiTommaso, T., Cottle, D. L., Pearson, H. B., Schluter, H., Kaur, P., Humbert, P. O., & Smyth, I. M. (2014). Keratin 76 is required for tight junction function and maintenance of the skin barrier. *PLoS Genetics, 10*(10), e1004706. https://doi.org/10.1371/journal.pgen.1004706.

Duan, S., Wanke, K., Wawrzyniak, P., Meng, Y., Kast, J. I., Ruckert, B., et al. (2016). Platelet-activating factor decreases skin keratinocyte tight junction barrier integrity. *The Journal of Allergy and Clinical Immunology, 138*(6), 1725–1728.E3 https://doi.org/10.1016/j.jaci.2016.05.037.

El-Darzi, E., Bazzi, S., Daoud, S., Echtay, K. S., & Bahr, G. M. (2017). Differential regulation of surface receptor expression, proliferation, and apoptosis in HaCaT cells stimulated with interferon-γ, interleukin-4, tumor necrosis factor-a, or muramyl dipeptide. *International Journal of Immunopathology and Pharmacology, 30*(2), 130–145. https://doi.org/10.1177/0394632017707611.

Elhaji, Y., Sasseville, D., Pratt, M., Asai, Y., Matheson, K., McLean, W. H. I., & Hull, P. R. (2019). Flaggrin gene loss-of-function mutations constitute a factor in patients with multiple contact allergens. *Contact Dermatitis, 80*(6), 354–358. https://doi.org/10.1111/cod.13268.

Enomoto, H., Hirata, K., Otsuka, K., Kawai, T., Takahashi, T., Hirota, T., et al. (2008). Filaggrin null mutations are associated with atopic dermatitis and elevated levels of IgE in Japanese population: A family and case-control study. *Journal of Human Genetics, 53*, 615–621. https://doi.org/10.1007/s10038-008-0293-z.

Eyerich, K., Pennino, D., Scarponi, C., Foerster, S., Nasorri, F., Behrendt, H., et al. (2009). IL-17 in atopic eczema: Linking allergen-specific adaptive and microbial-triggered innate immune response. *The Journal of Allergy and Clinical Immunology, 123*(1), 59–66. https://doi.org/10.1016/j.jaci.2008.10.031.

Fleckman, P., Dale, B. A., & Holbrook, K. A. (1985). Profilaggrin, a high-molecular-weight precursor of filaggri in human epidermis and cultured keratinocytes. *The Journal of Investigative Dermatology, 85*(6), 507–512.

Fuller, B. W., Nishmura, T., & Noelle, R. J. (2002). The selective triggering of CD40 on keratinocytes in vivo enhances cell-mediated immunity. *European Journal of Immunology, 32*(3), 895–902.   10.1002/1521-4141(200203)32:3<895::AID-IMMU895>3.0.CO:2-A.

Furuse, M., Hata, M., Furuse, K., Yoshida, Y., Haratake, A., Sugitani, Y., et al. (2002). Claudin-based tight junctions are crucial for the mammalian epidermal barrier: A lesson from claudin-1-deficient mice. *The Journal of Cell Biology, 156*(6), 1099–1111. https://doi.org/10.1083/jcb.200110122.

Garcia, M., Alout, H., Diop, F., Damour, A., Bengue, M., Weill, M., et al. (2018). Innate immune response of primary human keratinocytes to West Nile virus infection and its modulation by mosquito saliva. *Frontiers in Cellular and Infection Microbiology, 8*, 387. https://doi.org/10.3389/fcimb.2018.00387.

Giudice, G. J., Emery, D. J., & Diaz, L. A. (1992). Cloning and primary structural analysis of the bullous pemphigoid autoantigen BP180. *The Journal of Investigative Dermatology, 99*(3), 243–250.

Gruber, R., Bornchen, C., Rose, K., Daubmann, A., Volksdorf, T., Wladykowski, E., et al. (2015). Diverse regulation of claudin-1 and claudin-4 in atopic dermatitis. *The American Journal of Pathology, 185*(10), 2777–2789. https://doi.org/10.1016/j.ajpath.2015.06.021.

Gschwandtner, M., Mildner, M., Mlitz, V., Gruber, F., Eckhart, L., Werfel, T., et al. (2013). Histamine suppresses epidermal keratinocyte differentiation and impairs skin barrier function in a human skin model. *Allergy, 68*(1), 37–47. https://doi.org/10.1111/all.12051.

Handa, S., Khullar, G., Pal, A., Kamboj, P., & De, D. (2019). Filaggrin gene mutations in hand eczema patients in the Indian subcontinent: A prospective case-control study. *Contact Dermatitis, 80*(6), 359–364. https://doi.org/10.1111/cod.13233.

Hanifin, J. M., & Rajka, G. (1980). Diagnostic features of atopic dermatitis. *Acta Dermatovener (Stockholm), 60*, 44–47.

Has, C., Nystrom, A., Saeidian, A. H., Bruckner-Tuderman, L., & Jouni Uitto, J. (2018). Epidermolysis bullosa: Molecular pathology of connective tissue components in the cutaneous basement membrane zone. *Matrix Biology, 71-72*, 313–329. https://doi.org/10.1016/j.matbio.2018.04.001.

Hatano, Y., Adachi, Y., Elias, P. M., Crumrine, D., Sakai, T., Kurahashi, R., et al. (2013). The Th2 cytokine, interleukin-4, abrogates the cohesion of normal stratum corneum in mice: Implications for pathogenesis of atopic dermatitis. *Experimental Dermatology, 22*(1), 30–35. https://doi.org/10.1111/exd.12047.

Herve, P. L., Dhelft, V., Plaquet, C., Rousseaux, A., Bouzereau, A., Gaulme, L., et al. (2019). Epidermal micro-perforation potentiates the efficacy of epicutaneous vaccination. *Journal of Controlled Release, 298*, 12–26. https://doi.org/10.1016/j.conrel.2019.02.004.

Hidaka, T., Ogawa, E., Kobayashi, E. H., Suzuki, T., Funayama, R., Nagashima, T., et al. (2017). The aryl hydrocarbon receptor AhR links atopic dermatitis and air pollution via induction of the neurotrophic factor artemin. *Nature Immunology, 18*(1), 64–73. https://doi.org/10.1038/ni.3614.

Howell, M. D., Boguniewicz, M., Pastore, S., Novak, N., Bieber, T., Girolomoni, G., & Leung, D. Y. M. (2006b). Mechansims of HBD-3 deficinecy in atopic dermatitis. *Clinical Immunology, 121*(3), 332–338. https://doi.org/10.1016/j.clim.2006.08.008.

Howell, M. D., Fairchild, H. R., Kim, B. E., Bin, L., Boguniewicz, M., Redzic, J. S., et al. (2008). Th2 cytokines act on S100/A11 to downregulate keratinocyte differentiation. *The Journal of Investigative Dermatology, 128*(9), 2248–2258. https://doi.org/10.1038/jid.2008.74.

Howell, M. D., Gallo, R. L., Boguniewicz, M., Jones, J. F., Wong, C., Streib, J. E., & Leung, D. Y. M. (2006a). Cytokine milieu of atopic dermatitis skin subverts the innate immune response to vaccinia virus. *Immunity, 24*(3), 341–348. https://doi.org/10.1016/j.immuni.2006.02.006.

Howell, M. D., Novak, N., Bieber, T., Pastore, S., Girolomoni, G., Boguniewicz, M., et al. (2005). Interleukin-10 downregulates anti-microbial peptide expression in atopic dermatitis. *The Journal of Investigative Dermatology, 125*(4), 738–745. https://doi.org/10.1111/j.0022-202X.2005.23776.x.

Ikeda-Miyagawa, Y., Kobayashi, K., Yamanaka, H., Okubo, M., Wang, S., Dai, Y., et al. (2015). Peripherally increased artemin is a key regulator of TRPA1/V1 expression in primary afferent neurons. *Molecular Pain, 11*, 8. https://doi.org/10.1186/s12990-015-0004-7.

Jonkman, M. F., de Jong, M. D. J. M., Heeres, K., Pas, H. H., van der Meer, J. B., Owaribe, K., et al. (1995). 180-kD bullous pemphigoid antigen (BP180) is deficient in generalized atrophic benign epidermolysis bullosa. *The Journal of Clinical Investigation, 95*(3), 1345–1352.

Junghans, V. (1996). Human keratinocytes constitutively express IL-4 receptor molecules and respond to IL-4 with an increase in B7/BB1 expression. *Experimental Dermatology, 5*(6), 316–324.

Kagami, S., Sacki, H., Komine, M., Kakinuma, T., Tsunemi, Y., Nakamura, K., et al. (2005). Interleukin-4 and interleukin-13 enhance CCL26 production in a human keratinocyte cell line, HaCaT cells. *Clinical and Experimental Immunology, 141*(3), 459–466. https://doi.org/10.1111/j.1365-2249.2005.02875.x.

Kim, B. E., Leung, D. Y. M., Boguniewicz, M., & Howell, M. D. (2008). Loricrin and involucrin expression is down-regulated by Th2 cytokines through STAT-6. *Clinical Immunology, 126*(3), 332–337. https://doi.org/10.1016/j.clim.2007.11.006.

Kim, H. O., Kim, J. H., Chung, B. Y., Choi, M. G., & Park, C. W. (2014). Increased expression of the aryl hydrocarbon receptor in patients with chronic inflammatory skin diseases. *Experimental Dermatology, 23*(4), 278–281. https://doi.org/10.1111/exd.12350.

Kirschner, N., Haftek, M., Niessen, C. M., Behne, M. J., Furuse, M., Moll, I., & Brandner, J. M. (2011). CD44 regulates tight-junction assembly and barrier function. *The Journal of Investigative Dermatology, 131*(4), 932–943. https://doi.org/10.1038/jid.2010.390.

Kirtschig, G., Marinkovich, M. P., Burgeson, R. E., & Yancey, K. B. (1995). Anti-basement membrane autoantibodies in patients with anti-epilligrin cicatricial pemphigoid bind the alpha subunit of laminin 5. *The Journal of Investigative Dermatology, 105*(4), 543–548. https://doi.org/10.1111/1523-1747.ep12323431.

Kitajima, Y., Eguchi, K., Ohno, T., Mori, S., & Yaoita, H. (1983). Tight junctions of human keratinocytes in primary culture: A freeze-fracture study. *Journal of Ultrastructure Research, 82*(3), 309–313.

Klicznik, M. M., Szenes-Nagy, A. B., Campbell, D. J., & Gratz, I. K. (2018). Taking the lead – How keratinocytes orchestrate skin T cell immunity. *Immunology Letters, 200*, 43–51. https://doi.org/10.1016/j.imlet.2018.06.009.

Kuhn, R., Rajewsky, K., & Muller, W. (1991). Generation and analysis of interleukin-4 deficient mice. *Science, 254*(5032:), 707–710.

Luo, J., Feng, J., Yu, G., Yang, P., Mack, M., Du, J., et al. (2018). TRPV4-expressing macrophages and keratinocytes contribute differentially to allergic and non-allergic chronic itch. *The Journal of Allergy and Clinical Immunology, 141*(2), 608–619.E7. https://doi.org/10.1016/j.jaci.2017.05.051.

Manti, S., Amorini, M., Cuppari, C., Salpietro, A., Porcino, F., Leonardi, S., et al. (2017). Filaggrin mutations and molluscum contagiosum skin infection in patients with atopic dermatitis. *Annals of Allergy, Asthma and Immunology, 119*(5), 446–451. https://doi.org/10.1016/j.anai.2017.07.019.

Margolis, D. J., Mitra, N., Gochnauer, H., Wubbenhorst, B., D'Andrea, K., Kraya, A., et al. (2018). Uncommon filaggrin variants are associated with persistent atopic dermatitis in African Americans. *Journal of Investigative Dermatology, 138*(7), 1501–1506. https://doi.org/10.1016/j.jid.2018.01.029.

Marinkovich, M. P., Lunstrum, G. P., & Burgeson, R. E. (1992). The anchoring filament protein kalinin is synthesized and secreted as a high molecular weight precursor. *The Journal of Biological Chemistry, 267*(25), 17900–17906.

Matsumoto, A., Murota, H., Terao, M., & Katayama, I. (2018). Attenuated activation of homeostatic glucocorticoid in keratinocytes induces allokness via aberrant artemin production. *The Journal of Investigative Dermatology, 138*(7), 1491–1500. https://doi.org/10.1016/j.jid.2018.02.010.

McLean. W. H. (2016). Filaggrin failure – from ichthyosis vulgaris to atopic eczema and beyond. *British Journal of Dermatology, 175*(suppl. 2), 4–7. https://doi.org/10.1111/bjd.14997.

Meister, M., Tounsi, A., Gaffal, E., Bald, T., Papatriantafyllou, M., Ludwig, J., et al. (2015). Self-antigen presentation by keratinocytes in the inflamed adult skin modulates T-cell auto-reactivity. *The Journal of Investigative Dermatology, 135*(8), 1996–2004. https://doi.org/10.1038/jid.2015.130.

Mertens, A. E. E., Rygiel, T. P., Olivo, C., van der Kammen, R., & Collard, J. G. (2005). The Rac activator Tiam 1 controls tight junction biogenesis in keratinocytes through binding to and activation of the Par polarity complex. *The Journal of Cell Biology, 170*(7), 1029–1037. https://doi.org/10.1083/jcb.200502129.

Nadeau, P., Henehan, M., & De Benedetto, A. (2018). Activation of protease-activated receptor 2 leads to impairment of keratinocyte tight junction integrity. *The Journal of Allergy and Clinical Immunology, 142*(1), 281–284.E7. https://doi.org/10.1016/j.jaci.2018.01.007.

Niyonsaba, F., Kiatsurayanon, C., & Ogawa, H. (2016). The role of human β-defensins in allergic diseases. *Clinical and Experimental Allergy, 46*(12), 1522–1530. https://doi.org/10.1111/cea.12843.

Palmer, C. N. A., Irvine, A. D., Terron-Kwiatkowski, A., Zhao, Y., Liao, H., Lee, S. P., et al. (2006). Common loss-of-function variants of the epidermal barrier protein filaggrin are a major predisposing factor for atopic dermatitis. *Nature Genetics, 38*(4), 441–446. https://doi.org/10.1038/ng1767.

Parente, M. G., Chung, L. C., Ryynanen, J., Woodley, D. T., Wynn, K. C., Bauer, E. A., et al. (1991). Human type VII collagen: cDNA cloning and chromosomal mapping of the gene. *Proceedings of the National Academy of Sciences of the United States of America*, *88*(16), 6931–6935.

Perez, W. B. E., Ventrella, R., Kaplan, N., Cable, C. J., Thomas, P. M., & Getsios, S. (2017). EphA2 proteomics in human keratinocytes reveals a novel association with afadin and epidermal tight junctions. *Journal of Cell Science*, *130*(1), 111–118. https://doi.org/10.1242/jcs.188169.

Petersen, T. H., Jee, M. H., Gadsboll, A. -S. O., Schmidt, J. D., Sloth, J. J., Sonnenberg, G. F., et al. (2018). Mice with epidermal filaggrin deficiency show increased immune reactivity to nickel. *Contact Dermatitis*, *80*(3), 139–148. https://doi.org/10.1111/cod.13153.

Pierard, G. E., Goffin, V., Hermanns-Le, T., & Pierard-Franchimont, C. (2000). Corneocyte desquamation. *International Journal of Molecular Medicine*, *6*(2), 217–221. https://doi.org/10.3892/ijmm.6.2.217.

Pigors, M., Common, J. E. A., Wong, X. F. C. C., Malik, S., Scott, C. A., Tabarra, N., et al. (2018). Exome sequencing and rare variant analysis reveals multiple filaggrin mutations in Bangladeshi families with atopic eczema and additional risk genes. *The Journal of Investigative Dermatology*, *138*(12), 2674–2677. https://doi.org/10.1016/j.jid.2018.05.013.

Prens, E., Hegmans, J., Lien, R. C. A., Debets, R., Troost, R., van Joost, T., & Benner, R. (1996). Increased expression of interleuk-4 receptors on psoriatic epidermal cells. *The American Journal of Pathology*, *148*(5), 1493–1502.

Presland, R. B., Boggess, D. S., Lewis, S. P., Hull, C., Fleckman, P., & Sundberg, J. P. (2000). Loss of normal profilaggrin and filaggrin in flaky tail (ft/ft) mice: An animal model for the filaggrin-deficient skin disease ichthyosis vulgaris. *The Journal of Investigative Dermatology*, *115*(6), 1072–1081. https://doi.org/10.1046/j.1523-1747.2000.00178.x.

Pummi, K., Malminen, M., Aho, H., Karvonen, S. -L., Peltonen, J., & Peltonen, S. (2001). Epidermal tight junctions: ZO-1 and occluding are expressed in mature, developing, and affected skin and in vitro differentiating keratinocytes. *The Journal of Investigative Dermatology*, *117*(7), 1050–1058.

Rahn, E., Their, K., Petermann, P., Rubsam, M., Staeheli, P., Iden, S., et al. (2017). Epithelial barriers in murine skin during herpes simplex virus 1 infection: The role of tight junction formation. *The Journal of Investigative Dermatology*, *137*(4), 884–893. https://doi.org/10.1016/j.jid.2016.11.027.

Rahrig, S., Dettmann, J. M., Brauns, B., Lorenz, V. N., Buhl, T., Kezic, S., et al. (2019). Transient epidermal barrier deficiency and lowered allergic threshold in filaggrin-hornerin (FlgHrnr-/-) double-deficient mice. *Allergy*, *74*(7), 1327–1339. https://doi.org/10.1111/all.13756.

Raiko, L., Siljamaki, E., Mahoney, M. G., Putaala, H., Suominen, E., Peltonen, J., & Peltonen, S. (2012). Hailey-Hailey disease and tight junctions: Caludins 1 and 4 are regulated by ATP2C1 gene encoding Ca(2+)/Mn(2+) ATPase SPCA1 in cultured keratinocytes. *Experimental Dermatology*, *21*(8), 586–591. https://doi.org/10.1111/j.1600-0625.2012.01520.x.

Richmond, J. M., Bangari, D. S., Essien, K. I., Currimbhoy, S. D., Groom, J. R., Pandya, A. G., et al. (2017). Keratinocyte-derived chemokines orchestrate T-cell positioning in the epidermis during vitiligo and may serve as a biomarkers of disease. *The Journal of Investigative Dermatology*, *137*(2), 350–358. https://doi.org/10.1016/j.jid.2016.09.016.

Rodrigues, M., Kosaric, N., Bonham, C. A., & Gurtner, G. C. (2019). Wound healing: A cellular perspective. *Physiological Reviews*, *99*(1), 665–706. https://doi.org/10.1152/physrev.00067.2017.

Roziomiy, V. L., & Markov, A. G. (2010). Effect of interleukin-1b on the expression of tight junction proteins in the culture of HaCaT keratinocytes. *Bulletin of Experimental Biology and Medicine*, *149*(3), 280–283.

Ryu, W. -I., Lee, H., Bae, H. C., Jeon, J., Ryu, H. J., Kim, J., et al. (2018). IL-33 down-regulates CLDN1 expression through the ERK/STAT3 pathway in keratinocytes. *Journal of Dermatological Science*, *90*(no, 3), 313–322. https://doi.org/10.1016/j.j.dermsci.2018.02.017.

Sayedyahossein, S., Rudkouskaya, A., Leclerc, V., & Dagnino, L. (2016). Integrin-linked kinase is indispensable for keratinocyte differentiation and epidermal barrier function. *The Journal of Investigative Dermatology*, *136*(2), 425–435. https://doi.org/10.1016/j.jid.2015.10.056.

Schauber, J., & Gallo, R. L. (2008). Antimicrobial peptides and the skin immune defense system. *The Journal of Allergy and Clinical Immunology*, *122*(2), 261–266. https://doi.org/10.1016/j.jaci.2008.03.027.

Seguchi, T., Cui, C. Y., Kusuda, S., Takahashi, M., Aisu, K., & Tezuka, T. (1996). Decreased expression of filaggrin in atopic skin. *Archives of Dermatological Research*, *288*(6), 442–446.

Seneschal, J., Clark, R. A., Gehad, A., Baecher-Allan, C. M., & Kupper, T. S. (2012). Human epidermal Langerhans cells maintain immune homeostasis in skin by activating skin resident regulatory T cells. *Immunity*, *36*(5), 873–884. https://doi.org/10.1016/j.immuni.2012.03.018.

Shi, X., Wang, L., Clark, J. D., & Kingery, W. S. (2013). Keratinocytes express cytokines and nerve growth factor in response to neuropeptide activation of the ERK1/2 and JNK MARK transcription pathways. *Regulatory Peptides*, *10*(186), 92–103. https://doi.org/10.1016/j.regpep.2013.08.001.

Shin, J. W., Choi, Y. J., Choi, H. R., Na, J. I., Kim, K. H., Park, I. A., et al. (2014). Defective basement membrane in atopic dermatitis and possible role of IL-13. *Journal of the European Academy of Dermatology and Venereology*, *29*(10), 2060–2062. https://doi.org/10.1111/jdv.12596.

Shinkuma, S., McMillan, J. R., & Shimizu, H. (2011). Ultrastructure and molecular pathogenesis of epidermolysis bullosa. *Clinics in Dermatology*, *29*(4), 412–419. https://doi.org/10.1016/j.clindermatol.2011.01.010.

Shiraki, Y., Ishibashi, Y., Hiruma, M., Nishikawa, A., & Ikeda, S. (2006). Cytokine secretion profiles of human keratinocytes during *Trichophyton tonsurans* and *Arthroderma benhamiae* infection. *Journal of Medical Microbiology*, *55*(9), 1175–1185. https://doi.org/10.1099/jmm.0.46632.

Smith, F. J. D., Irvine, A. D., Terron-Kwiatkowski, A., Sandilands, A., Campbell, L. E., Zhao, Y., et al. (2006). Loss-of-function mutations in the gene encoding filaggrin cause ichthyosis vulgaris. *Nature Genetics*, *38*(3), 337–342. https://doi.org/10.1038/ng1743.

Spindler, V., Eming, R., Schmidt, E., Amagai, M., Grando, S., Jonkman, M. F., et al. (2018). Mechanisms causing loss of keratinocyte cohesion in pemphigus. *The Journal of Investigative Dermatology*, *138*(1), 32–37.

Sugita, K., Kabashima, K., Atarashi, K., Shimauchi, T., Kobayashi, M., & Tokura, Y. (2007). Innate immunity mediated by epidermal keratinocytes promotes acquired immunity involving Langerhans cells and T cells in the skin. *Clinical and Experimental Immunology*, *147*(1), 176–183. https://doi.org/10.1111/j.1365-2249.2006.03258.x.

Takahashi, T., & Gallo, R. L. (2017). The critical and multifunctional roles of antimicrobial peptides in dermatology. *Dermatologic Clinics*, *35*(1), 39–50. https://doi.org/10.1016/j.det.2016.07.006.

Talagas, M., & Misery, L. (2019). Role of keratinocytes in sensitive skin. *Frontiers in Medicine (Lausanne)*, 6, 108. https://doi.org/10.3389/fmed.2019.00108.

Tamoutounour, S., Han, S. -J., Deckers, J., Constantinides, M. G., Hurabielle, C., Harrison, O. J., et al. (2019). Keratinocyte-intrinsic MHCII expression controls microbiota-induced Th1 cell responses. *Proceedings of the National Academy of Sciences of the United States of America*, 116(47), 23643–23652. https://doi.org/10.1073/pnas.1912432116.

Tauchi, M., Hida, A., Negishi, T., Katsuoka, F., Noda, S., Mimura, J., et al. (2005). Constitutive expression of aryl hydrocarbon receptor in keratinocytes causes inflammatory skin lesions. *Molecular and Cellular Biology*, 25(21), 9360–9368. https://doi.org/10.1128/MCB.25.21.9360-9368.2005.

Tohgasaki, T., Ozswa, N., Yoshino, T., Ishiwatari, S., Matsukuma, S., Yanagi, S., & Fukuda, H. (2018). Enolase-1 expression in the stratum corneum is elevated with parakeratosis of atopic dermatitis and disrupts the cellular tight junction barrier in keratinocytes. *International Journal of Cosmetic Science*, 40(2), 178–186. https://doi.org/10.1111/ics.12449.

Tran, Q. T., Kennedy, L. H., Carrion, S. L., Bodreddigan, S., Goodwin, S. B., Sutter, C. H., & Sutter, T. R. (2012). EGFR regulation of epidermal barrier function. *Physiological Genomics*, 44(8), 455–469. https://doi.org/10.1152/physiolgenomics.00176.2011.

Ujiie, H., Sasaoka, T., Izumi, K., Nishie, W., Shinkuma, S., Natsuga, K., et al. (2014). Bullous pemphigoid autoantibodies directly induce blister formation without complement activation. *Journal of Immunology*, 193(9), 4415–4428. https://doi.org/10.4049/jimmunol.1400095.

Vidal, F., Aberdam, D., Miquel, C., Christiano, A. M., Pulkkinen, L., Uitto, J., et al. (1995). Integrin β4 mutations associated with junctional epidermolysis bullosa with pyloric aresia. *Nature Genetics*, 10(2), 229–234. https://doi.org/10.1038/ng0695-229.

Vockel, M., Breitenbach, U., Kreienkamp, H. -J., & Brandner, J. M. (2010). Somatostatin regulates tight junction function and composition in human keratinocytes. *Experimental Dermatology*, 19(10), 888–894. https://doi.org/10.1111/j.1600-0625.2010.01101.x.

Volksdorf, T., Heilmann, J., Eming, S. A., Schawjinski, K., Zorn-Kruppa, M., Ueck, C., et al. (2017). Tight junction proteins claudin-1 and occludin are important for cutaneous wound healing. *The American Journal of Pathology*, 187(6), 1301–1312. https://doi.org/10.1016/j.ajpath.2017.02.006.

Woodley, D. T., Burgeson, R. E., Lunstrum, G., Bruckner-Tuderman, L., Reese, M. J., & Briggaman, R. A. (1988). Epidermolysis bullosa acquisita antigen is the global carboxyl terminus of type VII procollagen. *The Journal of Clinical Investigation*, 81(3), 683–687. https://doi.org/10.1172/JCI113373.

Yokouchi, M., & Kubo, A. (2018). Maintenance of tight junction barrier integrity in cell turnover and skin diseases. *Experimental Dermatology*, 27(8), 876–883. https://doi.org/10.1111/exd.13742.

Yosipovitch, G., Berger, T., & Fassett, M. S. (2020). Neuroimmune interactions in chronic itch of atopic dermatitis. *Journal of the European Academy of Dermatology and Venereology*, 34(2), 239–250. https://doi.org/10.1111/jdv.15973.

Yuki, T., Yoshida, H., Akazawa, Y., Komiya, A., Sugiyama, Y., & Inoue, S. (2011). Activation of TLR2 enhances tight junction barrier in epidermal keratinocytes. *Journal of Immunology*, 187(6), 3230–3237. https://doi.org/10.4049/jimmunol.1100058.

Yuki, T., Toblishi, M., Kusaka-Kikushima, A., Ota, Y., & Tokura, Y. (2016). Impaired tight junctions in atopic dermatitis skin and in a skin equivalent model treated with interleukin-17. *PLoS One*, 11(9), e0161759. https://doi.org/10.1371/journal.pone.0161759.

Zhao, Y., Bao, L., Chan, L. S., DiPietro, L. A., & Chen, L. (2016). Aberrant wound healing in an epidermal interleukin-4 transgenic mouse model of atopic dermatitis. *PLoS One*, 11(1), e0146451. https://doi.org/10.1371/journal.pone.0146451.

12

Microvasculature

LAWRENCE S. CHAN

KEY POINTS

- Cutaneous microcirculation, a type of microvasculature situated just below the epidermis, is composed of major components of blood vessels (arterioles and venules) and lymphatic vessels.
- The cutaneous blood vessels are organized into a superficial plexus near the dermal-epidermal junction and a lower plexus near the dermal-subcutaneous junction. Cutaneous arteriole delivers oxygen and nutrients to the skin. It is also the conduit from which the immune system sent their armies of white blood cells to counter invasive microorganisms that enter into the skin. Importantly, the cutaneous arteriole is the key to mobilize immune components to the skin in case of allergic events, such as in atopic dermatitis. The most important segment in this regard is the postcapillary venule, site of leukocyte transmigration from vascular space into the tissue site.
- The cutaneous lymphatic system is comprised of larger draining vessels and is organized into two plexuses. The major function of the cutaneous lymphatic system is maintenance of interstitial fluid balance and immune recognition, but it can also become a pathway of cancer metastasis.
- Cutaneous microcirculation, due to its essential immunologic roles, plays an important part in the skin inflammatory process of atopic dermatitis. This specific role is illustrated in the keratin-14/IL4 transgenic mice, an animal model of atopic dermatitis in which cutaneous blood vessels exhibit angiogenesis and leakage, with resulting prominent skin infiltration of inflammatory cells. Similarly, the lymphatic vessels of this animal model exhibit prominent lymphangiogenesis and evidence of compromised integrity, providing another support in its role in atopic dermatitis development and sustainment.
- Understanding of the roles of cutaneous vasculature in the development of atopic dermatitis will pave the way to future targeted treatments.

Introduction

The cutaneous microvasculature situated at the dermis just below the epidermis is the major instrument for skin microcirculation. The cutaneous vasculature has three major components: arteriole, venule, and lymphatic vessels (Braverman, 1997, 2000; Skobe & Detmar, 2000). In the

sections that follow, the basic structures and common functions of blood vessels and lymphatic vessels are delineated. Having described these functional structures, we then discuss the roles of cutaneous microvasculature played in the inflammatory skin disease atopic dermatitis.

Cutaneous blood vessels: Structures

Since there is a close relationship between cutaneous blood vessels and cutaneous lymphatic vessels, the structures of cutaneous blood vessels are better depicted in conjunction with cutaneous lymphatic vessels. Fig. 12.1 illustrates a schematic picture of the structural proximity between these vessels (Skobe & Detmar, 2000). More details on the structures of cutaneous blood vessels are discussed in other publications (Braverman, 1997, 2000).

The cutaneous microcirculation is organized into two horizontal plexuses. *Plexus*, derived from a Latin word meaning "braid," denotes a branching network of blood vessels or nerves. The upper plexus is located just 1 to 1.5 mm below the stratum corneum, whereas the lower plexus is situated along the dermal-subcutaneous junction. Connecting the upper and lower plexuses are the pairing ascending arterioles and the descending venules. Arising from the upper horizontal plexus are the capillary loops. From an ultrastructural perspective, arterioles distinguish from capillaries and venules by the presence of an internal elastic lamina, capillaries are unique for their thin vascular wall containing pericytes (a special type cell of vessel wall) on the outer surface, and venules are characterized by their thicker vessel walls without elastic fibers. The papillary dermal arterioles have an outer diameter ranging from 17 to 26 μm and vessel wall with two layers of smooth muscle cells surrounding the endothelial cells at the lumen, and elastic fibers. As the arterioles move toward the capillary loop, their diameters, smooth muscle, and elastic fibers all reduce in caliber. When the vessels reach a size of 15 μm in outer diameter, the smooth muscles, which are identified by their dense bodies and myofilaments, are no longer present. At the point where the blood vessels turn into 10- to 12-μm outer diameter in size, all elastic fibers disappear, and this segment is now the beginning of arterial capillary. In the capillaries, pericytes, which also have contractile functions, replace smooth muscles and form tight junctions

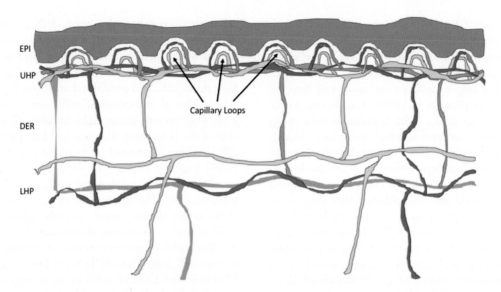

• **Fig. 12.1** Schematic presentation of cutaneous microcirculation, depicting the relationship between arterioles *(red)*, venules *(blue)*, and lymphatics *(yellow)* and their relationship to epidermis *(EPI)*. This presentation illustrates the close proximity of these vessels and the parallel arrangement of these vessels. The upper horizontal plexus *(UHP)* is located in upper dermis *(DER)*, whereas the lower horizontal plexus *(LHP)* is located in the dermis-subcutaneous interface. The capillary loops extending upward from the upper horizontal plexus into the papillary dermis provide the nutrition supplies to the skin. (From Skobe, M., & Detmar, M. [2000]. Structure, function, and molecular control of the skin lymphatic system. *Journal of Investigative Dermatology, 5*[1], 14–19; Braverman, I. M. [2000]. The cutaneous microcirculation. *Journal of Investigative Dermatology, 5*[1], 3–9.)

with endothelial cells. They have an important role in maintaining capillary integrity (Bergers & Song, 2005). The next segment is venous capillary, which has one layer of pericytes around the vessel wall. Venous capillary then connects to the next segment of the postcapillary venule, which usually has an external diameter ranging from 18 to 23 μm at the papillary dermis level, a thicker wall of 3.5 to 5 μm, and two to three layers of pericytes around the vessel wall. The papillary dermal blood vessels are composed entirely of terminal arterioles, arterial and venous capillaries, and postcapillary venules, with the latter being the major component. The vessel sizes are generally larger at the lower part of the dermis. At the lower third of the dermis, arterioles and collecting venules can reach external diameter ranging from 40 to 50 μm, with vessel wall thickness ranging from 10 to 16 μm, and four to five layers of pericytes surrounding the vessel wall (Braverman, 2000).

Cutaneous blood vessels: Functions

One of the important functions of a cutaneous blood vessel is to provide nutrients to the skin. The capillary loops arise from the upper horizontal plexus, which is the primary avenue for nutrient delivery. The lower horizontal plexus, however, is responsible to supply life-sustaining substances for the hair bulbs, sweat glands, and other dermal glands (Braverman, 2000). The control of cutaneous blood flow is achieved by vasodilatation (increase) and vasoconstriction (decrease) through the smooth muscles directed by the sympathetic branch of the central nervous system (Blessing, McAllen, & McKinley, 2016; Johnson, Minson, & Kellogg, 2014). Vasodilation, itself, also serves as an

effective mechanism for thermal regulation (i.e., heat loss) (Francisco & Minson, 2018). The upper horizontal plexus acts as a thermal radiator (Braverman, 2000). Interestingly, physical exercise training can modify cutaneous microvascular reactivity to different stimuli (Lanting, Johnson, Baker, Caterson, & Chuter, 2017).

Another major function of cutaneous blood vessel is to provide immune support to the skin. As such, the microvascular system is always involved when there is an inflammatory event (Pober & Sessa, 2015). From a physiologic perspective, the postcapillary venules are the most important as they are the primary sites where inflammatory cells transmigrate from the vascular space into the target tissue sites. It is in this vessel segment that endothelial cells, in response to inflammatory signals, commonly develop intercellular gaps leading to increased vascular permeability (Braverman, 2000). Endothelial cells in the cutaneous blood vessel, when encountering appropriate triggers, such as stimulation by immunoglobulin-1 (IL1), tumor necrosis factor-α (TNF-α), or B-spectrum ultraviolet light, upregulate expressions on their cell surfaces of several adhesion molecules that facilitate the binding and the subsequent transportation of inflammatory cells out of the cutaneous blood vessels into the tissue location of the inflammatory targets. These adhesion molecules include intercellular adhesion molecule-1 (ICAM-1) (CD54), vascular cell adhesion molecule-1 (VCAM-1) (CD106), endothelial leukocyte adhesion molecule-1 (ELAM-1) (new term E-selectin, CD62E), and P-selectin (CD62P) (Cornelius et al., 1994; Kyan-Aung, Haskard, Poston, Thornhill, & Lee, 1991; Picker, Kishmoto, Smith, Warnock, & Butcher, 1991; Rossiter et al., 1994; Tonnesen, 1989). The inflammatory cells, with the adhesion molecules such as cutaneous lymphocyte antigen (CLA), the very late antigen-4 (VLA-4, integrin α4β1) β1 subunit (CD29), or lymphocyte function-associated antigen-1 (LFA-1) α subunit (CD11a) expressed on their surfaces, can interact with ICAM-1, VCAM-1, or ELAM-1 and thus help to facilitate the movement into the tissue inflamed sites (Berg et al., 1991; Caughman, Li, & Degitz, 1992; Rossiter et al., 1994; Santamaria Babi et al., 1995). In addition, junctional adhesion molecules (JAMs), the proteins located at the borders of endothelial cells that take part in the final step of leukocyte extravasation, are also important for the transmigration of leukocytes from cutaneous blood vessels into the inflamed skin sites, although their expressions are unaltered by the inflammatory process (Ludwig et al., 2005). Moreover, the expression of CD40 in endothelial cells, a costimulatory protein typically found in antigen-presenting cells, raises another possible role of cutaneous blood vessels in the skin inflammation (Pober, Kluger, & Schechner, 2001; Singh, Casper, Summers, & Swerlick, 2001).

Another inflammation-related function of cutaneous blood vessels is documented in an animal model of wound healing. Mice lacking in both P- and E-selectins by genetic knockout showed a substantial reduction of inflammatory cell (neutrophils and macrophages) recruitment into the wounding site, resulting in impairment of wound closure (Subramaniam et al., 1997).

Cutaneous blood vessels can be examined in skin frozen sections by labeling with antibodies against common endothelial cell markers such as E-selectin or PAL-E (Skobe & Detmar, 2000). Cutaneous blood vessels and blood flow can be assessed by different noninvasive methods, including laser-based techniques such as laser Doppler flowmetry or laser speckle contrast imaging (LSCI), and more recently by optical coherence tomography and photoacoustic imaging methodologies (Braverman, Schechner, Silverman, & Keh-Yen, 1992; Chan, 2019a, 2019b; Cracowski & Roustit, 2016; Deegan et al., 2018; Matsumoto et al., 2018).

Cutaneous blood vessels: Roles in atopic dermatitis

It is intuitively obvious that blood vessel is involved in transporting those inflammatory cells into the site of skin inflammation. Atopic dermatitis, a chronic inflammatory skin disease, is no exception. Next, we will discuss the roles of angiogenesis in atopic dermatitis as documented in a mouse model and in human patients affected by this disease.

Cutaneous blood vessels in the keratin-14/IL4 transgenic mice

To generate a mouse model of atopic dermatitis, a prominent Th2 cytokine IL4 that is upregulated in human atopic dermatitis skin was artificially expressed in the basal layer of epidermis through a keratin-14 promoter. The IL4 transgenic mice showed substantial changes in cutaneous blood vessels, in parallel with prominent dermal inflammatory

cell infiltration (Chan, Robinson, & Xu, 2001; Chen et al., 2008). All the keratin-14/IL4 transgenic mice, but none of nontransgenic littermates, developed chronic inflammatory skin lesions primarily on their hairless skin surfaces, ears, face, neck, tails, and periorbital areas (see Fig. 11.5). Heavy infiltrations of mononuclear cells, mast cells, and eosinophils were present under light microscopy on the lesional skin of the IL4 transgenic mice (see Fig. 11.6) (Chan et al., 2001). These substantial infiltrations of inflammatory cells would logically require the support of cutaneous microcirculation for delivering these immune cells to the site of inflammation. The findings of clinical disease progression (from before disease onset), to early skin lesion (within 1 week of onset), to chronic skin lesion (>3 weeks of onset), paralleled with progressive increase in the amount of inflammatory cell infiltration (CD3+, CD4+, CD8+, IA-IE+, CD11a+, and CD23+ cells) in the transgenic mouse skin, provided another indirect evidence of cutaneous microcirculation involvement in delivering these inflammatory cells to the target sites (Chen et al., 2005). To obtain direct evidence for the roles of cutaneous circulation, particularly the blood vessels, in the development and progression of atopic dermatitis, blood vessels and their promoting factors in these IL4 transgenic mice skin were investigated in greater details (Chen et al., 2008). Skin samples were obtained from nontransgenic mice, the transgenic mice at different disease stages: before onset, early skin lesion, and late skin lesion. When transmission and scanning electron microscopy methods were used to visualize the cutaneous blood vessels in these mice, substantial ultrastructural changes were present in the transgenic mice by electron microscopy, providing solid evidences of the occurrence of angiogenesis (Fig. 12.2) (Agha-Majzoub, Becker, Schraufnagel, & Chan, 2005).

When the frozen sections of these skin samples were labeled with vascular endothelial cell marker CD31 and analyzed by computer-assisted photometric analysis, a significant increase of the number of blood vessels and area occupied by dermal vessels were present, compared to the nontransgenic mice. In addition, the diameters of the dermal blood vessels, as determined by the positive CD31 labeling, also increased in the transgenic mice skin. When these skin samples were extracted for RNA and reverse transcription real-time polymerase chain reaction (PCR) was performed, we found an upregulation of the CD31 mRNAs in the transgenic mice skin, compared to that of nontransgenic mice (Fig. 12.3) (Chen et al., 2008). Thus we documented that in this animal model of human atopic dermatitis, blood vessels increased in number and diameter, suggesting the occurrence of an angiogenesis process (Chen et al., 2008). To delineate the possible involvement of an angiogenic process, these skin sections were labeled by an antibody against vascular endothelial growth factor receptor-2 (VEGFR2), the receptor on the endothelial cell surfaces responsible for receiving signal from vascular endothelial growth factor (VEGF), a potential angiogenic factor, and for initiating cell proliferation and migration (Ruhrberg, 2003). The increasingly positive VEGFR2

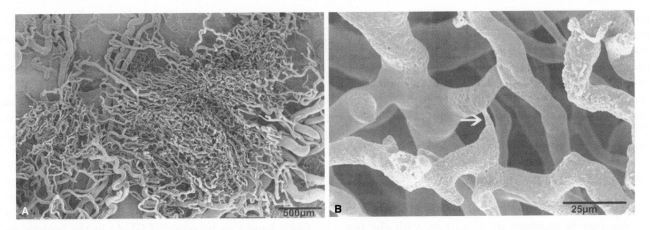

• **Fig. 12.2** Ultrastructure of cutaneous vasculature in keratin-14/IL4 transgenic mice depicting features of angiogenesis. Scanning electron microscopy of an early skin lesion showed abundance and disorganization of capillaries and general tortuosity of arterials and venules (A), and at high magnification showed capillaries' rough surface with sprouting *(arrow)* evidence of angiogenesis (B). (Reproduced with permission from Agha-Majzoub, R., Becker, R. P., Schraufnagel, D. E., & Chan, L. S. [2005]. Angiogenesis: The major abnormality of the keratin-14 IL-4 transgenic mouse model of atopic dermatitis. *Microcirculation, 12*[6], 455–476. doi:10.1080//10739660591003297.)

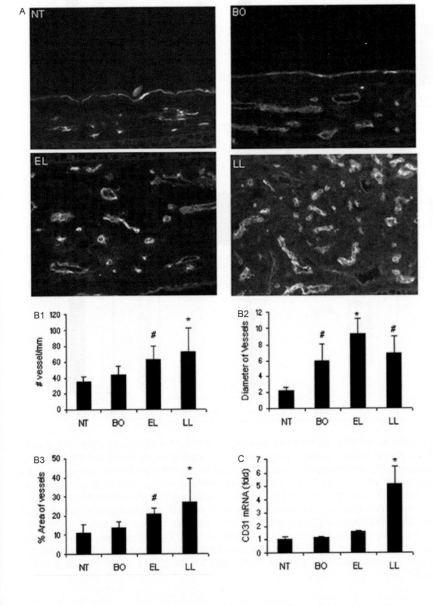

• **Fig. 12.3** In the keratin-14/IL4 transgenic mice skin, the increases of CD31 expressions parallel the progression of skin inflammation. (A) The progressive increase of CD31 labeling is visualized in the transgenic mice skin before skin lesion developed *(BO)*, early skin lesion *(EL)*, and late skin lesion *(LL)*, in comparison to nontransgenic mice *(NT)*. By computerized measurement, the number of vessels per high-power field (B1), diameter of the vessels (B2), and the percent of dermis area occupied by the CD31+ vessels (B3) illustrate a general trend of increase as the disease progresses. These physical blood vessel increases correspond well to the parallel increase in CD31 mRNA (C). (Reproduced with permission from Chen, L., Marble, D. J., Agha, R., Peterson, J. D., Becker, R. P., Jin, T., et al. [2008]. The progression of inflammation parallels the dermal angiogenesis in a keratin 14 IL-4-transgenic model of atopic dermatitis. *Microcirculation, 15*[1], 49–64. doi:10.1080/10739680701418416.) #p<0.05, *p<0.01 vs NT.

protein labeling and mRNA expression, not surprisingly, paralleled the increase in CD31 labeling and had a general trend of progressive increase, as the disease progressed from before disease onset to early skin lesion, and then to late skin lesion (Chen et al., 2008). Thus the determined parallel increase of VEGFR2 and CD31+ vessels and disease progression further supports a role of angiogenesis in atopic dermatitis. These parallel events of increased inflammation and increased blood vessel density are consistent with the findings that occurred in other cutaneous inflammatory processes (Tellechea et al., 2013).

To access the underlying mechanism of the angiogenic process, we examined proangiogenic factors known to take part in angiogenesis. Consistent with the progressive increase in skin endothelial cell marker CD31 and VEGFR2, there were also progressive increases of a potent proangiogenic factor VEGF-A skin mRNAs, skin-extracted proteins, and serum proteins (Fig. 12.4) (Chen et al., 2008). On the skin mRNA level, the prominent upregulations were detected for VEGF-A120 and VEGF-A188 isoforms. VEGF-A120 isoform and the VEGF-A164 isoform are the two predominant forms, capable of inducing proliferation of endothelial cells and in vivo angiogenesis process (Chen et al., 2008; Nakamura, Abe, & Tokunaga, 2002). In the skin and serum protein levels, the immunoreactive VEGF-A concentrations progressively elevated as the disease progressed from before onset stage, to early lesion stage, and then to late lesion stage (see Fig. 12.4). The upregulation of IL6 and interferon-gamma (IFN-γ) (both known to promote VEGF-A) in the protein and mRNA levels in the skin of transgenic mice supported the angiogenic role of these cytokines on atopic skin. In

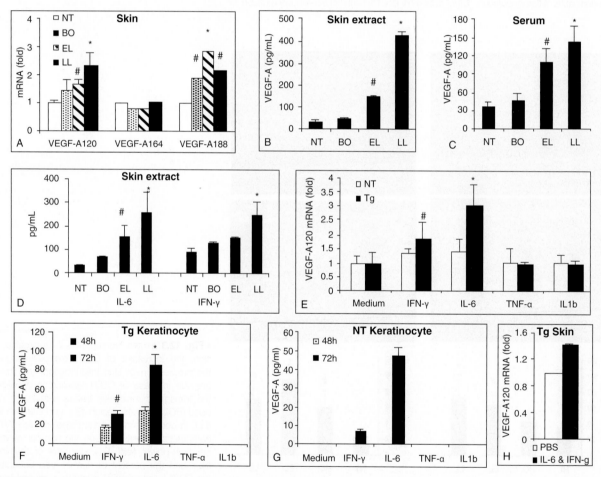

• **Fig. 12.4** Upregulation of a potent proangiogenic factor VEGF-A and VEGF-A–promoting cytokines observed in the skin and peripheral blood samples of the keratin-14/IL4 transgenic mice. Skin samples (A, B) and serum samples (C) collected from nontransgenic mice *(NT)* and the transgenic mice at the stages of before disease onset *(BO)*, early skin lesion *(EL)*, and late skin lesion *(LL)* were prepared for mRNA analysis by reverse transcription PCR (A) and protein assays by ELISA (B, C). The examination of potential sources of VEGF-A–promoting cytokines determined upregulation of IL6 and IFN-γ protein in the skin of transgenic mice (D). Direct evidence of the ability of IL6 and IFN-γ in enhancing VEGF-A120 mRNA expressions of keratinocyte cultured from transgenic mice skin, comparing to nontransgenic mice skin (E). The releases of VEGF-A proteins from primary cultured keratinocyte of transgenic mice (F) and nontransgenic mice (G) were stronger at 72 hours of IL6 and IFN-γ stimulation. The mRNA level of VEGF-A120 expression in the skin of transgenic mice was upregulated upon intradermal administration of IL6 and INF-γ (H). (Reproduced with permission from Chen, L., Marble, D. J., Agha, R., Peterson, J. D., Becker, R. P., Jin, T., et al. [2008]. The progression of inflammation parallels the dermal angiogenesis in a keratin 14 IL-4-transgenic model of atopic dermatitis. *Microcirculation, 15*[1], 49–64. doi:10.1080/10739680701418416.) #p<0.05, *p<0.01, comparing to NT (A, B, C, D) and to medium only (E and F).

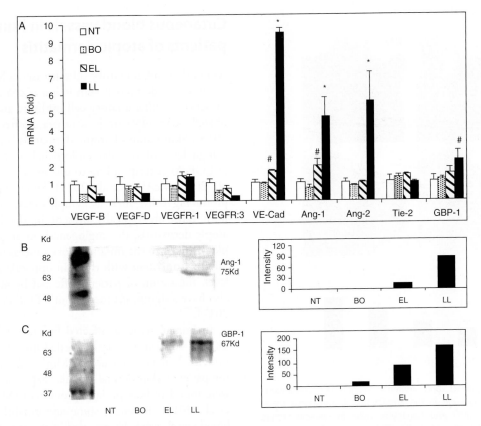

• **Fig. 12.5** Upregulation of mRNA and protein levels of other angiogenic factors in the skin of transgenic mice in the disease stages of before onset *(BO)*, early skin lesion *(EL)*, and late skin lesion *(LL)*, compared to that of nontransgenic mice *(NT)*. RNA samples extracted from the skin were reversely transcribed, followed by semiquantitative real-time PCR (A). Protein samples extracted from the skin were electrophoresed followed by Western blotting to detect Ang-1 (B, *left side*) and GBP-1 (C, *left side*), and scanning for intensity of the immunoreactive protein bands (B, C, *right side*). (Reproduced with permission from Chen, L., Marble, D. J., Agha, R., Peterson, J. D., Becker, R. P., Jin, T., et al. [2008]. The progression of inflammation parallels the dermal angiogenesis in a keratin 14 IL-4-transgenic model of atopic dermatitis. *Microcirculation, 15*[1], 49–64. doi:10.1080/10739680701418416.) #$p<0.05$, *$p<0.01$, vs NT. GBP-1, guanylate-binding protein-1.

addition, primary keratinocytes cultured from skin of nontransgenic and transgenic mice exhibited upregulation of VEGF-A protein and mRNA expressions upon stimulation by IL6 and INF-γ, with transgenic keratinocytes showing greater enhancement. Moreover, VEGF-A120 mRNA was upregulated in the skin of transgenic mice upon intradermal administration of IL6 and IFN-γ (see Fig. 12.4) (Chen et al., 2008).

To determine if proangiogenic factors other than VEGF-A might also be involved in the process of atopic dermatitis, we analyzed mRNA levels of the skin of both nontransgenic mice and transgenic mice in different disease stages for these angiogenic factors: VEGF-B, VEGF-D, VEGFR1, VEGFR3, VE-Cadherin, angiopoietin-1 (Ang-1), Ang-2, Tie-2 (endothelium-specific receptor tyrosine kinase, a ligand for which Ang-1), and guanylate-binding protein-1 (GBP-1). We found that there were substantial upregulations on VE-cadherin, Ang-1, Ang-2, and GBP-1, especially at the late lesion stage of disease in transgenic mice compared to nontransgenic mice. Similarly, in the same samples we also demonstrated increased protein levels of Ang-1 and GBP-1 in the skin of transgenic mice

compared to that of nontransgenic mice by Western blot analysis (Fig. 12.5) (Chen et al., 2008).

To evaluate if the prominent angiogenesis of the blood vessels in the mice affected by atopic dermatitis negatively modify the function of these blood vessels, we performed leakage study to answer this question. In parallel to the increase of skin inflammation in the transgenic mice, there was a progressive increase of leakage of intravenous administrated Evans blue dye into the skin matrices of transgenic mice, as determined by the increased blue intensities in the ear by standardized exposure photographs and by the higher concentrations of Evans blue by unit weight (Fig. 12.6) (Chen et al., 2008).

More recently, the important atopic dermatitis–related cytokine IL4 has shown its direct effect on cutaneous blood vessel by its upregulating of VEGF expressions in keratinocyte (Bao, Shi, & Chan, 2013). Together, the study results of this keratin-14/IL4 transgenic mouse model of atopic dermatitis establish a powerful link between cutaneous microvascular angiogenesis and atopic dermatitis. Next we illustrate the proposed immunologic mechanism of angiogenesis involvement in skin inflammation of this atopic dermatitis model (Fig. 12.7).

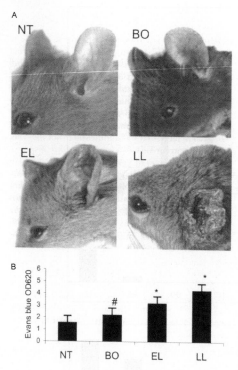

• **Fig. 12.6** Photographic and material weight documentations of dermal vascular leakage in the keratin-14/IL4 transgenic mice. Nontransgenic mice *(NT)* and transgenic mice at disease stages of before onset *(BO)*, early skin lesion *(EL)*, and late skin lesion *(LL)* were administered intravenously with Evans blue dye and photographed in 5 minutes postadministration of dye (A). The skin sections from these mice postadministration of dye were collected, and the dye extracted for concentration measurement (OD at 620 nm) (B). (Reproduced with permission from Chen, L., Marble, D. J., Agha, R., Peterson, J. D., Becker, R. P., Jin, T., et al. [2008]. The progression of inflammation parallels the dermal angiogenesis in a keratin 14 IL-4-transgenic model of atopic dermatitis. *Microcirculation, 15*[1], 49–64. doi:10.1080/10739680701418416.) #p<0.05 vs NT, *p<0.01 vs NT.

Cutaneous blood vessels in human patients of atopic dermatitis

As in other inflammatory skin diseases, a histology picture in an atopic dermatitis skin lesion is characterized by the presence of inflammatory cell infiltrate and some features of angiogenesis (Varricchi, Granata, Loffredo, & Genovese, 2015). Skin lesion of atopic dermatitis is characterized by a high level of vascular endothelial growth factor alpha (VEGF-A) corresponding to disease severity (Genovese et al., 2012; McAleer et al., 2019). Since angiogenic factor-producing cells, such as lymphocytes, eosinophils, and mast cells, are typically present in the lesional skin of atopic dermatitis, the angiogenesis in atopic dermatitis is likely linked to the inflammatory process (Genovese et al., 2012). Consistent with the skin upregulation of VEGF-A level, the serum of patients affected by atopic dermatitis also have a significant increase of VEGF-A (Brunner et al., 2017).

In human patients affected by atopic dermatitis, their lesional skin extracts have revealed upregulation of VEGF proteins (Zhang, Matsuo, & Morita, 2006). In addition, the patients' skin dermal vascular expressions of E-selectin were found to be especially prominent (Marinovic Kulisic et al., 2010). Recently, some abnormalities of cutaneous blood vessels were also revealed in the erythematous skin of human patients affected by atopic dermatitis. Specifically, researchers, using 2-photon microscopy in living tissues, found that skin from patients affected by atopic dermatitis exhibits "thickened, flexuous" blood vessels, suggesting increased blood flow in the erythematous skin areas (Tsutsumi et al., 2016). In addition, the prominent presence of mast cells, which has documented effects on angiogenesis and vascular leakage, in skin lesions of atopic dermatitis,

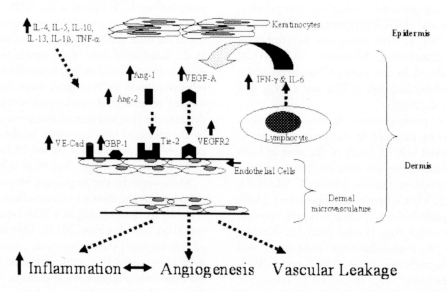

• **Fig. 12.7** Schematic illustration of pathophysiology of atopic dermatitis from the perspective of cutaneous blood vessels involvements. (Reproduced with permission from Chen, L., Marble, D. J., Agha, R., Peterson, J. D., Becker, R. P., Jin, T., et al. [2008]. The progression of inflammation parallels the dermal angiogenesis in a keratin 14 IL-4-transgenic model of atopic dermatitis. *Microcirculation, 15*[1], 49–64. doi: 10.1080/10739680701418416.)

may also contribute to the overall inflammatory process of the disease (Kritas et al., 2013). Overall, the findings in human atopic dermatitis patients are consistent with that found in the keratin-14/IL4 transgenic mouse, an animal model of the disease.

Cutaneous lymphatic vessels: Structures

Several publications have depicted details of general and cutaneous lymphatic structures (Petrova & Koh, 2018; Rovenska & Rovensky, 2011; Sallustio et al., 2000; Schwager & Detmar, 2019; Skobe & Detmar, 2000). Although it has originally been viewed as a passive channel for fluid and cellular transport, lymphatic vessels are now recognized as an active participant of homeostasis and physiologic functions, including inflammation, and lymphatic vessels are organ-specific (Petrova & Koh, 2018; Schwager & Detmar, 2019). Lymphatic vessels are absent from certain tissues such as cornea, lens, and cartilage but are abundantly present in skin (other than epidermis) and mucous membranes (other than epithelium). Like cutaneous blood vessels, the cutaneous lymphatic system also organizes in two plexuses. The superficial lymphatic plexus locates around the subpapillary arterial network and extends into the dermal papillae. In these areas, the lymphatic vessels have smaller diameters and no valves. Branching vessels from the superficial plexus drain vertically down to larger vessels in the lower dermis and the superficial zone of subcutaneous tissue. The lower lymphatic plexus locates below the second arterial network and contains larger lymphatic vessels with valves. In general, the lymphatic vessels have a uniform shape in firm and thick skin areas but have a variable shape in thin and loose skin areas (Skobe & Detmar, 2000). Lymphatic capillaries, the likely segment of lymphatic vessels where the resorption of fluid and macromolecules takes place, have several distinct features in comparison to arterial capillaries, and these differences are stated in Table 12.1.

TABLE 12.1 Feature comparisons of capillaries of arterial and lymphatic vessels

Feature	Arterial capillary	Lymphatic capillary
Vessel lumen	Smaller, regular shape (outer diameter 17–22 µm)	Wider, irregular shape (outer diameter up to 60 µm)
Vessel wall Thickness	Thicker, 3.5–5 µm	Thinner, 50–100 nm
Endothelial	Normal appearance	Extremely attenuated
Cytoplasm	No longitudinal filaments	Numerous longitudinal filaments
Basal lamina	Well developed	Poorly developed or absence
Pericyte	Encircled the vessel	Absence
Tight junctions/ major adherence junctions	Present	Infrequent present
Endothelium-matrix Connection	No connection	Anchoring filament attaching cell surface to connective tissues
Interendothelial Junctions	No overlapping junction	Extensive superimposing overlapping junctions

From Skobe, M., & Detmar, M. (2000). Structure, function, and molecular control of the skin lymphatic system. *Journal of Investigative Dermatology, 5*(1), 14–19.

Cutaneous lymphatic vessels: Functions

The understanding of the functions, and to some extent the structures, of cutaneous lymphatic vessels has been minimum until recently, in part because of the absence of molecular markers that we can use to distinguish blood vessels from lymphatic vessels. With the available knowledge and antibodies specific to the lymphatic vessel components and prolymphangiogenic factors, we now have greater opportunity to develop a clearer picture of how cutaneous lymphatic vessels take part in the biologic functions. Although blood and lymphatic vessels are structurally different and functionally distinct, they work in concert in keeping the skin in healthy conditions. We illustrate the proximal relationship between these vessels in Fig. 12.1. Besides the more commonly acknowledged function of extracellular tissue fluid homeostasis, we now recognize the lymphatic system as an important factor in

regulating other tissue homeostasis and immune responses in hypertension, obesity, neoplasm, wound healing, and inflammation (Coso, Bovay, & Petrova, 2014; Sallustio et al., 2000; Wilting, Becker, Buttler, & Weich, 2009; Lutter & Makinen, 2014). Failure of the lymphatic system will inevitably lead to compromised immune functions, fibrosis, and recurrent infections (Ryan, 1989). The lymphatic system is also a participant of genesis of blood vessels and lymphatic vessels (i.e., angiogenesis and lymphangiogenesis, respectively) (Jeltsch, Tammela, Alitalo, & Wilting, 2003; Scavelli et al., 2004). Several molecular markers (VEGFR3, LYVE-1 [lymphatic vessel endothelial receptor-1], and podoplanin [PDPN]) that are positively present in lymphatic vessels but negatively present in blood vessels enable molecular distinction between lymphatic and blood vessels (Skobe & Detmar, 2000).

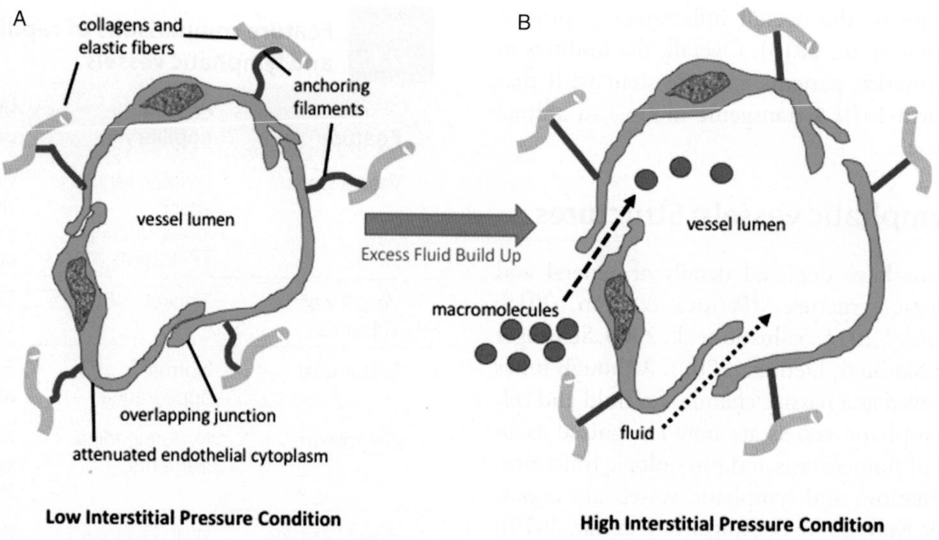

• **Fig. 12.8** Schematic illustration of the functional anatomy of a dermal lymphatic capillary. When the pressure of interstitial pressure is low, the overlapping junctions of endothelial cells are closed (A). When there is excessive fluid in the interstitial tissue, this induces the increase of interstitial pressure. The higher pressure results in increase of tension and stretching of the anchoring filaments connecting the lymphatic endothelial cells and its collagen and elastic fibers in the surrounding tissue, leading to the pulling of endothelial cells away from the vessel lumens and thus the opening of overlapping junctions. These openings will then allow fluid and macromolecules to enter into the lymphatic vessel lumen (B). (From Skobe, M., & Detmar, M. [2000]. Structure, function, and molecular control of the skin lymphatic system. *Journal of Investigative Dermatology, 5*[1], 14–19.)

Prolymphangiogenic factors VEGF-C and VEGF-D are now determined to be essential for lymphatic vessel development through binding of and triggering VEGFR3 signaling pathway, and many skin cell types are expressing VEGF-C, including melanocytes, keratinocytes, fibroblasts, and endothelial cells (Coso et al., 2014; Lund, Medler, Leachman, & Coussens, 2016; Scavelli et al., 2004; Skobe & Detmar, 2000). In addition, cytokines that promote or enhance these prolymphangiogenic factors have also been delineated, including IL1, TNF-α, and transforming growth factor-α (TGF-α) (Skobe & Detmar, 2000).

The importance of tissue fluid homeostasis is illustrated by the fact that on a single day, about 50% of the total proteins in the blood circulation escapes into the tissues and cannot return directly to the blood vessels. It is therefore essential for these macromolecules and the accompanied fluid to return to the blood, so as to prevent tissue pressure increase, to maintain a proper plasma volume in the blood, and to ensure adequate nutrition delivery by keeping a minimum distance between the capillaries and the target cells (Skobe & Detmar, 2000). The functional anatomy of lymphatic vessels in returning macromolecules and fluid is illustrated in Fig. 12.8. The lymphatic role in extracellular tissue fluid balance is easily demonstrated from a clinical perspective when its function is compromised as in patients with primary (genetically determined) or secondary (due to other disease) lymphedema, which can occur not only in the common sites of extremities but also in head and neck regions (Feely, Olsen, Gamble, Davis, & Pittelkow, 2012; Hirakawa & Detmar, 2004; Saaristo, Karkkainen, & Alitalo, 2002). In an issue relating to fluid hemostasis, lymphatic vessel is also recognized as an essential component of proper wound healing, as edematous tissue inhibits proper wound healing (Boyce & Lalley, 2018).

Lymphatic vessel's role in cancer is also well documented. Melanoma, one of the skin cancers with high mortality if detected in a late stage, commonly spread through the lymphatic system, as about half of first distant melanoma metastases are detected in lymph nodes (Leiter, Meier, Schittek, & Garbe, 2004). Thus sentinel lymph node biopsy has been utilized as a part of melanoma management strategy based on the primary melanoma cancer histologic depth level (Gonzalez, 2018; Trinidad, Torres-Cabala, Curry, Prieto, & Aung, 2019). Similarly, management of squamous cell carcinoma and Merkel cell carcinoma, which also have the tendency to metastasize through lymphatic system, may include sentinel lymph node biopsy and dissection (Baum et al., 2018; Gunaratne, Howle, & Veness, 2016). Some research results also suggest that active lymphangiogenesis may be induced by melanoma and other cancers (Dadras & Detmar, 2004; Lund et al., 2016; Raica, Jitariu, & Cimpean, 2016). The extracellular matrix, in turn, regulates the lymphangiogenesis (Lutter & Makinen, 2014).

From the perspective of inflammation, lymphatic is an important contributing component (Braverman, 1983; Cueni & Detmar, 2006; Dieterich, Seidel, & Detmar, 2014; Lund et al., 2016). Cutaneous lymphatic vessels are important conduits for antigen-presenting cell migration from skin to regional lymph node where these immune cells could initiate the adaptive immune functions governing cutaneous immune encounters. In fact, the actual migration of these living cells can be visualized and analyzed by multiphoton excitation microscopy (Roediger, Ng, Smith,

Fazeka de St Groth, & Weninger, 2008). The lymphatic system is essential for resolving inflammation, which inevitably induces extravasation of macromolecules, fluid, and inflammatory cells into the inflamed tissue. Thus the body depends on the lymphatic system to return the excess of macromolecules and fluid back to the blood vascular system after an inflammatory event. On the other hand, the inflammatory process could alter the lymphatic vessels in both structural and functional aspects. Structurally, chronic inflammation can induce lymphangiogensis, and functionally chronic inflammation could induce lymphatic leakage. The resulting altered lymphatic vessels may negatively affect the cutaneous homeostasis in a variety of ways.

The visualization of lymphatic vessels, in distinction from blood vessels, can be achieved in frozen skin sections with double immune labeling of the tissue utilizing antibodies against molecular markers LYVE-1 and PAL-E that bind only to lymphatic and blood vessels, respectively (Skobe & Detmar, 2000). Visualization of lymphatic vessels in vivo can be accomplished by specially equipped fluorescence microscopy conducted 30 minutes postdermal injection of FITC-labeled tracer dextran, a high-molecular-weight (MW = 500,000) molecule that could enter lymphatic vessels but not blood vessels (Skobe & Detmar, 2000).

Cutaneous lymphatic vessels: Roles in atopic dermatitis

Regarding the roles of the cutaneous lymphatic system in the disease of atopic dermatitis, there is currently no detailed report of human patient studies. One report resulted from a study in a mouse model of atopic dermatitis that will be utilized to imply its roles (Shi, Bao, & Chan, 2012; Zhang, Shi, & Chan, 2017).

Cutaneous lymphatic vessels in the keratin-14/IL4 transgenic mice

In this mouse model of atopic dermatitis, generated by transgenically expressing a prominent Th2 cytokine IL4 in the basal layer of epidermis through a keratin-14 promoter, significant angiogenesis, in parallel with prominent dermal inflammatory cell infiltration, was documented (Chan et al., 2001; Chen et al., 2008). To analyze the lymphatic vessels in this mouse model of atopic dermatitis, immunofluorescence microscopy, Evans Blue lymphatic flow and uptake, keratinocyte cell culture, quantitative real-time RT-PCR, and Western blot analysis were employed (Shi et al., 2012). Fig. 12.9 illustrates the prominent lymphatic proliferation in parallel with the progression of disease.

Having determined the atopic dermatitis skin's significant lymphangiogenesis, we next look for factors that might contribute to this process. Recognizing the fact that VEGF-C, VEGF-D, and other factors could participate in this process, we analyzed the expressions of mRNAs and proteins in selected factors and markers (Fig. 12.10). Total RNAs and

proteins were extracted from the ears of four groups of mice. Their mRNAs were determined by reverse transcription followed by RT-PCR, and the proteins were assayed by Western blot analyses. While no significant elevation in VEGF-D was found, there was a significant upregulation of VEGF-C mRNAs in the early and late skin lesions, compared to nontransgenic mice control skin samples. Consistently, the mRNA expressions of receptor for VEGF-C, VEGFR3, were also significantly upregulated in the early and late skin lesions. In addition, the mRNA expressions of Ang-1, Ang-2, PDPN, and LYVE-1 also significantly increased in early and late skin lesions. Interestingly, the mRNAs of Ang-2, PDPN, and LYVE-1 showed significant elevation even in transgenic mouse skin before their disease onset, supporting a notion that these markers might be involved some way in the initial phase of the disease. Correspondingly, the protein levels of VEGFR3, PDPN, and LYVE-1 significantly increased in the skin of transgenic mice before disease onset, and in early and late lesions.

Since the animal model of atopic dermatitis is developed under the initiation of a transgene, IL4, we next wanted to investigate what factors in epidermal cells influenced by IL4 might be relevant in the lymphangiogenesis of this mouse model. Toward that end, an immortal keratinocyte cell line (HaCAT) was experimentally stimulated with IL4, and their mRNA expressions were examined by a lymphangiogenesis-related gene PCR array method. As depicted in Fig. 12.11, the array determined that several factors were elevated by IL4 by at least twofold: ANG-1, ANGL4 (angiopoietin like-4), CXCL6 (granulocyte chemotactic protein-2), IGF1 (insulin growth factor-1), NOTCH4 (neurogenic locus notch homolog protein-4), PFG (placenta growth factor), and THBS1 (thrombospondin-1). Many factors, on the other hand, were downregulated by twofold or more. Significantly, the mRNAs of two known suppressors of lymphangiogenesis were decreased by IL4: interferon-alpha-1 (IFNA1) and TNF. Thus this downregulation supports a notion that IL4, by suppressing these negative regulators of lymphangiogenesis, is in fact prolymphangiogenic (Liu & He, 1997; Shao & Liu, 2006; Shi et al., 2012). However, IL4 did not increase the level of VEGF-C in a keratinocyte cell line. Thus we looked for other potential cell sources of VEGF-C upregulation. We hypothesized that IL4 could, by indirect pathway, influence VEGF-C elevation. Since macrophages are a cell type known to produce VEGF-C, we analyzed the possibility that IL4 could take part in macrophage recruitment by stimulating keratinocytes.

Toward that end, we found that IL4, indeed, could stimulate keratinocytes to increase a macrophage recruiting cytokine, MCP-1 (monocyte chemotactic protein-1), in a dose-dependent manner (Shi et al., 2012). Thus these data would suggest that IL4 could, by increasing MCP-1 production in keratinocytes, recruit macrophages to be the actual VEGF-C contributor for lymphangiogenesis in this atopic dermatitis model.

Confirming IL4's capability in upregulating keratinocyte-produced macrophage recruitment chemokine MCP-1

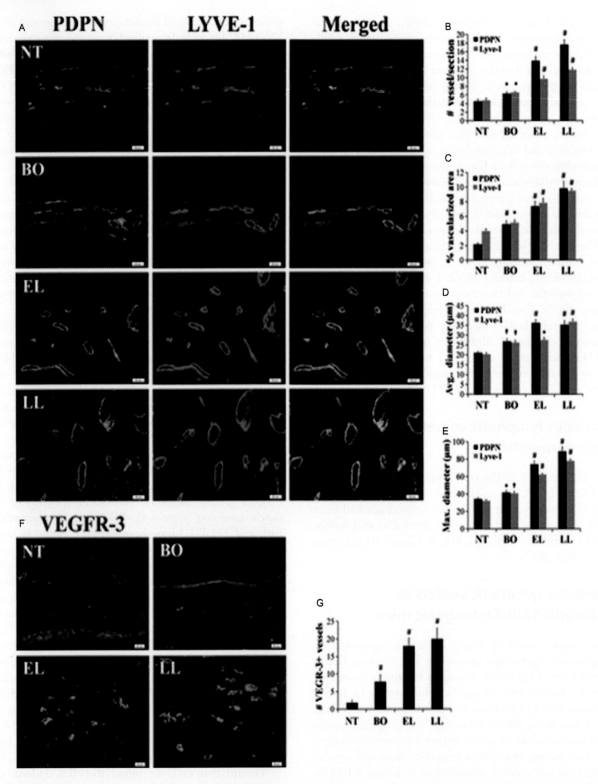

• **Fig. 12.9** Dermal lymphatic hyperproliferation parallel the progression of skin inflammation. (A) Immunofluorescence microscopy was performed on frozen sections of ear skin obtained from nontransgenic control mice *(NT)*, transgenic before disease onset *(BO)*, early lesion *(EL)*, and chronic/late lesion *(LL)* by labeling with antibodies to PDPN *(left column)*, LYVE-1 *(middle column)*. The right column showed the merged images of both left and middle columns. (B) The computer-assisted method calculated numbers of PDPN+ and LYVE-1+ vessels for each skin section. (C) The computer-assisted method determined percent area of skin occupied by labeled vessels. (D, E) The computer-assisted method identification of average diameter and maximum diameter of the labeled vessels, respectively. (F) The VEGFR3-labeled immunofluorescence microscopy, and (G) calculated the numbers of VEGFR3+ vessels per unit skin by computer-assisted method. N = 10 for all experiments. Data represent mean ± SD. *$P < 0.05$; +$P < 0.01$; #$P < 0.001$ statistical significance vs. NT group. (Reprinted with permission from Shi, V. Y., Bao, L., & Chan, L. S. [2012]. Inflammation-driven dermal lymphangiogenesis in atopic dermatitis is associated with CD11b+ macrophage recruitment and VEGF-C up-regulation in the IL-4-transgenic mouse model. *Microcirculation, 19*[7], 567–579. doi:10.1111/j.1549-8719.2012.00189xShi.)

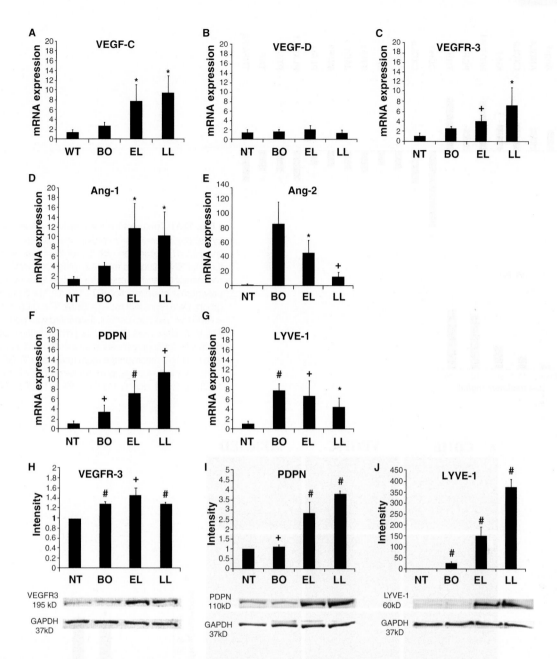

• **Fig. 12.10** Increased mRNA (A-G) and protein (H-J) expressions of factors and markers of lymphangiogenesis as detected in the skin of keratin-14/IL4 transgenic mice. Ear skin samples were obtained from four groups of mice: nontransgenic mice control (*NT*), transgenic mice before disease onset (*BO*), early lesion (*EL*), and late lesion (*LL*). Total RNAs and proteins extracted were assayed by reverse transcription followed by real-time polymerase chain reaction (RT-PCR) and Western blotting, respectively. GAPDH was used as an internal control. N = 5 for each group. *$P < 0.05$; +$P < 0.01$; #$P < 0.001$ vs. NT. (Reprinted with permission from Shi, V. Y., Bao, L., & Chan, L. S. [2012]. Inflammation-driven dermal lymphangiogenesis in atopic dermatitis is associated with CD11b+ macrophage recruitment and VEGF-C up-regulation in the IL-4-transgenic mouse model. *Microcirculation, 19*[7], 567–579. doi:10.1111/j.1549-8719.2012.00189xShi.)

led us to set out to validate experimentally that macrophages were in fact involved in this lymphangiogenic process. Toward that end, we used immunofluorescence microscopy to examine the presence of macrophages in the skin lesions of the keratin-14/IL4 transgenic mice and the locations of VEGF-C in these skin lesions. We verified that the CD11b+ macrophages were present in a sizable amount in the skin of transgenic mice, particularly in the early and late skin lesions. And most of the VEGF-C–labeled cells were

colocalized with the CD11b+ macrophages (Fig. 12.12). Thus we delineate that in our keratin-14/IL4 transgenic mouse model of atopic dermatitis, the lymphangiogenesis process is at least in part driven by IL4. This pathway is through stimulating keratinocyte to increase production of MCP-1, a strong chemokine for macrophages. The production of VEGF-C by the recruited macrophages may in fact be an important, if not the sole, cellular source in inducing lymphangiogenesis.

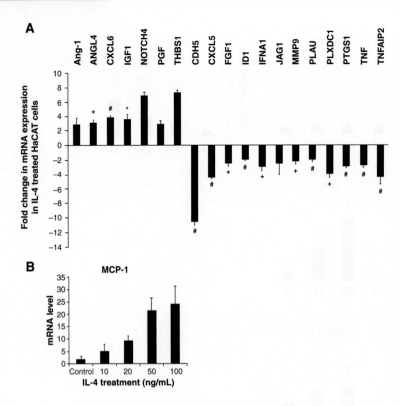

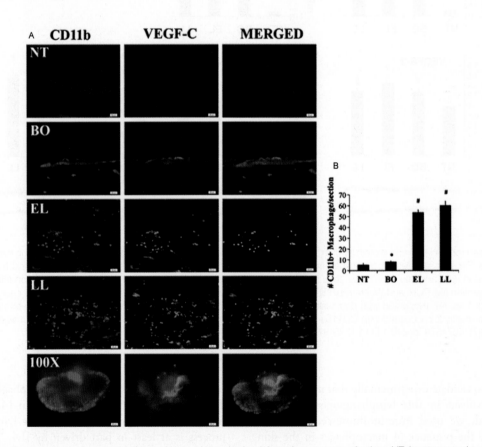

• **Fig. 12.11** The cytokine IL4 positively influences keratinocytes' participation in lymphangiogenesis. Keratinocyte cell line *(HaCaT)*, incubated with IL4 for 24 hours, was harvested for total RNA, and the mRNA expressions were assayed by microarray (A) and reverse transcription followed by real-time polymerase chain reaction (RT-PCR) (B). N = 3 per experiment group. Data represent mean ± SEM. *P < 0.05; +P < 0.01; #P < 0.001 vs. medium control. (Reprinted with permission from Shi, V. Y., Bao, L., & Chan, L. S. [2012]. Inflammation-driven dermal lymphangiogenesis in atopic dermatitis is associated with CD11b+ macrophage recruitment and VEGF-C up-regulation in the IL-4-transgenic mouse model. *Microcirculation, 19*[7], 567–579. doi:10.1111/j.1549-8719.2012.00189xShi.)

• **Fig. 12.12** Immunofluorescence microscopy of ear skin sections obtained from four groups of mice: *NT* (nontransgenic control), *BO* (before disease onset), *EL* (early lesion), and *LL* (late lesion). (A) The skin sections' images recorded were labeled with CD11b *(left column)*, VEGF-C *(middle column)*, and merged images of left and middle columns *(right column)*. (B) The numbers of CD11b+ cells per skin section as determined by computer-assisted photometric analysis. N = 5 per group. Data represents mean ± SD. *P < 0.05; +P < 0.01; #P < 0.001 vs. NT group. (Reprinted with permission from Shi, V. Y., Bao, L., & Chan, L. S. [2012]. Inflammation-driven dermal lymphangiogenesis in atopic dermatitis is associated with CD11b+ macrophage recruitment and VEGF-C up-regulation in the IL-4-transgenic mouse model. *Microcirculation, 19*[7], 567–579. doi:10.1111/j.1549-8719.2012.00189xShi.)

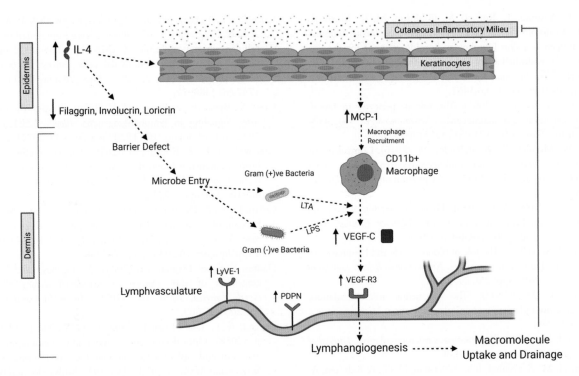

• **Fig. 12.13** Schematic illustration of the involvement of IL4 in the process of lymphangiogenesis. IL4, through the stimulation of MCP-1 in keratinocytes, can participate in macrophage recruitment. In addition, IL4, through the inhibitory act on skin barrier proteins filaggrin, involucrin, and loricrin, can provide easy penetration of bacteria, which could in turn stimulate macrophages to release VEGF-C by their components such as lipopolysaccharide (*LPS*) and lipoteichoic acid (*LTA*). VEGF-C can then become the proangiogenic factor for lymphatic vessels. *Red line* indicates negative influence. MCP-1, monocyte chemotatic protein 1.

To summarize the involvement of lymphangiogenesis in atopic dermatitis, Fig. 12.13 is presented to illustrate the potential participants in this process. As discussed throughout this chapter, the Th2 cytokine IL4 is in fact the essential trigger. In addition to the recruitment of macrophages by MCP-1 from keratinocyte under the influence of IL4, bacterial components such as lipopolysaccharide (LPS) and lipoteichoic acid (LTA) can also induce dermal macrophages to release VEGF-C.

Summary

Having analyzed the structures and functions of cutaneous microvasculature in relationship to the development of the chronic inflammatory skin disease atopic dermatitis, it is now clear that microcirculation has a significant role in this disease's development and progression. We now have a better understanding regarding how the inflammatory process present in atopic dermatitis would affect the vasculature, and how the altered vasculature's structure (as resulted in angiogenesis and lymphangiogenesis) and function (as resulted in vessel leakage) would contribute to the progression and sustaining of this chronic disease. In particular, specific factors that are involved in promoting the microvasculature alterations are well documented, and this important information would pave pathways for future pharmacologic intervention.

Further Reading

Abramson, D. I., & Dobrin, P. B. (Eds.), (2012). *Blood vessels and lymphatics in organ systems*. Academic Press.

Bikfalvi. A. (2018). *A brief history of blood and lymphatic vessels*. Springer.

Feige, J. -J., Pages, G., & Soncin, F. (Eds.), (2014). *Molecular mechanisms of angiogenesis: From ontogenesis to oncogenesis*. Springer.

Gigg, W. D., & Folkman, J. (Eds.), (2008). *Angiogenesis: An integrative approach from science to medicine*. Springer.

References

Agha-Majzoub, R., Becker, R. P., Schraufnagel, D. E., & Chan, L. S. (2005). Angiogenesis: The major abnormality of the keratin-14 IL-4 transgenic mouse model of atopic dermatitis. *Microcirculation*, 12(6), 455–476. https://doi.org/10.1080/10739680591003297.

Bao, L., Shi, V. Y., & Chan, L. S. (2013). IL-4 up-regulates epidermal chemotactic, angiogenic, and pro-inflammatory genes and down-regulates antimicrobial genes in vivo and in vitro: Relevant in the pathogenesis of atopic dermatitis. *Cytokine*, 61(2), 419–425. https://doi.org/10.1016/j.cyto.2012.10.031.

Baum, C. L., Wright, A. C., Martinez, J. C., Arpey, C. J., Brewer, J. D., Roenigk, R. K., & Otley, C. C. (2018). A new evidence-based risk stratification system for cutaneous squamous cell carcinoma into low, intermediate, and high risk groups with implications for management. *Journal of the American Academy of Dermatology*, 78(1), 141–147. https://doi.org/10.1016/j.jaad.2017.07.031.

Berg, E. L., Yoshino, T., Rott, L. S., Robinson, M. K., Warnock, R. A., Kishmoto, T. K., et al. (1991). The cutaneous lymphocyte antigen is a skin lymphocyte homing receptor for the vascular lectin endothelial cell-leukocyte adhesion molecule 1. *The Journal of Experimental Medicine, 174*(6), 1461–1466. https://doi.org/10.1084/jem.174.6.1461.

Bergers, G., & Song, S. (2005). The role of pericytes in blood-vessel formation and maintenance. *Neuro-oncology, 7*(4), 452–464. https://doi.org/10.1215/S1152851705000232.

Blessing, W., McAllen, R., & McKinley, M. (2016). Control of the cutaneous circulation by the central nervous system. *Comprehensive Physiology, 6*(3), 1161–1197. https://doi.org/10.1002/cphy.c150034.

Boyce, S. T., & Lalley, A. L. (2018). Tissue engineering of skin and regenerative medicine for wound care. *Burns & Trauma, 6*, 4. https://doi.org/10.1186/s41038-017-0103-y.

Braverman. I. M. (1983). The role of blood vessels and lymphatics in cutaneous inflammatory processes: An overview. *British Journal of Dermatology, 109*(Suppl 25), 89–98.

Braverman. I. M. (1997). The cutaneous microcirculation: Ultrastructure and microanatomical organization. *Microcirculation, 4*(3). 329–240.

Braverman. I. M. (2000). The cutaneous microcirculation. *Journal of Investigative Dermatology, 5*(1), 3–9.

Braverman, I. M., Schechner, J. S., Silverman, D. G., & Keh-Yen, A. (1992). Topographic mapping of the cutaneous microcirculation using two outputs of laser-Doppler flowmetry: Flux and the concentration of moving blood cells. *Microvascular Research, 44*(1), 33–48.

Brunner, P. M., Suarez-Farinas, M., He, H., Malik, K., Wen, H.-C., Gonzalex, J., et al. (2017). The atopic dermatitis blood signature is characterized by increases in inflammatory and cardiovascular risk proteins. *Scientific Reports, 7*, 8707. https://doi.org/10.1038/s41598-017-09207-z.

Caughman, S. W., Li, L. J., & Degitz, K. (1992). Human intercellular adhesion molecule-1 gene and its expression in the skin. *Journal of Investigative Dermatology, 98*(6 suppl), 61s–65s.

Chan. L. S. (2019a). Emerging biomedical imaging: Optical coherence tomography. In L. S. Chan & W. C. Tang (Eds.), *Engineering-medicine: Principles and applications of engineering in medicine.* Boca Raton: CRC Press..

Chan. L. S. (2019b). Emerging biomedical imaging: Photoacoustic imaging. In L. S. Chan & W. C. Tang (Eds.), *Engineering-medicine: Principles and applications of engineering in medicine.* Boca Raton: CRC Press.

Chan, L. S., Robinson, N., & Xu, L. (2001). Expression of interleukin-4 in the epidermis of transgenic mice results in a pruritic inflammatory skin disease: An experimental animal model to study atopic dermatitis. *Journal of Investigative Dermatology, 117*(4), 977–983. https://doi.org/10.1046/j.0022-202x.2001.01484.x.

Chen, L., Martinez, O., Venkataramani, P., Lin, S.-X., Prabhakar, B. S., & Chan, L. S. (2005). Correlation of disease evolution with progressive inflammatory cell activation and migration in the IL-4 trasgneic mouse model of atopic dermatitis. *Clinical and Experimental Immunology, 139*(2), 189–201. https://doi.org/10.1111/j.1365-2249.2004.02691.x.

Chen, L., Marble, D. J., Agha, R., Peterson, J. D., Becker, R. P., Jin, T., et al. (2008). The progression of inflammation parallels the dermal angiogenesis in a keratin 14 IL-4-transgenic model of atopic dermatitis. *Microcirculation, 15*(1), 49–64. https://doi.org/10.1080/10739680701418416.

Cornelius, L. A., Sepp, N., Li, L.-J., Degitz, K., Swerlick, R. A., Lawley, T. J., & Caughman, S. W. (1994). Selective upregulation of intercellular adhesion molecule (ICAM)-1 by ultraviolet B in human dermal microvascular endothelial cells. *Journal of Investigative Dermatology, 103*(1), 23–28. https://doi.org/10.1111/1523-1747.ep12388971.

Coso, S., Bovay, E., & Petrova, T. V. (2014). Pressing the right buttons: Signaling in lymphangiogenesis. *Blood, 123*(17), 2614–2624. https://doi.org/10.1182/blood-2013-12-297317.

Cracowski, J. L., & Roustit, M. (2016). Current method to assess human cutaneous blood flow: An updated focus on laser-based-technologies. *Microcirculation, 23*(5), 337–344. https://doi.org/10.1111/micc.12257.

Cueni, L. N., & Detmar, M. (2006). New insights into the molecular control of the lymphatic vascular system and its role in disease. *Journal of Investigative Dermatology, 126*(10), 2167–2177. https://doi.org/10.1038/sj.jid.5700464.

Dadras, S. S., & Detmar, M. (2004). Angiogenesis and lymphangiogenesis of skin cancers. *Hematology/Oncology Clinics of North America, 18*(5), 1059–1070. https://doi.org/10.1016/j.hoc.2004.06.009.

Deegan, A. J., Talebi-Liasi, F., Song, S., Li, Y., Xu, J., Men, S., et al. (2018). Optical coherence tomography angiography of normal skin and inflammatory dermatologic conditions. *Lasers in Surgery and Medicine, 50*(3), 183–193. https://doi.org/10.1002/lsm.22788.

Dieterich, L. C., Seidel, C. D., & Detmar, M. (2014). Lymphatic vessels: New targets for the treatment of inflammatory diseases. *Angiogenesis, 17*(2), 359–371. https://doi.org/10.1007/s10456-013-9406-1.

Feely, M. A., Olsen, K. D., Gamble, G. L., Davis, M. D., & Pittelkow, M. R. (2012). Cutaneous lymphatic and chronic lymphedema of the head and neck. *Clinical Anatomy, 25*(1), 72–85. https://doi.org/10.1002/ca.22009.

Francisco, M. A., & Minson, C. T. (2018). Cutaneous active vasodilation as a heat loss thermoeffector. *Handbook of Clinical Neurology, 156*, 193–209. https://doi.org/10.1016/B978-0-444-63912-7.00012-6.

Genovese, A., Detoraki, A., Granata, F., Galdiero, M. R., Spadaro, G., & Marone, G. (2012). Angiogenesis, lymphangiogenesis and atopic dermatitis. *Chemical Immunology and Allergy, 96*, 50–60. https://doi.org/10.1159/000331883.

Gonzalez. A. (2018). Sentinel lymph node biopsy: Past and present implications for the management of cutaneous melanoma with nodal metastasis. *American Journal of Clinical Dermatology, 19*(suppl no. 1), 24–30. https://doi.org/10.1007/s40257-018-0379-0.

Gunaratne, D. A., Howle, J. R., & Veness, M. J. (2016). Sentinel lymph node biopsy in Merkel cell carcinoma: A 15-year institutional experience and statistical analysis of 721 reported cases. *British Journal of Dermatology, 174*(2), 273–281. https://doi.org/10.1111/bjd.14240.

Hirakawa, S., & Detmar, M. (2004). New insights into the biology and pathology of the cutaneous lymphatic system. *Journal of Dermatological Science, 35*(1), 1–8. https://doi.org/10.1016/j.jdermsci.2003.10.006.

Jeltsch, M., Tammela, T., Alitalo, K., & Wilting, J. (2003). Genesis and pathogenesis of lymphatic vessels. *Cell and Tissue Research, 314*(1), 69–84.

Johnson, J. M., Minson, C. T., & Kellogg, D. L., Jr. (2014). Cutaneous vasodilator and vasoconstrictor mechanisms in temperature regulation. *Comprehensive Physiology, 4*(1), 33–89. https://doi.org/10.1002/cphy.c130015.

Kritas, S. K., Saggini, A., Varvara, G., Murmura, G., Caraffa, A., Antinolfi, P., et al. (2013). Impact of mast cells on the skin. *International Journal of Immunopathology and Pharmacology, 26*(4), 855–859. https://doi.org/10.1177/039463201302600403.

Kyan-Aung, U., Haskard, D. O., Poston, R. N., Thornhill, M. H., & Lee, T. H. (1991). Endothelial keukocyte adhesion molecule-1 and intercellular adhesion molecule-1 mediate the adhesion of eosinophils to endothelial cells in vitro and are expressed by endothelium in allergic cutaneous inflammation in vivo. *Journal of Immunology, 146*(2), 521–528.

Lanting, S. M., Johnson, N. A., Baker, M. K., Caterson, I. D., & Chuter, V. H. (2017). The effect of exercise training on cutaneous microvascular reactivity: A systematic review and meta-analysis. *Journal of Science and Medicine in Sport, 20*(2), 170–177. https://doi.org/10.1016/j.jsams.2016.04.002.

Leiter, U., Meier, F., Schittek, B., & Garbe, C. (2004). The natural course of cutaneous melanoma. *Journal of Surgical Oncology, 86*(4), 172–178. https://doi.org/10.1002/jso.20079.

Liu, N. F., & He, Q. L. (1997). The regulatory effects of cytokines on lymphatic angiogenesis. *Lymphology, 30*, 3–12.

Ludwig, R. J., Zollner, T. M., Santoso, S., Hardt, K., Gille, J., Baatz, H., et al. (2005). Junctional adhesion molecules (JAM)-B and -C contribute to leukocyte extravasation to the skin and mediate cutaneous inflammation. *The Journal of Investigative Dermatology, 125*(5), 969–976. https://doi.org/10.1111/j.0022-202X.2005.23912.x.

Lund, A. W., Medler, T. R., Leachman, S. A., & Coussens, L. M. (2016). Lymphatic vessels, inflammation, and immunity in skin cancer. *Cancer Discovery, 6*(1), 22–35. https://doi.org/10.1158/2159-8290.CD-15-0023.

Lutter, S., & Makinen, T. (2014). Regulation of lymphatic vasculature by extracellular matrix. *Advances in Anatomy, Embryology and Cell Biology, 214*, 55–65. https://doi.org/10.1007/978-3-7091-1646-3_5.

Marinovic Kulisic, S., Lipozencic, J., Gregorovic, G., Lackovic, G., & Junc-Lekic, G. (2010). Expression of e-selectin in the skin of patients with atopic dermatitis: Morphometric study. *Acta Dermatovenerologica Croatica, 18*(3), 141–145.

Matsumoto, Y., Asao, Y., Yoshikawa, A., Sekiguchi, H., Takada, M., Furu, M., et al. (2018). Label-free photoacoustic imaging of human palmar vessels: A structural morphological analysis. *Scientific Reports, 8*, 786. https://doi.org/10.1038/s41598-018-19161-z.

McAleer, M. A., Jakasa, I., Hurault, G., Sarvari, P., McLean, W. H. I., Tanaka, R. J., et al. (2019). Systemic and stratum corneum biomarkers of severity in infant atopic dermatitis include markers of innate and T helper cell-related immunity and angiogenesis. *British Journal of Dermatology, 180*(3), 586–596. https://doi.org/10.1111/bjd.17088.

Nakamura, M., Abe, Y., & Tokunaga, T. (2002). Pathological significance of vascular endothelial growth factor A isoform expression in human cancer. *Pathology International, 52*(5-6), 331–339.

Petrova, T. V., & Koh, G. Y. (2018). Organ-specific lymphatic vasculature: From development to pathophysiology. *The Journal of Experimental Medicine, 215*(1), 35–49. https://doi.org/10.1084/jem.20171868.

Picker, L. J., Kishmoto, T. K., Smith, C. W., Warnock, R. A., & Butcher, E. C. (1991). ELAM-1 is an adhesion molecur for skin–homing T cells. *Nature, 349*(6312), 796–799. https://doi.org/10.1038/349796a0.

Pober, J. S., Kluger, M. S., & Schechner, J. S. (2001). Human endothelial cell presentation of antigen and the homing of memory/effector T cells. *Annals of the New York Academy of Sciences, 941*, 12–25.

Pober, J. S., & Sessa, W. C. (2015). Inflammation and the blood microvascular system. *Cold Spring Harbor Perspectives in Biology, 7*(1), a016345. https://doi.org/10.1101/cshperspect.a016345.

Raica, M., Jitariu, A. A., & Cimpean, A. M. (2016). Lymphangiogenesis and anti-lymphangiogenesis in cutaneous melanoma. *Anticancer Research, 36*(9), 4427–4435. https://doi.org/10.21873/anticanres.10986.

Roediger, B., Ng, L. G., Smith, A. L., Fazeka de St Groth, B., & Weninger, W. (2008). Visualizing dendritic cells migration within the skin. *Histochemistry and Cell Biology, 130*(6), 1131–1146. https://doi.org/10.1007/s00418-008-0531-7.

Rossiter, H., van Reijsen, F., Mudde, G. C., Kalthoff, F., Carla Bruijnzeel-Koomen, A. F. M., Picker, L. J., & Kupper, T. S. (1994). Skin disease-related T cells bind to endothelial selectins: Expression of cutaneous lymphocyte antigen (CLA) predicts E-selectin but not P-selectin binding. *European Journal of Immunology, 24*(1), 205–210. https://doi.org/10.1002/eji.1830240132.

Rovenska, E., & Rovensky, J. (2011). Lymphatic vessels: Structure and function. *The Israel Medical Association Journal, 13*(12), 762–768.

Ruhrberg. C. (2003). Growing and shaping the vascular tree: Multiple roles for VEGF. *BioEssays, 25*(11), 1052–1060. https://doi.org/10.1002/bies.10351.

Ryan. T. J. (1989). Structure and function of lymphatics. *Journal of Investigative Dermatology, 93*, 18s–24s.

Saaristo, A., Karkkainen, M. J., & Alitalo, K. (2002). Insights into the molecular pathogenesis and targeted treatment of lymphedema. *Annals of the New York Academy of Sciences, 979*, 94–110.

Shao, X., & Liu, C. (2006). Influence of IFN-alpha and IFN-gamma on lymphangiogenesis. *Journal of Interferon and Cytokine Research, 26*, 568–574.

Sallustio, G., Giangregorio, C., Cannas, L., Vricella, D., Celi, G., & Rinaldi, P. (2000). Lymphatic system: Morphofunctional considerations. *Rays, 25*(4), 419–427.

Santamaria Babi, L. F., Moser, R., Perez Soler, M. T., Picker, L. J., Blaser, K., & Hauser, C. (1995). Migration of skin-homing T cells across cytokine-activated human endothelial cell layers involves interaction of the cutaneous lymphocyte-associated antigen (CLA), the very late antigen-4 (VLA-4), and the lymphocyte function-associated antigen-1 (LFA-1). *Journal of Immunology, 154*(4), 1543–1550.

Scavelli, C., Weber, E., Agliano, M., Cirulli, T., Nico, B., Vacca, A., & Ribatti, D. (2004). Lymphatics at the crossroads of angiogenesis and lymphangiogenesis. *Journal of Anatomy, 204*(6), 433–449.

Schwager, S., & Detmar, M. (2019). Inflammation and lymphatic function. *Frontiers in Immunology, 10*, 308. https://doi.org/10.3389/fimmu.2019.00308.

Shi, V. Y., Bao, L., & Chan, L. S. (2012). Inflammation-driven dermal lymphangiogenesis in atopic dermatitis is associated with CD11b+ macrophage recruitment and VEGF-C up-regulation in the IL-4-transgenic mouse model. *Microcirculation, 19*(7), 567–579. https://doi.org/10.1111/j.1549-8719.2012.00189.x.

Singh, S. R., Casper, K., Summers, S., & Swerlick, R. A. (2001). CD40 expression and function on human dermal microvascular endothelial cells: Role in cutaneous inflammation. *Clinical and Experimental Dermatology, 26*(5), 434–440. https://doi.org/10.1046/j.1365-2230.2001.00853.x.

Skobe, M., & Detmar, M. (2000). Structure, function, and molecular control of the skin lymphatic system. *Journal of Investigative Dermatology, 5*(1), 14–19.

Subramaniam, M., Saffaripour, S., van de Water, L., Frenette, P. S., Mayadas, T. N., Hynes, R. O., & Wagner, D. D. (1997). Role of endothelial selectins in wound repair. *The American Journal of Pathology, 150*(5), 1701–1709.

Tellechea, A., Kafanas, A., Leal, E. C., Tecilazich, F., Kuchibhotla, S., Auster, M. E., et al. (2013). Increased skin inflammation and blood vessel density in human and experimental diabetes. *The International Journal of Lower Extremity Wounds, 12*(1), 4–11. https://doi.org/10.1177/1534734612474303.

Tonnesen. M. G. (1989). Neutrophil-endothelial cell interactions: Mechanisms of neutrophil adherence to vascular endothelium. *Journal of Investigative Dermatology, 93*(2 suppl), 53s–58s.

Trinidad, C. M., Torres-Cabala, C. A., Curry, J. L., Prieto, V. G., & Aung, P. P. (2019). Update on eighth edition American Joint Committee on Cancer Classification for Cutaneous Melanoma and overview of potential pitfalls in histological examination of staging parameters. *Journal of Clinical Pathology, 72*(4), 265–270. https://doi.org/10.1136/clinpath-2018-205417.

Tsutsumi, M., Fukuda, M., Kumamoto, J., Goto, M., Denda, S., Yamasaki, K., et al. (2016). Abnormal morphology of blood vessels in erythematous skin from atopic dermatitis. *The American Journal of Dermatopathology, 38*(5), 363–364. https://doi.org/10.1097/DAD.0000000000000373.

Varricchi, G., Granata, F., Loffredo, S., & Genovese, A. (2015). Angiogenesis and lymphangiogenesis in inflammatory skin disorders. *Journal of the American Academy of Dermatology, 73*(1), 144–153. https://doi.org/10.1016/j.jaad.2015.03.041.

Wilting, J., Becker, J., Buttler, K., & Weich, H. A. (2009). Lymphatics and inflammation. *Current Medicinal Chemistry, 16*(34), 4581–4592.

Zhang, H., Shi, V. Y., & Chan, L. S. (2017). Potential role of angiogenesis and lymphangiogenesis in atopic dermatitis: evidence from human studies and lessons from an animal model of human disease. In J. L. Arbiser (Ed.), *Angiogenesis-based dermatology* (pp. 95–122). London: Springer.

Zhang, Y., Matsuo, H., & Morita, E. (2006). Increased production of vascular endothelial growth factor in the lesions of atopic dermatitis. *Archives of Dermatological Research, 297*, 425–429. https://doi.org/10.1007/s00403-006-0641-9.

13

Humoral Factors

HARUYO NAKAJIMA-ADACHI, KHIEM A. TRAN, AND MICHIKO SHIMODA

KEY POINTS

- Allergen-specific B cells are differentiated into plasma cells producing immunoglobulin E (IgE) antibodies. Through binding to the receptors (FcɛRI and FcɛRII), IgE induces cytokine and chemokine production from immune cells.
- Intrinsic atopic dermatitis is T-cell mediated, involving Th2 cytokines that cause skin inflammation and pruritus.
- Extrinsic atopic dermatitis is IgE mediated, involving allergen-specific IgE, including autoreactive IgE.
- Cytokines and chemokines that play a key role in the inflammatory lymphocytes' infiltration into skin can be potent biomarkers and therapeutic targets.

Introduction

Humoral factors (i.e., IgE antibodies, cytokines, and chemokines) play a key communication role in the development of atopic dermatitis (AD) that involves various types of immune and nonimmune cells. They also play a driving role in amplifying the inflammatory response during the disease transition from the acute to chronic phase. IgE antibodies are produced by skin B cells, whereas cytokines and chemokines are produced essentially by all types of cells involved in AD, including keratinocytes, epidermal-derived immune cells, as well as migrating lymphocytes and granulocytes from the skin draining lymph nodes and the circulation. Following skin barrier disruption, keratinocytes start secreting chemokines and cytokines such as thymic stromal lymphopoietin (TSLP), leading the maturation and migration of antigen-presenting cells such as epidermal Langerhans cells and dermal dendritic cells. Those antigen-presenting cells carry skin-associated antigens (including allergens and microbiota) to the skin draining lymph nodes. In the lymph nodes, they activate B cells and T cells, leading adoptive humoral response with IgE production, as well as Th2 cellular response with Th2-type cytokine production. Accordingly, AD has been classified into intrinsic and extrinsic phenotypes on the basis of serum IgE levels, IgE-mediated sensitization, and personal and family history of AD. Intrinsic AD is mostly T-cell mediated and represents 10% to 20% of AD. Extrinsic AD is IgE mediated,

representing 80% of the patients. Importantly, cytokine profiles that contribute to the pathophysiology of AD are distinct, in intrinsic versus extrinsic types of diseases, children versus adults, and in acute versus chronic diseases. In this chapter, the roles of cytokines and chemokines are discussed with consideration of phenotypic variations of AD. Cellular responses in AD are discussed in Chapter 14. Please refer to Figures 14.1 and 14.2, which illustrate the immune pathophysiology of AD that involves both humoral and cellular responses.

IgE antibodies in atopic dermatitis

B cells as the IgE producer

As a major part of the humoral response, B cells are lymphocytes specialized in differentiating into plasma cells (PCs) that produce antibodies. While B cells provide defense against infections via antibody production, they also adversely mediate autoimmune diseases and allergies such as AD. During development in the bone marrow, through the *VDJ* gene recombination mechanism, each B cell is programmed to express immunoglobulin (Ig) with a unique single specificity as its B-cell receptor (BCR). Similar to T-cell selection, B cells expressing a BCR with strong self-reactivity are eliminated by a variety of mechanisms. Selected immature B cells migrate to the peripheral tissues and lymphoid organs such as the spleen, to further differentiate into several B-cell subsets (Hardy & Kyoko 2001).

Upon binding to specific antigens via BCR, innate type B cells such as B-1 cells with conserved pathogen-specific Ig repertoire can mount rapid T-independent response with polyreactive IgM and IgA production. On the other hand, conventional B-2 cells capture antigens and present peptides to CD4[+] T cells in MHC-II–restricted manner. The cognate T-B interaction, in turn, supports B-cell differentiation into either short-lived PCs producing low-affinity antibodies or germinal center (GC) B cells that further differentiate into memory B cells and long-lived PCs carrying BCR with improved higher affinity to cognate antigens. Within GC, B cells undergo BCR affinity maturation via somatic mutation. They also undergo BCR class switching from IgM to another isotype such as IgG, IgA, and IgE, which allows acquisition of different effector properties while maintaining the same antigen specificity (McHeyzer-Williams & McHeyzer-Williams, 2005; Wu & Zarrin, 2014). In AD, B cells are thought to play a driving role in skin inflammation by producing IgE antibodies. Also, as discuss in the Chapter 14, some B cells can regulate inflammatory response by secreting IL10. B-cell accumulation is evident in inflamed skin. Higher B-cell activation status reflects accumulative antigen exposure and the ability to contribute to T-cell activation, leading to pathogenic IgE production (Czarnowicki, et al. 2016), which can be destructive to skin tissues especially in the case of IgE autoantibody production.

Mechanisms of IgE production

IgE is the immunoglobulin isotype providing a first-line defense against parasite infection. However, in response to allergen exposures IgE adversely mediates type I hypersensitivity reactions, including anaphylactic reaction by sensitizing mast cells and basophils for rapid degranulation. Although the mechanisms leading to IgE production remain poorly defined, evidence suggests that IgE production is tightly regulated by multiple mechanisms. In healthy humans, the concentration of free serum IgE is maintained at 50 to 200 ng/mL, which is extremely low compared to other Ig isotypes that range from 1 to 10 mg/mL. The half-life of IgE in humans is the shortest of all Ig isotypes, which is ~2 days compared to ~20 days for IgG (Dullaers et al., 2012). However, elevated levels of total serum IgE in association with various environmental allergens and autoantigens are reported in approximately 80% of the patients with severe AD (Kasperkiewicz, Schmidt, Ludwig, & Zillikens, 2018; Weidinger & Novak, 2016). In the patients with severe extrinsic AD, the concentration of total IgE was correlated with the severity of the disease (Jaworek, Szafraniec, Jaworek, Hałubiec, & Wojas-Pelc, 2019).

IgE is produced by B cells through class-switch recombination (CSR) mediated by Th2 type cytokines such as IL4. In the Ig gene locus, constant region genes for isotypes are localized in the order of IgM (Cμ), IgG1 (Cγ1), IgA (Cα), and IgE (Cε). The Cε locus is farthest from the Cμ, which may limit the direct CSR from IgM to IgE. In theory, B cells can also sequentially rearrange the constant region gene to another downstream isotype, such as first from Cμ to Cγ1, and then to Cε. However, analysis of Ig rearrangement in B cells from patients with AD showed no evidence of sequential CSR (van der Stoep, Korver, & Logtenberg, 1994).

The mechanisms of IgE B-cell differentiation have been mainly studied in mouse models in which either transcription or translation of membrane IgE is tagged with fluorescent protein (He et al., 2015; Talay et al., 2012; Yang, Sullivan, & Allen, 2012; also reviewed in Wu & Zarrin, 2014). Based on these studies, IgE GC response is transient. As a result, IgE antibody repertoire shows less diverse specificities and lower affinity than that of IgG1 (Erazo

et al., 2007; Yang et al., 2012). The latter is thought to be due to lower expression levels of IgE BCR, which limits BCR-mediated signaling required for survival and affinity maturation in GCs. Overall, IgE response is shifted toward short-lived extrafollicular PC generation rather than GC pathway. In fact, IgE B cells express higher levels of Blimp1 compared to IgG1 B cells, which likely predisposes IgE B cells to differentiate into PCs over GC pathway (Yang et al., 2012). In mice, IgG GC B cells have been shown to give rise to both IgG1 and IgE memory cells, and a small number of long-lived IgE PCs are detected in the bone marrow (He et al., 2015; Talay et al., 2012; Yang et al., 2012; also reviewed in Wu & Zarrin, 2014). However, more studies are needed for better understanding human IgE memory B cells.

Effector properties of IgE

IgE exhibits its effector properties through binding to two types of IgE receptors on immune cells. The high-affinity IgER (FcεRI) carrying immunoreceptor tyrosine-based activation motif (ITAM) is expressed on mast cells and basophils as a tetramer (α, β, γ, γ), the activation of which mediates degranulation, eicosanoid production, and cytokine production (Wu & Zarrin, 2014). In humans, FcεRI is also expressed by DCs and macrophages as a trimer (α, γ, γ), the activation of which mediates the internalization, processing, and presentation of IgE-bound antigens, leading to cytokine production supporting Th2 type immune responses (Wu & Zarrin, 2014). The low-affinity IgER (FcεRII or CD23) is a C-type lectin, expressed on B cells, which regulates IgE production, antigen processing, and presentation (Acharya et al., 2010). A study with B-cell–deficient mouse model indicates that FcεRII regulates the levels of free IgE in the blood by passively binding to IgE (Cheng, Wang, & Locksley, 2010). FcεRII is also expressed on macrophages and epithelial cells, and is involved in uptake of IgE-antigen complexes (Acharya et al., 2010).

Regarding specificities of IgE antibodies, a recent large-scale meta-analysis provided an important conclusion that AD is associated with IgE-autoreactivity (Tang, Bieber, & Williams, 2012). In fact, patients with severe AD show signs of multiple allergen-sensitizations, including aero, food, and microbial antigens (Roesner & Werfel, 2019; Sonesson et al., 2013; Tang et al., 2012; Virtanen et al., 1995). Furthermore, significant percentage of AD patients carry IgE antibodies cross-reacting with human proteins and fungal proteins (i.e., autoallergens) (reviewed by Roesner & Werfel, 2019). However, clinical trials with anti-IgE monoclonal antibody omalizumab showed limited efficacy in the control of AD symptoms (Heil, Maurer, Klein, Hultsch, & Stingl, 2010; Iyengar et al., 2013; Wang, Li, & Huang, 2016), suggesting that IgE reactivity in AD patients may be a result of other allergies often seen in the patients with severe AD.

Cytokines in atopic dermatitis: An overview

Roles of cytokines

AD is thought to arise because of barrier dysfunction of the skin and aberrant activation of Th2 responses. Characteristics of AD patients—especially patients with extrinsic AD (see later)—include elevated serum levels of total IgE and IgE specific to environmental or food allergens (Furue et al., 2017; Tokura, 2010). However, AD has recently been considered a T-cell–mediated disease, involving excessive activation and imbalance of T-cell subsets (Honda, Nomura, & Kabashima, 2017). Recent studies analyzing gene expression have shown that excessive Th1, Th17, and Th22 responses tend to build pathophysiology of AD, although Th-cell polarization into Th2 responses parallels activation of the other Th phenotypes. Understanding the contribution of each cytokine in this complex and integral (systemic as well as localized) disease has been markedly advanced by the use of cytokine inhibitors, such as anticytokine antibodies, administered in clinical trials of targeted therapeutics (Brunner, Guttman-Yassky, & Leung, 2017). The success of dupilumab, an anti-IL4 receptor (IL4R) monoclonal antibody, in blocking both IL4 and IL13 signals through binding to their common receptor expressed on the target cells, has advanced new therapies and clarified key roles of Th2 responses as critical mediators in controlling the skin disease (Beck et al., 2014). As mentioned, the cytokine profile that contributes to the development of AD is distinct (e.g., in intrinsic vs. extrinsic disease, children vs. adults, and acute vs. chronic disease). Clarifying and defining the phenotypes of AD in accordance with the status of AD patients should lead to more personalized AD treatment in the future (Brunner, Suárez-Fariñas, He, Malik, Wen, Gonzalez, & Guttman-Yassky, 2017). Cytokines are produced by epithelial cells (including keratinocytes) and epidermal-derived immune cells; cells infiltrate the skin region in response to chemokines or other chemical substances, such as prostanoids (lipid mediators that include leukotrienes) (Honda & Kabashima, 2019). It is also important to understand the types of cells involved in cytokine responses.

Cytokine effects on phenotypes of AD

Acute and chronic

In the acute phase of AD, Th2, and Th22 responses are augmented by Th17 response; these responses contribute to the further impairment of barrier function and activate epithelial cells, especially keratinocyte, increasing the severity of the disease and promoting its chronicity. Th1 skewing toward the Th2/Th22 response plays an important role in the progression of the disease (i.e., chronicity).

Mutation in the *FLG* gene is a strong risk factor for inducing barrier dysfunction in AD patients. Barrier defects promote cutaneous penetration of allergens and bacterial or viral products, which then stimulate the production of epithelial cell–derived proinflammatory cytokines such as TSLP, IL33, and IL25 (Cabanillas et al., 2017). These events further impair barrier function and potentiate inflammatory responses of epidermal infiltration of inflammatory cells, activation of Th2 cells and innate lymphoid cells (ILCs), and expansion of multicytokine responses (Th2, Th22, and Th17) in the acute phase. Abnormal cytokine responses are observed in both lesional and nonlesional skin of AD patients. In chronic AD, unlike in acute AD, Th1 (but not Th17) attends to the expansion of Th2/Th22 responses and the upregulation of IgE-mediated responses, but the mechanism remains to be clarified. The profound Th2 response stimulates cutaneous neuronal itch response via IL31. Pruritus exacerbates AD by promoting scratching and sleep deprivation, which decrease the quality of life of AD patients.

Children and adults

Our understanding of the transition in AD phenotype from the acute to the chronic state relies on recent data obtained by analyzing the skin of adults who have suffered chronic AD since the first 5 years of life. To characterize the changes in skin immunity and barrier function that occur from the onset of the disease, several researchers have investigated the cytokine phenotype of early pediatric lesional and nonlesional AD skin, comparing it with age-matched healthy individual skin and adult skin with AD (Brunner et al., 2017; Cabanillas et al. 2017; Czarnowicki et al., 2015; Esaki et al., 2016; Kim et al., 2016). Such analysis has enabled us to advance targeted treatments for children with AD. The cytokine phenotype differs between early pediatric AD skin and adult moderate-to-severe AD skin. Similar to that in the acute phase of adult AD, the lesional skin in pediatric AD is characterized by strong Th2 (IL13, IL31, CCL17) and Th22 (IL22) activation, with some IL9, IL33, and Th17 skewing (IL17A, IL19, CCL20). In pediatric skin, IL8, IL17A, and antimicrobial peptides (AMP) produced by commensal bacteria to protect against *Staphylococcus aureus* are increased, reflecting a response to infectious agents in children without fully acquired immunity. However, these inflammatory responses further injure epithelial cells and promote Th2/Th1 imbalance, contributing to AD pathophysiology. In pediatric skin, IL19 is upregulated in lesional and nonlesional skin. Because IL19 amplifies the effects of IL17 on keratinocytes, it indirectly promotes Th2 activation. Thus IL19 is thought to bridge the Th2 and Th17 responses in AD. In addition, in the nonlesional skin of pediatric AD patients, abnormalities and inflammatory responses are enhanced (keratinocyte hyperactivation; increased TSLP, IL17, and IL19 production), indicating a disease-initiation state. Therefore, to prevent AD chronicity in pediatric AD patients, treatment targeted to various cytokines distinct from targeted approaches in adult AD may be necessary (Esaki et al., 2016).

Intrinsic and extrinsic

The phenotype of AD has been classified into intrinsic and extrinsic types on the basis of total and specific serum IgE levels, IgE-mediated sensitization, and personal and family history of AD (Suárez-Fariñas et al., 2014). Intrinsic AD (also known as pure or nonallergic type) is thought to be T-cell mediated and represents 10% to 20% of AD. Extrinsic type (also known as mixed or allergic type) is IgE mediated; 80% of the patients are classified as having this type. Analysis of mRNA expression in skin lesions showed that Th2 cytokine (IL4, IL5, IL13, and IL31) expressions were augmented in both AD phenotypes, whereas higher IFN-γ levels are detected in only intrinsic-type AD compared with extrinsic AD. Intrinsic AD is thought to be closely linked to metal allergy, and IFN-γ plays a role in contact sensitivity (Tokura, 2010). In addition, Th17 and Th22 subsets are activated in intrinsic AD, and 61.3% of patients report allergy in response to one or more metals, including nickel, cobalt, or chrome. In some cases, AD patients with known allergies to nickel may not tolerate eating nickel-containing foods, such as chocolate. (Suárez-Fariñas et al., 2014; Tokura, 2010; Yamaguchi et al., 2013). Food allergies and intolerance are further discussed in Chapter 8.

Cytokines: Detail analysis

Epithelial cell–derived cytokines

AD pathogenesis is characterized by Th2 skewing and barrier dysfunction. TSLP, IL33, and IL25 are regarded as inducers of excess production of Th2 cytokines in the lesional skin of AD patients. The mechanism by which these cytokines are upregulated in epidermal keratinocytes remains unknown. Scratching or signals through human intelectin-1 (ITLN1), which is a soluble lectin on keratinocytes that recognizes galactofuranose of bacterial cell wall, are candidate upregulators of epithelial cell–derived cytokine expression in the lesional skin of AD patients (Yi et al., 2017).

TSLP is a cytokine that has been suggested to be an initiator of Th2 response. Keratinocytes and Langerhans cells function as antigen-presenting cells and were reported to express high levels of TSLP through the OX-40 ligand pathway in the injured skin of AD patients (Wang & Liu, 2009). TSLP transduces signals to different cells via its heterodimeric receptor that comprises the IL7 receptor α-chain and the TSLP receptor (TSLPR). Dendritic cells are primary targets of TSLP (Liu et al., 2007). By binding to TSLP, dendritic cells (in this instance, dermal Langerhans cells) express OX40L, CD80, and CD86 on their surfaces and produce IL4, IL5, and IL13, which cause naïve T cells to differentiate into the Th2 phenotype. TSLP also promotes Th2 cytokine production by mast cells, ILCs, epithelial cells, macrophages, and basophils (Han, Roan, & Ziegler, 2017), thus exacerbating Th2 immune activation. In contrast, the cytokines produced by keratinocytes activate regulatory T cells, leading to inhibition of excessive inflammatory

responses (Kashiwagi et al., 2017). In infantile AD, analysis of the expression of several epidermal proteins has revealed that TSLP may be an effective biomarker for predicting the development of AD (Kim et al., 2016).

IL33 is a member of the IL1 family and binds to a heterodimer of ST2 (suppression of tumorigenecity 2) and its coreceptor of IL1RAcP (IL1 receptor accessory protein). Because IL33 is produced in response to tissue damage, stress, and scratching of the skin, it is classified as one of the alarmins, which are also known as endogenous substance in danger-associated molecular patterns (DAMPs). DAMPs are released during cell necrosis, transduce danger signals, and are associated with Th2 skewing. IL33 is constitutively released by human tissues (Han et al., 2017), but in the skin of AD patients its expression is further increased, especially in children compared with adults (Cabanillas et al. 2017). Keratinocytes are producers of IL33, and IL33 can decrease filaggrin (FLG) expression at the gene and protein levels in keratinocytes from the skin of AD patients (Seltmann, Roesner, von Hesler, Wittmann, & Werfel, 2015). IL33 is specifically expressed in the skin and is associated with Th2 cells and ILC2 (group 2 innate lymphoid cells, which produce Th2 cytokines) infiltration, activation, as well as with Th2 cytokine production (Morita, Moro, & Koyasu, 2016). In addition, IL33 affects mast cells in that it colocalizes with IL2-producing mast cells in chronically inflamed skin (Salamon et al., 2017).

IL25 (also known as IL17E) is a member of the IL17 family and binds to a heterodimeric receptor complex of IL17RA and IL17RB (Han et al. 2017). It is important in inducing Th2-skewing immune responses, and it is produced by epithelial cells (including keratinocytes) and endothelial cells, as well as by DCs. Its level is elevated in the skin of AD patients and negatively affects FLG expression at the gene and protein levels (Hvid et al., 2011). IL25 links impaired skin barrier function with Th2-mediated skin inflammation in AD patients. Because ILC2 expresses IL17RB as well as ST2 or TSLPR in human injured skin, IL25 can activate ILC2, but the functions of IL33 and TSLP to ILC2 differ from IL25. For example, KLRG1 (killer cell lectin-like receptor G1), which is a marker of ILC2 and highly expressed on these cells in AD patients, is upregulated by IL33 and TSLP, but not by IL25 (Morita et al., 2016). In addition to ILC2, mast cells, basophils, and eosinophils are activated by IL25. The interaction among TSLP, IL33, and IL25 and the mechanism responsible for the differences in their roles remain to be clarified, but it is clear that Th2 cells and ILC2 respond to these cytokines and further exacerbate the lesional skin in AD.

Th2 cytokines

IL4, IL13, IL5, and IL31 are Th2 cytokines that play critical roles in the pathogenesis of AD. The importance of Th2 responses in the pathophysiology of patients with moderate-to-severe AD has been demonstrated by the marked improvement in skin barrier function, skin lesions, pruritus, and serum biomarker levels obtained following treatment with dupilumab (a human anti-IL4Rα antibody that blocks signals via both IL4 and IL13). IL4 and IL13, in particular, play central roles in development of AD pathogenesis. They bind a common heterodimeric receptor composed of the IL4Rα and IL13Rα1; IL4 also binds a heterodimeric receptor complex composed by IL4Rα and γC (Wang & Secombes, 2015). IL4 and IL13 are thought to be produced by mainly Th2 cells and ILC2. Mast cells, basophils, and eosinophils can also produce these cytokines. The receptor is expressed on DCs, keratinocytes, and eosinophils (Cabanillas et al., 2017). Keratinocytes differentiated under high IL4 and IL13 conditions show reduced *FLG* gene expression, even in the absence of *FLG* gene mutations. Binding of *S. aureus* and AMP production by keratinocytes trigger dysfunction of the skin barrier, promote TSLP production, and facilitate the Th2 injury responses in AD. This Th2 response induces IgE production. IL5 acts on eosinophil chemotaxis and activation. In the lesional skin and blood of AD patients, eosinophil numbers are increased (Brunner et al., 2017).

Other cytokines

IL31 belongs to the IL6 family. IL31 is produced by mainly activated Th2 CD4+ T cells and has proinflammatory and barrier-disrupting roles (Takamori et al., 2018). Granulocytes and mast cells are the additional sources of IL31 in AD patients (Nakashima, Otsuka, & Kabashima, 2018). IL31 gene expression and production are induced by IL4 and further promoted by IL33. IL31 signals to and functions in cutaneous nerves, dorsal root ganglia (DRG), epithelial cells, and keratinocytes through IL31 heterodimeric receptor complex, which is comprised of IL31 receptor A (IL31RA) and the oncostatin M receptor. Staphylococcal enterotoxin B is a potent inducer of IL31 from peripheral mononuclear cells of both healthy individuals and AD patients. IL31 binds IL31 receptor expressed on sensory nerves, facilitates the elongation and branching of the nerves, and causes pruritus. IL31 also stimulates the expression of IL-1β and the Th2-specific chemokine of CCL17 or CCL22, and decreases FLG expression, thus contributing to AD pathology. Control of the severe itching sensation that disturbs the sleep of AD patients can be improved by subcutaneous injection of anti-IL31RA antibody nemolizumab. Other targets for inhibition of IL31 activation include potential molecules of JAK (Janus kinase) inhibitors (targeting the signal pathway from IL31R engaged by IL31 in Th2 cells), dupilumab (an anti-IL4 receptor-α antibody), and EPAS1 (endothelial PAS domain–containing protein 1, a transcription factor that binds to the promotor region of the IL31 gene) (Furue, Yamamura, Kido-Nakahara, Nakahara, & Fukui, 2018).

The IL17 cytokine family, produced by Th17-type helper T cells, contributes to host protection against infectious pathogens, but it also promotes the pathology of autoimmune diseases. IL17A (and its receptor IL17RA/IL17RC) is a founding member of this family (Gaffen, 2009) and plays a major role in AD phenotype development. IL17A expression in the skin of AD patients is increased, especially in the acute phase, in pediatric patients, and in Asian AD patients (Brunner et al., 2017). In moderate-to-severe psoriasis showing similar pathogenesis with AD, IL17 also contributes to cause the pathophysiology. Ustekinumab, an IL12/IL23p40 blocker that inhibits Th1 and Th17/Th22 responses, effectively treats psoriasis. IL17A produced by Th17 cells affects keratinocytes to induce TSLP and CCL17, and is involved in the critical upregulation of IL4 signaling in mouse model (Nakajima et al., 2014).

IL22 is a member of the IL10 family and binds a heterodimeric complex with IL22R1 and IL10R2. The main producers of IL22 are thought to be CD4+ T cells, CD8+ T cells, and mast cells in AD patients (Fujita, 2013). Recent studies have shown that a newly discovered, unique phenotype of Th22 cells can produce IL22, not IL4, IFN-γ, and IL17 (Trifari, Kaplan, Tran, Crellin, & Spits, 2009). Functional IL22 receptors are expressed on nonhematopoietic cells (i.e., epithelial cells) (Fujita, 2013; Mashiko et al., 2015) most highly in the skin. Keratinocytes produce higher levels of AMPs (β-defensins, lipocalin, LL37, S100A7, 8, 9) in response to IL22 in AD patients than in their healthy counterparts or in psoriasis patients, leading to enhanced proliferation of epithelial cells and induction of epidermal hyperplasia. Although AMP production is effective in protecting the skin from microbial invasion, excess AMP production promotes skin barrier dysfunction, leading to severe and chronic AD. In one study, the blood of adult AD patients had significantly higher levels of IL22-producing T cells expressing the skin-homing receptor cutaneous lymphocyte antigen (CLA) (IL22+CLA+ T cells) than did control adult or pediatric AD patients (Czarnowicki et al., 2015); there was no difference in IL22+CLA+ T-cell numbers between healthy adults and pediatric AD patients. AD in infants and young children is thought to represent the initiation of AD pathology, with patients exhibiting the acute phenotype of adult AD, thus fewer IL22+CLA+ T cells in pediatric AD patients would suggest a role for IL22 in the progress of chronicity of AD, not its initiation.

Chemokines

Chemokines in atopic dermatitis: An overview

The pathophysiology of AD is characterized by inflammatory cell infiltration into the enflamed skin. Chemokines play a key role in promoting these infiltration events, and excess chemokines production can be observed in the skin lesions. Chemokines are cytokines with chemotaxis activity; they have a low molecular weight (8–14 kDa) and are divided into four classes (CC, C, CXC, CX3C) on the basis of their N-terminal conserved cysteine residue (Abboud & Hanson, 2017). Chemokines are produced by various cell types; in AD they are produced mainly by epithelial cells, including keratinocytes, Langerhans cells, lymphocytes, vascular endothelial cells, and fibroblast. They bind to receptors expressed on target cells and induce chemotaxis. Chemotaxis is the migration of cells induced by chemical substances; by chemotaxis, cells can move toward or away from the source.

Many chemokines, such as CCL1 (I-309), CCL2 (MCP-1), CCL3 (MIP-1α), CCL4 (MIP-1β), CCL5 (RANTES), CCL11 (eotaxin), CCL24 (eotaxin-2), CCL26 (eotaxin-3), CCL13 (MCP-4), CCL17 (TARC), CCL18 (PARC), CCL20 (LARC/MIP-3α), CCL22 (MDC), CCL27 (CTACK), CXCL12 (SDF-1α), CXCL9 (Mig), CXCL10 (IP-10), CXCL11 (ITAC), and CX3CL1 (fractalkine), are associated with the pathophysiology of AD (Abboud & Hanson, 2017; Ahmadi, Hassanshahi, Khorramdelazad, Zainodini, & Koochakzadeh, 2016; Brunner et al., 2017; Esaki et al., 2016; Giustizieri et al., 2001; Gombert et al., 2005; Gros, Bussmann, Bieber, Förster, & Novak, 2009; Kaburagi et al., 2001; Kanda, Shimizu, Tada, & Watanabe, 2007; Kim et al., 2012; Nakayama et al., 2001; Nakazato et al., 2008; Suárez-Fariñas et al., 2013) (Table 13.1).

TABLE 13.1 Chemokines associated with atopic dermatitis

Chemokines	Receptor	Production	Target cells	Reference
CCL1 (I-309)	CCR8	DC, Mc, EC	Activated T cells, LC	Gombert et al., 2005; Giustizieri et al., 2001
CCL2 (MCP-1)	CCR2	KC/lymphocytes	Mo/DC/memory T cells	Kaburagi et al., 2001; Giustizieri et al., 2001
CCL3 (MIP-1α)	CCR1/CCR5	Lymphocytes	Mo/lymphocytes/Th1 cells	Giustizieri et al., 2001
CCL4 (MIP-1β)	CCR5	Lymphocytes	Mo/lymphocytes/Th1 cells	Kaburagi et al., 2001
CCL5 (RANTES)	CCR3	KC/TC/EC/DC/fibroblast	Eo/Mo/DC/T cells	Giustizieri et al., 2001
CCL11 (eotaxin)	CCR3	KC/TC/EC/fibroblast	Eo	Ahmadi et al., 2016
CCL13 (MCP-4)	CCR2/CCR3	KC/Mq/T cells	Eo, Mo, T cells/ DC precurser	Gros et al., 2009; Kim et al., 2012
CCL17 (TARC)	CCR4	KC/EC/DC/Fib	Th2 cells	Thijs et al., 2015; Nakazato et al., 2008
CCL18 (PARC)	CCR8	KC/DC/Mq	CLA+T cells/naïve T cells	Gros et al., 2009; Kim et al., 2012
CCL20 (LARC/MIP-3α)	CCR6	KC	Immature DC/Th17 cells	Nakayama et al., 2001; Esaki et al., 2016
CCL22 (MDC)	CCR4	DC/activated B cells	Th2 cells	Thijs et al., 2015; Nakazato et al., 2008
CCL24 (eotaxin-2)	CCR3	Mo/Mq	Eo	Ahmadi et al., 2016
CCL26 (eotaxin-3)	CCR3	KC/EC/VEC /Fib	Eo/T cells	Ahmadi et al., 2016
CCL27 (CTACK)	CCR10	KC	CLA+T cells	Thijs et al., 2015; Nakazato et al., 2008
CXCL9 (Mig)	CXCR3	KC	Th1 cells	Kanda et al., 2007
CXCL10 (IP-10)	CXCR3	KC	Th1 cells	Kanda et al., 2007
CXCL11 (ITAC)	CXCR3	KC	Th1 cells	Kanda et al., 2007
CXCL12 (SDF-1)	CXCR4/CXCRR7	BC/TC/EC/Fib	Immature LC/NK cell/Mq/BC/TC	Gombert et al., 2005
CX3CL1	CX3CR1	EC/VEC	T cells/NK cells/Mo/DC	Brunner et al., 2017

DC, Dendritic cells; *EC*, epithelial cells; *Eo*, eosinophils; *Fib*, fibroblasts; *KC*, keratinocyte; *LC*, Langerhans cells; *MC*, mononuclear cells; *Mq*, macrophage; *TC*, T cells; *VEC*, vascular endothelial cells.

Adapted from Abboud, D., & Hanson, J. (2017). Chemokine neutralization as an innovative therapeutic strategy for atopic dermatitis. *Drug Discovery Today*, 22(4), 702–711. https://doi.org/10.1016/j.drudis.2016.11.023.

Chemotaxis activity, target cells, and biomarkers

The roles of chemokines in AD can be divided in accordance with their chemotaxis activity toward various kinds of target cells, such as Th2, Th1, and others (Furue et al., 2017). Recent studies have attempted to measure serum chemokine levels or mRNA expressions in the lesional and nonlesional skin and to analyze correlation of the levels with severity of AD. In regard to the importance of chemokine with its Th2 chemotaxis activity, CCL17 is currently considered to be the most reliable biomarker reflecting the disease severity of AD (Abboud & Hanson, 2017; Nakazato et al., 2008; Thijs et al., 2015) and is produced by various cells, especially keratinocytes, and dendritic cells activated by IL13 produced by group 2 innate lymphoid cells (ILC2) (Morita et al., 2016). Both CCL17 and CCL22 attract Th2 cells by binding CCR4 (CC chemokine receptor 4) (Abboud & Hanson, 2017). CCL5, CCL11, CCL13, CCL24, CCL26 are enhanced in the skin lesions of AD patients (Kaburagi et al., 2001). They are mainly produced by keratinocytes, T cells, and endothelial cells; bind CCR3; and play a role in eosinophil migration (Ahmadi et al., 2016). Eosinophils, which are differentiated by IL5, produce brain-derived neurotrophic factor (BDNF) and contribute to disease severity (Fölster-Holst et al., 2016). Especially, CCL11 was reported to be elevated in serum and injured skin of AD patients, and IL4-induced CCL11 in dermal fibroblasts attracts eosinophils and corresponds to their localization in the skin (Abboud & Hanson, 2017). In recent reports, CCL26 seems to more associate with pathogenesis of AD compared with CCL24 (Kagami, et al. 2003).

CCL1 binds to CCR8 thereby linking adaptive and innate immune functions. CCL1 is abundantly produced by dendritic cells, mast cells, and dermal endothelial cells via FcεRI engagement with allergens, and allergens as *S. aureus*–derived products. CCL1 may play a key role in the recruitment of Langerhans cells in AD by synergizing with CXCL12 and works by linking with CCL17 and contributing at least in part to Th2-induced skin inflammation (Gombert et al., 2005). CCR8 is expressed on dendritic cells, Langerhans cells, and monocytic precursors and affects Langerhans cell maturation (Abboud & Hanson, 2017). CXCL12 is produced by dermal fibroblasts and promotes Langerhans cell maturation via its receptor, CXCR4 (Abboud & Hanson, 2017). CCL18 (pulmonary and activation-regulated chemokine [PARC]), CCL27 (cutaneous T cell-attracting chemokine [CTACK]), and MDC (CCL22) are promised as biomarkers for AD. MDC is produced by dendritic cells or macrophage and induces Th2 cell migration, whereas CTACK is produced by mainly keratinocytes and attract CLA+T cells (Nakazato et al., 2008; Thijs et al., 2015).

With chemotaxis activity toward Th1 and the others, CXCL9, CXCL10, and CXCL11 are produced by keratinocytes and promote infiltration of IFN-γ–producing Th1 cells toward the skin lesions, which are enhanced by IL18 (Kanda et al., 2007). The roles of the IL18 and IL1 families have been well studied, and in particular IL18 has been shown to

be a useful biomarker (Thijs et al., 2015). CCL18 produced by dendritic cells and macrophage has chemotactic activity to naïve T cells (Gros et al., 2009). Levels of CX3CL1 (fractalkine) and CCL8, as atherosclerosis maker (Brunner et al., 2017), increase in the serum of only AD patients compared with psoriasis and healthy controls. Augmented levels of CCL2, CCL3, CCL4, and CCL5 were observed in peripheral mononuclear cells from AD patients compared with normal controls. CCL2 produced by endothelial cells, and CCL3 and CCL4 from lymphocytes, are strong chemoattractants for monocytes and lymphocytes (Kaburagi et al., 2001). Recently, the role of Th22 has gained attention in AD pathophysiology. Th22 expresses CCR4 and CCR10 on its cell surface (Fujita, 2013). CCL20 produced by keratinocytes attracts Th17 cells in especially lesional skin of children (Esaki et al., 2016; Nakayama et al., 2001).

Chemokine inhibitor as potential therapeutics

Although neutralizing receptors have been studied as part of the effort to develop new treatments and to further our understanding of the pathophysiology of AD, there are few reports showing that chemokine inhibitors are effective in terms of improving the clinical score or state of AD. In some cases, chemokines share a single receptor on target cells to exert their biologic effect (chemotaxis activity); for example, CCL5, CCL11, CCL13, and CCL26 all bind CCR3, especially that expressed on Th2 cells, eosinophils, mast cells, and basophils, and transduce signals (Ahmadi et al., 2016). Similarly, CCL17 and CCL22 share CCR4 (Abboud & Hanson, 2017). Consequently, these chemokines function redundantly at target cells and make it difficult to regulate AD pathophysiology by inhibiting cell responses to chemokines via their receptors. To inhibit AD by blocking chemokine signaling pathway, we may need strategies other than neutralizing their receptors like chemokine ligands (chemicals; tick-producing evasin 4, etc.), the effects of which have been investigated (Abboud & Hanson, 2017; Déruaz, et al. 2013).

Summary

As a mediator of cellular communications, soluble factors, including IgE, cytokines, and chemokines, play essential roles in the development and pathology of AD. Introduction of sophisticated animal models significantly improved our understanding of how rare IgE-producing antibodies are generated during the allergic immune response. Characterization of various cytokines and chemokines in AD patients also contributed to identifying useful biomarkers and targets for therapies. Complexed cytokine/chemokine profiling in the biopsies of AD patients may help to differentiate several variants in AD, which would be useful for future personalized therapies. Additionally, it is important identity molecules to simultaneously target multiple cytokines/chemokines implicated in AD pathogenesis. In this context, JAK/STAT inhibitors have been introduced as oral and topical therapies for AD to target biologic effects of multiple cytokines, with encouraging results (He & Guttman-Yassky, 2019). On the other hand, the efficacy of neutralizing IgE therapy was so far minimal in AD patients, suggesting that more research is needed for better targeting of IgE in AD. The involvement of autoreactive IgE antibodies in AD patients suggests that therapeutic approaches to treat autoimmune diseases may be required in cases of severe AD. A recent high-throughput proteomic study revealed that the AD blood signature was largely different compared to psoriasis, with dysregulation of inflammatory and cardiovascular risk markers, suggesting that AD is a systemic disease beyond atopic/allergic association (Brunner et al., 2017). As such, multiparametric omics (e.g., proteomic, genomic, glycomic) characterization and unbiased analysis of biopsies from AD patients will improve our understanding of AD and aid in therapeutic development.

Uncited references

Salamon et al. (2017)

Further readings

Cabanillas, B., Brehler, A. -C., & Novak, N. (2017). Atopic dermatitis phenotypes and the need for personalized medicine. *Current Opinion in Allergy and Clinical Immunology, 17*(4), 309–315. Author note: In AD treatment, targeted therapies by using biologics are expected to open a new area, but the treatments have not been sufficiently achieved. This review explains key molecules of immune responses affecting AD and discusses the importance of strategies establishing targeted, phenotype-specific therapies for AD by focusing on the individual pathogenesis, especially from pediatrics.

Gowthaman, U., Chen, J. S., Zhang, B., Flynn, W. F., Lu, Y., Song, W., et al. (2019). Identification of a T follicular helper cellsubset that drives anaphylactic IgE. *Science, 365*(6456). https://doi.org/10.1126/science.aaw6433, eaaw6433.

Roesner, L. M., & Werfel, T. (2019). Autoimmunity (or not) in atopic dermatitis. *Frontiers in Immunology, 10*, 2128. https://doi.org/10.3389/fimmu.2019.02128.

Schwartz, C., Moran, T., Saunders, S. P., Kaszlikowska, A., Floudas, A., Bom, J., et al. (2019). Spontaneous atopic dermatitis in mice with a defective skin barrier is independent of ILC2 and mediated by IL-1β. *Allergy: European Journal of Allergy and Clinical Immunology, 74*(10), 1920–1933. Author note: Th2 responses induced by ILC2 as well as Th2 cells have been considered to play critical roles in the pathogenesis of AD. This topic indicates a novel mechanism inducing AD-like skin inflammation in mice model; mice with mutation in a gene of filaggrin affecting the integrity of skin barrier develop AD-like skin inflammation independently of ILC2, but dependently of an interplay between pathogenic microbiome present in neonates and IL1β responding mast cells. Further investigation will be required, but this discusses a key factor to prevent AD-like inflammation in adults; that is to clarify pathophysiology, including microbiome in young children.

Wu, L. C., & Zarrin, A. A. (2014). The production and regulation of IgE by the immune system. *Nature Reviews Immunology, 14*(4), 247–259. https://doi.org/10.1038/nri3632.

References

Abboud, D., & Hanson, J. (2017). Chemokine neutralization as an innovative therapeutic strategy for atopic dermatitis. *Drug Discovery Today, 22*(4), 702–711. https://doi.org/10.1016/j.drudis.2016.11.023.

Acharya, M., Borland, G., Edkins, A. L., Maclellan, L. M., Matheson, J., Ozanne, B. W., & Cushley, W. (2010). CD23/FcεRII: Molecular multi-tasking. *Clinical & Experimental Immunology, 162*(1), 12–23. https://doi.org/10.1111/j.1365-2249.2010.04210.x.

Ahmadi, Z., Hassanshahi, G., Khorramdelazad, H., Zainodini, N., & Koochakzadeh, L. (2016). An overlook to the characteristics and roles played by eotaxin network in the pathophysiology of food allergies: Allergic asthma and atopic dermatitis. *Inflammation, 39*(3), 1253–1267. https://doi.org/10.1007/s10753-016-0303-9.

Beck, L. A., Thaçi, D., Hamilton, J. D., Graham, N. M., Bieber, T., Rocklin, R., et al. (2014). Dupilumab treatment in adults with moderate-to-severe atopic dermatitis. *New England Journal of Medicine, 371*(2), 130–139. https://doi.org/10.1056/NEJMoa1314768.

Brunner, P. M., Guttman-Yassky, E., & Leung, D. Y. M. (2017). The immunology of atopic dermatitis and its reversibility with broad-spectrum and targeted therapies. *The Journal of Allergy and Clinical Immunology, 139*(4), S65–S76. https://doi.org/10.1016/j.jaci.2017.01.011.

Brunner, P. M., Suárez-Fariñas, M., He, H., Malik, K., Wen, H. -C., Gonzalez, J., et al. (2017). The atopic dermatitis blood signature is characterized by increases in inflammatory and cardiovascular risk proteins. *Scientific Reports, 7*(1), 8707. https://doi.org/10.1038/s41598-017-09207-z.

Cabanillas, B., Brehler, A. C., & Novak, N. (2017). Atopic dermatitis phenotypes and the need for personalized medicine. *Current Opinion in Allergy and Clinical Immunology, 17*(4), 309–315. https://doi.org/10.1097/ACI.0000000000000376.

Cheng, L. E., Wang, Z. -E., & Locksley, R. M. (2010). Murine B cells regulate serum IgE levels in a CD23-dependent manner. *Journal of Immunology, 185*(9), 5040–5047. https://doi.org/10.4049/jimmunol.1001900.

Czarnowicki, T., Esaki, H., Gonzalez, J., Malajian, D., Shemer, A., Noda, S., et al. (2015). Early pediatric atopic dermatitis shows only a cutaneous lymphocyte antigen (CLA)+ TH2/TH1 cell imbalance, whereas adults acquire CLA+ TH22/TC22 cell subsets. *The Journal of Allergy and Clinical Immunology, 136*(4), 941–951. https://doi.org/10.1016/j.jaci.2015.05.049. E3.

Czarnowicki, T., Gonzalez, J., Bonifacio, K. M., Shemer, A., Xiangyu, P., Kunjravia, N., et al. (2016). Diverse activation and differentiation of multiple B-cell subsets in patients with atopic dermatitis but not in patients with psoriasis. *The Journal of Allergy and Clinical Immunology, 137*(1), 118–129. https://doi.org/10.1016/j.jaci.2015.08.027. E5.

Déruaz, M., Bonvin, P., Severin, I. C., Johnson, Z., Krohn, S., Power, C. A., & Proudfoot, A. E. I. (2013). Evasin-4, a tick-derived chemokine-binding protein with broad selectivity can be modified for use in preclinical disease models. *FEBS Journal, 280*(19), 4876–4887. https://doi.org/10.1111/febs.12463.

Dullaers, M., De Bruyne, R., Ramadani, F., Gould, H. J., Gevaert, P., & Lambrecht, B. N. (2012). The who, where, and when of IgE in allergic airway disease. *The Journal of Allergy and Clinical Immunology, 129*(3), 635–645. https://doi.org/10.1016/j.jaci.2011.10.029.

Erazo, A., Kutchukhidze, N., Leung, M., Christ, A. P. G., Urban, J. F., Jr., Curotto de Lafaille, M. A., & Lafaille, J. J. (2007). Unique maturation program of the IgE response in vivo. *Immunity*, 26(2), 191–203. https://doi.org/10.1016/j.immuni.2006.12.006.

Esaki, H., Brunner, P. M., Renert-Yuval, Y., Czarnowicki, T., Huynh, T., Tran, G., et al. (2016). Early-onset pediatric atopic dermatitis is TH2 but also TH17 polarized in skin. *The Journal of Allergy and Clinical Immunology*, 138(6), 1639–1651. https://doi.org/10.1016/j.jaci.2016.07.013.

Fölster-Holst, R., Papakonstantinou, E., Rüdrich, U., Buchner, M., Pite, H., Gehring, M., et al. (2016). Childhood atopic dermatitis-brain-derived neurotrophic factor correlates with serum eosinophil cationic protein and disease severity. *Allergy: European Journal of Allergy and Clinical Immunology*, 71(7), 1062–1065. https://doi.org/10.1111/all.12916.

Fujita, H. (2013). The role of IL-22 and Th22 cells in human skin diseases. *Journal of Dermatological Science*, 72(1), 3–8. https://doi.org/10.1016/j.jdermsci.2013.04.028.

Furue, M., Yamamura, K., Kido-Nakahara, M., Nakahara, T., & Fukui, Y. (2018). Emerging role of interleukin-31 and interleukin-31 receptor in pruritus in atopic dermatitis. *Allergy: European Journal of Allergy and Clinical Immunology*, 73(1), 29–36. https://doi.org/10.1111/all.13239.

Furue, M., Chiba, T., Tsuji, G., Ulzii, D., Kido-Nakahara, M., Nakahara, T., et al,(2017). Atopic dermatitis: Immune deviation, barrier dysfunction, IgE autoreactivity and new therapies. *Allergology International*, 66(3), 398–403. https://doi.org/10.1016/j.alit.2016.12.002.

Gaffen. S. L. (2009). Structure and signaling in the IL-17 receptor family. *Nature Reviews. Immunology*, 9(8), 556–567. https://doi.org/10.1038/nri2586.

Giustizieri, M. L., Mascia, F., Frezzolini, A., De Pità, O., Chinni, L. M., Giannetti, A., et al. (2001). Keratinocytes from patients with atopic dermatitis and psoriasis show a distinct chemokine production profile in response to T cell-derived cytokines. *Journal of Allergy and Clinical Immunology*, 107(5), 871–877. https://doi.org/10.1067/mai.2001.114707.

Gombert, M., Dieu-Nosjean, M. -C., Winterberg, F., Bünemann, E., Kubitza, R. C., Da Cunha, L., et al. (2005). CCL1-CCR8 interactions: An axis mediating the recruitment of T cells and Langerhans-type dendritic cells to sites of atopic skin inflammation. *The Journal of Immunology*, 174(8), 5082–5091. https://doi.org/10.4049/jimmunol.174.8.5082.

Gros, E., Bussmann, C., Bieber, T., Förster, I., & Novak, N. (2009). Expression of chemokines and chemokine receptors in lesional and nonlesional upper skin of patients with atopic dermatitis. *The Journal of Allergy and Clinical Immunology*, 124(4), 14–16. https://doi.org/10.1016/j.jaci.2009.07.004.

Han, H., Roan, F., & Ziegler, S. F. (2017). The atopic march: Current insights into skin barrier dysfunction and epithelial cell-derived cytokines. *Immunological Reviews*, 278(1), 116–130. https://doi.org/10.1111/imr.12546.

Hardy, R. R., & Kyoko, H. (2001). B cell development pathways. *Annual Review of Immunology*, 19, 595–621. https://doi: 10.1146/annurev.immunol.19.1.595.

He, H., & Emma, G. -Y. (2019). JAK inhibitors for atopic dermatitis: An update. *American Journal of Clinical Dermatology*, 20(2), 181–192. https://doi.org/10.1007/s40257-018-0413-2.

He, J. -S., Narayanan, S., Subramaniam, S., Ho, W. Q., Lafaille, J. J., & Curotto de Lafaille, M. A. (2015). Biology of IgE production: IgE cell differentiation and the memory of IgE responses. *Current Topics in Microbiology and Immunology*, 388, 1–19. https://doi.org/10.1007/978-3-319-13725-4-1.

Heil, P. M., Maurer, D., Klein, B., Hultsch, T., & Stingl, G. (2010). Omalizumab therapy in atopic dermatitis: Depletion of IgE does not improve the clinical course - a randomized, placebo-controlled and double blind pilot study. *Journal der Deutschen Dermatologischen Gesellschaft=Journal of the German Society of Dermatology*, 8(12), 990–998. https://doi.org/10.1111/j.1610-0387.2010.07497.x.

Honda, T., & Kabashima, K. (2019). Prostanoids and leukotrienes in the pathophysiology of atopic dermatitis and psoriasis. *International Immunology*, 31(9), 589–595. https://doi.org/10.1093/intimm/dxy087.

Honda, T., Nomura, T., & Kabashima, K. (2017). Advances in atopic dermatitis and urticarial in 2016. *The Journal of Allergy and Clinical Immunology*, 140(2), 369–376. https://doi.org/10.1016/j.jaci.2017.06.005.

Hvid, M., Vestergaard, C., Kemp, K., Christensen, G. B., Deleuran, B., & Deleuran, M. (2011). IL-25 in atopic dermatitis: A possible link between inflammation and skin barrier dysfunction. *Journal of Investigative Dermatology*, 131(1), 150–157. https://doi.org/10.1038/jid.2010.277.

Iyengar, S. R., Hoyte, E. G., Loza, A., Bonaccorso, S., Chiang, D., Umetsu, D. T., & Nadeau, K. C. (2013). Immunologic effects of omalizumab in children with severe refractory atopic dermatitis: A randomized, placebo-controlled clinical trial. *International Archives of Allergy and Immunology*, 162(1), 89–93. https://doi.org/10.1159/000350486.

Jaworek, A. K., Szafraniec, K., Jaworek, M., Hałubiec, P., & Wojas-Pelc, A. (2019). The level of total immunoglobulin E as an indicator of disease grade in adults with severe atopic dermatitis. *Polish Medical Journal*, 47(282), 217–220.

Kaburagi, Y., Shimada, Y., Nagaoka, T., Hasegawa, M., Takehara, K., & Sato, S. (2001). Enhanced production of CC-chemokines (RANTES, MCP-1, MIP-1alpha, MIP-1beta, and eotaxin) in patients with atopic dermatitis. *Archives of Dermatological Research*, 293(7), 350–355. https://doi.org/10.1007/s004030100230.

Kagami, S., Kakinuma, T., Saeki, H., Tsunemi, Y., Fujita, H., Nakamura, K., et al. (2003). Significant elevation of serum levels of eotaxin-3/CCL26, but not eotaxin-2/CCL24, in patients with atopic dermatitis: Serum eotaxin-3/CCL26 levels reflect the disease activity of atopic dermatitis. *Clinical and Experimental Immunology*, 134(2), 309–313. https://doi.org/10.1046/j.1365-2249.2003.02273.x.

Kanda, N., Shimizu, T., Tada, Y., & Watanabe, S. (2007). IL-18 enhances IFN-γ-induced Production of CXCL9, CXCL10, and CXCL11 in human keratinocytes. *European Journal of Immunology*, 37(2), 338–350. https://doi.org/10.1002/eji.200636420.

Kashiwagi, M., Hosoi, J., Lai, J. F., Brissette, J., Ziegler, S. F., Morgan, B. A., & Georgopoulos, K. (2017). Direct control of regulatory T cells by keratinocytes. *Nature Immunology*, 18(3), 334–343. https://doi.org/10.1038/ni.3661.

Kasperkiewicz, M., Schmidt, E., Ludwig, R. J., & Zillikens, D. (2018). Targeting IgE antibodies by immunoadsorption in atopic dermatitis. *Frontiers in Immunology*, 19(9), 254. https://doi.org/10.3389/fimmu.2018.00254.

Kim, H. O., Cho, S. I., Chung, B. Y., Ahn, H. K., Park, C. W., & Lee, C. H. (2012). Expression of CCL1 and CCL18 in atopic dermatitis and psoriasis. *Clinical and Experimental Dermatology*, 37(5), 521–526. https://doi.org/10.1111/j.1365-2230.2011.04295.x.

Kim, J., Kim, B. E., Lee, J., Han, Y., Jun, H. Y., Kim, H., et al. (2016). Epidermal thymic stromal lymphopoietin predicts the development of atopic dermatitis during Infancy. *The Journal of Allergy and Clinical Immunology*, 137(4), 1282–1285. https://doi.org/10.1016/j.jaci.2015.12.1306. E4.

Liu, Y. -J., Soumelis, V., Watanabe, N., Ito, T., Wang, Y. -H., de Malefyt, R. W., et al. (2007). TSLP: An epithelial cell cytokine that regulates T cell differentiation by conditioning dendritic cell maturation. *Annual Review of Immunology*, 25, 193–219. https://doi.org/10.1146/annurev.immunol.25.022106.141718.

Mashiko, S., Bouguermouh, S., Rubio, M., Baba, N., Bissonnette, R., & Sarfati, M. (2015). Human mast cells are major IL-22 producers in patients with psoriasis and atopic dermatitis. *The Journal of Allergy and Clinical Immunology*, 136(2), 351–359. https://doi.org/10.1016/j.jaci.2015.01.033. E1.

McHeyzer-Williams, L. J., & McHeyzer-Williams, M. G. (2005). Antigen-specific memory B cell development. *Annual Review of Immunology*, 23, 487–513. https://doi.org/10.1146/annurev.immunol.23.021704.115732.

Morita, H., Moro, K., & Koyasu, S. (2016). Innate lymphoid cells in allergic and nonallergic inflammation. *The Journal of Allergy and Clinical Immunology*, 138(5), 1253–1264. https://doi.org/10.1016/j.jaci.2016.09.011.

Nakajima, S., Kitoh, A., Egawa, G., Natsuaki, Y., Nakamizo, S., Moniaga, C. S., et al. (2014). IL-17A as an inducer for Th2 immune responses in murine atopic dermatitis models. *Journal of Investigative Dermatology*, 134(8), 2122–2130. https://doi.org/10.1038/jid.2014.51.

Nakashima, C., Otsuka, A., & Kabashima, K. (2018). Interleukin-31 and interleukin-31 receptor: New therapeutic targets for atopic dermatitis. *Experimental Dermatology*, 27(4), 327–331. https://doi.org/10.1111/exd.13533.

Nakayama, T., Fujisawa, R., Yamada, H., Horikawa, T., Kawasaki, H., Hieshima, K., et al. (2001). Inducible expression of a CC chemokine liver- and activation-regulated chemokine (LARC)/macrophage inflammatory protein (MIP)-3α/CCL20 by epidermal keratinocytes and its role in atopic dermatitis. *International Immunology*, 13(1), 95–103. https://doi.org/10.1093/intimm/13.1.95.

Nakazato, J., Kishida, M., Kuroiwa, R., Fujiwara, J., Shimoda, M., & Shinomiya, N. (2008). Serum levels of Th2 chemokines, CCL17, CCL22, and CCL27, were the important markers of severity in infantile atopic dermatitis. *Pediatric Allergy and Immunology*, 19(7), 605–613. https://doi.org/10.1111/j.1399-3038.2007.00692.x.

Roesner, L. M., & Werfel, T. (2019). Autoimmunity (or Not) in atopic dermatitis. *Frontiers in Immunology*, 10(10), 2128. https://doi.org/10.3389/fimmu.2019.02128.

Salamon, P., Shefler, I., Moshkovits, I., Munitz, A., Horwitz Klotzman, D., Mekori, Y. A., & Hershko, A. Y. (2017). IL-33 and IgE stimulate mast cell production of IL-2 and regulatory T cell expansion in allergic dermatitis. *Clinical and Experimental Allergy*, 47(11), 1409–1416. https://doi.org/10.1111/cea.13027.

Seltmann, J., Roesner, L. M., von Hesler, F. W., Wittmann, M., & Werfel, T.et al. (2015). IL-33 impacts on the skin barrier by downregulating the expression of filaggrin. *The Journal of Allergy and Clinical Immunology*, 135(6), 1659–1961.E4. https://doi.org/10.1016/j.jaci.2015.01.048.

Sonesson, A., Bartosik, J., Christiansen, J., Roscher, I., Nilsson, F., Schmidtchen, A., & Bäck, O. (2013). Sensitization to skin-associated microorganisms in adult patients with atopic dermatitis is of importance for disease severity. *Acta Dermato-Venereologica*, 93(3), 340–345. https://doi.org/10.2340/00015555-1465.

Suárez-Fariñas, M., Dhingra, N., Gittler, J., Shemer, A., Cardinale, I., de Guzman Strong, C., et al. (2013). Intrinsic atopic dermatitis (AD) shows similar Th2 and higher Th17 immune activation compared to extrinsic AD. *The Journal of Allergy and Clinical Immunology*, 132(2), 361–370. https://doi.org/10.1016/j.jaci.2013.04.046.

Takamori, A., Nambu, A., Sato, K., Yamaguchi, S., Matsuda, K., Numata, T., et al. (2018). IL-31 is crucial for induction of pruritus, but not inflammation, in contact hypersensitivity. *Scientific Reports*, 8(1), 1–11. https://doi.org/10.1038/s41598-018-25094-4.

Talay, O., Yan, D., Brightbill, H. D., Straney, E. E. M., Zhou, M., Ladi, E., et al. (2012). IgE⁺ memory B cells and plasma cells generated through a germinal-center pathway. *Nature Immunology*, 13(4), 396–404. https://doi.org/10.1038/ni.2256.

Tang, T. S., Bieber, T., & Williams, H. C. (2012). Does "autoreactivity" play a role in atopic dermatitis? *The Journal of Allergy and Clinical Immunology*, 129(5), 1209–1215. https://doi.org/10.1016/j.jaci.2012.02.002. E2.

Thijs, J., Krastev, T., Weidinger, S., Buckens, C. F., De Bruin-Weller, M., Bruijnzeel-Koomen, C., et al. (2015). Biomarkers for atopic dermatitis: A systematic review and meta-analysis. *Current Opinion in Allergy and Clinical Immunology*, 15(5), 453–460. https://doi.org/10.1097/ACI.0000000000000198.

Tokura. Y. (2010). Extrinsic and intrinsic types of atopic dermatitis. *Journal of Dermatological Science*, 58(1), 1–7. https://doi.org/10.1016/j.jdermsci.2010.02.008.

Trifari, S., Kaplan, C. D., Tran, E. H., Crellin, N. K., & Spits, H. (2009). Identification of a human helper T cell population that has abundant production of interleukin 22 and Is distinct from TH-17, TH1 and TH2 cells. *Nature Immunology*, 10(8), 864–871. https://doi.org/10.1038/ni.1770.

van der Stoep, N., Korver, W., & Logtenberg, T. (1994). In vivo and in vitro IgE isotype switching in human B lymphocytes: Evidence for a predominantly direct IgM to IgE class switch program. *European Journal of Immunology*, 24(6), 1307–1311. https://doi.org/10.1002/eji.1830240610.

Virtanen, T., Maggi, E., Manetti, R., Piccinni, M. P., Sampognaro, S., Parronchi, P., et al. (1995). No relationship between skin-infiltrating TH2-like cells and allergen-specific IgE response in atopic dermatitis. *The Journal of Allergy and Clinical Immunology*, 96(3), 411–420. https://doi.org/10.1016/s0091-6749(95)70061-7.

Wang, H. -H., Li, Y. -C., & Huang, Y. -C. (2016). Efficacy of omalizumab in patients with atopic dermatitis: A systematic review and meta-analysis. *The Journal of Allergy and Clinical Immunology*, 138(6), 1719–1722.E1. https://doi.org/10.1016/j.jaci.2016.05.038.

Wang, T., & Secombes, C. J. (2015). The evolution of IL-4 and IL-13 and their receptor subunits. *Cytokine*, 75(1), 8–13. https://doi.org/10.1016/j.cyto.2015.04.012.

Wang, Y. -H., & Liu, Y. -J. (2009). Thymic stromal lymphopoietin, OX40-ligand, and interleukin-25 in allergic responses. *Clinical and Experimental Allergy*, 39(6), 798–806. https://doi.org/10.1111/j.1365-2222.2009.03241.x.

Weidinger, S., & Novak, N. (2016). Atopic dermatitis. *Lancet*, 387(10023), 1109–1122. https://doi.org/10.1016/S0140-6736(15)00149-X.

Wu, L. C., & Zarrin, A. A. (2014). The production and regulation of IgE by the immune system. *Nature Reviews Immunology*, 14(4), 247–259. https://doi.org/10.1038/nri3632.

Yamaguchi, H., Kabashima-Kubo, R., Bito, T., Sakabe, J. I., Shimauchi, T., Ito, T., et al. (2013). High frequencies of positive nickel/cobalt patch tests and high sweat nickel concentration in patients with intrinsic atopic dermatitis. *Journal of Dermatological Science, 72*(3), 240–245. https://doi.org/10.1016/j.jdermsci.2013.07.009.

Yang, Z., Sullivan, B. M., & Allen, C. D. C. (2012). Fluorescent in vivo detection reveals that IgE(+) B cells are restrained by an intrinsic cell fate predisposition. *Immunity, 36*(5), 857–872. https://doi:10.1016/j.immuni.2012.02.009.

Yi, L., Cheng, D., Zhang, K., Huo, X., Mo, Y., Shi, H., et al. (2017). Intelectin contributes to allergen-induced IL-25, IL-33, and TSLP expression and type 2 response in asthma and atopic dermatitis. *Mucosal Immunology, 10*(6), 1491–1503. https://doi.org/10.1038/mi.2017.10.

14

Cellular Factors

MICHIKO SHIMODA, KHIEM A. TRAN, AND MASAKO TODA

KEY POINTS

- Atopic dermatitis (AD) is a complex disease with various types of leukocytes involved in its pathology.
- Multiple subsets of CD4+ helper T cells, which are sensitized, activated, and differentiated by antigen presenting cells (i.e., Langerhans cells and dendritic cells) in damaged skin and *Staphylococcus aureus* infection, lead to acute and chronic inflammation in AD.
- Mast cells, granulocytes (basophils and eosinophils), and group 2 innate lymphoid cells (ILC2) contribute to the onset and development of skin inflammation.
- Advanced knowledge about cellular factors in AD pathology may lead to novel strategies for treatment of such disease.

Introduction

Atopic dermatitis (AD), also known as atopic eczema, is a chronic inflammatory skin disease characterized by impaired skin barrier function, marked inflammatory infiltration of activated leukocytes, intense itching, and eczematous lesions. AD is a heterogeneous disease with several subtypes, involving multiple CD4+ helper T-cell (Th) subsets and inflammatory cells. The pathologic mechanism of AD is divided into three phases: sensitization, acute inflammation, and chronic inflammation. During sensitization, specific T cells and immunoglobulin E (IgE) antibodies are produced in response to allergen(s). The first step of sensitization is allergen capture by antigen presenting cells (APCs), such as epidermal Langerhans cells (LCs) and dermal dendritic cells (DCs), which are mainly located in epidermis and dermis, respectively. This induces the activation of Th2, Th22 cells, and follicular Th (Tfh) cells, which are subsets of CD4+ Th cells (Fig. 14.1). The cytokines produced by Th2 and Tfh cells, as a result of T cell–B cell interaction, trigger IgE production in B cells and elicit acute inflammation in adult AD patients (Fig. 14.2). Evidence has suggested that Th2 cells also play a role in itching sensation and scratching behavior. Th22 cells cause diffuse epidermal hyperplasia. In acute inflammation, a complex interplay among several inflammatory cells, such as mast cells, granulocytes (basophils and eosinophils), and group 2 innate lymphoid cells (ILC2), is

induced by both IgE-associated and -nonassociated mechanisms (see Fig. 14.2). In chronic inflammation, multiple subsets of CD4+ Th cells, including Th1, Th2, Th17, and/or Th22 cells, together with inflammatory cells, are accumulated in the lesional tissues (see Fig. 14.2). Th1 and Th17 cells aggravate inflammation and tissue remodeling, whereas Th22 cells deteriorate diffuse epidermal hyperplasia. Notably, recent studies have suggested that Th17 cells are also involved in the onset of acute inflammation in pediatric patients, indicating that pathology of AD is complex (Weidinger, Beck, Bieber, Kabashima, & Irvine, 2018). In this chapter we will review how these T-cell subsets, APCs, and inflammatory cells contribute to the development of AD. Humoral factors are reviewed in Chapter 13.

Antigen presenting cells

APCs are a group of immune cells that are capable of processing and presenting antigens for recognition by T cells to initiate the adaptive cellular immune responses. Professional APCs in human skin include DCs, LCs, and B cells. Dermal DCs and LCs are central to the skin APC networks by physically interacting with neighboring cells, including keratinocytes, mast cells, and sensory nerve fibers for antigen acquisition and transfer, as well as signal activation and delivery, which collectively translate into skin T-cell responses. In AD, those APCs play a key role in the induction of pathogenic inflammatory T cells.

Dendritic cells

DCs are derived from hematopoietic progenitor cells in the bone marrow. They express various types of receptors for pathogen-associated pattern recognition molecules (PAMPs) for dictating pathogenic insults. Once they are activated by PAMPs, DCs upregulate major histocompatibility complex (MHC) molecules and costimulatory receptors, and act as the major professional APCs in establishing immunity against pathogens. Alternatively, upon sensing certain ligands such as those binding to C-type lectins carrying an immunoreceptor tyrosine-based inhibitory motif (ITIM) (e.g., DC-SIGN), they mature into suppressive DCs actively inducing tolerance against self-components,

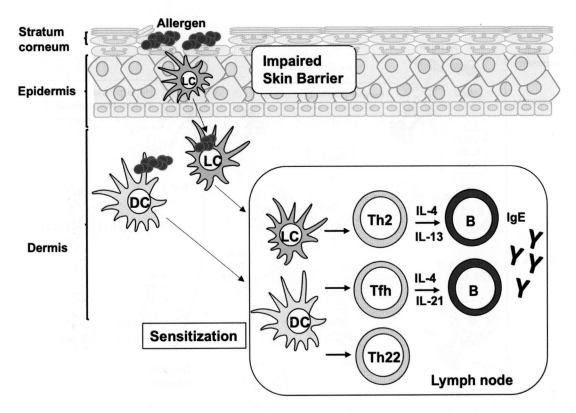

• **Fig. 14.1** Mechanism of sensitization in atopic dermatitis. The first cells to capture allergens in cutaneous tissues are epidermal Langerhans cells and dermal dendritic cells. These antigen presenting cells induce activation and differentiation of Th2, Th22, and Tfh cells. Cytokines produced by Th2 and Tfh cells induce IgE production by B cells. *B*, B cell; *DC*, dendritic cell; *IL*, interleukin; *LC*, Langerhans cell; *Tfh*, follicular T helper cell; *Th*, T helper cell.

commensal microbacteria, and environmental antigens (Brown, Willment, & Whitehead, 2018). Recent high-dimensional phenotypic mapping of human DCs revealed that human dermal DC subsets are distinct from blood and lymphoid tissues, exhibiting interindividual variation (Alcántara-Hernández et al., 2017). Dermal DCs are grouped into multiple phenotypic and distinct functions, which include conventional DC1s (cDC1s), cDC2s, and monocyte-derived DCs (Kashem, Haniffa, & Kaplan, 2017). Based on the genetic ablation approach in mouse models, primary functions of DC subsets have been defined. cDC1s (CD141+ DCs) are essential for cross-priming and Th1 responses, whereas cDC2s (CD1c+ DCs) promote Th2 immune responses (Kashem et al., 2017). Under inflammatory conditions, monocyte-derived DCs are differentiated in the epidermis and act as local APCs along with LCs (see next section) (Doebel, Voisin, Nagao, 2017). Dermal DCs not only locally can activate tissue resident T cells within the skin but also carry acquired antigens to skin-draining lymph nodes where they prime naïve and memory T cells.

In AD, DCs mature in the presence of a cytokine, thymic stromal lymphopoietin (TSLP), which plays a prominent role in the induction of inflammatory Th2 responses. TSLP is highly expressed by keratinocytes in AD lesions, which is also associated with LCs activation and migration (Ziegler, 2012). In vitro, TSLP strongly up-regulates the expression of MHC class II and costimulatory molecules, including OX40L on DCs (Ito et al., 2005). TSLP-matured DCs produce CC chemokine ligand 17 (CCL17; also known as thymus and activation-regulated chemokine [TARC]) and CCL22, which recruit pathogenic Th2 cells in AD but fail to produce Th1 polarizing cytokine interleukin-12 (IL12) or proinflammatory cytokines (Ito et al., 2005; Liu, 2006). Furthermore, TSLP-matured DCs can induce robust proliferation of naïve CD4+ T cells, which subsequently differentiated into Th2 cells that produce allergy-associated cytokines IL4, IL5, IL13, and tumor necrosis factor (TNF), but not IL10 and interferon-gamma (IFN-γ) (Ito et al., 2005; Soumelis et al., 2002; Ziegler, 2012).

Langerhans cells

LCs are highly unique professional APCs that reside in the epidermis under steady conditions, and make up 3% to 5% of all nucleated cells in the epidermis (Deckers, Hammad, & Hoste, 2018). LCs originate from tissue-resident macrophage precursor cells that directly seeded to the epidermis during embryonic development (Deckers et al., 2018; Doebel et al., 2017) and are maintained by self-renewal mechanism via autocrine transforming growth factor-β (TGF-β) production (Kaplan et al., 2007). Despite their

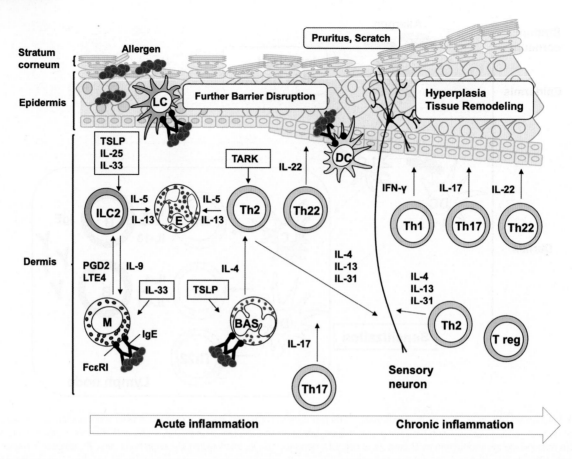

• Fig. 14.2 Mechanism of acute and chronic inflammation in atopic dermatitis. Multiple cells are involved in development of acute and chronic inflammation by secreting inflammatory and pruritic cytokines and chemokines. *B*, B cell; *BAS*, basophil; *DC*, dendritic cell; *E*, eosinophil; *LC*, Langerhans cells; *IFN-γ*, interferon gamma; *IL*, interleukin; *ILC2*, type 2 innate lymphoid cell; *M*, mast cell; *TARC*, thymus- and activation-regulated chemokine; *Th*, T helper cell; *TSLP*, thymic stromal lymphopoietin.

macrophage origin as defined by a lineage-specific transcription factor *Mafb* expression, LCs share many phenotypic features with cDCs. For example, they have migratory capacity to draining lymph nodes via CC chemokine receptor (CCR) 7–mediated signals and express MHC class II as well as CD1a and CD1c that are MHC class I–related molecules involved in lipid antigen presentation (Kashem et al., 2017). A recent lineage tracking study indeed shows that LCs express Zbtb46, the transcription factor enforcing cDC identity (Wu et al., 2016).

Under homeostatic conditions, LCs are thought to constantly migrate to the lymph nodes and present self antigen to establish immune tolerance (Ghigo et al., 2013; Gosselin et al., 2014). Also, as a part of the first line of defense to pathogens, they protrude their dendrites via tight junctions toward the stratum corneum and can acquire antigens across epidermis (Deckers et al., 2018; Doebel et al., 2017). After barrier disruption, such as in the case of AD or in patients with filaggrin deficiency, LCs exhibit activated phenotype with increased proliferation and expression of costimulatory molecules: CD80, CD86 (Leitch et al., 2016; Schuller et al., 2001), and FcεRI (Bruynzeel-Koomen, van Wichen, Toonstra, Berrens, & Bruynzeel, 1986), the high-affinity IgE receptor that binds allergen-specific IgE thereby promoting

allergen deposition and uptake (Novak & Bieber, 2003). In subsequent bacterial infection in the AD lesions, LCs likely mediate Th17 responses to certain bacteria. For example, in a mouse model of AD, infiltrating γδT cells and Th17 cells in response to *Staphylococcus aureus* were abrogated when mice lacked LCs (Kobayashi et al., 2015). Human LCs have also been shown to induce IL22 production by γδT cells, clearing *S. aureus* infection (Malhotra et al., 2016).

B cells

As discussed in Chapter 13, B cells act as APCs to support differentiation of Tfh cells, leading to high-affinity allergen-specific IgE production. In addition, B cells can modulate immune response through cytokine productions. Evidence suggests the existence of skin-specific B-cell subsets with restricted usage of heavy chain V gene and lower representation of IgG1 compared to bloodborne counterparts. These B cells may play a role in skin homeostasis by regulating wound healing and cutaneous microbiome through production of various cytokines such as IL6, granulocyte macrophage colony-stimulating factor (GM-CSF), IFN-γ, IL4, and IL10 (Shen & Fillatreau, 2015). Evidence has suggested the existence of skin-specific B-cell subsets that may play a role in skin homeostasis by regulating wound healing and cutaneous microbiome through production of cytokines such as IL6, IL10, TGF-β, platelet-derived growth factor, and basic fibroblast growth factor (Debes & McGettigan, 2019). In addition, skin-associated B1-like regulatory B cells have emerged as critical negative regulators of skin inflammation via IL10 production.

T cells

T cells are a subset of lymphocytes generated in the thymus, playing a central role in the adaptive immune system. They express T-cell receptor (TCR) with diverse specificities and recognize antigenic peptides bound to MHC presented by antigen presenting cells. In the thymus, the self-tolerance mechanism ensures elimination of high-affinity autoreactive T cells that recognize self antigens (Klein, Kyewski, Allen, & Hogquist, 2014). T cells (CD4+ and CD8+ T cells) that survived through the selection enter the peripheral T-cell pool or reside in peripheral lymph nodes and tissues, including the skin. There, naïve CD4+ T cells differentiate into functionally distinct and diverse effector T cells (such as Th1, Th2, Th17, and Tfh cells), in response to polarizing immunologic milieus set by a combination of specific TCR signaling strength, and costimulatory and cytokine signals provided by APCs.

AD is considered a T-cell–driven disease carrying a complex immune signature with phenotypic variations depending on the stage, age, and race (Biedermann, Skabytska, Kaesler, & Volz, 2015; Brunner, Guttman-Yassky, & Leung, 2017; Trautmann, Akdis, Bröcker, Blaser, & Akdis, 2001; Werfel et al., 2016). Once sensitized, the T-cell–mediated immune reaction is progressive. The acute phase, especially in childhood, is predominantly driven by an inflammatory Th2 phenotype with production of Th2 (IL4, IL5, IL13, IL31, and CCL18) and Th22 (IL22 and S100A proteins) cytokines (Brunner et al., 2017; Czarnowicki, Krueger, & Guttman-Yassky, 2014; Oliva, Renert-Yuval, & Guttman-Yassky, 2016; Weidinger et al., 2018). Infiltration of activated CD45RO+ (a memory marker) cutaneous lymphocyte-associated antigen (CLA+) T cells around the perivascular area of postcapillary venules in the upper dermis is a hallmark of acute eczematous lesions (Leung & Bieber, 2003; Trautmann et al., 2001). This inflammatory Th2 type response is later shifted toward Th1 and Th17 dominant responses in the chronic stage with increased chemokine (C-X-C motif) ligand 10 (CXCL10) and IFN-γ production (Brunner et al., 2017; Czarnowicki et al., 2014; Oliva et al., 2016; Weidinger et al., 2018). In addition, Tfh cells that help to produce IgE and regulatory T cells (Treg) to suppress T-cell responses are also likely involved in AD.

Inflammatory Th2 and Th22 cells

AD has been classically thought to be a Th2 dominant disease. Th2 cells that accumulate in the upper dermis and later penetrate the basal membrane into the epidermal keratinocytes layer are mainly mediated by Th2 cytokines such as IL4, IL5, IL13, IL31, and IL33. IL4 and IL13 induce IgE production by B cells, whereas IL4, IL5, IL13, and IL33 are maturation, activation, and/or migration factors for mast cells, basophils, and eosinophils. These Th2 cytokines as well as IL22 from Th22 cells have been shown to influence keratinocyte differentiation by inducing keratinocyte apoptosis and reducing filaggrin and tight junction proteins (such as claudins), which collectively results in skin barrier defect (Eyerich, Pennino, et al., 2009; Eyerich, Eyerich, et al., 2009; Guttman-Yassky, Nograles, & Krueger, 2011; Gutowska-Owsiak, Schaupp, Salimi, Taylor, & Ogg, 2011; Howell et al., 2006; Nomura et al., 2003; Ong et al., 2002; Trautmann et al., 2001). These Th2 and Th22 cytokines also inhibit skin production of antimicrobial peptides (Cho, Strickland, Boguniewicz, & Leung, 2001; Cho, Strickland, Tomkinson et al., 2001) and initial development of Th1 and Th17 response effective for preventing infections (Biedermann et al., 2001; Ghoreschi et al., 2003; Guenova et al., 2015; O'Connor, Zenewic, & Flavell, 2010), which accelerates the epidermal barrier disruption and enhances the risk of S. aureus infection in AD skin.

Th22 cells are identified as IL22+IFN-γ−IL4− and IL17−CD4+ T-cell subset with expression of CCR6 as well as skin homing receptors CCR4 and CCR10 (Duhen, Geiger, Jarrossay, Lanzavecchia, & Sallusto, 2009; Trifari, Kaplan, Tran, Crellin, & Spits, 2009). Significant increase in IL22 levels is reported in acute legion of AD (Gittler et al., 2012). In addition, the numbers of Th22 (CD4+IL22+IL17A−IFN-γ−) cells as well as Tc22 cells (CD8+IL22+IL17A−IFN-γ−) in the chronic lesional skin are significantly increased compared to those seen in psoriasis disease (Nograles et al., 2009). A recent study has shown that Th22 cells inhibit staphylococcal enterotoxins, whereas Tc22 cells exhibit an enhanced response to the bacterial stimuli, indicating the relevance of CD8+ T cells modulated by staphylococcal enterotoxins in adult AD patients causing the immunologic imbalance (Orfali et al., 2018).

How biased Th2 differentiation is induced in the first place remains unclear. It is likely multiple genetic, cellular, and cytokine/chemokine factors, including TSLP, are involved in conditioning Th2 differentiation (Ziegler, 2012). A recent study shed light on the role of ionic checkpoints, such as sodium chloride (NaCl) and potassium, as cutaneous microenvironmental checkpoint factors that may influence the Th2 polarization in AD (Matthias et al., 2019).

Based on cytokine profile, the Th2 response seen in patients with AD is an "inflammatory" Th2 type, different from conventional Th2 response (Liu, 2006). The initial acute inflammatory Th2 response in AD is marked by high levels of TNF and conventional Th2 cytokines (IL4, IL5, and IL13) but little or no IL10 (Soumelis et al., 2002). The inflammatory Th2 response is driven by DCs and LCs matured in the presence of TSLP that is highly expressed by keratinocytes, mast cells, epithelial cells, and fibroblasts in

AD lesions. In addition, TLSP-stimulated DC and LC promote production of CCL17 and CCL22 that recruit pathogenic Th2 cells. CCL17 and CCL22 are also expressed by dermal endothelial cells (Fuhlbrigge, Kieffer, Armerding, & Kupper, 1997; Hirahara et al., 2006). CCR4 and its ligands are regarded as potential therapeutic targets for AD (see Chapter 13).

Finally, Th2 cells play a key role in AD-related pruritus through IL4, IL13, and IL33 production. These Th2 cytokines directly activated both human and mouse sensory neurons to transmit itch signal from the peripheral to central nervous system (Oetjen et al., 2017). Transgenic mouse models overexpressing IL4 and IL13 exhibited pruritic dermatitis along with symptoms associated with AD such as thickening lesions and increase in IgE (Chan, Robinson, & Xu, 2001; Zheng et al., 2009). Neurosensory mechanisms in AD are further discussed in Chapter 16.

Th1 and Th17 cells

In the later chronic stage of adult AD patients, T-cell response is shifted toward Th1 and Th17 response. Th1 cells, marked by the expression of T-bet, are polarized from naïve T cells in the presence of DCs secreting large amounts of IL12p70. Th1 cells that produce IFN-γ are seen infiltrating in chronic lesions colonized by *S. aureus* and cause skin tissue damages. Skin-colonized *S. aureus* produces lipoteichoic acid, a toll-like receptor 2 (TLR2) agonist (Travers, 2014). DCs matured with lipoteichoic acid plus IL4 in vitro produce IL12p70 and IL23 to promote Th1 and Th17 priming, respectively (Volz et al., 2010). Th17 cells are characterized to produce IL17 and IL22 (Harrington et al., 2005). In AD, the numbers of IL17- producing T cells in peripheral blood and lesions correlates with disease severity (Toda et al., 2003). IL17 production by Th17 cells requires staphylococcal superantigen stimulation, indicating the role of bacterial exposure in triggering a Th17 response in AD (Eyerich, Pennino, et al., 2009; Eyerich, Eyerich, et al., 2009). Collectively, these studies suggest that IL12, which is often produced by microbial infections, plays a critical role in the shift toward Th1/Th17 response by overriding the OX40L-induced inflammatory Th2 response driven by TSLP (Liu, 2006). Notably, Esaki et al. (2016) showed that accumulation of Th17 cells was observed in AD patients aged 3 months to 5 years with early onset in the previous 6 months and moderate-to-severe disease. The same research group showed the significant Th17/Th22 skewing in pediatric AD with early onset but lacked the Th1 upregulation that characterizes adult AD (Brunner et al., 2018). Taken together, the pathologic mechanism for onset and development of AD appears different in pediatric and adult patients and has to be elucidated in more detail.

T follicular helper cells

Tfh cells marked by high levels of CXCR5, PD-1, and Bcl-6 expression are specialized to support B-cell response in germinal centers that are essential for class switching recombination and somatic hypermutation for the generation of high-affinity antibody producing plasma cells and memory B cells (Crotty, 2014; Tangye, Ma, Brink, & Deenick, 2013). By supporting humoral response, Tfh cells are involved in clearing infections but are adversely linked to autoimmunity. In AD, Tfh cells are thought to support allergen-specific IgE production. Notably, recent studies have suggested that IgG1 and IgE response is mainly supported by IL4 produced by Tfh cells but not by Th2 cells (Kubo, 2017). In addition, a recent study showed that differentiation of Tfh cells are promoted by TSLP-matured DCs via OX40L, but not ICOS, costimulation. Such TSLP-DC differentiated Tfh cells are capable of helping IgE secretion by memory B cells through production of IL4, IL21, and CXCL13 (Pattarini et al., 2017). Evidently blood-circulating Tfh cells are increased in AD compared to healthy children, but not adults, implying that the role of Tfh cells in children and adults is different (Szabó et al., 2017).

Regulatory T cells

Tregs are identified as CD4+CD25hiFoxp3+ cells that establish and maintain immune homeostasis by suppressing immune responses (Panduro, Benoist, & Mathis, 2016). Tregs are generated during thymic T-cell development as a subset of self-reactive T cells under transcription factor Foxp3 regulation. Tregs are specialized in regulating inflammatory responses by utilizing tissue-dependent distinct mechanisms such as IL10 secretion and TGF-β–mediated contact dependent suppression. In skin, Foxp3+ Tregs are one of the largest immune cell subsets; they localize to hair follicles where commensal bacteria reside (Ali & Rosenblum, 2017; Rodriguez et al., 2014). Accordingly, the frequency of Tregs fluctuates 20% to 80% of total CD4+ T cells at steady state along with the hair follicle cycle (Kalekar & Rosenblum, 2019). Skin-resident Tregs express skin-homing receptors CLA (Psgl-1), CCR4, and CCR6 as do pathogenic Th2 cells in AD. The ligands for CCR4 (i.e., CCL17 and CCL22) are expressed by dermal endothelial cells (Fuhlbrigge et al., 1997; Hirahara et al., 2006). Although the role of Tregs in AD disease is not entirely clear, it is conceivable that they play a critical role in regulating abnormal inflammatory Th2 response based on the spontaneous development of AD-like eczematous dermatitis in patients with the IPEX syndrome that have dysfunctional Tregs due to the mutations in the *Foxp3* gene (Halabi-Tawil et al., 2009; Van Gool et al., 2019). In a mouse model of AD, retinoic acid receptor–related orphan receptor-α (ROR-α)–expressing Tregs (Malhotra et al., 2018) and IRF4-expressing Tregs (Noval & Chatila, 2016) in skin were shown to be important in regulating type 2 immune responses. Finally, dysregulation of Tregs functions has been suggested in AD. The frequency of Tregs is elevated in both mouse models and human patients and correlates with AD severity, indicating that Tregs in AD are unable to appropriately downregulate the ongoing inflammatory response (Roesner et al., 2015).

Autoreactive T cells

Recently, the pathologic role of autoreactive T cells in AD has been suggested (Balaji et al., 2011; Boehncke & Brembilla, 2019; Tang, Bieber, & Williams, 2012). Although at low frequencies (1–10 in 10^6 T cells), harmful autoreactive T cells that escaped central tolerance in thymus are detectable in the peripheral T-cell pool (Yu et al., 2015). Their response is normally suppressed via multiple mechanisms, including anergy, ignorance, and suppression by Tregs (Mueller, 2010). However, a combination of genetic and environmental factors may trigger their inappropriate activation, resulting in autoimmune responses (Rosenblum, Remedio, & Abbas, 2015). In fact, autoreactivity has been known in inflammatory skin diseases, including AD, but the role of autoreactive T cells differs among diseases (Boehncke & Brembilla, 2019). In the case of vitiligo, autoreactive T cells are directly involved as effector T cells by attacking the target in skin or as memory cells (i.e., tissue resident memory T cells [T_{RM}]) that are thought to be responsible for relapsing disease. In pemphigus and pemphigoid, autoreactive T cells help B cells to produce pathogenic autoantibodies to cause skin damage. Autoreactive T cells in AD have both functions. The presence of autoreactive IgE antibodies is seen in about 30% of the AD patients (Tang et al., 2012). Several IgE-binding keratinocyte-associated antigens show homology with environmental antigens, indicating that molecular mimicry may be a mechanism of autoantibody production in skin diseases (Zeller et al., 2009). Also, IFN-γ and IL4 secreting effector CD8$^+$ T cells specific to Hom s 2, the α-chain of the nascent polypeptide-associated complex (α-NAC), are found at higher numbers in AD patients compared to non-AD controls (Roesner et al., 2016).

Mast cells

Mast cells are long-lived, tissue-resident cells with one nucleolus and many granules. Mast cells express tetrameric αβγ2 form of the high-affinity IgE receptor FcεRI on the cell surface. Degranulated mast cells are observed in lesional skin of patients with acute AD. Moreover, the number of the degranulated cells is often increased in chronic AD, suggesting that IgE-mediated pathology may be a driving force of AD (Liu, Goodarzi, & Chen, 2011). The association of allergen with IgE bound to FcεRI triggers degranulation and activation of mast cell degranulation and activation. Mast cell degranulation is characterized by the release of bioactive chemical mediators (e.g., histamine, serotonin, substance P, and heparin) and mast cell–specific proteases (e.g., tryptases, chymases, and matrix metalloproteases, in particular 1 and 4) (Galli & Tsai, 2012). In addition, activated mast cells release de novo synthesized proinflammatory lipid mediators (e.g., prostaglandin D2, leukotriene C4, leukotriene B4, and platelet-activating factor). These mast cell–derived components cause itching, redness, tissue damage, and skin dryness in AD patients (Liu et al., 2011). Given the fact that histamine levels are also highly elevated in inflamed skin, it is likely that histamine plays a relevant role in disease pathology. However, antagonists that block histamine H$_1$ or H$_2$ receptors are largely ineffective in reducing chronic symptoms in AD. Recent clinical studies have reported that H$_4$ receptor antagonists display antipruritic and antiinflammatory effects and might be a novel therapeutic option in AD treatment (Schaper-Gerhardt et al., 2018).

FcεRI-engaged mast cells also produce a large variety of (i) cytokines, including interleukins (IL1β, IL3, IL4, IL5, IL6, IL8, IL9, IL10, IL11, IL12, IL13, IL15, IL16, IL18, IL22, IL25, and IL33), TNF-α, TGF-β, and GM-CSF; (ii) growth factors, including fibroblast growth factor 2, vascular endothelial growth factor, and nerve growth factor; and (iii) CC and CXC chemokines, including CCL2 (monocyte chemotactic protein 1) and CCL3 (macrophage inflammatory protein-1α) (Mukai, Tsai, Saito, & Galli, 2018). Mast cell–derived cytokines and chemokines cause activation and trafficking of inflammatory cells such as eosinophils and Th2 cells into the AD sites.

In addition to FcεRI, mast cells express various types of receptors, including pattern recognition receptors (e.g., TLRs), complement receptors, cytokine receptors, and immunoglobulin receptors, all of which are involved in the activation of mast cells (Redegeld, Yu, Kumari, Charles, & Blank, 2018). In the inflamed skin of patients with chronic AD, S. aureus superficially colonizes and activates mast cells via TLR2 and TLR4 (Nakamura et al., 2013; Redegeld et al., 2018). IL33, an alarmin cytokine released upon epithelial barrier disruption (e.g., by allergens with protease activity, granule components released by mast cells and granulocytes, and other stimuli in allergic condition), activates mast cells via ST2 receptor (Olivera, Beaven, & Metcalfe, 2018). Such TLR or ST2 receptor engagement augments FcεRI-mediated mast cell degranulation, induces cytokine/chemokine production even in the absence of IgE stimulation, and promotes inflammation.

Basophils

Basophils principally circulate in peripheral blood and represent less than 1% of circulating leukocytes under homeostatic conditions. Like mast cells, basophils have many granules and express FcεRI on their cell surface. Their granules contain chemical mediators (e.g., histamine, chondroitin sulfate, and substance P) and other basophil-specific proteins (e.g., basogranulin). FcεRI engagement triggers degranulation, de novo synthesis of lipid mediators (e.g., leukotriene C4 and platelet-activating factor), and production of cytokines and chemokines in the cells (Schwartz, Eberle, & Voehringer, 2016). In comparison to mast cells, basophils produce a limited variety of lipid mediators, cytokines, and chemokines (Varricchi, Raap, Rivellese, Marone, & Gibbs, 2018). Although basophils have recently been implicated in the pathogenesis of murine AD-like disease, their precise role in human disease remains to be further elucidated.

Basophils produce high amounts of IL4 and are considered initiators and accessory cells for the Th2 cell polarization in AD (Siracusa, Kim, Spergel, & Artis, 2013). Recent studies have shown that basophil-derived IL4 promotes IL5 and IL13 secretion by ILC2, leading to eosinophilia in a murine model of AD (Kim et al., 2014). (Detailed discussion of ILC2 is in the last section of this chapter.) Increased levels of basophils, ILC2, and/or Th2 cells in skin of AD patients has also been observed (Mashiko, Mehta, Bissonnette, & Sarfati, 2017). In addition, basophils proliferate and migrate into tissues to promote type 2 immune responses upon stimulation with TSLP, a key cytokine released by keratinocytes involved in the pathogenesis of AD (Siracusa et al., 2011). However, basophil-deficient mice showed only modest attenuation in the development of AD-like inflammation (Siracusa et al., 2013); this observation might be attributed to a limited variety of cytokine/chemokine production and a short lifespan of the cells. Mast cells have a long lifespan of 20 to 30 days, whereas basophils have a lifespan of only 2 to 3 days. Moreover, IgE is a survival factor for mast cells but not for basophils (Varricchi et al., 2018). Therefore the contribution of IgE- and/or TSLP-activated basophils to the pathogenesis of AD still needs to be elucidated.

Eosinophils

Eosinophils represent 1% to 6% of circulating leukocytes in blood and do not migrate to the skin under normal physiologic conditions. However, increased blood and tissue eosinophilia are often associated with disease severity of AD (Simon, Braathen, & Simon, 2004). Eosinophil degranulation and deposits of granular proteins in lesional skin of AD patients have been observed (Simon et al., 2004). Secretory granules of eosinophils contain mainly five cytotoxic proteins, including the eosinophil major basic protein, eosinophil-cationic protein (ECP), eosinophil protein X (EPX), eosinophil-derived neurotoxin (EDN), and eosinophil peroxidase (EPO). These cytotoxic proteins are implicated in cytotoxicity, tissue damage, and mediation of AD since several studies showed that their levels in sera and urine samples correlate with disease progression in AD patients (Liu et al., 2011).

Cytokines and chemokines that are involved in the development of skin eosinophilia include IL3, IL5, IL13, IL33, GM-CSF, CCL11 (eotaxin-1), CCL24 (eotaxin-2), and CCL26 (eotaxin-3) (Chan, Lam, Tam, & Wong, 2019; Rothenberg & Hogan, 2006). Increased expression of IL5, IL13, IL33, CCL11, CCL24, and/or CCL26 in lesional skin of AD patients has been reported. Among the chemoattractants, IL5 exhibits the most potent eosinophil-specific properties to induce maturation, migration, activation (that leads to release of granules), proliferation, and survival of the cells. Several studies have shown the association of IL5 expression levels with eosinophilia in lesional skin (Liu et al., 2011). However, two single doses of 750 mg mepolizumab,

an antibody against IL5, did not meet clinical expectations in a short-term pilot study in patients with modest to severe AD, although a significant decrease of blood eosinophils was reached (Brunner et al., 2017; Oldhoff et al., 2005). These data trigger the debate whether eosinophils could serve as therapeutic targets for treatment of AD. To address the long-term risk:benefit ratio of mepolizumab, new studies have been undertaken in a subset of patients with modest to severe AD and increased eosinophil counts (Kang et al., 2019).

ILC2

ILCs are the most recently identified immune lymphoid cells that are phenotypically similar to Th subsets but lacking T- or B-cell receptors (Spits et al., 2013). There are three main subsets of ILCs: ILC1, ILC2, and ILC3, which produce IFN-γ, IL5/IL9/IL13, and IL17A/IL22, respectively. These ILC subsets are considered to mirror the profile of cytokine production of Th1, Th2, and Th17 cells. Although ILC population is rare, the cells are capable of producing significantly higher amounts of cytokines than T cells. Evidence has suggested that ILC2 plays a crucial role in the development of AD by producing IL5, IL9, and IL13. The levels of ILC2 are increased in lesional skin, but not in peripheral blood, of adult AD patients, when compared to healthy subjects and patients with psoriasis (Salimi et al., 2013).

ILC2 expands and produces cytokines upon stimulation with IL25, IL33, and TSLP individually, or in combination (Roediger, Kyle, Le Gros, & Weninger, 2014). These cytokines are alarmin cytokines released by damaged epithelial cells and keratinocytes in AD condition. Increased numbers of ILC2 were associated with expression levels of IL25, IL33, and TSLP in the AD tissues (Salimi et al., 2013). IL25- and IL33-induced cytokine production of ILC2 is augmented by prostaglandin D2 and leukotriene E4 derived from mast cells. IL4 derived from basophils also promotes the cytokine production of ILC2 (Salimi, Stöger, & Liu, 2017; Xue et al., 2014).

The depletion of murine ILCs significantly ameliorates skin inflammation in a model of AD-like inflammation, suggesting that ILC2 plays an essential role in promoting skin inflammation (Imai et al., 2019). The potential of ILC2 to produce IL5 and IL13 implies a role in induction of eosinophilia, barrier dysfunction, and causing an itching sensation in AD. ILC2 is also a key source of IL9, a mast cell growth factor, suggesting that these cells may affect disease severity by regulating mast cell number and/or function in the skin. Live imaging studies showed a proximity of dermal ILC2 with skin-resident mast cells in mice (Roediger et al., 2013). However, the majority of studies investigating the functions of this cell population have been based on murine models. Detailed characterization of ILC2 in lesional tissues of AD patients is essential to deepen our insights into pathologic mechanisms of AD and to establish a novel strategy for AD treatment.

Summary

AD was initially recognized as a Th2-driven skin inflammatory disease. However, accumulating studies have revealed that AD is a more complex and heterogeneous disease with several subtypes, involving multiple CD4$^+$ T-cell subsets (e.g., Th1, Th2, Th17, and Th22), APCs (e.g., DCs, LCs, and B cells), innate inflammatory cells, keratinocytes, and possibly neuronal cells for pruritus. Several classes of newly identified cells exist, of which roles need to be clarified. For example, the relevance of Tfh cells in AD needs to be addressed in relationship to IgE production. The presence of autoreactive T cells in AD patients raises a possibility that AD is associated with autoimmune diseases. ILCs, which have been identified in mice, need to be characterized in AD patients. It is also crucial to identify T-cell phenotypes in pediatric AD since they appear to be different from those in adult patients. Current advances in technologies, such as the single cell sequencing approach, may further allow characterization of key cellular components in AD patients and relevant mouse models, which would improve the understanding of the pathophysiology of AD. In the meantime, a large-scale transcriptome analysis and machine-learning data mining may help identify essential signaling pathways shared among multiple cell types in AD as therapeutic targets.

Further readings

Brunner. P. M. (2019). Early immunologic changes during the onset of atopic dermatitis. *Annals of Allergy, Asthma & Immunology, 123*, 152–157. Author note: One of the most important aspects in AD treatment is to intervene the onset and development in infants and young children by controlling emergence of sensitization and skin inflammation at the earliest time point. This review discusses the necessity of a detailed profiling of early-onset AD, including immunologic characterization to establish prophylactic and therapeutic strategies of AD treatment.

Brunner, P. M., Guttman-Yassky, E., & Leung, D. Y. (2017). The immunology of atopic dermatitis and its reversibility with broad-spectrum and targeted therapies. *Journal of Allergy and Clinical Immunology, 139*, S65–S76. Author note: Since AD is a heterogeneous disease with several subtypes, where multiple T-cell subsets and inflammatory cells are involved, a more personalized approach to AD treatment has been anticipated. This review discusses the immune pathway of AD progression that would lead to personalized treatment of patients.

Kennedy, K., Heimall, J., & Spergel, J. M. (2018). Advances in atopic dermatitis in 2017. *Journal of Allergy and Clinical Immunology, 142*, 1740–1747. Author note: *Journal of Allergy and Clinical Immunology*, the top-ranking journal in the allergy category, annually releases review articles about AD. It encompasses relevant scientific and clinical advances in AD.

Lunjani, N., Hlela, C., & O'Mahony, L. (2019). Microbiome and skin biology. *Current Opinion in Allergy and Clinical Immunology, 19*, 328–333. Author note: Microbial dysbiosis has been observed in the skin and gut of AD patients. The role of specific microbes in the development of AD has been intensively investigated. This review discusses the association of altered microbiome-host interaction and immune dysfunction in AD and potential strategies of disease treatment.

Weidinger, S., Beck, L. A., Bieber, T., Kabashima, K., & Irvine, A. D. (2018). Atopic dermatitis. *Nature Reviews Disease Primers, 4*, 1. Author note: This article offers a global overview of the epidemiology, immunologic aspects, clinical features, and translational research of AD.

References

Alcántara-Hernández, M., Leylek, R., Wagar, L. E., Engleman, E. G., Keler, T., Marinkovich, P. M., et al. (2017). High-dimensional phenotypic mapping of human dendritic cells reveals interindividual variation and tissue specialization. *Immunity, 47*(6). https://doi.org/10.1016/j.immuni.2017.11.001. 1037-1050.E6.

Ali, N., & Rosenblum, M. D. (2017). Regulatory T cells in skin. *Immunology, 152*(3), 372–381. https://doi.org/10.1111/imm.12791.

Balaji, H., Heratizadeh, A., Wichmann, K., Niebuhr, M., Crameri, R., Scheynius, A., & Werfel, T. (2011). *Malassezia Sympodialis* thioredoxin-specific T cells are highly cross-reactive to human thioredoxin in atopic dermatitis. *The Journal of Allergy and Clinical Immunology, 128*(1). https://doi.org/10.1016/j.jaci.2011.02.043. 92-99.E4.

Biedermann, T., Zimmermann, S., Himmelrich, H., Gumy, A., Egeter, O., Sakrauski, A. K., et al. (2001). IL-4 instructs TH1 responses and resistance to *Leishmania major* in susceptible BALB/c mice. *Nature Immunology, 2*(11), 1054–1060. https://doi.org/10.1038/ni725.

Biedermann, T., Skabytska, Y., Kaesler, S., & Volz, T. (2015). Regulation of T cell immunity in atopic dermatitis by microbes: The Yin and Yang of cutaneous inflammation. *Frontiers in Immunology, 6*, 353. https://doi.org/10.3389/fimmu.2015.00353.

Boehncke, W.-H., & Brembilla, N. C. (2019). Autoreactive T-lymphocytes in inflammatory skin diseases. *Frontiers in Immunology, 10*, 1198. https://doi.org/10.3389/fimmu.2019.01198.

Brown, G. D., Willment, J. A., & Whitehead, L. (2018). C-type lectins in immunity and homeostasis. *Nature Reviews Immunology, 18*(6), 374–389. https://doi.org/10.1038/s41577-018-0004-8.

Brunner, P. M., Guttman-Yassky, E., & Leung, D. Y. (2017). The immunology of atopic dermatitis and its reversibility with broad-spectrum and targeted therapies. *The Journal of Allergy and Clinical Immunology, 139*(4S), S65–S76. https://doi.org/10.1016/j.jaci.2017.01.011.

Brunner, P. M., Israel, A., Zhang, N., Leonard, A., Wen, H.-C., Huynh, T., et al. (2018). Early-onset pediatric atopic dermatitis is characterized by T(H)2/T(H)17/T(H)22-centered inflammation and lipid alterations. *The Journal of Allergy and Clinical Immunology, 141*(6), 2094–2106. https://doi.org/10.1016/j.jaci.2018.02.040.

Bruynzeel-Koomen, C., van Wichen, D. F., Toonstra, J., Berrens, L., & Bruynzeel, P. L. (1986). The presence of IgE molecules on epidermal Langerhans cells in patients with atopic dermatitis. *Archives of Dermatological Research, 278*(3), 199–205. https://doi.org/10.1007/BF00412924.

Chan, B. C. L., Lam, C. W. K., Tam, L.-S., & Wong, C. K. (2019). IL33: Roles in allergic inflammation and therapeutic perspectives. *Frontiers in Immunology, 10*, 364. https://doi.org/10.3389/fimmu.2019.00364.

Chan, L. S., Robinson, N., & Xu, L. (2001). Expression of interleukin-4 in the epidermis of transgenic mice results in a pruritic inflammatory skin disease: An experimental animal model to study atopic dermatitis. *The Journal of Investigative Dermatology, 117*(4), 977–983. https://doi.org/10.1046/j.0022-202x.2001.01484.x.

Cho, S. H., Strickland, I., Boguniewicz, M., & Leung, D. Y. M. (2001). Fibronectin and fibrinogen contribute to the enhanced binding of *Staphylococcus aureus* to atopic skin. *The Journal of Allergy and Clinical Immunology, 108*(2), 269–274. https://doi.org/10.1067/mai.2001.117455.

Cho, S.-H., Strickland, I., Tomkinson, A., Fehringer, A. P., Gelfand, E. W., & Leung, D. Y. M. (2001). Preferential binding of *Staphylococcus aureus* to skin sites of Th2-mediated inflammation in a murine model. *The Journal of Investigative Dermatology, 116*(5), 658–663. https://doi.org/10.1046/j.0022-202x.2001.01331.x.

Crotty. S. (2014). T follicular helper cell differentiation, function, and roles in disease. *Immunity, 41*(4), 529–542. https://doi.org/10.1016/j.immuni.2014.10.004.

Czarnowicki, T., Krueger, J. G., & Guttman-Yassky, E. (2014). Skin barrier and immune dysregulation in atopic dermatitis: an evolving story with important clinical implications. *The Journal of Allergy and Clinical Immunology, 2*(4), 371–379. https://doi.org/10.1016/j.jaip.2014.03.006. quiz 380-1.

Debes, G. F., & McGettigan, S. E. (2019). Skin-associated B cells in health and inflammation. *Journal of Immunology, 202*(6), 1659–1666. https://doi.org/10.4049/jimmunol.1801211.

Deckers, J., Hammad, H., & Hoste, E. (2018). Langerhans cells: Sensing the environment in health and disease. *Frontiers in Immunology, 9*, 93. https://doi.org/10.3389/fimmu.2018.00093.

Doebel, T., Benjamin, V., & Keisuke, N. (2017). Langerhans cells - The macrophage in dendritic cell clothing. *Trends in Immunology, 38*(11), 817–828. https://doi.org/10.1016/j.it.2017.06.008.

Duhen, T., Geiger, R., Jarrossay, D., Lanzavecchia, A., & Sallusto, F. (2009). Production of interleukin 22 but not interleukin 17 by a subset of human skin-homing memory T cells". *Nature Immunology, 10*(8), 857–863. https://doi.org/10.1038/ni.1767.

Esaki, H., Brunner, P. M., Renert-Yuval, Y., Czarnowicki, T., Huynh, T., Tran, G., et al. (2016). Early-onset pediatric atopic dermatitis is T(H)2 but also T(H)17 polarized in skin. *The Journal of Allergy and Clinical Immunology, 138*(6), 1639–1651. https://doi.org/10.1016/j.jaci.2016.07.013.

Eyerich, K., Pennino, D., Scarponi, C., Foerster, S., Nasorri, F., Behrendt, H., et al. (2009). IL-17 in atopic eczema: Linking allergen-specific adaptive and microbial-triggered innate immune response. *The Journal of Allergy and Clinical Immunology, 123*(1). https://doi.org/10.1016/j.jaci.2008.10.031. 59-66.E4.

Eyerich, S., Eyerich, K., Pennino, D., Carbone, T., Nasorri, F., Pallotta, S., et al. (2009). Th22 cells represent a distinct human T cell subset involved in epidermal immunity and remodeling. *The Journal of Clinical Investigation, 119*(12), 3573–3585. https://doi.org/10.1172/JCI40202.

Fuhlbrigge, R. C., Kieffer, D. J., Armerding, D., & Kupper, T. S. (1997). Cutaneous lymphocyte antigen is a specialized form of PSGL-1 expressed on skin-homing T cells. *Nature, 389*(6654), 978–981. https://doi.org/10.1038/40166.

Galli, S. J., & Tsai, M. (2012). IgE and mast cells in allergic disease. *Nature Medicine, 18*(5), 693–704. https://doi.org/10.1038/nm.2755.

Ghigo, C., Mondor, I., Jorquera, A., Nowak, J., Wienert, S., Zahner, S. P., et al. (2013). Multicolor fate mapping of Langerhans cell homeostasis. *The Journal of Experimental Medicine, 210*(9), 1657–1664. https://doi.org/10.1084/jem.20130403.

Ghoreschi, K., Thomas, P., Breit, S., Dugas, M., Mailhammer, R., van Eden, W., et al. (2003). Interleukin-4 therapy of psoriasis induces Th2 responses and improves human autoimmune disease. *Nature Medicine, 9*(1), 40–46. https://doi.org/10.1038/nm804.

Gittler, J. K., Shemer, A., Suárez-Fariñas, M., Fuentes-Duculan, J., Gulewicz, K. J., Wang, C. Q., et al. (2012). Progressive activation of T(H)2/T(H)22 cytokines and selective epidermal proteins characterizes acute and chronic atopic dermatitis. *The Journal of Allergy and Clinical Immunology, 130*(6), 1344–1354. https://doi.org/10.1016/j.jaci.2012.07.012.

Gosselin, D., Link, V. M., Romanoski, C. E., Fonseca, G. J., Eichenfield, D. Z., Spann, N. J., et al. (2014). Environment drives selection and function of enhancers controlling tissue-specific macrophage identities. *Cell, 159*(6), 1327–1340. https://doi.org/10.1016/j.cell.2014.11.023.

Guenova, E., Skabytska, Y., Hoetzenecker, W., Weindl, G., Sauer, K., Tham, M., et al. (2015). IL-4 abrogates T(H)17 cell-mediated inflammation by selective silencing of IL-23 in antigen-presenting cells. *Proceedings of the National Academy of Sciences of the United States America, 112*(7), 2163–2168. https://doi.org/10.1073/pnas.1416922112.

Gutowska-Owsiak, D., Schaupp, A. L., Salimi, M., Taylor, S., & Ogg, G. S. (2011). Interleukin-22 downregulates filaggrin expression and affects expression of profilaggrin processing enzymes. *The British Journal of Dermatology, 165*(3), 492–498. https://doi.org/10.1111/j.1365-2133.2011.10400.x.

Guttman-Yassky, E., Nograles, K. E., & Krueger, J. G. (2011). Contrasting pathogenesis of atopic dermatitis and psoriasis--part II: Immune cell subsets and therapeutic concepts. *The Journal of Allergy and Clinical Immunology, 127*(6), 1420–1432. https://doi.org/10.1016/j.jaci.2011.01.054.

Halabi-Tawil, M., Ruemmele, F. M., Fraitag, S., Rieux-Laucat, F., Neven, B., Brousse, N., et al. (2009). Cutaneous manifestations of immune dysregulation, polyendocrinopathy, enteropathy, X-linked (IPEX) syndrome. *The British Journal of Dermatology, 160*(3), 645–651. https://doi.org/10.1111/j.1365-2133.2008.08835.x.

Harrington, L. E., Hatton, R. D., Mangan, P. R., Turner, H., Murphy, T. L., Murphy, K. M., & Weaver, C. T. (2005). Interleukin 17-producing CD4+ effector T cells develop via a lineage distinct from the T helper type 1 and 2 lineages. *Nature Immunology, 6*(11), 1123–1132. https://doi.org/10.1038/ni1254.

Hirahara, K., Liu, L., Clark, R. A., Yamanaka, K., Fuhlbrigge, R. C., & Kupper, T. S. (2006). The majority of human peripheral blood CD4+CD25highFoxp3+ regulatory T cells bear functional skin-homing receptors. *Journal of Immunology, 177*(7), 4488–4494. https://doi.org/10.4049/jimmunol.177.7.4488.

Howell, M. D., Gallo, R. L., Boguniewicz, M., Jones, J. F., Wong, C., Streib, J. E., & Leung, D. Y. M. (2006). Cytokine milieu of atopic dermatitis skin subverts the innate immune response to vaccinia virus. *Immunity, 24*(3), 341–348. https://doi.org/10.1016/j.immuni.2006.02.006.

Imai, Y., Yasuda, K., Nagai, M., Kusakabe, M., Kubo, M., Nakanishi, K., & Yamanishi, K. (2019). IL-33-induced atopic dermatitis-like inflammation in mice is mediated by Group 2 innate lymphoid cells in concert with basophils. *The Journal of Investigative Dermatology, 139*(10), 2185–2194. https://doi.org/10.1016/j.jid.2019.04.016.

Ito, T., Wang, Y.-H., Duramad, O., Hori, T., Delespesse, G. J., Watanabe, N., et al. (2005). TSLP-activated dendritic cells induce an inflammatory T helper type 2 cell response through OX40 ligand. *The Journal of Experimental Medicine, 202*(9), 1213–1223. https://doi.org/10.1084/jem.20051135.

Kalekar, L. A., Cohen, J. N., Prevel, N., Sandoval, P. M., Mathur, A. N., Moreau, J. M., et al. (2019). Regulatory T cells in skin are uniquely poised to suppress profibrotic immune responses. *Science Immunology, 4*(39), eaaw2910. https://doi.org/10.1126/sciimmunol.aaw2910.

Kalekar, L. A., & Rosenblum, M. D. (2019). Regulatory T cells in inflammatory skin disease: From mice to humans. *International*

Immunology, *31*(7), 457–463. https://doi.org/10.1093/intimm/dxz020.

Kang, E. G., Narayana, P. K., Pouliquen, I. J., Lopez, M. C., Celeste-Ferreira-Cornwell, M., & Getsy, J. A. (2019). Efficacy and safety of mepolizumab administered subcutaneously for moderate to severe atopic dermatitis. *Allergy*, *75*(4), 950–953. https://doi.org/10.1111/all.14050.

Kaplan, D. H., Li, M. O., Jenison, M. C., Shlomchik, W. D., Flavell, R. A., & Shlomchik, M. J. (2007). Autocrine/paracrine TGFbeta1 is required for the development of epidermal Langerhans cells. *The Journal of Experimental Medicine*, *204*(11), 2545–2552. https://doi.org/10.1084/jem.20071401.

Kashem, S. W., Haniffa, M., & Kaplan, D. H. (2017). Antigen-presenting cells in the skin. *Annual Review of Immunology*, *35*, 469–499. https://doi.org/10.1146/annurev-immunol-051116-052215.

Klein, L., Kyewski, B., Allen, P. M., & Hogquist, K. A. (2014). Positive and negative selection of the T cell repertoire: What thymocytes see (and don't see). *Nature Reviews Immunology*, *14*(6), 377–391. https://doi.org/10.1038/nri3667.

Kim, B. S., Wang, K., Siracusa, M. C., Saenz, S. A., Brestoff, J. R., Monticelli, L. A., et al. (2014). Basophils promote innate lymphoid cell responses in inflamed skin. *Journal of Immunology*, *193*(7), 3717–3725. https://doi.org/10.4049/jimmunol.1401307.

Kobayashi, T., Glatz, M., Horiuchi, K., Kawasaki, H., Akiyama, H., Kaplan, D. H., et al. (2015). Dysbiosis and staphylococcus aureus colonization drives inflammation in atopic dermatitis. *Immunity*, *42*(4), 756–766. https://doi.org/10.1016/j.immuni.2015.03.014.

Kubo. M. (2017). T follicular helper and T(H)2 cells in allergic responses. *Allergology International: Official Journal of the Japanese Society of Allergology*, *66*(3), 377–381. https://doi.org/10.1016/j.alit.2017.04.006.

Leitch, C. S., Natafji, E., Yu, C., Abdul-Ghaffar, S., Madarasingha, N., Venables, Z. C., et al. (2016). Filaggrin-null mutations are associated with increased maturation markers on Langerhans cells. *The Journal of Allergy and Clinical Immunology*, *138*(2). https://doi.org/10.1016/j.jaci.2015.11.040. 482-490.E7.

Leung, D. Y., & Bieber, T. (2003). Atopic dermatitis. *Lancet*, *361*(9352), 151–160. https://doi.org/10.1016/S0140-6736(03)12193-9.

Liu, F.-T., Goodarzi, H., & Chen, H.-Y. (2011). IgE, mast cells, and eosinophils in atopic dermatitis. *Clinical Reviews in Allergy and Immunology*, *41*, 298–310. https://doi.org/10.1007/s12016-011-8252-4.

Liu. Y.-J. (2006). Thymic stromal lymphopoietin: master switch for allergic inflammation. *The Journal of Experimental Medicine*, *203*(2), 269–273. https://doi.org/10.1084/jem.20051745.

Malhotra, N., Leyva-Castillo, J. M., Jadhav, U., Barreiro, O., Kam, C., O'Neill, N. K., et al. (2018). RORα-expressing T regulatory cells restrain allergic skin inflammation. *Sci Immunol*, *3*(21). https://doi.org/10.1126/sciimmunol.aao6923. aao6923.

Malhotra, N., Yoon, J., Leyva-Castillo, J. M., Galand, C., Archer, N., Miller, L. S., & Geha, R. S. (2016). IL-22 derived from γδ T cells restricts *Staphylococcus aureus* infection of mechanically injured skin. *The Journal of Allergy and Clinical Immunology*, *138*(4). https://doi.org/10.1016/j.jaci.2016.07.001. 1098-1107.E3.

Mashiko, S., Mehta, H., Bissonnette, R., & Sarfati, M. (2017). Increased frequencies of basophils, type 2 innate lymphoid cells and Th2 cells in skin of patients with atopic dermatitis but not psoriasis. *Journal of Dermatological Science*, *88*(2), 167–174. https://doi.org/10.1016/j.jdermsci.2017.07.003.

Matthias, J., Maul, J., Noste, R., Meinl, H., Chao, Y. -Y., Gerstenberg, H., et al. (2019). Sodium chloride is an ionic checkpoint for human T(H)2 cells and shapes the atopic skin microenvironment. *Science Translational Medicine*, *11*(480). https://doi.org/10.1126/scitranslmed.aau0683. aau0683.

Mueller. D. L. (2010). Mechanisms maintaining peripheral tolerance. *Nature Immunology*, *11*(1), 21–27. https://doi.org/10.1038/ni.1817.

Mukai, K., Tsai, M., Saito, H., & Galli, S. J. (2018). Mast cells as sources of cytokines, chemokines and growth factors. *Immunological Reviews*, *282*(1), 121–150. https://doi.org/10.1111/imr.12634.

Nakamura, Y., Oscherwitz, J., Cease, K. B., Chan, S. M., Muñoz-Planillo, R., Hasegawa, M., et al. (2013). Staphylococcus δ-toxin induces allergic skin disease by activating mast cells. *Nature*, *503*(7476), 397–401. https://doi.org/10.1038/nature12655.

Nograles, K. E., Zaba, L. C., Shemer, A., Fuentes-Duculan, J., Cardinale, I., Kikuchi, T., et al. (2009). IL-22-producing "T22" T cells account for upregulated IL-22 in atopic dermatitis despite reduced IL-17-producing TH17 T cells. *The Journal of Allergy and Clinical Immunology*, *123*(6). https://doi.org/10.1016/j.jaci.2009.03.041. 1244-52.E2.

Nomura, I., Goleva, E., Howell, M. D., Hamid, Q. A., Ong, P. Y., Hall, C. F., et al. (2003). Cytokine milieu of atopic dermatitis, as compared to psoriasis, skin prevents induction of innate immune response genes. *Journal of Immunology*, *171*(6), 3262–3269. https://doi.org/10.4049/jimmunol.171.6.3262.

Novak, N., & Bieber, T. (2003). Allergic and nonallergic forms of atopic diseases. *The Journal of Allergy and Clinical Immunology*, *112*(2), 252–262. https://doi.org/10.1067/mai.2003.1595.

Noval, M. R., & Chatila, T. A. (2016). Regulatory T cells in allergic diseases. *The Journal of Allergy and Clinical Immunology*, *138*(3), 639–652. https://doi.org/10.1016/j.jaci.2016.06.003.

O'Connor, W., Jr, Zenewic, L. A., & Flavell, R. A. (2010). The dual nature of T(H)17 cells: Shifting the focus to function. *Nature Immunology*, *11*(6), 471–476. https://doi.org/10.1038/ni.1882.

Oetjen, L. K., Mack, M. R., Feng, J., Whelan, T. M., Niu, H., Guo, C. J., et al. (2017). Sensory neurons co-opt classical immune signaling pathways to mediate chronic itch. *Cell*, *171*(1). https://doi.org/10.1016/j.cell.2017.08.006. 217-228.E13.

Oldhoff, J. M., Daesow, U., Werfel, T., Katzer, K., Wulf, A., Laifaoui, J., Hijnen, D.J., et al. (2005). Anti-IL-5 recombinant humanized monoclonal antibody (mepolizumab) for the treatment of atopic dermatitis. *Allergy*, *60*(5), 693–696. https://doi.org/10.1111/j.1398-9995.2005.00791.x.

Oliva, M., Renert-Yuval, Y., & Guttman-Yassky, E. (2016). The 'omics' revolution: Redefining the understanding and treatment of allergic skin diseases. *Current Opinion in Allergy and Clinical Immunology*, *16*(5), 469–476. https://doi.org/10.1097/ACI.0000000000000306.

Olivera, A., Beaven, M. A., & Metcalfe, D. D. (2018). Mast cells signal their importance in health and disease. *The Journal of Allergy and Clinical Immunology*, *142*(2), 381–393. https://doi.org/10.1016/j.jaci.2018.01.034.

Ong, P. Y., Ohtake, T., Brandt, C., Strickland, I., Boguniewicz, M., Ganz, T., et al. (2002). Endogenous antimicrobial peptides and skin infections in atopic dermatitis. *The New England Journal of Medicine*, *347*(15), 1151–1160. https://doi.org/10.1056/NEJMoa021481.

Orfali, R. L., da Silva Oliveira, L. M., de Lima, J. F., de Carvalho, G. C., Ramos, Y. A. L., Pereira, N. Z., et al. (2018). *Staphylococcus aureus* enterotoxins modulate IL-22-secreting cells in adults with atopic dermatitis. *Scientific Reports*, *8*, 6665. https://doi.org/10.1038/s41598-018-25125-0.

Panduro, M., Benoist, C., & Mathis, D. (2016). Tissue Tregs. *Annual Review of Immunology, 34,* 609–633. https://doi.org/10.1146/annurev-immunol-032712-095948.

Pattarini, L., Trichot, C., Bogiatzi, S., Grandclaudon, M., Meller, S., Keuylian, Z., et al. (2017). TSLP-activated dendritic cells induce human T follicular helper cell differentiation through OX40-ligand. *The Journal of Experimental Medicine, 214*(5), 1529–1546. https://doi.org/10.1084/jem.20150402.

Redegeld, F. A., Yu, Y., Kumari, S., Charles, N., & Blank, U. (2018). Non-IgE mediated mast cell activation. *Immunological Reviews, 282*(1), 87–113. https://doi.org/10.1111/imr.12629.

Roediger, B., Kyle, R., Le Gros, G., & Weninger, W. (2014). Dermal group 2 innate lymphoid cells in atopic dermatitis and allergy. *Current Opinion in Immunology, 31,* 108–114. https://doi.org/10.1016/j.coi.2014.10.008.

Roediger, B., Kyle, R., Yip, K. H., Sumaria, N., Guy, T. V., Kim, B. S., et al. (2013). Cutaneous immunosurveillance and regulation of inflammation by group 2 innate lymphoid cells. *Nature Immunology, 14*(6), 564–573. https://doi.org/10.1038/ni.2584.

Roesner, L. M., Floess, S., Witte, T., Olek, S., Huehn, J., & Werfel, T. (2015). Foxp3+ regulatory T cells are expanded in severe atopic dermatitis patients. *Allergy, 70*(12), 1656–1660. https://doi.org/10.1111/all.12712.

Roesner, L. M., Heratizadeh, A., Wieschowski, S., Mittermann, I., Valenta, R., Eiz-Vesper, B., et al. (2016). α-NAC-specific autoreactive CD8+ T cells in atopic dermatitis are of an effector memory type and secrete IL-4 and IFN-γ. *The Journal of Immunology, 196*(8), 3245–3252. https://doi.org/10.4049/jimmunol.1500351.

Rodriguez, R. S., Pauli, M. L., Neuhaus, I. M., Yu, S. S., Arron, S. T., Harris, H. W., et al. (2014). Memory regulatory T cells reside in human skin. *The Journal of Clinical Investigation, 124*(3), 1027–1036. https://doi.org/10.1172/JCI72932.

Rosenblum, M. D., Remedio, K. A., & Abbas, A. K. (2015). Mechanisms of human autoimmunity. *The Journal of Clinical Investigation, 125*(6), 2228–2233. https://doi.org/10.1172/JCI78088.

Rothenberg, M. E., & Hogan, S. P. (2006). The eosinophil. *Annual Review of Immunology, 24,* 147–174. https://doi.org/10.1146/annurev.immunol.24.021605.090720.

Salimi, M., Barlow, J. L., Saunders, S. P., Xue, L., Gutowska-Owsiak, D., Wang, X., et al. (2013). A role for IL-25 and IL-33-driven type-2 innate lymphoid cells in atopic dermatitis. *The Journal of Experimental Medicine, 210*(13), 2939–2950. https://doi.org/10.1084/jem.20130351.

Salimi, M., Stöger, L., Liu, W., Go, S., Pavord, I., Klenerman, P., et al. (2017). Cysteinyl leukotriene E4 activates human group 2 innate lymphoid cells and enhances the effect of prostaglandin D2 and epithelial cytokines. *The Journal of Allergy and Clinical Immunology, 140*(4). https://doi.org/10.1016/j.jaci.2016.12.958. 1090-1100.E11.

Schaper-Gerhardt, K., Rossbach, K., Nikolouli, E., Werfel, T., Gutzmer, R., & Mommert, S. (2018). The role of the histamine H4 receptor in atopic dermatitis and psoriasis. *British Journal of Pharmacology, 177*(3), 465–712. https://doi.org/10.1111/bph.14550.

Schuller, E., Teichmann, B., Haberstok, J., Moderer, M., Bieber, T., & Wollenberg, A. (2001). In situ expression of the costimulatory molecules CD80 and CD86 on langerhans cells and inflammatory dendritic epidermal cells (IDEC) in atopic dermatitis. *Archives of Dermatological Research, 293*(9), 448–454. https://doi.org/10.1007/s004030100263.

Schwartz, C., Eberle, J. U., & Voehringer, D. (2016). Basophils in inflammation. *European Journal of Pharmacology, 778,* 90–95. https://doi.org/10.1016/j.ejphar.2015.04.049.

Shen, P., & Fillatreau, S. (2015). Antibody-independent functions of B cells: A focus on cytokines. *Nature Reviews Immunology, 15*(7), 441–451. https://doi.org/10.1038/nri3857.

Simon, D., Braathen, L. R., & Simon, H. U. (2004). Eosinophils and atopic dermatitis. *Allergy, 59*(6), 561–570. https://doi.org/10.1111/j.1398-9995.2004.00476.x.

Siracusa, M. C., Kim, B. S., Spergel, J. M., & Artis, D. (2013). Basophils and allergic inflammation. *The Journal of Allergy and Clinical Immunology, 132*(4), 789–801. https://doi.org/10.1016/j.jaci.2013.07.046.

Siracusa, M. C., Saenz, S. A., Hill, D. A., Kim, B. S., Headley, M. B., Doering, T. A., et al. (2011). TSLP promotes interleukin-3-independent basophil haematopoiesis and type 2 inflammation. *Nature, 477,* 229–233. https://doi.org/10.1038/nature10329.

Soumelis, V., Reche, P. A., Kanzler, H., Yuan, W., Edward, G., Homey, B., et al. (2002). Human epithelial cells trigger dendritic cell mediated allergic inflammation by producing TSLP. *Nature Immunology, 3*(7), 673–680. https://doi.org/10.1038/ni805.

Spits, H., Artis, D., Colonna, M., Diefenbach, A., Di Santo, J. P., Eberl, G., et al. (2013). Innate lymphoid cells—A proposal for uniform nomenclature. *Nature Reviews Immunology, 13*(2), 145–149. https://doi.org/10.1038/nri3365.

Szabó, K., Gáspár, K., Dajnoki, Z., Papp, G., Fábos, B., Szegedi, A., & Zeher, M. (2017). Expansion of circulating follicular T helper cells associates with disease severity in childhood atopic dermatitis. *Immunology Letters, 189,* 101–108. https://doi.org/10.1016/j.imlet.2017.04.010.

Tang, T. S., Bieber, T., & Williams, H. C. (2012). Does "autoreactivity" play a role in atopic dermatitis? *The Journal of Allergy and Clinical Immunology, 129*(5). https://doi.org/10.1016/j.jaci.2012.02.002. 1209-1215.E2.

Tangye, S. G., Ma, C. S., Brink, R., & Deenick, E. K. (2013). The good, the bad and the ugly – TFH cells in human health and disease. *Nature Reviews Immunology, 13*(6), 412–426. https://doi.org/10.1038/nri3447.

Trautmann, A., Akdis, M., Bröcker, E. B., Blaser, K., & Akdis, C. A. (2001). New insights into the role of T cells in atopic dermatitis and allergic contact dermatitis. *Trends in Immunology, 22*(10), 530–532. https://doi.org/10.1016/s1471-4906(01)02004-x.

Travers. J. B. (2014). Toxic interaction between Th2 cytokines and *Staphylococcus aureus* in atopic dermatitis. *The Journal of Investigative Dermatology, 134*(8), 2069–2071. https://doi.org/10.1038/jid.2014.122.

Trifari, S., Kaplan, C. D., Tran, E. H., Crellin, N. K., & Spits, H. (2009). Identification of a human helper T cell population that has abundant production of interleukin 22 and is distinct from T(H)-17, T(H)1 and T(H)2 cells. *Nature Immunology, 10*(8), 864–871. https://doi.org/10.1038/ni.1770.

Toda, M., Leung, D. Y., Molet, S., Boguniewicz, M., Taha, R., Christodoulopoulos, P., et al. (2003). Polarized in vivo expression of IL-11 and IL-17 between acute and chronic skin lesions. *The Journal of Allergy and Clinical Immunology, 111*(4), 875–881. https://doi.org/10.1067/mai.2003.1414.

Van Gool, F., Nguyen, M. L. T., Mumbach, M. R., Satpathy, A. T., Rosenthal, W. L., Giacometti, S., et al. (2019). A mutation in the transcription factor Foxp3 drives T helper 2 effector function in regulatory T cells. *Immunity, 50*(2). https://doi.org/10.1016/j.immuni.2018.12.016. 362-377.E6.

Varricchi, G., Raap, U., Rivellese, F., Marone, G., & Gibbs, B. F. (2018). Human mast cells and basophils—How are they similar how are they different? *Immunological Reviews, 282*(1), 8–34. https://doi.org/10.1111/imr.12627.

Volz, T., Nega, M., Buschmann, J., Kaesler, S., Guenova, E., Peschel, A., et al. (2010). Natural *Staphylococcus aureus*-derived peptidoglycan fragments activate NOD2 and act as potent costimulators of the innate immune system exclusively in the presence of TLR signals. *The FASEB Journal: Official Publication of the Federation of American Societies for Experimental Biology, 24*(10), 4089–4102. https://doi.org/10.1096/fj.09-151001.

Weidinger, S., Beck, L. A., Bieber, T., Kabashima, K., & Irvine, A. D. (2018). Atopic dermatitis. *Nature Reviews Disease Primers, 4*(1), 1. https://doi.org/10.1038/s41572-018-0001-z.

Werfel, T., Allam, J. -P., Biedermann, T., Eyerich, K., Gilles, S., Guttman-Yassky, E., et al. (2016). Cellular and molecular immunologic mechanisms in patients with atopic dermatitis. *The Journal of Allergy and Clinical Immunology, 138*(2), 336–349. https://doi.org/10.1016/j.jaci.2016.06.010.

Wu, X., Briseño, C. G., Durai, V., Albring, J. C., Haldar, M., Bagadia, P., et al. (2016). Mafb lineage tracing to distinguish macrophages from other immune lineages reveals dual identity of Langerhans cells. *The Journal of Experimental Medicine, 213*(12), 2553–2565. https://doi.org/10.1084/jem.20160600.

Xue, L., Salimi, M., Panse, I., Mjösberg, J. M., McKenzie, A. N. J., Spits, H., et al. (2014). Prostaglandin D2 activates group 2 innate lymphoid cells through chemoattractant receptor-homologous molecule expressed on TH2 cells. *The Journal of Allergy and Clinical Immunology, 133*(4), 1184–1194. https://doi.org/10.1016/j.jaci.2013.10.056.

Yu, W., Jiang, N., Ebert, P. J. R., Kidd, B. A., Müller, S., Lund, P. J., et al. (2015). Clonal deletion prunes but does not eliminate self-specific αβ CD8(+) T lymphocytes. *Immunity, 42*(5), 929–941. https://doi.org/10.1016/j.immuni.2015.05.001.

Zeller, S., Rhyner, C., Meyer, N., Schmid-Grendelmeier, P., Akdis, C. A., & Crameri, R. (2009). Exploring the repertoire of IgE-binding self-antigens associated with atopic eczema. *The Journal of Allergy and Clinical Immunology, 124*(2). https://doi.org/10.1016/j.jaci.2009.05.015. 278–285.E7.

Zheng, T., Oh, M. H., Oh, S. Y., Schroeder, J. T., Glick, A. B., & Zhu, Z. (2009). Transgenic expression of interleukin-13 in the skin induces a pruritic dermatitis and skin remodeling. *The Journal of Investigative Dermatology, 129*(3), 742–751. https://doi.org/10.1038/jid.2008.295.

Ziegler. S. F. (2012). Thymic stromal lymphopoietin and allergic disease. *The Journal of Allergy and Clinical Immunology, 130*(4), 845–852. https://doi.org/10.1016/j.jaci.2012.07.010.

15

Skin-Gut-Lung Epithelial Permeability

YANA KOST, TIAN HAO ZHU, TIAN RAN ZHU, AND VIVIAN Y. SHI

KEY POINTS

- The atopic march is a phenomenon characterized by progressive development of atopic dermatitis, food allergy, allergic rhinitis, and later asthma.
- The mechanism by which atopic dermatitis advances toward gastrointestinal or airway disease remains to be fully elucidated, but current evidence points to multiorgan epithelial breakdown contributing to pathogenesis.
- Initial disruption in the skin epidermal barrier permits allergen sensitization and colonization by pathogens.
- Allergen sensitization and pathogen colonization induce T helper 2 inflammatory response and a thymic stromal lymphopoietin-mediated pathway that further promote barrier breakdown at distant sites.
- Several factors contribute to epithelial permeability in the skin, gut, and lungs, including structural and junction defects, cytokine dysregulation, microbial dysbiosis, and the itch-scratch response in skin.

Introduction

Childhood onset of atopic dermatitis is often followed by sequential development of food allergy, allergic rhinitis, and later asthma, a phenomenon commonly known as atopic march (Bantz et al., 2014). While the cutaneous disease process has been the subject of extensive research, the mechanism by which atopic dermatitis progresses toward gastrointestinal or airway disease remains to be elucidated. Recent findings suggest that both inherited and acquired defects at epithelial barrier surfaces permit enhanced allergen penetration, immunoglobulin E (IgE) sensitization, and systemic T helper 2 (Th2) response (Leung & Guttman-Yassky, 2014). In addition, levels of regulatory T cells (Tregs) in the skin, gut, and lung epithelia are diminished or ineffective at modulating the inflammatory response (Huang et al., 2017; Loxham & Davies, 2017; Penders et al., 2007). When the barrier of the epidermal skin surface fails, there is increased epicutaneous absorption of environmental allergens and a dysregulated immune response that predisposes to development of food allergy and asthma (Weidinger & Novak, 2016). The initial insult to the skin may explain why atopic dermatitis is often the first disease to manifest in the atopic

triad (Zhu, Zhu, Tran, Sivamani, & Shi, 2018). The chapter will highlight functions of the epithelial permeability barrier in the skin, gastrointestinal tract, and respiratory tract, and discuss how epithelial dysfunction linking microbiome alteration and immune dysregulation can predispose to development of atopic march.

Skin permeability

The epidermal barrier is composed of the stratum corneum and tight junctions (TJs) (Baldwin, Bhatia, Friedman, Eng, & Seite, 2017). Epidermal barrier impairment in atopic dermatitis can result from altered lipid composition, dysfunctional and decreased structural proteins, increased skin pH, and reduced skin microbiome diversity. Cutaneous permeability defects can be assessed by measuring transepidermal water loss, which correlates with disease severity (Hon, Leung, & Barankin, 2013; Weidinger & Novak, 2016).

Lipid alterations

Ceramides, free fatty acids, and cholesterol comprise the main stratum corneum lipids, of which ceramides are the most abundant (Li et al., 2016; Pappas, 2009). Ceramides are a critical component of the lipid matrix that aids in preventing transepidermal water loss (Jungersted & Agner, 2013). In atopic dermatitis there is decreased total ceramide content and alteration in ceramide chain length (Hon et al., 2013). Specifically, short-chain ceramides are increased and long-chain ceramides are diminished, disrupting structural conformation and allowing increased transepidermal water loss (Danso et al., 2017; Janssens et al., 2012; Meckfessel & Brandt, 2014). Studies have shown that inflammatory cytokines decrease levels of long-chain ceramides by downregulating expression of key ceramide synthesizing enzymes such as elongases (ELOVL) and ceramide synthases (CerS), which are necessary for proper lipid formation (Danso et al., 2017; Tawada et al., 2014).

Similarly, free fatty acid chain length also influences conformational ordering of the lipid matrix. Long-chain fatty acids help maintain stratum corneum structure, whereas short-chain fatty acids induce less densely packed hexagonal lipid organization and disrupt the typical orthorhombic organization of the lipid lattice (van Smeden et al., 2014). Lipid imbalance within atopic dermatitis lesions has been shown to be caused by downregulation of elongase (ELOVL), a key enzyme in fatty acid extension, which is often a result of systemic Th2 response (Park et al., 2012; van Smeden et al., 2014). Atopic dermatitis lesions generated with Th2 cytokines in human skin equivalents show reduced levels of ELOVL, indicating that Th2 response may cause changes in lipid composition in atopic dermatitis (Danso et al., 2017).

Furthermore, sebaceous lipids are secreted onto the skin surface and function to lubricate the skin, prevent dehydration, provide antimicrobial support, and deliver antioxidants in the form of vitamin E (De Luca & Valacchi, 2010; Ricketts, Squire, & Topley, 1951). In atopic dermatitis there is a reduction in sebum content (squalene and wax esters), suggesting an association between decreased sebaceous gland activity leading to skin barrier dysfunction and increased permeability (Mustakallio, Kiistala, Piha, & Nieminen, 1967; Rajka, 1974; Wheatley, 1965).

Filaggrin deficiency

Filaggrin (FLG) is a structural protein that is fundamental in forming the cornified cell envelope and maintaining intercellular cohesion (De Benedetto, Kubo, & Beck, 2012; Lee & Lee, 2014). Breakdown of FLG generates alanine, pyrrolidone carboxylic acid, and urocanic acid, natural moisturizing factors that preserve hydration, lower surface pH, and contribute to skin antimicrobial defense (Baldwin et al., 2017; Linehan et al., 2018). FLG deficiency leads to increased epidermal pH, which promotes serine protease activity to degrade stratum corneum desmosomes and inhibits ceramide production (Hon et al., 2013; Thyssen & Kezic, 2014). Inherited loss-of-function mutation in one or both FLG alleles results in either a reduced (heterozygous) or complete absence (homozygous) of epidermal FLG (Thyssen & Kezic, 2014). In mouse models with *FLG–/–* genotype there is expansion of innate lymphoid cells type 2 (ILC2) in the skin and airway, leading to atopic dermatitis and pulmonary inflammation, respectively (Saunders et al., 2016). FLG expression can also be downregulated by Th2 cytokines (interleukin-4 [IL4] and IL13) and environmental factors (low humidity, ultraviolet [UV] radiation, and external irritant) (Howell et al., 2009; Thyssen & Kezic, 2014). Studies have shown that individuals with reduced FLG levels due to loss of function mutations exhibit early-onset atopic dermatitis that is often more persistent and closely associated with asthma and food allergy than those with normal FLG levels (Leung & Guttman-Yassky, 2014). Fig. 15.1 illustrates physiologic alterations as a result of FLG defect.

Tight junction defects

TJs are composed of transmembrane proteins—claudins, occludins, and junctional adhesion molecules—localized to the paracellular spaces of the stratum granulosum (Sugawara et al., 2013; Yokouchi et al., 2015). Claudin-1 and claudin-4 are responsible for intercellular sealing and formation of the liquid-liquid interface barrier within the epidermis (Kubo, Nagao, & Amagai, 2012; Lee & Lee, 2014). TJ disruption weakens barrier function by altering lipid and profilaggrin processing (Yuki et al., 2013). Allergens gain rapid entry across a disrupted TJ, engage Langerhans cells, and prime the systemic inflammatory response (Fig. 15.2) (Shi et al., 2015). Fine structures of TJs are detailed in the Chapter 11.

Proteases

Various environmental allergens, such as house dust mite, cockroach, fungi, and pollen, contain cysteine and serine proteases (Lee & Lee, 2014; Shimura et al., 2016). The proteolytic allergens can bind protease-activated receptor on keratinocytes, triggering epidermal degradation, resulting in increased permeability and Th2-mediated inflammation (Lee & Lee, 2014; Shimura et al., 2016). Reduction in serine protease inhibitors, such as serine protease inhibitor Kazal type-5, has been shown to further enhance protease-activated pathways and contribute to disease aggravation (Leung & Guttman-Yassky, 2014).

Itch and scratch

Among the many symptoms experienced by patients with atopic dermatitis, itch is nearly universal and leads to unremitting scratching that can erode the epithelial barrier (Chamlin et al., 2005). Although the exact mechanism has not been elucidated, it has been purported that endogenous and exogenous triggers such as histamine, proteases, substance P, various ILs (e.g., IL31), and environmental allergens can signal through specific itch pathways (such as histamine 1 receptor, protease-activated receptor 2, neurokinin 1 receptor, IL31 receptor, and transient receptor potential cation channel ankyrin subtype 1) present on nerve fiber endings (Furue, Yamamura, Kido-Nakahara, Nakahara, & Fukui, 2018; Hermanns, 2015).

Following breaks in the skin, allergens and pathogens gain entry across the epidermis and activate a Th2 allergic inflammatory response, which increases lymphovascular permeability allowing for the additional recruitment of pruritic initiators to the site of injury. Vigorous scratching in response to the itch can further erode the skin barrier and trigger secondary bacterial infection, perpetuating the cycle.

Recently, IL31 has emerged as a key player and potential drug target in the pathogenesis of atopic dermatitis. IL31 is primarily secreted by Th2 T cells following stimulation by IL4 and to a lesser extent by dendritic cells, mast cells, eosinophils, and basophils (see Fig. 15.2) (Furue et al., 2018; Nemoto et al., 2016; Ruzicka et al., 2017). IL31 primarily modulates cell-mediated immunity in the skin through perception of itch in the peripheral nervous system, in the lung through increased airway inflammation, and in the intestine through defense against microbes (Hermanns, 2015; Perrigoue, Zaph, Guild, Du, & Artis, 2009).

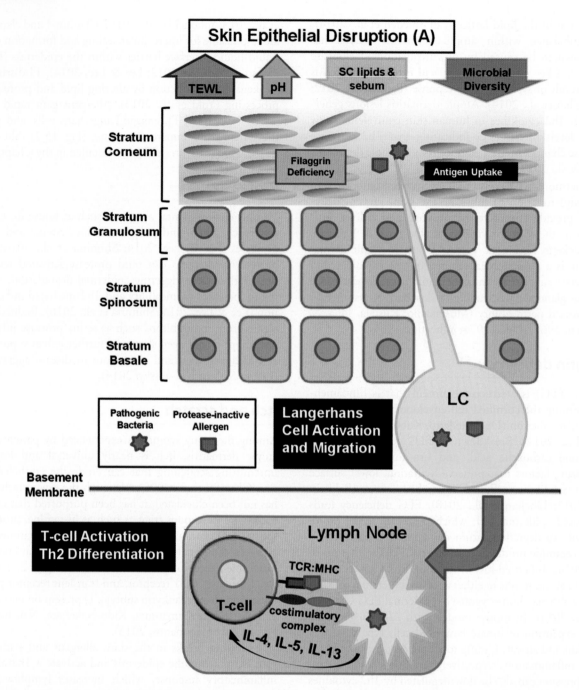

• **Fig. 15.1** Skin barrier disruption. In atopic dermatitis, stratum corneum (*SC*) barrier damage often occurs as a result of a decrease in surface microbial diversity, filaggrin (*FLG*) expression, antimicrobial peptide production, and SC lipid synthesis (measured by increased skin pH and transepidermal water loss [*TEWL*]). After SC breakdown, protease-inactive allergens and bacterial molecules are taken up by resident Langerhans cells (*LCs*), which migrate to draining lymph nodes to trigger an adaptive immune response. Engagement of the T-cell receptor (*TCR*) with major histocompatibility complex (*MHC*) containing antigen and concomitant engagement of costimulatory complex activate the naive T cell. Additional factors secreted by LCs include interleukin-4 (IL4), IL5, and IL13, which induce T helper 2 (*Th2*) differentiation.

Regulatory cytokines such as transforming growth factor-β (TGF-β) can downregulate IL31 levels, whereas bacteria toxins such as staphylococcal α-toxin or enterotoxin B can augment IL31 levels (Furue et al., 2018). Selectively targeting the IL31 signaling pathway is a promising strategy to treat patients with moderate-to-severe pruritus associated with atopic dermatitis for whom conventional medical management has not

been successful. Two phase II randomized, double-blind, placebo-controlled clinical trials demonstrated that monoclonal antibodies directed against the IL31 receptor can safely and effectively decrease itch and sleep disturbance, improve skin lesions, and minimize the use of topical steroids (Nemoto et al., 2016; Ruzicka et al., 2017). Fig. 15.3 illustrates the itch and scratch cycle and its relationship to skin barrier alteration.

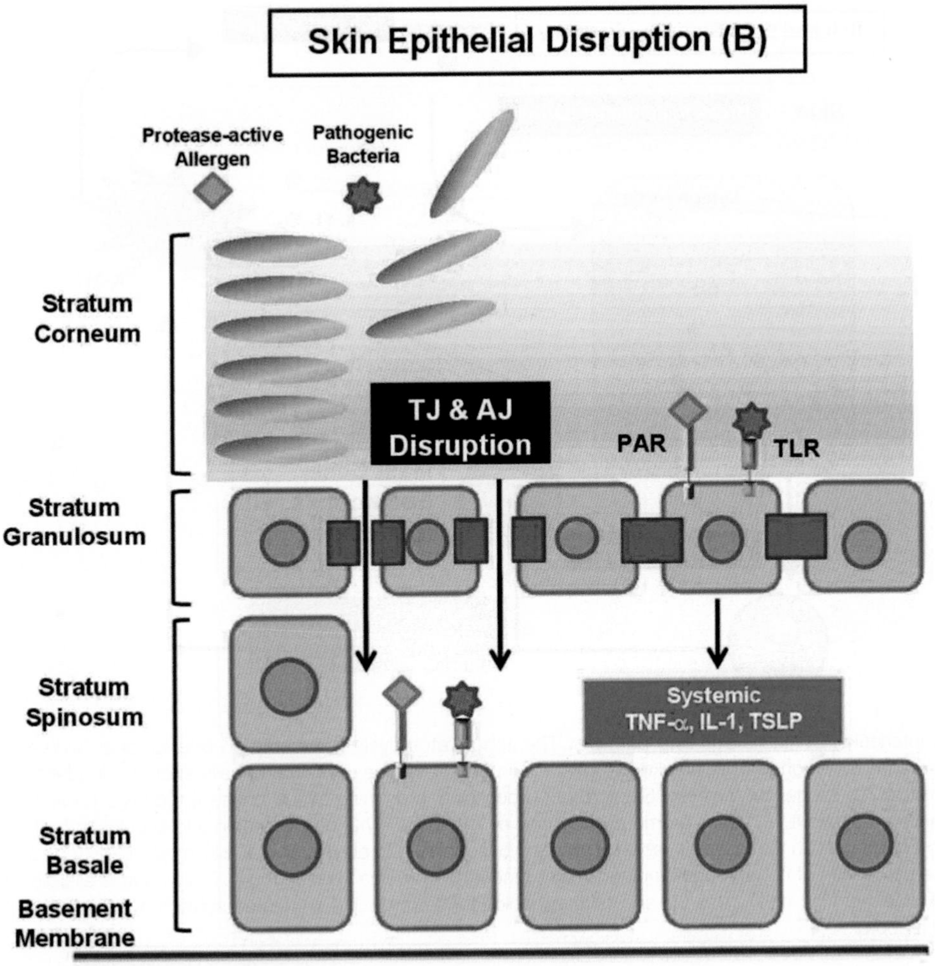

• **Fig. 15.2** Skin barrier disruption. Tight junction (*TJ*) and adherens junction (*AJ*) disruption in the stratum granulosum can also result from a decrease in surface microbial diversity, filaggrin (*FLG*) expression, antimicrobial peptide production, and stratum corneum (*SC*) lipid synthesis. Protease-active antigens can directly cause SC breakdown and activate protease-activated receptors (*PARs*) and toll-like receptors (*TLRs*) on keratinocytes (*black arrows*), triggering production of proinflammatory cytokines, including tumor necrosis factor-α (*TNF-α*), interleukin-1 (*IL1*), and thymic stromal lymphopoietin (*TSLP*), which can mediate permeability defects at other sites such as the intestinal and respiratory tracts.

Skin microbiome alteration

The skin provides an ecologic niche for a wide range of microorganisms that influence the pathogenesis of inflammatory dermatoses (Bjerre, Bandier, Skov, Engstrand, & Johansen, 2017). A diverse skin microbiota has been shown to promote normal skin homeostasis through induction of Th17 cell immune response and secretion of antimicrobial peptides that nourish commensal flora and prevent growth of pathogenic species (Linehan et al., 2018). For example, *Staphylococcus epidermidis* is a commensal bacterium that suppresses inflammation after skin injury and enhances innate immunity (Nakatsuji et al., 2016). *S. epidermidis* also restricts growth and reproduction of pathogenic gram-positive species through competition for resources and secretion of antimicrobial peptides (Baldwin et al., 2017; Linehan et al., 2018). Conversely, *Staphylococcus aureus* colonization leads to skin breakdown and increased risk of atopic dermatitis development (Li et al., 2017). Serine proteases

derived from *S. aureus* are capable of physically digesting the epithelial barrier, releasing enterotoxins, and inducing proinflammatory cytokines such as IL4, IL12, and IL22 (Leung & Guttman-Yassky, 2014; Nakatsuji et al., 2016). Furthermore, studies show that *S. aureus* is found on the skin of 90% of patients with atopic dermatitis and produces ceramidases, which result in breakdown of important structural components of skin (Baldwin et al., 2017). Dysbiosis, the imbalance between commensal and pathogenic microbes, is a hallmark of atopic dermatitis (Bjerre et al., 2017; Huang et al., 2017). During atopic dermatitis flares, skin bacterial diversity is lowered, with increased *S. aureus* and diminished *S. epidermidis* (Bjerre et al., 2017). Periods of remission are associated with increased bacterial diversity, with more *S. epidermidis* and species of *Streptococcus, Corynebacterium,* and *Propionibacterium* (Kong et al., 2012). This temporal shift in skin microflora may be related to skin structural barrier defects that permit penetration by pathogenic species and loss of protective species

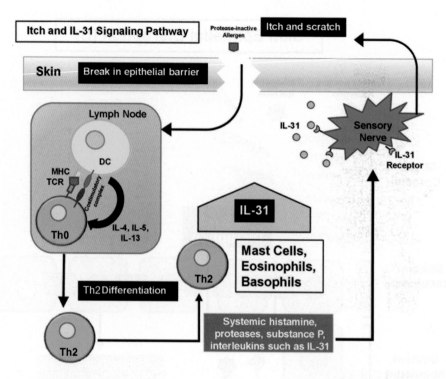

• **Fig. 15.3** Itch and interleukin-31 (IL31) signaling pathway. The itch-scratch cycle is a common phenomenon whereby scratching behavior induced by itch sensory transmission causes breakdown of the skin barrier. Antigen presenting cells such as dendritic cells (*DCs*) and macrophages are then sensitized to exogenous antigen. Subsequent processing in draining lymph nodes engages a naive T cell (*Th0*) with the DC. The DC also secretes IL4, IL5, and IL13, which promotes induction of T helper 2 (*Th2*) differentiation and circulation to the target organs. IL31 is secreted by activated Th2 in addition to mast cells, eosinophils, and basophils. IL31 plays a pivotal role in cell-mediated immunity in the skin, lung, and intestine, and the perception of itch through binding to IL31 receptors on nerve fiber endings. The systemic allergic inflammatory response ultimately recruits additional pruritic initiators to the site of injury, which further propagates the itch-scratch cycle. *MHC*, Major histocompatibility complex; *TCR*, T-cell receptor.

(Baldwin et al., 2017). Cutaneous microbiome in atopic dermatitis is further discussed in Chapter 6.

Gut permeability

Gut epithelium forms a critical barrier that prevents entry of pathogens and noxious agents from the gastrointestinal lumen (Peterson & Artis, 2014). Recent studies utilizing the lactulose:mannitol ratio to measure gastrointestinal permeability have provided information on the degree of epithelial damage in individuals with atopic dermatitis (Odenwald & Turner, 2013).

Gut barrier defects

The intestinal barrier is lined with simple columnar epithelium interspersed with goblet cells, encased in a mucous layer that functions to shield the host from digestive enzymes and microorganism penetration (see Fig. 15.3). TJ barrier breakdown enables dendritic cell access to luminal antigens followed by uptake in the lamina propriae (Kubo et al., 2012). In contrast to claudin-1 in the skin, claudin-2, a pore-forming claudin, is associated with increased intestinal permeability in patients with atopic dermatitis (Georas

& Rezaee, 2014). IL4/IL13 pathway dysregulation in atopic dermatitis is thought to upregulate intestinal claudin-2 expression, supporting the notion that cutaneous inflammation influences permeability defects in other organs (Georas & Rezaee, 2014). Fig. 15.4 illustrates the disruption of gut barrier and its immunologic consequences.

Food allergy

Atopic dermatitis is closely associated with food allergy, an abnormal immune response to common foods such as milk, eggs, peanuts, tree nuts, wheat, soy, fish, and shellfish (Noti et al., 2014; Wesemann & Nagler, 2016). In healthy individuals, food allergen–specific Tregs produce IL22 to maintain intestinal immune tolerance at barrier surfaces (Peterson & Artis, 2014). The lamina propria also contains secretory IgA that aids in immune exclusion and reduces the ability of food allergens to enter the host. In individuals with atopic dermatitis there is a depletion of allergy-protective metabolites such as bacteria-derived short-chain fatty acids and an increase in allergen danger signals such as IL25 and IL33 (Wesemann & Nagler, 2016). Early introduction of peanuts to high-risk infants (with severe eczema, egg allergy, or both) has been shown to reduce the incidence

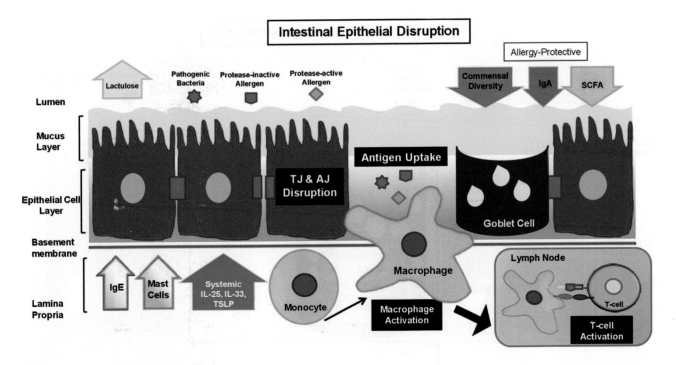

• **Fig. 15.4** Gut barrier disruption. Various factors can modulate gastrointestinal permeability and contribute to increased gut leakiness measured by increased luminal lactulose levels. Patients with atopic dermatitis have elevated reduction of luminal IgA, luminal commensal bacteria, and short-chain fatty acids (*SCFAs*). Normal gastrointestinal function and homeostasis are regulated by junctional complexes formed by tight junctions (*TJs*) and adherens junctions (*AJs*), mucus production by goblet cells, and the immune system within the intestinal laminal propria. Systemic inflammatory signals, including interleukin-25 (IL25), IL33, and thymic stromal lymphopoietin (*TSLP*) can promote monocyte migration, diapedesis, and activation into macrophage (*arrow*). Breaks in the barrier formed by the junctional complex allow luminal antigens access through the epithelial barrier where they are phagocytosed by macrophages and subsequently presented to T cells in draining lymph nodes (*arrowhead*) to trigger visceral T helper 2-dominant hypersensitivity. Patients with atopic dermatitis also demonstrate elevated IgE levels in the serum and lamina propria and increased mast cell number and function, which can contribute to food allergen sensitivity.

of peanut allergy significantly, which is likely to be due to dietary induction of antigen-specific Tregs (Du Toit et al., 2015; Wesemann & Nagler, 2016). These findings suggest that exposure to food allergens through a disrupted skin barrier is a risk factor for developing allergic inflammation in the gut but can be partially overcome by introduction of the allergen early in childhood.

Gut microbiome alteration

Intestinal bacterial communities evolve in response to host factors (pH, bile acids, and pancreatic enzymes), nonhost factors (nutrients, medications, and environmental allergens), and bacterial factors (toxins) (Penders et al., 2007). In developed countries, high-fat and sugar diet and routine antibiotic use may drive atopy by diminishing microbial diversity and depleting populations of gut bacteria with barrier-protective function (Wesemann & Nagler, 2016). Early exposure to commensal gut bacteria antigens, such as bacteriocins, confers protection against atopy by restricting growth of pathogenic bacteria (Gallo & Nakatsuji, 2011; West et al., 2015). Patients with atopic dermatitis have a significantly lower number of intestinal commensal *Bifidobacterium*, which correlates with disease severity (Watanabe et al., 2003). Conversely, infants with atopic dermatitis have higher numbers of pathogenic fecal *Clostridium*

difficile (Penders et al., 2007). In one large-scale prospective birth cohort study (KOALA), infants who developed atopic dermatitis had higher numbers of *Escherichia coli* and *C. difficile* colonization than those without atopic dermatitis (Penders et al., 2007). *E. coli* and *C. difficile* overgrowth was associated with a decrease in beneficial bacteria, loss of immune tolerance, and increased intestinal permeability through toxin production. In contrast, a well-balanced gut microflora in infants protects against the risk of developing atopic dermatitis and later food allergy. Gut microbiome in atopic dermatitis is further discussed in Chapter 6.

Lung permeability

The respiratory epithelium is the first site of contact with inhaled particles such as allergens, irritants, and microorganisms and is therefore essential for orchestrating appropriate inflammatory responses to eliminate foreign pathogens while limiting tissue injury (Kast et al., 2012).

Lung epithelium defects

The respiratory tract is made of pseudostratified epithelium, comprising ciliated cells, mucus-producing goblet cells, and undifferentiated basal cells (Fig. 15.5) (Loxham & Davies, 2017; Smits, van der Vlugt, von Mutius, & Hiemstra, 2016).

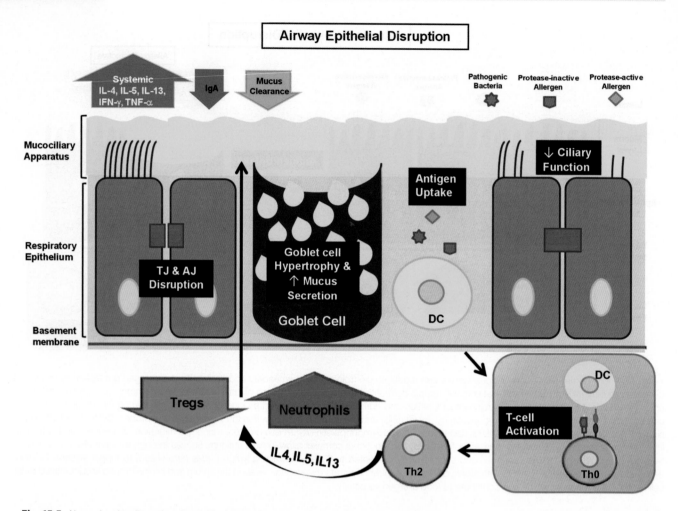

• **Fig. 15.5** Airway barrier disruption. In atopic dermatitis a vicious cycle operates in the upper respiratory airways, in which initial epidermal barrier dysfunction leads to elevated serum interleukin-4 (IL4), IL5, IL13, interferon-gamma (*IFN-γ*), and tumour necrosis factor-α (*TNF-α*). These proinflammatory cytokines cause abnormal mucociliary differentiation, goblet cell hypertrophy, tight junction (*TJ*) and adherens junction (*AJ*) breakdown, and IgA depletion (*vertical arrow*). Goblet cells secrete excess mucus, which, in conjunction with impaired cilia function, results in poor mucous clearance, reduced air-current mobility, and increased risk of colonization by respiratory pathogens. Uptake of antigens by dendritic cells (*DCs*) leads to T-cell activation and T helper 2 (*Th2*)-predominant immune response. This leads to further cytokine release in addition to neutrophil chemotaxis and downregulation of regulatory T cells (*Tregs*) that further perpetrate tissue damage and airway epithelial leakiness.

The mucosal layer contains mucins, defensins, IgA, and antioxidants, which form an integral part of the innate immune response (Loxham & Davies, 2017). In the asthmatic airway, the mucociliary apparatus becomes remodeled toward increased mucin secretion and decreased ciliary function, resulting in mucous plugging and ultimately airway obstruction (Loxham & Davies, 2017). Respiratory epithelium reprogramming toward a hypersecretory phenotype has been linked to increased activity of IL4, IL12, interferon-c, and tumor necrosis factor-α (TNF-α) (Loxham & Davies, 2017).

Lung epithelium junctional defects

Multiprotein subunits (claudins, occludin, zona occludens [ZOs], and junctional adhesion molecules) comprise the respiratory TJs that regulate permeability, promote cell-cell adhesion, and maintain barrier integrity (Georas & Rezaee, 2014). In asthmatic airways, claudin-1, claudin-4, and claudin-18 are suppressed by the IL13/Th2 pathway, which results in increased paracellular leakiness and respiratory hyperresponsiveness (Loxham & Davies, 2017; Steelant et al., 2016; Sweerus et al., 2017). Occludins and ZOs, particularly ZO-1, are reduced in upper airway epithelial cells, permitting neutrophil activation and cytotoxic cytokine release, causing local tissue damage (Loxham & Davies, 2017). Junctional adhesion molecule abnormalities enhance viral particle binding and uptake in the basolateral space (Georas & Rezaee, 2014). Finally, epithelial junctional complexes as a whole can be disrupted, leading to inhalation of proteolytic substances, including air pollutants, cigarette smoke, and toxins (Loxham & Davies, 2017; Steelant et al., 2016).

Below the TJ are adherens junctions (AJs), composed of cadherins and catenins, which are important for epithelial adhesion, wound repair, gene regulation, and cell differentiation (Steelant et al., 2016). Internal forces, such as IL4, IL13, and histamine, directly inhibit surface expression of E-cadherin and b-catenin, while external forces, such as house dust mite, indirectly downregulate E-cadherin expression (Georas & Rezaee, 2014). In addition, chronic inflammation downregulates caveolin-1, a stabilizer of AJs, reducing E-cadherin and b-catenin expression (Georas & Rezaee, 2014; Loxham & Davies, 2017). These findings suggest a vicious cycle operating in asthmatic airways, in which barrier dysfunction leads to allergen sensitization, followed by Th2 polarization and secretion of cytokines that further perpetrate airway epithelial leakiness.

Airway microbiome alteration

The neonatal period represents the most vulnerable window for allergen-induced allergic inflammation, a susceptibility that diminishes after the development of respiratory microbiome in the first 3 weeks of life (Huang et al., 2017). Living in an environment with diverse microbial flora reduces the incidence of allergic disease (Ege et al., 2011). Disturbances in microbial balance shift toward overgrowth of *Haemophilus, Moraxella, Neisseria,* and *Streptococcus* (Smits et al., 2016; Thomas & Fernandez-Penas, 2017). In addition, *Pseudomonas* and *Staphylococcus* are frequent colonizers of sinus tracts in patients with chronic rhinosinusitis, which predisposes to the development of asthma (Lan, Zhang, Gevaert, Zhang, & Bachert, 2016). Upon pathogen entry, a systemic inflammatory response upregulates TNF, IL1, IL6, and IL8, which have been shown to promote epithelial barrier dysfunction by decreasing expression of occludin, claudins, E-cadherin, and catenin (Steelant et al., 2016). Upper airway disease may also be influenced by gastrointestinal microflora. Bacterial fermentation of dietary fibers produces short-chain fatty acids that can mitigate allergic responses and improve respiratory function (Huang et al., 2017). Microbiome-derived short-chain fatty acids, such as propionate, butyrate, and acetate, dampen the Th2 inflammatory response in the lung by directly inducing Treg upregulation and exerting epigenetic modifications in the forkhead box P3 pathway (Huang et al., 2017). Studies examining a high-fiber diet in patients with atopy have suggested a role for short-chain fatty acids in promoting tolerance to antigen exposure in the lungs (Trompette et al., 2014).

The skin-gut-lung model

Although atopic dermatitis is fundamentally a dermatologic condition, cumulative evidence has supported a skin-gut-lung model of disease pathogenesis in the atopic march. Insight from immunologic studies has provided a significant breakthrough in understanding how defects in the skin could affect distant organ systems. Furthermore, microbial communities from various organs can modulate disease course and present opportunities for therapeutic intervention (Table 15.1).

TABLE 15.1 Characteristics of skin, gut, and lung changes in atopic dermatitis

	Biophysical changes	Barrier dysfunction	Microbiome alteration	Immune dysregulation
Skin	⬇ CER content ⬇ Long-chain CER and LCFA ⬇ Sebum ⬆ Short-chain CER and SCFA ⬆ Surface pH, TEWL	⬇ Filaggrin ⬇ TJ barrier proteins (claudin-1, claudin-4, occludins) ⬆ Protease activity	⬇ *Staphylococcus epidermidis, Corynebacterium* ⬆ *Propionibacterium acnes, Staphylococcus aureus*	⬇ Cathelicidin and β-defensins ⬆ IL4, IL5, IL13, IL22, IL31, IgE ⬆ TSLP
Gut	⬆ Permeability ⬆ Enterocyte loss and damage	⬇ TJ barrier proteins (occludins) ⬇ AJ barrier proteins (E-cadherin and β-catenin) ⬆ TJ pore proteins (claudin-2)	⬇ *Bifidobacteria, Lactobacillus* ⬆ *Escherichia coli, Clostridium difficile*	⬇ Treg cells, IgA, SCFA ⬆ IL25, IL33, basophils
Lung	⬇ Ciliary function ⬆ Goblet cells ⬆ Mucin secretion	⬇ TJ barrier proteins (claudin-1, claudin-4, claudin-18, ZO-1) ⬇ AJ barrier proteins (E-cadherin and β-catenin, caveolin) ⬆ Protease activity	⬆ *Haemophilus, Moraxella, Neisseria, Streptococcus, Pseudomonas,* and *Staphylococcus*	⬇ IgA ⬆ IL4, IL5, IL12, IL13, IL31, IFN-γ, TNF-α ⬆ IgE, IgG, eosinophils

AJ, Adherens junction; *CER,* ceramide; *IL,* interleukin; *LCFA,* long-chain fatty acid; *SCFA,* short-chain fatty acid; *TEWL,* transepidermal water loss; *Treg,* regulatory T cells; *TJ,* tight junction; *TSLP,* thymic stromal lymphopoietin; *ZO-1,* zonula occludens-1.

A compromised barrier promotes a hyperactive immune system

Epithelial cells sense pathogen-associated molecular patterns by expressing pattern-recognition receptors, including toll-like receptors, protease-activated receptors, and Nod-like receptors (Steelant et al., 2016). In atopic dermatitis, skin barrier dysfunction enhances allergen exposure (sensitization phase) and activates innate immune defenses. Antigen acquisition by Langerhans cells further activates adaptive immune cells (Kubo et al., 2012). In atopic dermatitis mouse models, epicutaneous sensitization with allergen promotes a local and systemic Th2-predominant response, characterized by increased IL4, IL5, IL13, and IgE (De Benedetto et al., 2012). The combination of papain (a proteolytic antigen) and mechanical barrier damage caused by tape stripping synergistically promote dermatitis and antigen-specific IgE response (Shimura et al., 2016). Following epicutaneous sensitization, airway challenge then leads to systemic inflammation characterized by IL33-mediated activation of ILC2, robust eosinophilia, and IgE/IgG1 production (Shimura et al., 2016). Systemic levels of Th2 cytokines (IL4, IL13, IL31) directly suppress FLG production (Leung & Guttman-Yassky, 2014). This chronic inflammation impairs lipid synthesis, reduces junctional adhesiveness, increases pathogenic colonization, and compromises epithelial barrier function across multiple organ systems (Georas & Rezaee, 2014; Steelant et al., 2016; Wesemann & Nagler, 2016). Thus epicutaneous sensitization on barrier-disrupted skin is sufficient to induce systemic Th2 allergic inflammation at distant sites, including intestinal tract and lower respiratory airways, and is believed to be the inciting event for the atopic march (De Benedetto et al., 2012).

Thymic stromal lymphopoietin (TSLP) has emerged as a key mediator by which epicutaneous sensitization can maintain chronic lung inflammation and intestinal food allergy (Leyva-Castillo, Hener, Jiang, & Li, 2013). TSLP is an IL7-like cytokine produced by keratinocytes following epidermal breakdown (De Benedetto et al., 2012; Demehri, Morimoto, Holtzman, & Kopan, 2009). When released into the circulation, TSLP enhances maturation and proliferation of dendritic cells and B cells, stimulating the production of Th2 cytokines IL13 and IL31 (Lee & Lee, 2014). In atopic dermatitis, TSLP overexpression in lesional keratinocytes promotes allergic sensitization and bronchial hyperresponsiveness (Leyva-Castillo et al., 2013). Conversely, diminished TSLP levels result in attenuated Th2 response and airway inflammation (Leyva-Castillo et al., 2013). Antigen-induced allergic inflammation in the gastrointestinal tract is also influenced by a TLSP-basophil pathway (Noti et al., 2014). Epicutaneous sensitization to ovalbumin or peanut on an atopic dermatitis–like skin lesion followed by intragastric antigen challenge directly increases TSLP-elicited basophils in the skin, which leads to elevated antigen-specific serum IgE levels and the accumulation of mast cells in the intestine (Noti et al., 2014). These findings suggest that inhibiting TSLP production in the skin can be useful in preventing or limiting allergen sensitization and halting progression of atopic march.

Another route of dysregulation involves IL17, a key tissue signaling cytokine that provides protection and regeneration of barrier organs such as the skin, lung, and gastrointestinal system (Eyerich, Dimartino, & Cavani, 2017). Studies have shown that IL17 orchestrates protection against infections by enhancing the epithelial release of antimicrobial peptides and neutrophil chemoattractants, in addition to directly inducing claudin expression in the formation of TJs, thus ensuring mucosal barrier integrity (Eyerich et al., 2009, 2017). Under natural exposure conditions, superantigens derived from *S. aureus*, such as staphylococcal enterotoxin B, directly induces IL17 expression that triggers keratinocyte production of human beta-defensin (HBD) (Eyerich, Eyerich, & Biedermann, 2015). However, in atopic dermatitis, IL17 is substantially impaired in the presence of type 2 cytokines (Eyerich et al., 2015, 2017). The Th2 skin immune milieu contains abundant IL4 and IL13, which partially inhibits the IL17/HBD axis. This may partially explain why patients with atopic dermatitis have difficulty clearing *S. aureus* colonization. Finally, it is important to note that factors involved in the development of atopic dermatitis and associated disorders are likely different from those involved in the flares and/or maintenance of these disorders, although it is likely that there is an overlap. For example, TLSP modulation may help prevent disease recurrence or progression of the march, but may have more modest effects on the disease activity itself (Demehri et al., 2009; Leyva-Castillo et al., 2013).

"Chicken or the egg" conundrum

Parents of individuals with atopic dermatitis often share a common concern regarding the prognosis of their child's skin disease: Who will go on to develop other manifestations of atopy such as asthma and/or allergic rhinitis and when? To answer this question, it's important to recognize that atopic dermatitis is characterized clinically by a wide spectrum of phenotypes, from very mild forms of xerosis to keratosis pilaris–like follicular prominence to papular eczema to classic scaly edematous papules and plaques to the uncommon severely erythrodermic variant, each carrying a different risk for systemic involvement. In addition, the age at which an individual exhibits the first signs and symptoms of atopy may influence the probability of extracutaneous atopic disease (Lee & Hong, 2019). Emerging work on phenotypic profiling of atopic dermatitis patients has examined the significance of atopic dermatitis onset and associative risk toward progressing to atopic march. A 1000-patient cohort study identified several atopic dermatitis phenotypes, including early-transient (early onset within age 2 and no further symptoms after age 4), early-persistent (onset within age 2 and persistence of symptoms until age 6), and a late phenotype (onset of atopic dermatitis after age 2) (Roduit et al., 2017). Children with early phenotypes were found to have an increased risk for developing asthma and food allergy, and the positve association was found to be stronger with the early-persistent phenotype (Roduit et al., 2017). The late phenotype was only associated with allergic rhinitis and not with asthma or food allergy (Roduit et al., 2017).

A cohort study in France found that atopic dermatitis with multiple sensitizations, defined as a specific serum IgE concentration against common inhalant or food allergens, and atopic dermatitis with familial history of asthma both convey higher risks of asthma during childhood (Amat et al., 2015). Furthermore, another study showed that early-onset atopic dermatitis with high atopy and high eosinophil levels is associated with an increased risk of childhood asthma but not of food allergy (Lee et al., 2016).

Despite the emerging progress in assessing correlation of atopic dermatitis phenotype to susceptibility of developing asthma, food allergy, and allergic rhinitis, the complexity of atopic diseases commonly invokes the argument as to whether immunogen (medications, stress, toxins, bacteria, food particles) entry through leaky gut or airways causes systemic atopic responses that include atopic dermatitis, or whether immunogen entry through leaky skin causes systemic atopic responses that include asthma and food allergies. Recent work suggests that only a small proportion of children (4%–25%) actually follow a trajectory profile similar to that of the atopic march (Lule et al., 2017). In addition, approximately 20% of patients do not have any evidence of IgE sensitization (based on skin prick tests), suggesting a degree of heterogeneity within the population (Lule et al., 2017). As not all individuals show sequential disease progression from atopic dermatitis to food allergy/intolerance to asthma to allergic rhinitis, perhaps instead of a linear sequence the two processes occur concomitantly, each reciprocally influencing the other. This may explain why some children do not follow the atopic march and why some children may eventually exit out of the march. Finally, current evidence of twin and sibling studies suggests the association between atopic dermatitis and asthma and hay fever may be independent of shared early-life environmental factors, suggesting that further causal risk factors remain to be discovered despite there being a clear sequential association and plausible biologic mechanisms to explain such an association (Khan, Dharmage, Matheson, & Gurrin, 2018).

Summary

This chapter aims to provide an overview of current evidence relating to the skin-gut-lung model of atopy. Abnormal epidermal epithelium serves as a site for allergic sensitization to antigens and colonization by bacteria. This induces a systemic Th2 response that facilitates barrier dysfunction at distant sites such as the intestinal and respiratory tracts. The typical sequence of clinical presentation is an initial atopic dermatitis that progresses to food allergy, allergic rhinitis, and later asthma. The causes of epidermal barrier abnormalities are complex and driven by a combination of structural, genetic, environmental, and immunologic factors. In addition, microbial diversity and dysbiosis influence disease severity, duration, and response to treatment. As there are no immediate cures for food allergy or asthma, the development of effective treatment for atopic dermatitis will prove to be an important strategy for prevention of the atopic march.

Further readings

Beck, L. A., Thaci, D., Hamilton, J. D., Graham, N. M., Bieber, T., Rocklin, R., et al. (2014). Dupilumab treatment in adults with moderate-to-severe atopic dermatitis. *New England Journal of Medicine, 371*(2), 130–139.

Elias, P. M. (2014). Lipid abnormalities and lipid-based repair strategies in atopic dermatitis. *Biochimica et Biophysica Acta, 1841*(3), 323–330.

Gueniche, A., Knaudt, B., Schuck, E., Volz, T., Bastien, P., Martin, R., et al. (2008). Effects of nonpathogenic gram-negative bacterium *Vitreoscilla filiformis* lysate on atopic dermatitis: A prospective, randomized, double-blind, placebo-controlled clinical study. *British Journal of Dermatology, 159*(6), 1357–1363.

Huang, J. T., Abrams, M., Tlougan, B., Rademaker, A., & Paller, A. S. (2009). Treatment of *Staphylococcus aureus* colonization in atopic dermatitis decreases disease severity. *Pediatrics, 123*(5), e808–e814.

Lee, D. E., Clark, A., K., Tran, K. A., & Shi, V. Y. (2018). New and emerging targeted systemic therapies: A new era for atopic dermatitis. *Journal of Dermatological Treatment, 29*(4), 364–374.

Niccoli, A. A., Artesi, A. L., Candio, F., Ceccarelli, S., Cozzali, R., Ferraro, L., et al. (2014). Preliminary results on clinical effects of probiotic *Lactobacillus salivarius* LS01 in children affected by atopic dermatitis. *Journal of Clinical Gastroenterology, 48*(1), S34–S36.

Nomura, T., & Kabashima, K. (2016). Advances in atopic dermatitis in 2015. *Journal of Allergy and Clinical Immunology, 138*(6), 1548–1555.

Shi, V. Y., Foolad, N., Ornelas, J. N., Hassoun, L. A., Monico, G., Takeda, N., et al. (2016). Comparing the effect of bleach and water baths on skin barrier function in atopic dermatitis: A split-body randomized controlled trial. *British Journal of Dermatology, 175*(1), 212–214.

Volz, T., Skabytska, Y., Guenova, E., Chen, K. M., Frick, J. S., Kirschning, C. J., et al. (2014). Nonpathogenic bacteria alleviating atopic dermatitis inflammation induce IL-10-producing dendritic cells and regulatory Tr1 cells. *Journal of Investigative Dermatology, 134*(1), 96–104.

References

Amat, F., Saint-Pierre, P., Bourrat, E., Nemni, A., Couderc, R., Boutmy-Deslandes, E., et al. (2015). Early-onset atopic dermatitis in children: Which are the phenotypes at risk of asthma? Results from the ORCA cohort. *PLoS One, 10*(6), e0131369. https://doi.org/10.1371/journal.pone.0131369. https://www.ncbi.nlm.nih.gov/pubmed/26107938.

Baldwin, H. E., Bhatia, N. D., Friedman, A., Eng, R. M., & Seite, S. (2017). The role of cutaneous microbiota harmony in maintaining a functional skin barrier. *Journal of Drugs in Dermatology, 16*(1), 12–18. https://www.ncbi.nlm.nih.gov/pubmed/28095528.

Bantz, S. K., Zhu, Z., & Zheng, T. (2017). The atopic march: Progression from atopic dermatitis to allergic rhinitis and asthma. *Journal of Clinical & Cellular Immunology, 5*(2). https://doi.org/10.4172/2155-9899.1000202. https://www.ncbi.nlm.nih.gov/pubmed/25419479.

Bjerre, R. D., Bandier, J., Skov, L., Engstrand, L., & Johansen, J. D. (2017). The role of the skin microbiome in atopic dermatitis: A systematic review. *British Journal of Dermatology, 177*(5), 1272–1278. https://doi.org/10.1111/bjd.15390. https://www.ncbi.nlm.nih.gov/pubmed/28207943.

Chamlin, S. L., Mattson, C. L., Frieden, I. J., Williams, M. L., Mancini, A. J., Cella, D., & Chren, M. M. (2005). The price of pruritus: Sleep disturbance and cosleeping in atopic dermatitis. *Archives of Pediatrics & Adolescent Medicine, 159*(8), 745–750. https://doi.org/10.1001/archpedi.159.8.745. https://www.ncbi.nlm.nih.gov/pubmed/16061782.

Danso, M., Boiten, W., van Drongelen, V., Gmelig Meijling, K., Gooris, G., El Ghalbzouri, A., et al. (2017). Altered expression of epidermal lipid bio-synthesis enzymes in atopic dermatitis skin is accompanied by changes in stratum corneum lipid composition. *Journal of Dermatological Science, 88*(1), 57–66. https://doi.org/10.1016/j.jdermsci.2017.05.005. https://www.ncbi.nlm.nih.gov/pubmed/28571749. https://www.jdsjournal.com/article/S0923-1811(16)30793-9/fulltext.

De Benedetto, A., Kubo, A., & Beck, L. A. (2012). Skin barrier disruption: A requirement for allergen sensitization? *Journal of Investigative Dermatology, 132*(3 Pt 2), 949–963. https://doi.org/10.1038/jid.2011.435. https://www.ncbi.nlm.nih.gov/pubmed/22217737. https://www.jidonline.org/article/S0022-202X(15)35605-0/pdf.

De Luca, C., & Valacchi, G. (2010). Surface lipids as multifunctional mediators of skin responses to environmental stimuli. *Mediators of Inflammation, 2010*, 321494. https://doi.org/10.1155/2010/321494. https://www.ncbi.nlm.nih.gov/pubmed/20981292.

Demehri, S., Morimoto, M., Holtzman, M. J., & Kopan, R. (2009). Skin-derived TSLP triggers progression from epidermal-barrier defects to asthma. *PLoS Biology, 7*(5), e1000067. https://doi.org/10.1371/journal.pbio.1000067. https://www.ncbi.nlm.nih.gov/pubmed/19557146.

Du Toit, G., Roberts, G., Sayre, P. H., Bahnson, H. T., Radulovic, S., Santos, A. F., et al. (2015). Randomized trial of peanut consumption in infants at risk for peanut allergy. *The New England Journal of Medicine, 372*(9), 803–813. https://doi.org/10.1056/NEJMoa1414850. https://www.ncbi.nlm.nih.gov/pubmed/25705822.

Ege, M. J., Mayer, M., Normand, A. C., Genuneit, J., Cookson, W. O., Braun-Fahrlander, C., et al. (2011). Exposure to environmental microorganisms and childhood asthma. *The New England Journal of Medicine, 364*(8), 701–709. https://doi.org/10.1056/NEJMoa1007302. https://www.ncbi.nlm.nih.gov/pubmed/21345099.

Eyerich, K., Dimartino, V., & Cavani, A. (2017). IL-17 and IL-22 in immunity: Driving protection and pathology. *European Journal of Immunology, 47*(4), 607–614. https://doi.org/10.1002/eji.201646723. https://www.ncbi.nlm.nih.gov/pubmed/28295238.

Eyerich, K., Eyerich, S., & Biedermann, T. (2015). The Multi-modal immune pathogenesis of atopic eczema. *Trends in Immunology, 36*(12), 788–801. https://doi.org/10.1016/j.it.2015.10.006. https://www.ncbi.nlm.nih.gov/pubmed/26602548.

Eyerich, K., Pennino, D., Scarponi, C., Foerster, S., Nasorri, F., Behrendt, H., et al. (2009). IL-17 in atopic eczema: Linking allergen-specific adaptive and microbial-triggered innate immune response. *The Journal of Allergy and Clinical Immunology, 123*(1), 59–66.e4. https://doi.org/10.1016/j.jaci.2008.10.031. https://www.ncbi.nlm.nih.gov/pubmed/19056110.

Furue, M., Yamamura, K., Kido-Nakahara, M., Nakahara, T., & Fukui, Y. (2018). Emerging role of interleukin-31 and interleukin-31 receptor in pruritus in atopic dermatitis. *Allergy, 73*(1), 29–36. https://doi.org/10.1111/all.13239. https://www.ncbi.nlm.nih.gov/pubmed/28670717.

Gallo, R. L., & Nakatsuji, T. (2011). Microbial symbiosis with the innate immune defense system of the skin. *Journal of Investigative Dermatology, 131*(10), 1974–1980. https://doi.org/10.1038/jid.2011.182. https://www.ncbi.nlm.nih.gov/pubmed/21697881.

Georas, S. N., & Rezaee, F. (2014). Epithelial barrier function: At the front line of asthma immunology and allergic airway inflammation. *The Journal of Allergy and Clinical Immunology, 134*(3), 509–520. https://doi.org/10.1016/j.jaci.2014.05.049. https://www.ncbi.nlm.nih.gov/pubmed/25085341.

Hermanns, H. M. (2015). Oncostatin M and interleukin-31: Cytokines, receptors, signal transduction and physiology. *Cytokine & Growth Factor Reviews, 26*(5), 545–558. https://doi.org/10.1016/j.cytogfr.2015.07.006. https://www.ncbi.nlm.nih.gov/pubmed/26198770.

Hon, K. L., Leung, A. K., & Barankin, B. (2013). Barrier repair therapy in atopic dermatitis: An overview. *Journal of the American Academy of Dermatology, 14*(5), 389–399. https://doi.org/10.1007/s40257-013-0033-9. https://www.ncbi.nlm.nih.gov/pubmed/23757122. https://link.springer.com/article/10.1007%2Fs40257-013-0033-9.

Howell, M. D., Kim, B. E., Gao, P., Grant, A. V., Boguniewicz, M., DeBenedetto, A., et al. (2009). Cytokine modulation of atopic dermatitis filaggrin skin expression. *The Journal of Allergy and Clinical Immunology, 124*(3 Suppl 2), R7–R12. https://doi.org/10.1016/j.jaci.2009.07.012. https://www.ncbi.nlm.nih.gov/pubmed/19720210. https://www.jacionline.org/article/S0091-6749(09)01122-1/pdf.

Huang, Y. J., Marsland, B. J., Bunyavanich, S., O'Mahony, L., Leung, D. Y., Muraro, A., & Fleisher, T. A. (2017). The microbiome in allergic disease: Current understanding and future opportunities-2017 PRACTALL document of the American Academy of Allergy, Asthma & Immunology and the European Academy of Allergy and Clinical Immunology. *The Journal of Allergy and Clinical Immunology, 139*(4), 1099–1110. https://doi.org/10.1016/j.jaci.2017.02.007. https://www.ncbi.nlm.nih.gov/pubmed/28257972. https://www.jacionline.org/article/S0091-6749(17)30327-5/pdf.

Janssens, M., van Smeden, J., Gooris, G. S., Bras, W., Portale, G., Caspers, P. J., et al. (2012). Increase in short-chain ceramides correlates with an altered lipid organization and decreased barrier function in atopic eczema patients. *Journal of Lipid Research, 53*(12), 2755–2766. https://doi.org/10.1194/jlr.P030338. https://www.ncbi.nlm.nih.gov/pubmed/23024286. https://www.ncbi.nlm.nih.gov/pmc/articles/PMC3494247/pdf/2755.pdf.

Jungersted, J. M., & Agner, T. (2013). Eczema and ceramides: An update. *Contact Dermatitis 69*(2), 65–71. https://doi.org/10.1111/cod.12073. https://www.ncbi.nlm.nih.gov/pubmed/23869725.

Kast, J. I., Wanke, K., Soyka, M. B., Wawrzyniak, P., Akdis, D., Kingo, K., et al. (2012). The broad spectrum of interepithelial junctions in skin and lung. *The Journal of Allergy and Clinical Immunology, 130*(2), 544–547.e4. https://doi.org/10.1016/j.jaci.2012.04.044. https://www.ncbi.nlm.nih.gov/pubmed/22704535.

Khan, S. J., Dharmage, S. C., Matheson, M. C., & Gurrin, L. C. (2018). Is the atopic march related to confounding by genetics and early-life environment? A systematic review of sibship and twin data. *Allergy, 73*(1), 17–28. https://doi.org/10.1111/all.13228. https://www.ncbi.nlm.nih.gov/pubmed/28618023.

Kong, H. H., Oh, J., Deming, C., Conlan, S., Grice, E. A., Beatson, M. A., et al. (2012). Temporal shifts in the skin microbiome associated with disease flares and treatment in children with atopic dermatitis. *Genome Research, 22*(5), 850–859. https://doi.org/10.1101/gr.131029.111. https://www.ncbi.nlm.nih.gov/pubmed/22310478.

Kubo, A., Nagao, K., & Amagai, M. (2012). Epidermal barrier dysfunction and cutaneous sensitization in atopic diseases. *Journal of Clinical Investigation, 122*(2), 440–447. https://doi.org/10.1172/JCI57416. https://www.ncbi.nlm.nih.gov/pubmed/22293182.

https://www.ncbi.nlm.nih.gov/pmc/articles/PMC3266780/pdf/JCI57416.pdf.

Lan, F., Zhang, N., Gevaert, E., Zhang, L., & Bachert, C. (2016). Viruses and bacteria in Th2-biased allergic airway disease. *Allergy, 71*(10), 1381–1392. https://doi.org/10.1111/all.12934. https://www.ncbi.nlm.nih.gov/pubmed/27188632.

Lee, E., & Hong, S. J. (2019). Phenotypes of allergic diseases in children and their application in clinical situations. *Korean Journal of Pediatrics, 62*(9), 325–333. https://doi.org/10.3345/kjp.2018.07395. https://www.ncbi.nlm.nih.gov/pubmed/31096745.

Lee, E., Lee, S. H., Kwon, J. W., Kim, Y. H., Cho, H. J., Yang, S. I., et al. (2016). Atopic dermatitis phenotype with early onset and high serum IL-13 is linked to the new development of bronchial hyperresponsiveness in school children. *Allergy, 71*(5), 692–700. https://doi.org/10.1111/all.12844. https://www.ncbi.nlm.nih.gov/pubmed/26797819.

Lee, Hae-Jin, & Lee, Seung-Hun (2014). Epidermal permeability barrier defects and barrier repair therapy in atopic dermatitis. *Allergy, Asthma & Immunology Research, 6*(4), 276–287.

Leung, D. Y., & Guttman-Yassky, E. (2014). Deciphering the complexities of atopic dermatitis: Shifting paradigms in treatment approaches. *The Journal of Allergy and Clinical Immunology, 134*(4), 769–779. https://doi.org/10.1016/j.jaci.2014.08.008. https://www.ncbi.nlm.nih.gov/pubmed/25282559. https://www.jacionline.org/article/S0091-6749(14)01159-2/pdf.

Leyva-Castillo, J. M., Hener, P., Jiang, H., & Li, M. (2013). TSLP produced by keratinocytes promotes allergen sensitization through skin and thereby triggers atopic march in mice. *Journal of Investigative Dermatology, 133*(1), 154–163. https://doi.org/10.1038/jid.2012.239. https://www.ncbi.nlm.nih.gov/pubmed/22832486.

Li, S., Ganguli-Indra, G., & Indra, AK. (2016). Lipidomic analysis of epidermal lipids: a tool to predict progression of inflammatory skin disease in humans. *Expert Rev Proteomic, 13*, 451–456.

Li, S., Villarreal, M., Stewart, S., Choi, J., Ganguli-Indra, G., Babineau, D. C., et al. (2017). Altered composition of epidermal lipids correlates with *Staphylococcus aureus* colonization status in atopic dermatitis. *British Journal of Dermatology, 177*(4), e125–e127. https://doi.org/10.1111/bjd.15409. https://www.ncbi.nlm.nih.gov/pubmed/28244066.

Linehan, J. L., Harrison, O. J., Han, S. J., Byrd, A. L., Vujkovic-Cvijin, I., Villarino, A. V., et al. (2018). Non-classical immunity controls microbiota impact on skin immunity and tissue repair. *Cell, 172*(4), 784–796.e18. https://doi.org/10.1016/j.cell.2017.12.033. https://www.ncbi.nlm.nih.gov/pubmed/29358051. https://www.cell.com/cell/pdf/S0092-8674(17)31513-1.pdf.

Loxham, M., & Davies, D. E. (2017). Phenotypic and genetic aspects of epithelial barrier function in asthmatic patients. *The Journal of Allergy and Clinical Immunology, 139*(6), 1736–1751. https://doi.org/10.1016/j.jaci.2017.04.005. https://www.ncbi.nlm.nih.gov/pubmed/28583446.

Lule, S. A., Mpairwe, H., Nampijja, M., Akello, F., Kabagenyi, J., Namara, B., et al. (2017). Life-course of atopy and allergy-related disease events in tropical sub-Saharan Africa: A birth cohort study. *Pediatric Allergy and Immunology, 28*(4), 377–383. https://doi.org/10.1111/pai.12719. https://www.ncbi.nlm.nih.gov/pubmed/28339128.

Meckfessel, M. H., & Brandt, S. (2014). The structure, function, and importance of ceramides in skin and their use as therapeutic agents in skin-care products. *Journal of the American Academy of Dermatology, 71*(1), 177–184. https://doi.org/10.1016/j.jaad.2014.01.891. https://www.ncbi.nlm.nih.gov/pubmed/24656726. https://www.jaad.org/article/S0190-9622(14)01022-6/fulltext.

Mustakallio, K. K., Kiistala, U., Piha, H. J., & Nieminen, E. (1967). Epidermal lipids in Besnier's prurigo (atopic eczema). *Annales medicinae experimentalis et biologiae Fenniae, 45*(3), 323–325. https://www.ncbi.nlm.nih.gov/pubmed/5583968.

Nakatsuji, T., Chen, T. H., Two, A. M., Chun, K. A., Narala, S., Geha, R. S., et al. (2016). *Staphylococcus aureus* exploits epidermal barrier defects in atopic dermatitis to trigger cytokine expression. *Journal of Investigative Dermatology, 136*(11), 2192–2200. https://doi.org/10.1016/j.jid.2016.05.127. https://www.ncbi.nlm.nih.gov/pubmed/27381887.

Nemoto, O., Furue, M., Nakagawa, H., Shiramoto, M., Hanada, R., Matsuki, S., et al. (2016). The first trial of CIM331, a humanized antihuman interleukin-31 receptor A antibody, in healthy volunteers and patients with atopic dermatitis to evaluate safety, tolerability and pharmacokinetics of a single dose in a randomized, double-blind, placebo-controlled study. *British Journal of Dermatology, 174*(2), 296–304. https://doi.org/10.1111/bjd.14207. https://www.ncbi.nlm.nih.gov/pubmed/26409172.

Noti, M., Kim, B. S., Siracusa, M. C., Rak, G. D., Kubo, M., Moghaddam, A. E., et al. (2014). Exposure to food allergens through inflamed skin promotes intestinal food allergy through the thymic stromal lymphopoietin-basophil axis. *The Journal of Allergy and Clinical Immunology, 133*(5), 1390–1399, 1399.e1-6. https://doi.org/10.1016/j.jaci.2014.01.021. https://www.ncbi.nlm.nih.gov/pubmed/24560412.

Odenwald, M. A., & Turner, J. R. (2013). Intestinal permeability defects: Is it time to treat? *Clinical Gastroenterology and Hepatology, 11*(9), 1075–1083. https://doi.org/10.1016/j.cgh.2013.07.001. https://www.ncbi.nlm.nih.gov/pubmed/23851019.

Pappas, A. (2009). Epidermal surface lipids. *Dermatoendocrinol, 1*, 72–76.

Park, Y. H., Jang, W. H., Seo, J. A., Park, M., Lee, T. R., Park, Y. H., et al. (2012). Decrease of ceramides with very long-chain fatty acids and downregulation of elongases in a murine atopic dermatitis model. *Journal of Investigative Dermatology, 132*(2), 476–479. https://doi.org/10.1038/jid.2011.333. https://www.ncbi.nlm.nih.gov/pubmed/22158556. https://www.jidonline.org/article/S0022-202X(15)35580-9/pdf.

Penders, J., Thijs, C., van den Brandt, P. A., Kummeling, I., Snijders, B., Stelma, F., et al. (2007). Gut microbiota composition and development of atopic manifestations in infancy: The KOALA Birth Cohort Study. *Gut, 56*(5), 661–667. https://doi.org/10.1136/gut.2006.100164. https://www.ncbi.nlm.nih.gov/pubmed/17047098. https://www.ncbi.nlm.nih.gov/pmc/articles/PMC1942165/pdf/661.pdf.

Perrigoue, J. G., Zaph, C., Guild, K., Du, Y., & Artis, D. (2009). IL-31-IL-31R interactions limit the magnitude of Th2 cytokine-dependent immunity and inflammation following intestinal helminth infection. *The Journal of Immunology, 182*(10), 6088–6094. https://doi.org/10.4049/jimmunol.0802459. https://www.ncbi.nlm.nih.gov/pubmed/19414760.

Peterson, L. W., & Artis, D. (2014). Intestinal epithelial cells: Regulators of barrier function and immune homeostasis. *Nature Reviews Immunology, 14*(3), 141–153. https://doi.org/10.1038/nri3608. https://www.ncbi.nlm.nih.gov/pubmed/24566914.

Rajka, G. (1974). Surface lipid estimation on the back of the hands in atopic dermatitis. *Archiv für dermatologische Forschung, 251*(1), 43–48. https://doi.org/10.1007/bf00561709. https://www.ncbi.nlm.nih.gov/pubmed/4282013.

Ricketts, C. R., Squire, J. R., & Topley, E. (1951). Human skin lipids with particular reference to the self-sterilising power of the skin. *Clinical Science, 10*(1), 80–110. https://www.ncbi.nlm.nih.gov/pubmed/24540677.

Roduit, C., Frei, R., Depner, M., Karvonen, A. M., Renz, H., Braun-Fahrlander, C., et al. (2017). Phenotypes of atopic dermatitis depending on the timing of onset and progression in childhood. *JAMA Pediatrics*, *171*(7), 655–662. https://doi.org/10.1001/jamapediatrics.2017.0556. https://www.ncbi.nlm.nih.gov/pubmed/28531273.

Ruzicka, T., Hanifin, J. M., Furue, M., Pulka, G., Mlynarczyk, I., Wollenberg, A., et al. (2017). Anti-interleukin-31 receptor a antibody for atopic dermatitis. *The New England Journal of Medicine*, *376*(9), 826–835. https://doi.org/10.1056/NEJMoa1606490. https://www.ncbi.nlm.nih.gov/pubmed/28249150.

Saunders, S. P., Moran, T., Floudas, A., Wurlod, F., Kaszlikowska, A., Salimi, M., et al. (2016). Spontaneous atopic dermatitis is mediated by innate immunity, with the secondary lung inflammation of the atopic march requiring adaptive immunity. *The Journal of Allergy and Clinical Immunology*, *137*(2), 482–491. https://doi.org/10.1016/j.jaci.2015.06.045. https://www.ncbi.nlm.nih.gov/pubmed/26299987. https://www.jacionline.org/article/S0091-6749(15)01022-2/pdf.

Shi, V. Y., Leo, M., Hassoun, L., Chahal, D. S., Maibach, H. I., & Sivamani, R. K. (2015). Role of sebaceous glands in inflammatory dermatoses. *Journal of the American Academy of Dermatology*, *73*(5), 856–863. https://doi.org/10.1016/j.jaad.2015.08.015. https://www.ncbi.nlm.nih.gov/pubmed/26386632. https://www.jaad.org/article/S0190-9622(15)02016-2/fulltext.

Shimura, S., Takai, T., Iida, H., Maruyama, N., Ochi, H., Kamijo, S., et al. (2016). Epicutaneous allergic sensitization by cooperation between allergen protease activity and mechanical skin barrier damage in mice. *Journal of Investigative Dermatology*, *136*(7), 1408–1417. https://doi.org/10.1016/j.jid.2016.02.810. https://www.ncbi.nlm.nih.gov/pubmed/26987428.

Smits, H. H., van der Vlugt, L. E., von Mutius, E., & Hiemstra, P. S. (2016). Childhood allergies and asthma: New insights on environmental exposures and local immunity at the lung barrier. *Current Opinion in Immunology*, *42*, 41–47. https://doi.org/10.1016/j.coi.2016.05.009. https://www.ncbi.nlm.nih.gov/pubmed/27254380.

Steelant, B., Seys, S. F., Boeckxstaens, G., Akdis, C. A., Ceuppens, J. L., & Hellings, P. W. (2016). Restoring airway epithelial barrier dysfunction: A new therapeutic challenge in allergic airway disease. *Rhinology*, *54*(3), 195–205. https://doi.org/10.4193/Rhin15.376. https://www.ncbi.nlm.nih.gov/pubmed/27316042.

Sugawara, T., Iwamoto, N., Akashi, M., Kojima, T., Hisatsune, J., Sugai, M., & Furuse, M. (2013). Tight junction dysfunction in the stratum granulosum leads to aberrant stratum corneum barrier function in claudin-1-deficient mice. *Journal of Dermatological Science*, *70*(1), 12–18. https://doi.org/10.1016/j.jdermsci.2013.01.002. https://www.ncbi.nlm.nih.gov/pubmed/23433550. https://www.jdsjournal.com/article/S0923-1811(13)00012-1/fulltext.

Sweerus, K., Lachowicz-Scroggins, M., Gordon, E., LaFemina, M., Huang, X., Parikh, M., et al. (2017). Claudin-18 deficiency is associated with airway epithelial barrier dysfunction and asthma. *The Journal of Allergy and Clinical Immunology*, *139*(1), 72–81.e1. https://doi.org/10.1016/j.jaci.2016.02.035. https://www.ncbi.nlm.nih.gov/pubmed/27215490.

Tawada, C., Kanoh, H., Nakamura, M., Mizutani, Y., Fujisawa, T., Banno, Y., & Seishima, M. (2014). Interferon-gamma decreases ceramides with long-chain fatty acids: Possible involvement in atopic dermatitis and psoriasis. *Journal of Investigative Dermatology*, *134*(3), 712–718. https://doi.org/10.1038/jid.2013.364. https://www.ncbi.nlm.nih.gov/pubmed/24008422. https://www.jidonline.org/article/S0022-202X(15)36691-4/pdf.

Thomas, C. L., & Fernandez-Penas, P. (2017). The microbiome and atopic eczema: More than skin deep. *Australasian Journal of Dermatology*, *58*(1), 18–24. https://doi.org/10.1111/ajd.12435. https://www.ncbi.nlm.nih.gov/pubmed/26821151. https://onlinelibrary.wiley.com/doi/abs/10.1111/ajd.12435.

Thyssen, J. P., & Kezic, S. (2014). Causes of epidermal filaggrin reduction and their role in the pathogenesis of atopic dermatitis. *The Journal of Allergy and Clinical Immunology*, *134*(4), 792–799. https://doi.org/10.1016/j.jaci.2014.06.014. https://www.ncbi.nlm.nih.gov/pubmed/25065719. https://www.jacionline.org/article/S0091-6749(14)00863-X/pdf.

Trompette, A., Gollwitzer, E. S., Yadava, K., Sichelstiel, A. K., Sprenger, N., Ngom-Bru, C., et al. (2014). Gut microbiota metabolism of dietary fiber influences allergic airway disease and hematopoiesis. *Nature Medicine*, *20*(2), 159–166. https://doi.org/10.1038/nm.3444. https://www.ncbi.nlm.nih.gov/pubmed/24390308.

van Smeden, J., Janssens, M., Kaye, E. C., Caspers, P. J., Lavrijsen, A. P., Vreeken, R. J., & Bouwstra, J. A. (2014). The importance of free fatty acid chain length for the skin barrier function in atopic eczema patients. *Experimental Dermatology*, *23*(1), 45–52. https://doi.org/10.1111/exd.12293. https://www.ncbi.nlm.nih.gov/pubmed/24299153. https://onlinelibrary.wiley.com/doi/abs/10.1111/exd.12293.

Watanabe, S., Narisawa, Y., Arase, S., Okamatsu, H., Ikenaga, T., Tajiri, Y., & Kumemura, M. (2003). Differences in fecal microflora between patients with atopic dermatitis and healthy control subjects. *The Journal of Allergy and Clinical Immunology*, *111*(3), 587–591. https://www.ncbi.nlm.nih.gov/pubmed/12642841.

Weidinger, S., & N. Novak. (2016). Atopic dermatitis. *Lancet 387*(10023), 1109–1122. https://doi.org/10.1016/S0140-6736(15)00149-X. https://www.ncbi.nlm.nih.gov/pubmed/26377142.

Wesemann, D. R., & Nagler, C. R. (2016). The microbiome, timing, and barrier function in the context of allergic disease. *Immunity*, *44*(4), 728–738. https://doi.org/10.1016/j.immuni.2016.02.002. https://www.ncbi.nlm.nih.gov/pubmed/27096316.

West, C. E., Ryden, P., Lundin, D., Engstrand, L., Tulic, M. K., & Prescott, S. L. (2015). Gut microbiome and innate immune response patterns in IgE-associated eczema. *Clinical & Experimental Allergy*, *45*(9), 1419–1429. https://doi.org/10.1111/cea.12566. https://www.ncbi.nlm.nih.gov/pubmed/25944283.

Wheatley, V. R. (1965). Secretions of the skin in eczema. *The Journal of Pediatrics*, *66*, 200–202. https://doi.org/10.1016/s0022-3476(65)80278-5. https://www.ncbi.nlm.nih.gov/pubmed/14246571.

Yokouchi, M., Kubo, A., Kawasaki, H., Yoshida, K., Ishii, K., Furuse, M., & Amagai, M. (2015). Epidermal tight junction barrier function is altered by skin inflammation, but not by filaggrin-deficient stratum corneum. *Journal of Dermatological Science*, *77*(1), 28–36. https://doi.org/10.1016/j.jdermsci.2014.11.007. https://www.ncbi.nlm.nih.gov/pubmed/25511077. https://www.jdsjournal.com/article/S0923-1811(14)00260-6/fulltext.

Yuki, T., Komiya, A., Kusaka, A., Kuze, T., Sugiyama, Y., & Inoue, S. (2013). Impaired tight junctions obstruct stratum corneum formation by altering polar lipid and profilaggrin processing. *Journal of Dermatological Science*, *69*(2), 148–158. https://doi.org/10.1016/j.jdermsci.2012.11.595. https://www.ncbi.nlm.nih.gov/pubmed/23273645.

Zhu, T. H., Zhu, T. R., Tran, K. A., Sivamani, R. K., & Shi, V. Y. (2018). Epithelial barrier dysfunctions in atopic dermatitis: A skin-gut-lung model linking microbiome alteration and immune dysregulation. *British Journal of Dermatology*, *179*(3), 570–581. https://doi.org/10.1111/bjd.16734. https://www.ncbi.nlm.nih.gov/pubmed/29761483.

16

Neurosensory Mechanisms

RACHEL SHIREEN GOLPANIAN, TAKASHI HASHIMOTO, AND GIL YOSIPOVITCH

KEY POINTS

- Both itch and pain are very frequent symptoms in patients with atopic dermatitis, with a prevalence of more than 50%.
- Patients with atopic dermatitis show neuronal sensitization to both itch and pain.
- Itch neuronal sensitization is associated with alloknesis (phenomena in which normal or nonpruritic stimuli are perceived as itchy) and hyperknesis (excessive itch perception to pruritic stimuli).
- Pain neuronal sensitization is associated with hyperalgesia (increased pain due to a normal noxious stimuli) and allodynia (a painful response to normally nonnoxious mechanical, tactile, or thermal stimuli).
- Neuronal sensitization to itch and pain can occur at any level of perception, including peripheral sensitization (in the skin and peripheral sensory neurons) and central sensitization (at neuronal circuits in the spinal cord, descending inhibitory pathways in the spinal cord, and the brain).

Introduction

Itch and pain are two main symptoms that play major roles in causing morbidities in patients affected by atopic dermatitis (AD). In addition, the persistence of these symptoms can significantly affect the general health of afflicted patients and even patients' family members. In this chapter we discuss the prevalence of these symptoms, the pathomechanisms of these symptoms, and the relationship between itch and pain as it occurs in AD.

Prevalence of itch and pain in atopic dermatitis

Itch is the predominant feature of AD. A study of 304 patients with AD revealed that itch occurred at least once a day in over 90% of patients with mean itch intensity of 8.3 out of 10 (Dawn et al., 2009). In another study of 170 members of the French Eczema Association, the worst pruritus intensity was 8.8 out of 10 (Huet et al., 2019).

Patient-reported outcomes collected at screening from a multinational, phase 2 clinical trial of dupilumab showed that 85% of patients reported itch with mean intensity of 6.5 out of 10 (Simpson et al., 2016).

Similar to itch, pain is one of the most frequent symptoms of AD. One study of 284 AD participants found that pain was the third most common symptom (58%) after itch (99%) and sleep difficulties (66%). Other studies also revealed a similar prevalence of pain (~50%) (Huet et al., 2019; Silverberg et al., 2019; Simpson et al., 2016). In a study of 365 AD patients, 22% of patients who reported pain rated pain intensity as 7 or greater (Silverberg et al., 2019). In a different study of 144 AD patients, 14% of patients reported severe or very severe pain (Vakharia et al., 2017).

AD patients often complain of both itch and pain, and itch and pain sensations were found to be highly correlated with one another (Dawn et al., 2009; Silverberg et al., 2019; Vakharia et al., 2017), suggesting a similarity between these phenomena. This chapter explains the neurosensory mechanisms of itch and pain in AD, focusing on neuronal sensitization, a phenomenon in which a minimal sensory stimulus results in an enhanced neural response (Yosipovitch, Berger, & Fassett, 2020).

Pathogenesis of itch in atopic dermatitis and neuronal sensitization

Pathogenesis of itch in atopic dermatitis

Itch begins at the skin when unmyelinated, itch-selective C fibers are activated by pruritogen(s) in the epidermis and dermal-epidermal junction. Pruritogens are substances or molecules that have the potential to cause itch (Table 16.1). These nerve fibers are categorized as histaminergic or nonhistaminergic depending on the receptors they express. Activation of these receptors results in the opening of ion channels, which leads to induction of an action potential. This signal is then transmitted to the spinal cord via the spinothalamic/spinoparabrachial tract, and is ultimately processed in the cerebral cortex of brain, which interprets and signals "itch" to the patient (Yosipovitch, Rosen, & Hashimoto, 2018).

<table>
<tr><td colspan="2">TABLE
16.1   **Major pruritogens in atopic dermatitis**</td></tr>
</table>

Category	Pruritogens
Neuropeptide	NGF Substance P, acetylcholine, GRP
Protease	Tryptase, cathepsin S, kallikreins
Amines	Histamine, serotonin, bradykinin, endothelin
Cytokines	IL2, IL4/IL13 IL31 IL33 TSLP IL17A, IL17C
Lipid mediators	PGE2, phospholipase A2

GRP, Gastrin-releasing peptide; *IL*, interleukin; *NGF*, nerve growth factor; *PGE2*, prostaglandin E2; *TSLP*, thymic stromal lymphopoietin.

Note that histaminergic and nonhistaminergic nerve fibers transmit itch via separate neural tracts in the peripheral and central nervous system (Yosipovitch et al., 2018, 2020).

Neuronal sensitization of itch

The perception threshold of itch is significantly lower in AD patients as compared with healthy controls. Itch neuronal sensitization is represented by two classically known phenomena: alloknesis and hyperknesis. Alloknesis is a phenomena in which normal or nonpruritic stimuli are perceived as itchy. Hyperknesis is excessive itch perception to pruritic stimuli (Andersen, Akiyama, et al., 2018). Neuronal sensitization can occur due to various factors acting at the peripheral level (i.e., the skin) or at the central level (i.e., the brain or spinal cord). Peripheral sensitization is characterized by hypersensitivity of sensory neurons to itch stimuli caused by inflammatory mediators. Central sensitization is promoted by upregulation of itch-related receptors and molecules, dysfunction of the inhibitor circuits in the spinal cord, attenuation of descending inhibitory pathways in the spinal cord, and functional and structural changes in the brain (Yosipovitch et al., 2018) (Fig. 16.1).

The epidermis, barrier dysfunction, and neuronal sensitization

The role of barrier dysfunction in AD-associated itch is multifactorial. Cross-talk between nerve fibers may be an explanation (Yosipovitch & Papoiu, 2008). Impaired barrier function can promote entry of pruritogens such as allergens and proteases into the skin. In addition, damage to the stratum corneum may lead to pruritogen release by keratinocytes (Yosipovitch, 2004). The acidity of the stratum corneum is important for barrier formation and defense

against bacteria, and skin pH in AD patients was shown to be elevated. High skin pH enhances the activity of proteases, which can act as pruritogens, thus contributing to itch in AD.

Nerve growth factor (NGF) is a neuropeptide that is secreted mainly by epidermal keratinocytes and promotes neural survival. Expression of NGF and its high-affinity receptor TrkA (tropomyosin receptor kinase A) is increased in AD. NGF may sensitize peripheral nerve endings through promotion of nerve sprouting and elongation (Ikoma, Steinhoff, Ständer, Yosipovitch, & Schmelz, 2006). NGF is also capable of increasing sensory nerve sensitivity to substance P and brain-derived neurotrophic factor (BDNF), which further contributes to the lowered itch threshold seen in AD patients.

Itch mediators in the skin and neuronal sensitization

Receptors

Unmyelinated C fibers transmit itch upon activation of specific receptors. The majority of these receptors are G protein–coupled receptors (GPCRs). A notable receptor within GPCRs is protease-activated receptor-2 (PAR2), which can be activated by various proteases such as tryptase (a secretary granule primarily by mast cells) and dust mites (Mollanazar, Smith, & Yosipovitch, 2016). AD patients exhibited increased levels of tryptase in lesional skin and PAR2 in both lesional and nonlesional skin (Steinhoff et al., 2003). Administration of a PAR2 agonist caused prolonged itching in AD patients (Steinhoff et al., 2003).

Ion channels

When pruritogens encounter their receptors on C nerve fibers, calcium influx through specific ion channels is required to generate action potentials and propagate the itch signal. These ion channels include the transient receptor potential (TRP) family, which is a main component of all sensory perception, including itch, and voltage-gated sodium ion channels (Na_v).

TRP vanilloid 1 (TRPV1) exhibited increased expression in AD lesions, and its activation results in inflammation and pruritus. TRP ankyrin 1 (TRPA1) is involved in the transmission of histamine-independent itch. TRPA1 expression is enhanced in lesional skin of AD compared to healthy controls (Oh et al., 2013). PAR2 can sensitize TRP channels, including TRPV1 and TRPA1 on peripheral nerve fibers, resulting in peripheral neuronal sensitization (Amadesi et al., 2006).

TRPV1/TRPA1 activates $Na_v1.7$, a subtype of the Na_v family. $Na_v1.7$ controls action potentials in itch mediation. $Na_v1.7$ mRNA expression is enhanced in pruritic skin lesion in AD (Nattkemper et al., 2018). In addition, a monoclonal antibody against $Na_v1.7$ attenuates itch sensation and pain

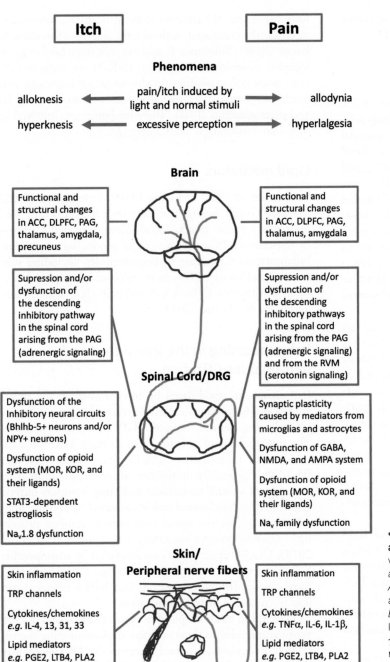

• **Fig. 16.1** Neuronal sensitization of itch and pain in atopic dermatitis. Neural sensitivity can be induced by various causes in the skin, dorsal root ganglia, spinal cord, and brain. *5-HT*, Serotonin; *ACC*, anterior cingulate cortex; *AMPA*, α-amino-3-hydroxy-5-methyl-4-isoxazolepropionic acid receptor; *BDNF*, brain-derived neurotrophic factor; *Bhlhb-5*, helix-loop-helix family member B5; *DLPFC*, dorso-lateral prefrontal cortex; *DRG*, dorsal root ganglion; *GABA*, γ-amino butyric acid; *KOR*, κ-opioid receptor; *LTB4*, leukot-riene B4; *MOR*, μ-opioid receptor; *NGF*, nerve growth factor; *NPY*, neuropeptide Y; *PAG*, periaqueductal gray matter; *PGE2*, prostaglandin E2; *PLA2*, phospholipase A2; *RVM*, rostroventral medulla; *SP*, substance P.

(Lee et al., 2014). Conversely, overactivity of $Na_v1.7$, which may be induced by skin inflammation, can lead to peripheral neuronal sensitization of itch.

Amines

Histamine is a prototype pruritogen that is involved in acute itch and released primarily by mast cells, basophils, and keratinocytes. However, psychophysiologic studies demonstrated that AD patients showed nonhistaminergic neuronal

itch sensitization (but not histaminergic itch sensitization) (Andersen, Elberling, Sharma et al., 2017) and that antihistamines are not effective in treating chronic itch in AD. Thus nonhistaminergic causes are now considered to play a central role in AD itch (Ikoma et al., 2006). Histamine may play a partial role in chronic itch of AD as studies involving blockers against H4R, a subtype of histamine receptor, have shown promising results (Murata et al., 2015).

Furthermore, serotonin and bradykinin, molecules which normally function as endogenous algogens (pain-inducing agents), can cause neuronal sensitization and serve as potent nonhistaminergic pruritogens in lesional skin of AD.

Cytokines

Th2-related cytokines, such as interleukin-4 (IL4), IL13, IL31, and IL33, are known to be involved in the pathogenesis of AD and also reported to be involved in peripheral neuronal sensitization in AD. IL4 and IL13 are canonical Th2-related cytokines that help to drive AD (Mollanazar et al., 2016), and their expression is increased in lesional skin of AD. IL13 was shown to be a potent stimulator of itch in murine AD model and to strongly stimulate TRPA1 expression on nerve fibers (Oh et al., 2013). In addition, IL4/IL13 can sensitize sensory neurons via IL4 receptor subunit α (IL4Rα). Dupilumab, an anti-IL4Rα monoclonal antibody, can greatly improve pruritus in AD even before the improvement of skin symptoms, indicating a promoting role of IL4/IL13 in the development of itch (Simpson et al., 2016).

IL31 is generated mainly by activated Th2 cells and has been coined the "itchy cytokine." IL31 receptor transcripts are abundantly expressed in dorsal root ganglia (Sonkoly et al., 2006). Lesional IL31 expression was increased in AD compared with controls. Serum IL31 levels were correlated with disease activity in AD. IL31 provokes pruritus through directly stimulating sensory neurons and may do so indirectly through its interaction with keratinocytes (Cevikbas et al., 2014). Additionally, IL31 was also shown to induce sensory nerve elongation and branching, resulting in peripheral neuronal sensitization (Feld et al., 2016). Nemolizumab, an anti-IL31 receptor A monoclonal antibody, dramatically improves itch in AD patients.

IL33 is a keratinocyte-derived cytokine. Lesional IL33 levels were increased in AD patients. Serum IL33 levels were correlated with disease severity (Tamagawa-Mineoka, Okuzawa, Masuda, & Katoh, 2014). IL33 can trigger Th2-associated inflammation and directly stimulate itch sensory neurons (Liu et al., 2016). IL33 also can contribute to peripheral neuron sensitization in immune inflammation responses (Fattori et al., 2017).

Thymic stromal lymphopoietin (TSLP) and IL17A are also implicated in AD-associated itch. They are reported to play a role in pain neuronal sensitization and may be involved itch neuronal sensitization; however, there is no direct evidence for this. TSLP is a Th2-related cytokine secreted by keratinocytes partially via PAR2 and is able to directly stimulate itch sensory neurons via TRPA1 (Wilson et al., 2013). IL17A is a Th17-related cytokine involved in the acute phase of AD. mRNA expression of IL17A and its related cytokine IL23A is enhanced in itchy AD lesions compared with nonitchy skin (Nattkemper et al., 2018).

Neuropeptides

Aside from NGF, substance P is another tachykinin neuropeptide implicated in AD itch. Plasma substance P levels were higher in AD patients than in healthy controls and significantly correlated with disease activity (Salomon & Baran, 2008). Substance P initiates itch once bound to its receptor neurokinin receptor-1 (NK-1) on various cells (e.g., mast cells), resulting in the release of histamine and nonhistaminergic itchy mediators such as leukotrienes (LTs) and prostaglandins (PGs). These mediators are involved in neuronal sensitization (see Chapter 2).

Lipid mediators

Production of PGs, including PGE2, is increased in AD lesions. PGs can directly stimulate their receptors expressed on sensory nerve fibers. In addition, activated C fibers in response to PGs are capable of producing neurogenic inflammation via release of neuropeptides, including substance P. In this way, PGs can be involved in peripheral neuronal sensitization to both itch and pain (Ji, Nackley, Huh, Terrando, & Maixner, 2018).

Itch processing in the spinal cord and neuronal sensitization

Itch signals are modulated by interneurons in the spinal cord (Fig. 16.2). Chemical itch is transmitted through gastrin-releasing peptide receptor (GRPR) positive neurons. The transmission of chemical itch through GRPR+ neurons can be inhibited by helix-loop-helix family member B5 (Bhlhb5)–positive inhibitory interneurons upon their secretion of several molecules, including γ-amino butyric acid (GABA). Mechanical itch is conveyed by another itch-related circuit in the spinal cord, which involves urocortin 3 (Ucn3)–positive excitatory interneurons (Pan et al., 2019). Ucn3+ interneurons are inhibited by neuropeptide Y (NPY)–positive neurons. Dysfunction of inhibitory neuronal circuits (Bhlhb5+ neurons and NPY+ neurons) can lead to enhanced neural sensitization.

Dynorphin binds κ-opioid receptors (KORs) on GRPR+ neurons and inhibits these neurons, thus attenuating chemical itch. In contrast, μ-opioid receptors (MORs) antagonize this inhibition (Yosipovitch et al., 2018). Thus an imbalance between KORs and MORs may result in exaggerated neuronal sensitization. AD patients have increased serum levels of endogenous μ-opioid agonists (i.e., β-endorphin) compared with controls, and these levels correlate with disease severity and itch intensity (Lee et al., 2006).

Astrocytes in the spinal cord act on GRPR+ interneurons through lipocalin-2 secretion, resulting in prolongation of itch sensation in a STAT3-dependent manner (Shiratori-Hayashi et al., 2015). Astrocytes are also activated through toll-like receptor 4 signaling, resulting in exacerbation of chronic itch.

The supraspinal areas of the spinal cord such as the periaqueductal gray (PAG) matter give rise to a descending inhibitory pathway of itch. This inhibition is mediated through α_2-adrenoreceptor on Bhlhb5+ neurons.

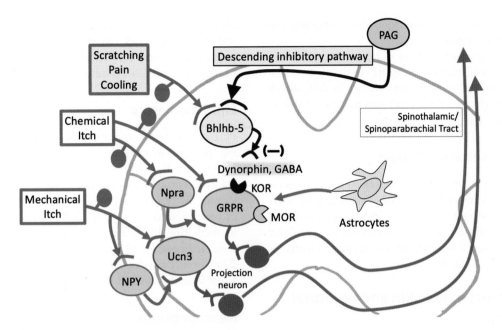

• **Fig. 16.2** The spinal neuronal circuit involved in itch perception in atopic dermatitis. Chemical itch is transmitted through gastrin-releasing peptide receptor *(GRPR)*–positive neurons. This transmission can be inhibited by helix-loop-helix family member B5 *(Bhlhb5)*–positive inhibitory interneurons upon secretion of several molecules, including γ-amino butyric acid *(GABA)* and dynorphin. Dynorphin binds κ-opioid receptors *(KORs)* on GRPR+ neurons and inhibits these neurons, thus attenuating chemical itch. In contrast, μ-opioid receptors *(MORs)* antagonize this inhibition. Astrocytes in the spinal cord act on GRPR+ interneurons. Mechanical itch is conveyed by another itch-related circuit in the spinal cord, which involves urocortin 3 *(Ucn3)*–positive excitatory interneurons. Ucn3+ interneurons are inhibited by neuropeptide Y *(NPY)*–positive neurons. The supraspinal areas of the spinal cord such as the periaqueductal gray *(PAG)* matter give rise to a descending inhibitory pathway of itch.

Suppression/dysfunction of this pathway may lead to neuronal hypersensitivity (Murota & Katayama, 2017).

Itch processing in the brain and neuronal sensitization

After undergoing modulation in the spinal cord, itch signals are transmitted to various brain areas. AD patients showed a more diffuse brain activation pattern associated with itch compared to healthy subjects (Ishiuji et al., 2009). There was a significant correlation between brain activity in the anterior cingulate cortex (ACC) and contralateral insula and histamine-induced itch intensity (Ishiuji et al., 2009). In addition, increased brain activity in these areas in addition to the dorsolateral prefrontal cortex (DLPFC) were also positively correlated with disease severity, suggesting that brain activity of acute itch in AD differs from that of healthy subjects. In another study, brain activity was significantly higher in the thalamus, precuneus, caudate, and pallidum of AD patients as compared to healthy controls (Schneider et al., 2008). Itch can be aggravated by chronic stress. Itch signals are projected into the amygdala, the center of emotion processing, from the thalamus and parabrachial nucleus. Chronic stress can induce hyperexcitability of the amygdala, and this may result in an increase in negative reaction, anxiety, and itch (Pavlenko & Akiyama, 2019). The PAG in the midbrain is part of the descending inhibitory pathway of itch in the spinal cord. Suppression/dysfunction of this pathway may lead

to neuronal hypersensitivity (Murota & Katayama, 2017). These brain changes may be responsible for neural sensitization to itch. In addition, these involved brain areas, including the thalamus, amygdala, ACC, and PAG, can be implicated in chronic pain, as patients with chronic pain show increases in excitability of these brain areas (Latremoliere & Woolf, 2009). This suggests that overactivity of these areas in AD-associated itch can attribute to itch and pain in AD.

Pathogenesis of pain in atopic dermatitis and neuronal sensitization

Pathogenesis of pain in atopic dermatitis

Similar to the sensation of itch, pain sensation is conducted by peripheral nerve fibers to the neuronal circuit in the spinal cord, and then ascends to the brain, where pain is processed. The term *nociceptor* indicates a specialized subset of sensory neurons that are involved in pain conduction. Nociceptor neurons have three subclasses: C fibers, Aβ neurons, and Aδ neurons. C fibers are nonmyelinated, slow-conducting fibers that are mostly capsaicin sensitive and often convey thermal pain. Aβ and Aδ neurons are myelinated, faster-conducting fibers that mediate mechanosensation and mechanical pain sensitivity. Nociceptors express various types of ion channels, receptors, and neuropeptides. Nociceptors are able to respond to mechanical, chemical, and/or thermal (both heat and cold) noxious stimuli through these receptors and channels. Activation of these receptors and channels generate action potentials required for conveying pain signals through nociceptor neurons.

Mediators uniquely involved in AD-associated pain have yet to be elucidated, but importantly, classic pain mediators are also involved in itch transmission in AD, which leads to the thought that these mediators may play a role in AD-related pain.

Neuronal sensitization of pain

Pain sensitization is defined as an increased responsiveness of nociceptor neurons to their normal or subthreshold afferent input. Hyperalgesia is defined as increased pain due to normal noxious stimuli, while allodynia means a painful response to normally nonnoxious mechanical, tactile, or thermal stimuli (see Fig. 16.1).

Pain mediators in the skin and neuronal sensitization

Ion channels

TRP channels are involved in the generation of action potential generation in nerve fibers. TRPV1 can be activated by capsaicin and heat stimuli (>42ºC), while TRPA1 is activated by allyl isothiocyanate (found in wasabi and mustard oils) and cold stimuli (<17ºC) (Moore et al., 2018).

Voltage-gated sodium ion channels ($Na_v1.7$, $Na_v1.8$, and $Na_v1.9$), which are activated by TRPA1/TRPV1, control action potentials. Loss of function of $Na_v1.7$ may lead to impaired pain perception. Gain of function of $Na_v1.7$, $Na_v1.8$, and $Na_v1.9$ may result in increased pain perception found in inherited erythromelalgia and painful neuropathy (Cardoso & Lewis, 2018). mRNA expression of $Na_v1.7$ and $Na_v1.9$ is enhanced in pruritic skin lesion in AD (Nattkemper et al., 2018). A monoclonal antibody that targets $Na_v1.7$ attenuates both itch and pain (caused by both inflammatory and neuropathic causes) (Lee et al., 2014). Inflammatory skin diseases such as AD may enhance the function of these channels, resulting in heightened pain sensitivity. Taken together, $Na_v1.7$ may be crucial in pain and itch in AD.

Amines

Nociceptor neurons express histamine receptors (H1 and H2). Activation of these receptors increase the expression of $Na_v1.8$, leading to sensitization to mechanical and thermal stimuli (Yu et al., 2013). Serotonin acts on nociceptor neurons via 5-HT2, a subtype of the serotonin receptor, and can increase pain sensitivity.

Cytokines

A variety of inflammatory cytokines are involved in chronic pain through directly activating nociceptor neurons via their receptors. These cytokines include TNF-α, IL6, and IL1β (mainly from mast cells, neutrophils, and macrophages), IL5 (mainly from mast cells), and IL17A (mainly from Th17 cells and γδT cells). They can also stimulate PG synthesis and potentiate activation of TRP and Na_v, resulting in rapid sensitization of nociceptors (Pinho-Ribeiro, Verri, & Chiu, 2017).

Lipid mediators

PGE2 can boost inflammatory pain through sensitizing nociceptor neurons via its receptors EP1 to EP4. Leukotriene B-4 (LTB4) can activate C fibers and Aδ fibers via its receptor BLT1 involved in pain. In pruritic AD skin lesions, mRNA expression of phospholipase A2 (PLA2) was increased (Nattkemper et al., 2018). PLA2 may be involved in mediating histamine-induced and SP-induced itch in C nerve fibers. PLA2 is also known to be involved in pain (Davidson & Giesler, 2010). Taken together, PLA2 can play a role in both pain and itch in AD.

Neuropeptides

NGF and its receptor TrkA cause axon terminal-sprouting of nociceptor neurons, resulting in pain sensitivity. TrkA-activation also can rapidly sensitize nociceptor neurons. SP is implicated in chronic pain through nociceptive sensitization.

Pain processing in the spinal cord and neuronal sensitization

In the spinal cord, nociceptors generate and release mediators, including cytokines (e.g., C-C motif chemokine [CCL2], TNF-α), neurotransmitters (e.g., calcitonin-related gene peptide, glutamate), neuropeptides (e.g., substance P), and growth factors (e.g., colony-stimulating factor-1). These mediators activate microglial cells and astrocytes. Microglial cells and astrocytes in turn release inflammatory mediators (including cytokines [e.g., IL1β, TNF-α, CCL2, CXCL1], growth factors [e.g., BDNF], and PGs [e.g., PGE2]), which promote synaptic plasticity and induce amplification of pain sensitivity (spinal sensitization) in peripheral nerve fibers and second-order neurons (interneurons). Glutamate N-methyl-D-aspartate (NMDA) receptors on postsynaptic neurons and insertion of α-amino-3-hydroxy-5-methyl-4-isoxazole propionic acid (AMPA) receptors in the plasma membrane, in addition to extracellular signal regulated kinase (ERK) activation in the postsynaptic neurons, are also involved in synaptic plasticity, which induces and maintains central pain sensitization (Ji et al., 2018; Latremoliere & Woolf, 2009). Both peripheral nerve fibers and interneurons express opioid receptors (especially MOR), and stimulation of MOR can inhibit neuronal activation and relieve pain.

Similar to itch, pain sensation can be inhibited by descending pathways. There are two types of descending inhibitory pathways emanating from the PAG in the brainstem. One pathway travels through the locus coeruleus to the spinal cord and involves norepinephrine/α₂-adrenoreceptor signaling. The other pathway descends via the rostroventral medulla (RVM) and involves serotonin/serotonin receptor signaling

(Yoshimura & Furue, 2006). In the RVM, neurons are regulated by opioids/μ-opioid receptors and GABA/GABA receptors (François et al., 2017). Attenuation of these descending inhibitory pathways may result in pain neuronal sensitization.

Pain processing in the brain and neuronal sensitization

After being processed in the spinal cord, pain sensation is conducted through the spinothalamic tract to the thalamus in the brain and subsequently projected to various brain areas. The ACC and insular cortex are reported to be the main brain structures involved in pain perception. Other areas also involved in pain processing include the somatosensory cortex, prefrontal cortex, posterior cingulate cortex, thalamus, amygdala, hippocampus, hypothalamus, ventral striatum, PAG, and cerebellum. These areas may show functional and/or structural changes caused by chronic pain conditions, which may be responsible for neuronal sensitization of AD pain. However, no papers are currently available on brain changes regarding pain in AD. However, as mentioned earlier, similar structures such as the thalamus, amygdala, ACC, and PAG are also overactivated in chronic itch in AD, and it may be likely that overactivity of these areas in AD-associated itch can attribute to pain in AD (Latremoliere & Woolf, 2009).

Association of itch and pain in atopic dermatitis

Several studies on pain in AD demonstrated that nociceptive symptoms are more evident in inflammatory itch rather than in neuropathic itch in chronic pruritus patients (Rosen, Fostini, Chan, Nattkemper, & Yosipovitch, 2018). It is also reported that about half of AD patients felt that pain occurred after scratching in itchy areas, fissures, or inflamed skin, or that their pain was attributable at least partially to scratching (Silverberg et al., 2019; Thyssen, Halling-Sønderby, Wu, & Egeberg, 2020; Vakharia et al., 2017). On the other hand, about 20% of patients reported their skin pain was part of their itch (Vakharia et al., 2017). Our group has reported that, compared with healthy individuals, AD patients perceived higher itch from cowhage (a beanlike plant native in the tropics) but not significantly from histamine in lesional and non-lesional skin. In addition, AD patients had decreased lesional mechanical detection thresholds and increased lesional and extralesional sensitivity to mechanical pain (hyperalgesia) provoked with pinprick. AD patients also showed intralesional and extralesional hyperknesis before itch provocations with histamine or cowhage, and augmented hyperknesis after itch provocations. This data suggest that these patients have increased susceptibility to mechanically evoked itch and pain (i.e., sensitization of mechanosensitive circuitry) (Andersen, Elberling, Sharma, et al., 2017).

In general, pain sensation inhibits itch sensation via the inhibitory neuronal circuit in the spinal cord; pain sensation conveyed by TRPV1/TPRA1+ nerves stimulates Bhlhb-5+ inhibitory interneurons, which suppress GRPR+ excitatory

interneurons (Andersen, Elberling, Sølvsten, et al., 2017; Yosipovitch et al., 2018). However, itch and pain in AD largely share similar neurosensory mechanisms, and they may coexist in a significant proportion of AD patients. The explanation for this is still uncertain, but one may consider that a maladaptive central processing of itch can lead to a blunting of normal pain-induced itch suppression (Andersen, Yosipovitch, & Arendt-Nielsen, 2018). Another explanation would be scratching pleasurability. Scratching not only relieves itch, but also can be rewarding and addictive. These phenomena are explained by activation of certain brain areas involved in the reward system (Ishiuji, 2019; Yosipovitch et al., 2018). The pleasure from scratching may cause further scratching even though patients feel scratch-induced pain.

Summary

Both itch and pain are common symptoms in AD patients, and AD patients may show neuronal sensitization to itch and pain. The mechanisms underlying neuronal sensitization to itch and pain share many similarities. These processes can occur at any level of perception, including the skin, peripheral sensory neurons, neuronal circuits in the spinal cord, descending inhibitory pathways in the spinal cord, and the brain.

Further readings

Carstens, E., & Akiyama, T. (Eds.). (2014). *Itch: Mechanisms and treatment*. CRC Press.
Ma, C., & Huang, Y. (Eds.), (2016). *Translational research in pain and itch*. Springer.
Yosipovitch, G., Greaves, M. W., Fleischer, A. B., & McGlone, F. (Eds.), (2004). *Itch: Basic mechanisms and therapy*. CRC Press.

References

Amadesi, S., Cottrell, G. S., Divino, L., Chapman, K., Grady, E. F., Bautista, F., et al. (2006). Protease-activated receptor 2 sensitizes TRPV1 by protein kinase Cε- and A-dependent mechanisms in rats and mice. *The Journal of Physiology*, *575*(2), 555–571.
Andersen, H. H., Akiyama, T., Nattkemper, L. A., van Laarhoven, A., Elberling, J., Yosipovitch, G., et al. (2018). Alloknesis and hyperknesis-mechanisms, assessment methodology, and clinical implications of itch sensitization. *Pain*, *159*(7), 1185–1197.
Andersen, H. H., Elberling, J., Sharma, N., Hauberg, L. E., Gazerani, P., & Arendt-Nielsen, L. (2017). Histaminergic and non-histaminergic elicited itch is attenuated in capsaicin-evoked areas of allodynia and hyperalgesia: A healthy volunteer study. *European Journal of Pain (United Kingdom)*, *21*(6), 1098–1109.
Andersen, H. H., Elberling, J., Sølvsten, H., Yosipovitch, G., & Arendt-Nielsen, L. (2017). Nonhistaminergic and mechanical itch sensitization in atopic dermatitis. *Pain*, *158*(9), 1780–1791.
Andersen, H. H., Yosipovitch, G., & Arendt-Nielsen, L. (2018). Pain inhibits itch, but not in atopic dermatitis? *Annals of Allergy, Asthma & Immunology*, *120*(5), 548–549.
Cardoso, F. C., & Lewis, R. J. (2018). Sodium channels and pain: From toxins to therapies. *The British Journal of Pharmacology*, *175*(12), 2138–2157.

Cevikbas, F., Wang, X., Akiyama, T., Kempkes, C., Savinko, T., Antal, A., et al. (2014). A sensory neuron-expressed IL-31 receptor mediates T helper cell-dependent itch: Involvement of TRPV1 and TRPA1. *The Journal of Allergy and Clinical Immunology, 133*(2), 448–460.

Davidson, S., & Giesler, G. J. (2010). The multiple pathways for itch and their interactions with pain. *Trends in Neurosciences, 33*(12), 550–558.

Dawn, A., Papoiu, A. D., Chan, Y. H., Rapp, S. R., Rassette, N., & Yosipovitch, G. (2009). Itch characteristics in atopic dermatitis: results of a web-based questionnaire. *British Journal of Dermatology, 160*(3), 642–644.

Fattori, V., Hohmann, M. S. N., Rossaneis, A. C., Manchope, M. F., Alves-Filho, J. C., Cunha, T. M., et al. (2017). Targeting IL-33/ST2 signaling: Regulation of immune function and analgesia. *Expert Opinion on Therapeutic Targets, 21*(12), 1141–1152.

Feld, M., Garcia, R., Buddenkotte, J., Katayama, S., Lewis, K., Muirhead, G., et al. (2016). The pruritus- and TH 2-associated cytokine IL-31 promotes growth of sensory nerves. *The Journal of Allergy and Clinical Immunology, 138*(2), 500–508. e24.

François, A., Low, S. A., Sypek, E. I., Christensen, A. J., Sotoudeh, C., Beier, K. T., et al. (2017). A brainstem-spinal cord inhibitory circuit for mechanical pain modulation by GABA and enkephalins. *Neuron, 93*(4), 822–839. e6.

Huet, F., Faffa, M. S., Poizeau, F., Merhand, S., Misery, L., & Brenaut, E. (2019). Characteristics of pruritus in relation to self-assessed severity of atopic dermatitis. *Acta Dermato-Venereologica, 99*(3), 279–283.

Ikoma, A., Steinhoff, M., Ständer, S., Yosipovitch, G., & Schmelz, M. (2006). The neurobiology of itch. *Nature Reviews Neuroscience, 7*(7), 535–547.

Ishiuji, Y. (2019). Addiction and the itch-scratch cycle. What do they have in common? *Experimental Dermatology, 28*(12), 1448–1454.

Ishiuji, Y., Coghill, R. C., Patel, T. S., Oshiro, Y., Kraft, R. A., & Yosipovitch, G. (2009). Distinct patterns of brain activity evoked by histamine-induced itch reveal an association with itch intensity and disease severity in atopic dermatitis. *The British Journal of Dermatology, 161*(5), 1072–1080.

Ji, R. R., Nackley, A., Huh, Y., Terrando, N., & Maixner, W. (2018). Neuroinflammation and central sensitization in chronic and widespread pain. *Anesthesiology, 129*(2), 343–366.

Latremoliere, A., & Woolf, C. J. (2009). Central sensitization: A generator of pain hypersensitivity by central neural plasticity. *The Journal of Pain: Official Journal of the American Pain Society, 10*(9), 895–926.

Lee, C. H., Chuang, H. Y., Shih, C. C., Jong, S. B., Chang, C. H., & Yu, H. S. (2006). Transepidermal water loss, serum IgE and β-endorphin as important and independent biological markers for development of itch intensity in atopic dermatitis. *The British Journal of Dermatology, 154*(6), 1100–1107.

Lee, J. H., Park, C. K., Chen, G., Han, Q., Xie, R. G., Liu, T., et al. (2014). A monoclonal antibody that targets a Na$_v$1.7 channel voltage sensor for pain and itch relief. *Cell, 157*(6), 1393–1404.

Liu, B., Tai, Y., Achanta, S., Kaelberer, M. M., Caceres, A. I., Shao, X., et al. (2016). IL-33/ST2 signaling excites sensory neurons and mediates itch response in a mouse model of poison ivy contact allergy. *Proceedings of the National Academy of Sciences of the United States of America, 113*(47), E7579–E7579.

Mollanazar, N. K., Smith, P. K., & Yosipovitch, G. (2016). Mediators of chronic pruritus in atopic dermatitis: Getting the itch out? *Clinical Reviews in Allergy and Immunology, 51*(3), 263–292.

Moore, C., Gupta, R., Jordt, S. E., Chen, Y., & Liedtke, W. B. (2018). Regulation of pain and itch by TRP channels. *Neuroscience bulletin, 34*(1), 120–142.

Murata, Y., Song, M., Kikuchi, H., Hisamichi, K., Xu, X. L., Greenspan, A., et al. (2015). Phase 2a, randomized, double-blind, placebo-controlled, multicenter, parallel-group study of a H4 R-antagonist (JNJ-39758979) in Japanese adults with moderate atopic dermatitis. *The Journal of Dermatology. Research & Development, Janssen Pharmaceutical KK, Tokyo, Japan: Japanese Dermatological Association, 42*(2), 129–139.

Murota, H., & Katayama, I. (2017). Exacerbating factors of itch in atopic dermatitis. *Allergology International: Official Journal of the Japanese Society of Allergology, 66*(1), 8–13.

Nattkemper, L. A., Tey, H. L., Valdes-Rodriguez, R., Lee, H., Mollanazar, N. K., Albornoz, C., et al. (2018). The genetics of chronic itch: Gene expression in the skin of patients with atopic dermatitis and psoriasis with severe itch. *The Journal of Investigative Dermatology, 138*(6), 1311–1317.

Oh, M.-H., Oh, S. Y., Lu, J., Lou, H., Myers, A. C., Zhu, Z., & Zheng, T. (2013). TRPA1-dependent pruritus in IL-13–induced chronic atopic dermatitis. *Journal of Immunology, 191*(11), 5371–5382.

Pan, H., Fatima, M., Li, A., Lee, H., Cai, W., Horwitz, L., et al. (2019). Identification of a spinal circuit for mechanical and persistent spontaneous itch. *Neuron, 103*(6), 1135–1149. e6.

Pavlenko, D., & Akiyama, T. (2019). Why does stress aggravate itch? A possible role of the amygdala. *Experimental Dermatology, 28*(12), 1439–1441.

Pinho-Ribeiro, F. A., Verri, W. A., & Chiu, I. M. (2017). Nociceptor sensory neuron–immune interactions in pain and inflammation. *Trends in Immunology, 38*(1), 5–19.

Rosen, J. D., Fostini, A. C., Chan, Y. H., Nattkemper, L. A., & Yosipovitch, G. (2018). A cross-sectional study of clinical distinctions between neuropathic and inflammatory pruritus. *Journal of the American Academy of Dermatology, 79*(6), 1143–1144.

Salomon, J., & Baran, E. (2008). The role of selected neuropeptides in pathogenesis of atopic dermatitis. *The Journal of the European Academy of Dermatology and Venereology, 22*(2), 223–228.

Schneider, G., Ständer, S., Burgmer, M., Driesch, G., Heuft, G., & Weckesser, M. (2008). Significant differences in central imaging of histamine-induced itch between atopic dermatitis and healthy subjects. *European Journal of Pain, 12*(7), 834–841.

Shiratori-Hayashi, M., Koga, K., Tozaki-Saitoh, H., Kohro, Y., Toyonaga, H., Yamaguchi, C., et al. (2015). STAT3-dependent reactive astrogliosis in the spinal dorsal horn underlies chronic itch. *Nature Medicine, 21*(8), 927–931.

Silverberg, J. I., Gelfand, J. M., Margolis, D. J., Boguniewicz, M., Fonacier, L., Grayson, M. H., et al. (2019). Pain is a common and burdensome symptom of atopic dermatitis in United States adults. *The Journal of Allergy and Clinical Immunology, 7*(8), 2699–2706.e7.

Simpson, E. L., Bieber, T., Eckert, L., Wu, R., Ardeleanu, M., Graham, N. M. H., et al. (2016). Patient burden of moderate to severe atopic dermatitis (AD): Insights from a phase 2b clinical trial of dupilumab in adults. *Journal of the American Academy of Dermatology, 74*(3), 491–498.

Sonkoly, E., Muller, A., Lauerma, A. I., Pivarcsi, A., Soto, H., Kemeny, L., et al. (2006). IL-31: A new link between T cells and pruritus in atopic skin inflammation. *The Journal of Allergy and Clinical Immunology, 117*(2), 411–417.

Steinhoff, M., Neisius, U., Ikoma, A., Fartasch, M., Heyer, G., Skov, P. S., et al. (2003). Proteinase-activated receptor-2 mediates itch: A novel pathway for pruritus in human skin. *The Journal of Neuroscience*, *23*(15), 6176–6180.

Tamagawa-Mineoka, R., Okuzawa, Y., Masuda, K., & Katoh, N. (2014). Increased serum levels of interleukin 33 in patients with atopic dermatitis. *The Journal of the American Academy of Dermatology*, *70*(5), 882–888.

Thyssen, J. P., Halling-Sønderby, A.-S., Wu, J. J., & Egeberg, A. (2020). Pain severity and use of analgesic medication in adults with atopic dermatitis: A cross-sectional study. *British Journal of Dermatology*, *182*(6), 1430–1436.

Vakharia, P. P., Chopra, R., Sacotte, R., Patel, K. R., Singam, V., Patel, N., et al. (2017). Burden of skin pain in atopic dermatitis. *Annals of Allergy, Asthma & Immunology*, *119*(6), 548–552.e3.

Wilson, S. R., Thé, L., Batia, L. M., Beattie, K., Katibah, G. E., McClain, S. P., et al. (2013). The epithelial cell-derived atopic dermatitis cytokine TSLP activates neurons to induce itch. *Cell*, *155*(2), 285–295.

Yoshimura, M., & Furue, H. (2006). Mechanisms for the antinociceptive actions of the descending noradrenergic and serotonergic systems in the spinal cord. *Journal of Pharmacological Sciences*, *101*(2), 107–117.

Yosipovitch, G. (2004). Dry skin and impairment of barrier function associated with itch - New insights. *International Journal of Cosmetic Science*, *26*(1), 1–7.

Yosipovitch, G., Berger, T., & Fassett, M. S. (2020). Neuroimmune interactions in chronic itch of atopic dermatitis. *The Journal of the European Academy of Dermatology and Venereology*, *34*(2), 239–250.

Yosipovitch, G., & Papoiu, A. D. P. (2008). What causes itch in atopic dermatitis? *Current Allergy and Asthma Reports*, *8*(4), 306–311.

Yosipovitch, G., Rosen, J. D., & Hashimoto, T. (2018). Itch: From mechanism to (novel) therapeutic approaches. *The Journal of Allergy and Clinical Immunology*, *142*(5), 1375–1390.

Yu, J., Fang, Q., Lou, G. D., Shou, W. T., Yue, J. X., Tang, Y. Y., et al. (2013). Histamine modulation of acute nociception involves regulation of $Na_v1.8$ in primary afferent neurons in mice. *CNS Neuroscience & Therapeutics*, *19*(9), 649–658.

17

Epigenetics

DAVID GRAND, JOHN W. FREW, AND JASON E. HAWKES

KEY POINTS

- There are three major types of epigenetic modifications: DNA methylation, microRNAs, and posttranslational histone modifications.
- DNA methylation and microRNAs alter the expression of atopic dermatitis-associated genes identified in multiple genomewide association studies.
- Epigenetic alterations also impact epidermal barrier function and immune activity, two critical components that contribute to the immunopathogenesis of atopic dermatitis.
- Epigenetic modifications provide a potential mechanism by which environmental factors associated with atopic dermatitis contribute to the skin manifestations of this inflammatory condition.
- The epigenetic modifications found in atopic dermatitis may also serve as novel biomarkers of disease activity and potential therapeutic targets for this chronic skin disease.

Introduction

Epigenetics is defined as the study of heritable changes in gene expression without alteration of the DNA sequence. DNA methylation, microRNAs (miRNAs), and posttranslational histone modifications represent three fundamental epigenetic mechanisms that alter gene expression within cells and tissues. Atopic dermatitis (AD) is a common, chronic, cyclic inflammatory skin disease frequently encountered in dermatology. Epigenetic alterations have been implicated in a variety of dermatologic conditions, including AD, plaque psoriasis, systemic lupus erythematosus (SLE), systemic sclerosis, and cutaneous malignancies (Bradbury, 2003; Lu, 2013). Epigenetic changes may occur as a result of a number of environmental stimuli or exposures, such as dietary changes and chemical or drug exposures. Given the association between AD, food/diet, and the environment, the potential role for epigenetic modifications in the onset of AD and other inflammatory skin conditions has generated significant interest.

Recent advancements in genetic and sequencing technologies, as well as ongoing investments into the Human Epigenome Project (Bradbury, 2003; Potaczek et al., 2017),

offer an unparalleled opportunity to more completely investigate the heritable genetic changes that may be contributing to complex dermatologic conditions. These epigenetic changes are likely to yield additional insights into the disease pathogenesis of AD beyond the rare single-gene mutations linked with this condition. Understanding the frequency and breadth of epigenetic alterations associated with AD, as well as the evidence surrounding their clinical relevance, will enhance our knowledge of the factors contributing to disease onset. Ultimately, these insights could lead to the identification of novel disease biomarkers and/or personalized, targeted therapies.

Current model of atopic dermatitis

AD is an inflammatory disease characterized by chronic, episodic, inflamed, eczematous skin lesions and intense itch. Histologically, the lesional (or involved) skin obtained from patients with AD reveals a thickened epidermal layer (acanthosis) with epidermal edema (spongiosis), increased scale (hyperkeratosis), dysregulated keratinocyte maturation (parakeratosis), and a mixed immune infiltrate in the epidermal and dermal compartments. A number of disease subtypes have been suggested, including childhood and adult-onset disease. Immune variations in distinct ethnic populations, such as individuals of Asian descent, have also been described. The current disease model for this condition involves two primary hallmarks: (1) epidermal barrier dysfunction and (2) immune cell activation and dysregulation. The skin barrier dysfunction in AD involves a loss of proteins that are essential to maintaining epidermal structural integrity, which results in physiologic alterations to the skin surface, such as alkalization of the skin pH and loss of key lipid components. As a result, AD skin is prone to epidermal water loss and subsequent colonization with pathogenic organisms leading to increased bacterial and viral skin infections (Weidinger & Novak, 2016).

The immune dysregulation found in AD skin involves the activation of specific helper T (Th) cell populations. These activated immune cell populations contribute to the clinical manifestations of this disease and lead to further alterations in the skin microbiome. While several variants and population subtypes of AD have been described, each share

Th2/Th22 polarization with smaller contributions from activated Th1 and Th17 cell populations (Czarnowicki, He, Krueger, & Guttman-Yassky, 2019). Genetic mutations and polymorphisms, such as loss-of-function mutations in genes required for epidermal structural integrity and gain-of-function mutations in genes central to Th2 axis polarization, play an integral role in giving rise to the clinical and microscopic features of AD mentioned earlier (Bin & Leung, 2016). There is a complex interplay between the skin, the immune response, and specific genetic alterations, which contributes to the pathogenesis of AD, but it is incompletely understood. Additionally, though many allergens such as animal/dust mites, a Western diet, tobacco exposure, and vitamin D deficiency have all been associated with AD, the precise relationship between these exposures and predisposing genetic alterations is not entirely clear (Liang, Chang, & Lu, 2016). Uncovering the mechanistic link between these environmental exposures, the skin, susceptibility loci, and/or specific gene polymorphisms will shed light on the immunopathogenesis of AD. Epigenetic modifications may also provide researchers with a potential mechanism that links AD to environmental exposures and predisposing genetic markers of disease. Epigenetic changes may also explain why a significant portion of patients lacking AD-associated gene mutations have clinical manifestations of the disease.

Three major types of epigenetic modifications

DNA methylation

Gene regulatory elements (or promoters) contain regions concentrated with cytosines followed by guanines, which are collectively known as CpG sites. CpG sites are more frequently found at promotor regions compared to other sites of the human genome. These areas of increased CpG sites are collectively known as CpG islands or clusters. The cytosine bases of CpG sites are subject to methylation by enzymes known as DNA methyltransferases (DNMTs). The addition of methyl groups to promoter-region CpG islands typically decreases gene expression, while the removal of methyl groups from these regions tends to increase gene expression (Potaczek et al., 2017). Conversely, intragenic (exonic or intronic) CpG methylation commonly results in genetic overexpression (Jjingo, Conley, Yi, Lunyak, & Jordan, 2012).

Alterations to multiple CpG sites have been implicated in the pathogenesis of AD. The major methylation changes in AD are summarized in Table 17.1. Nakamura et al. (2006) reported a role of differential CpG methylation patterns in AD by showing reduced expression of DNMT-1 in the peripheral blood mononuclear cells (PBMCs) of AD study

TABLE 17.1   Major DNA methylation changes in atopic dermatitis

Gene	Tissue	CpG site	CpG methylation	Gene expression
Epidermal structure				
FLG	Whole blood	Intragenic (exonic)	↑	NR
	Buccal cells	Promoter	↓	No change
	Skin	Promoter	No change	NR
Epidermal proliferation				
KRT6A	Skin	Intragenic (intronic)	↓	↑
Innate immune response				
hBD1	Skin	Promoter	↑	NR
NLRP2	Cord blood	Promoter	↑	↓
Adaptive immune response				
FCER1G	Monocytes	Promoter	↓	↑
TSLP	Skin	Promoter	↓	↑
IL4R	Cord tissue	Promoter	↑	NR
Tbet	Cord tissue	Promoter	↑	NR
NEU1	Skin	NR	↑	NR
OAS1/2/3	Skin	Intragenic (exonic)	↓	↑

NR, Not measured or reported.

participants compared to healthy controls. The frequency of these epigenetic findings across a wide range of study participants and ethnicities is unknown and will require additional subsequent studies to tease out whether these changes are truly causative or merely secondary changes in response to an activated, dysregulated immune response. Ongoing investigations and similar clinical studies are underway and may shed light on the impact of CpG methylation and demethylation on the onset and severity of AD.

microRNAs

miRNAs are short, single-stranded, noncoding RNA molecules that are 18 to 22 nucleotides in length and provide a novel mechanism of posttranscriptional control of genes within cells and tissues. miRNAs are transcribed by RNA polymerase II, undergo processing, and then become associated with protein complexes that bind to 3′ untranslated regions of target messenger RNA. The mechanism by which miRNAs disrupt translation or promote degradation of protein transcripts is well established, thereby confirming their importance in epigenetics (Specjalski & Jassem, 2019).

miRNAs have also been shown to participate in RNA activation, whereby miRNAs directly bind promoter elements to positively regulate gene transcription (Xiao et al., 2017).

Approximately 2500 miRNAs have been characterized in humans and can influence the expression of 30% of all genes. miRNAs play a critical role in cellular development, proliferation, apoptosis, immune regulation, and the stress response to trauma or infections (Specjalski & Jassem, 2019). Dysregulated miRNAs have been associated with most human diseases and dermatologic conditions, including cutaneous malignancies, AD, SLE, and psoriasis (Hawkes et al., 2016). Comparisons of miRNA expression profiles in skin and body fluids of AD participants versus healthy volunteers have implicated miRNAs in the pathogenesis of this inflammatory condition (Table 17.2). Importantly, sequencing and gene expression algorithms can easily be used to predict and identify the gene target(s) of specific dysregulated miRNAs in AD as shown in Table 17.2. These identified targets shed light on the immune perturbations driving the development of AD and represent an opportunity for novel therapeutic strategies via selective targeting of miRNAs as a means of restoring normal immune

TABLE 17.2 Dysregulated microRNAs (miRNAs) in AD and other allergic or inflammatory diseases

miRNA	Disease	Tissue	miRNA expression	Putative target(s)
miR-155	UC	Intestinal mucosa	↑	IL13RA
	FA	Intestinal mucosa	↑	IL10
	AD	Skin	↑	CTLA4
	AD	Skin	↑	SOCS1
miR-146a	Asthma	CD4/CD8 T cells	↓	NR
	Asthma	Plasma	↑	NR
	AR	PBMC	↓	NR
	AD	Skin	↑	CARD10, IRAK1, CCL5
miR-203	Ps	Skin	↑	SOCS3, TNFA, IL24
	EoE	Esophagus	↓	NR
	AR	Nasal mucosa	↑	NR
	AD	Serum	↑	NR
miR-10a-5p	Asthma	Bronchial epithelium	↑	NR
	AD	Skin	↑	HAS3
miR-143	AR	Nasal mucosal	↓	NR
	Asthma	Nasal mucosal	↑	NR
	AD	Skin	↓	IL13RA1
miR-151a	Ps	Exosomes	↑	NR
	AD	Skin	↑	IL12RB2

AD, atopic dermatitis; *AR*, allergic rhinitis; *EoE*, eosinophilic esophagitis; *FA*, food atopy, *NR*, not measured or reported; *PBMC*, peripheral blood mononuclear cell; *Ps*, psoriasis; *UC*, ulcerative colitis.

function. A number of clinical trials testing the efficacy of specific miRNAs for the treatment of a dermatologic condition are already underway in inflammatory conditions, such as cutaneous T-cell lymphoma (CTCL). Finally, miRNAs can be shared between cells and shuttled to distant body sites in the bloodstream via membrane-bound microvesicles called exosomes.

Posttranslational histone modifications

DNA associates with an octamer of proteins, known as histones, to form densely packed chromatin. Transcription of genes is determined by the degree of chromatin packing. When chromatin is open, transcriptional machinery can easily access DNA and initiate gene transcription. A greater degree of compaction, on the other hand, results in diminished gene expression. The degree of chromatic compaction is dictated by the posttranslational modification of the amino acids of the N-terminal tails of histones. Common modifications include methylation, acetylation, phosphorylation, and ubiquitination. Acetylation promotes chromatin opening. Histone acetyltransferase and histone deacetylases (HDAC) catalyze the addition or removal of acetyl groups from histones respectively. Histone methyltransferases catalyze histone methylation, which can either open or condense chromatin depending on the specific amino acid methylated and the number of methyl groups added (Alaskhar Alhamwe et al., 2018). To our knowledge, studies of histone modifications in allergic diseases have been limited to studies looking at the biologic role of HDAC and HDAC blockade in mice and in vitro studies. It is unclear if posttranslational histone modifications contribute to AD pathogenesis or whether HDAC blockade could result in the reversal of clinical symptoms affected by this condition.

Epigenetic mechanisms affecting AD

Predisposing genetic mutations can act via epigenetic mechanisms

Genomewide association studies have already linked a number of genetic mutations and single nucleotide polymorphisms (SNPs) to AD pathogenesis. The direct link between disease-associated polymorphisms and complex, chronic diseases such as psoriasis and AD has been elusive. However, recent research in AD has demonstrated that these genetic alterations may have consequences on an epigenetic level via their contribution to differential DNA methylation patterns. For example, Kumar et al. (2017) demonstrated that the T allele of SNP rs612529 on the promoter of the VSTM1 gene promotes demethylation of VSTM1 in monocytes. VSTM1 encodes a protein named SIRL-1, which acts as an inhibitor of innate immunity. As a result of the hypomethylation of VSTM1, SIRL-1 expression increases and lowers the risk for AD in individuals who carry the rs612529 T allele. Interestingly, increased risk of AD was associated with the C allele, which is not associated

with this demethylation event. Stevens et al. (2019) also demonstrated that two SNPs (rs2299007, rs11740584) in the KIF3A gene generate new methylated CpG sites in nasal airway cells that result in decreased KIF3A expression. KIF3A is required for skin barrier homeostasis, and loss-of-function mutations in this gene in a murine model demonstrated increased transepidermal water loss, increased epidermal thickness, and dysregulated filaggrin and claudin-1 protein expression. This research provides a nice link between KIF3A polymorphisms and the clinical features of AD. Similar translational research that provides an epigenetic mechanism by which specific SNPs can contribute to skin barrier dysfunction and/or a dysregulated immune response would bridge a major gap in the study of AD and other inflammatory skin diseases.

Epigenetic alterations may disrupt epidermal integrity

Preservation of the skin's allergen, microbial, and irritant barrier function requires adequate expression of epidermal structural and cell-cell adhesion proteins (Weidinger & Novak, 2016). Filaggrin is an intermediate filament-associated protein expressed in the stratum corneum. Absent or decreased expression of filaggrin has been implicated in the pathogenesis of AD (Bin & Leung, 2016). Filaggrin (FLG) gene loss-of-function mutations confer the strongest genetic risk of AD, though most patients with AD do not carry this mutation. Of the European population, 10% carry a null mutation in FLG, which results in mild ichthyosis vulgaris and a threefold increase in the risk of AD (Irvine, McLean, & Leung, 2011).

Filaggrin has been the subject of many DNA methylation investigations. Ziyab et al. (2013) reported that hypermethylation of an intragenic CpG methylation site of FLG in whole blood was associated with a higher risk of AD in a birth cohort. However, the study did not measure or correlate FLG methylation with its expression level, and it is unclear whether the methylation status of FLG changes as this AD cohort ages. Both are important research questions to be answered. In contrast, Tan et al. (2014) reported hypomethylation of a FLG promoter CpG site in buccal cells of AD participants compared to healthy controls. Filaggrin expression, however, did not significantly differ between the two groups. Rodriguez et al. (2014) did not discover methylation differences in the FLG promoter between AD participants and healthy controls in skin and blood samples. The variation in methylation status between these filaggrin studies may also be due in part to the heterogeneous participant cohorts and our current inability to tease out clinical subtypes of AD (e.g., early vs. late onset, mild vs. severe disease, flexural vs. nonflexural involvement).

CpG methylation differences have been observed in other genes involved in epidermal structural integrity. Quraishi et al. (2015) performed a large-scale screen of more than 450,000 CpG sites associated with 24,000 genes on the cord blood of an AD birth cohort. This team reported enriched methylation patterns of multiple genes involved in cell-to-cell adhesion, such as cadherins and tight junctions, in AD participants compared to healthy controls. Loss-of-function mutations in both cadherins and tight junctions have already been implicated in AD pathogenesis, so this finding is consistent with previous knowledge about the disease (De Benedetto et al., 2011; Faura Tellez, Nawijn, & Koppelman, 2014). Downregulation of tight junction proteins via methylation results in increased paracellular permeability and enhanced keratinocyte proliferation, which are key features of AD. Diminished cadherin expression would also contribute to epidermal edema (spongiosis) as noted in histologic studies of AD lesional skin (Ohtani et al., 2009). These early results suggest that the methylation status of AD-related genes may impact skin and/or alter epidermal structural integrity.

Epigenetic alterations regulate innate immune dysfunction in AD

Human β-defensins (hBD) make up a major class of antimicrobial peptides (AMP) that contribute to the innate immune defense of the skin. Three β-defensins (hBD-1, hBD-2, and hBD-3) are expressed in the skin. Inflammatory cytokines (e.g., interleukin-17 [IL17]), infections, and trauma/injury induce expression of hBD-2 and hBD-3, whereas hBD-1 is constitutively expressed (Clausen, Slotved, Krogfelt, Andersen, & Agner, 2016). Some studies suggest that hBD-1 is upregulated in AD skin lesions (Gambichler, Skrygan, Tomi, Altmeyer, & Kreuter, 2006), while others report that its expression is diminished (Gambichler et al., 2008). This inconsistency has been shown for multiple AMP, though the vast majority of studies show a global reduction in AMP compared to global increases in psoriasis. This reduction in AD is largely mediated by interferon-gamma (IFN-γ) with synergistic effects from Th2-related cytokines, such as IL4 and IL13. Reduction in AMP, such as β-defensins, in response to Th2 and IFN-related genes may explain why *Staphylococcus* species colonize the skin in ~90% AD patients (Abeck & Mempel, 1998; Noh, Lee, Seo, & Myung, 2018).

Diminished AMP levels in AD results in an increased risk for bacterial and viral infections, such as gram-positive bacteria and herpes or vaccinia viruses (De Benedetto, Agnihothri, McGirt, Bankova, & Beck, 2009). Noh et al. (2018) reported hypermethylation of promoter CpG sites of *DEFB1*, the gene encoding hBD1, in AD lesional skin samples compared to nonlesional and healthy control samples. Topical application of a DNMT inhibitor increased hBD-1 expression in normal human epidermal keratinocytes, which suggests that CpG hypermethylation could contribute to hBD-1 downregulation in skin and possibly AD lesions. The clinical testing of such inhibitors would be of interest in terms of its clinical efficacy on inflammatory skin lesions and/or the potential of reducing skin infections in this patient population.

IFN-γ and NF-κB intracellular signaling activity are two other hallmarks of the innate immune response. Their activation is observed in AD lesional skin (Cui, Chen, Wang, & Wang, 2014). miRNAs play an important regulatory role of IFN-γ and NF-κB intracellular signaling activity. miR-146a is a miRNA known for its general antiinflammatory activity, in contrast to the proinflammatory effects of miR-155 (Rebane & Akdis, 2013). Though dependent on NF-κB for its expression, miR-146a inhibits the NF-κB pathway by targeting IL1 receptor-associated kinase 1 (IRAK1) and tumor necrosis factor receptor-associated factor 6 (TRAF6). miR-146a is overexpressed in AD keratinocytes and targets the caspase recruitment domain-containing protein 10 (CARD10), IRAK1, and CCL5, which are known mediators of the proinflammatory NF-κB and IFN-γ cascades. The likely role of miR-146a in AD is the loss of its antiinflammatory effects via inhibition of the innate immune response (Rebane et al., 2014). Accordingly, the role of miR-155 in AD is to sustain activation of the upregulated innate immune response in lesional AD skin. miR-155 also likely promotes the secretion of Th2 cytokines (discussed in more detail later). Bacterial antigens (e.g., lipopolysaccharide and staphylococcal superantigens) and multiple environmental allergens used in patch testing have also been shown to induce miR-155 expression in inflamed skin (Quinn et al., 2014; Sonkoly et al., 2010). Interestingly, a number of miRNAs have also been found in significant concentrations in the breast milk and represent another understudied area in neonatal immunology that could lead to insights about the onset of AD (Simpson et al., 2015).

NLRP2 is a member of the NALP family of proteins that acts as an immunosuppressive signal by inhibiting NF-κB. NLRP2 is upregulated in IFN-γ–stimulated hair follicle-derived keratinocytes collected from AD participants (Yoshikawa et al., 2013). Thurmann et al. (2018) discovered promoter hypermethylation and decreased expression of NLRP2 in the cord blood of a birth cohort with early-onset AD (i.e., diagnosis of AD before age 2 years) compared with healthy controls. The authors concluded that NLRP2 expression blunts excess NF-κB activity. They also suggest that *NLRP2* gene hypermethylation and decreased protein expression lead to NF-κB overactivity resulting in an increased risk of AD. Selective blockade of NF-κB signaling could therefore have several indications for the treatment of multiple inflammatory conditions such as AD given the central role for NF-κB in the innate immune response.

Epigenetic alterations environmental allergen sensitivity

Active and passive exposure to tobacco smoke is associated with an increased prevalence of AD (Kantor, Kim, Thyssen, & Silverberg, 2016). Several studies show that tobacco smoke may act via several independent epigenetic mechanisms. Ferreira et al. (2017) associated smoking with hypermethylation and decreased expression of the PYK2-binding protein, PITPNM2, in patients with atopy (seasonal allergies, asthma, and/or AD) compared to healthy controls.

The exact role of PITPNM2 in inflammatory conditions is unclear, but early studies suggest that it may be involved in neutrophil function. Tobacco smoke has also been linked to the hypermethylation of *NLRP2*, discussed earlier (Thurmann et al., 2018). Hinz et al. (2012) also quantified the number of regulatory T cells (Treg) via demethylation of the TSDR (Treg-specific demethylated region) of *FOXP3* in cord blood. Maternal exposure to tobacco smoke during pregnancy was associated with lower Treg numbers, which was associated with an increased risk for AD during the first year of life. Decreased numbers of Treg cells in subsets of patients with AD could explain, in part, the hyperreactivity of the skin and the atopic march observed in patients.

Vitamin D deficiency is another environmental risk factor of AD (Kim, Kim, Lee, Choe, & Ahn, 2016). Cho et al. (2019) discovered that severe 25-hydroxyvitamin D deficiency in cord blood was associated with a higher risk of AD. Severe vitamin D deficiency was also associated with hypomethylation and overexpression of the *MICAL3* gene in leukocytes obtained from cord blood compared to healthy controls. *MICAL3* has previously been implicated in reactive oxygen species (ROS) production and several proinflammatory signals (Terman, Mao, Pasterkamp, Yu, & Kolodkin, 2002). The link between tobacco exposure, AD, and increased ROS was further supported by the finding of increased expression of *OGG1*, a gene strongly associated with oxidative stress. Epigenetic mechanisms as a potential link between certain environmental exposures and the proinflammatory events in AD patients is an attractive area of study given our current inability to mitigate the injurious environment effects on the skin of so many AD patients.

Th2/Th22 axis predominance is influenced by epigenetic changes

All three major epigenetic modifications have been linked to the overactivation of the Th2 axis in AD. AD lesions share a Th2/Th22 predominance with smaller contributions from Th1 and Th17 immune axes (Renert-Yuval & Guttman-Yassky, 2019). CD4+ Th cell populations play a central role in the adaptive immune response that characterizes the immunologic dysfunction observed in AD (Czarnowicki et al., 2019). miRNAs can further dysregulate the pathogenic T-lymphocyte populations in AD. Sonkoly et al. (2010) suggest that miR-155 promotes a proliferation in pathogenic T lymphocytes in AD skin. Their research demonstrates that miR-155 is highly overexpressed in lesional CD4+ T cells and targets CTLA4, an important costimulatory receptor of the T-cell receptor, which counterbalances T-cell proliferation (Hellings et al., 2002). This suggested mechanism was further supported by the observation that T-lymphocyte counts increased in response to miR-155 cell transfection experiments.

A number of other dysregulated miRNAs in AD have been linked to T-lymphocyte genes that further regulate the adaptive immune response (see Table 17.2). miR-151a and miR-143 are two of these miRNAs that contribute to Th2 polarization in AD. Chen et al. (2018) reported that miR-151a is upregulated in AD skin and targets *IL12RB2*, the gene encoding a subunit of the IL12 receptor. IL12-mediated signaling promotes Th1 differentiation and T-cell proliferation (Zou, Presky, Wu, & Gubler, 1997). miR-151a therefore inhibits the Th1 immune response as a result of its overexpression in T cells by diminishing the expression of IL2, IL12, and IFN-γ—three canonic Th1 cytokines (Chen et al., 2018). miR-151a–mediated downregulation of IL12R may also contribute to Th2 axis skewing since Th1/Th2 axes are known to counterregulate one another (Fishman & Perelson, 1994). Zeng, Nguyen, and Jin (2016) suggest miR-143 targets the IL13 receptor and is decreased in AD skin lesions. IL13-mediated inflammation induces IgE synthesis, eosinophilia (Pope et al., 2001), and downregulates the expression of epidermal barrier proteins (filaggrin, loricrin, and involucrin) in keratinocytes (Howell et al., 2008; Kim, Leung, Boguniewicz, & Howell, 2008). In healthy individuals, miR-143 expression in epidermal keratinocytes inhibits IL13-mediated repression of the epidermal barrier proteins (Zeng et al., 2016). However, this protective feature is lost in AD due to decreased expression of miR-143, which leads to increased IL13 signaling in inflamed skin.

DNA methylation has been shown to alter the expression of thymic stromal lymphopoietin (TSLP) and subunits of the IgE receptor, which contribute to Th2 polarization. TSLP is a pivotal cytokine that is highly expressed in acute and chronic eczematous lesions and promotes Th2 axis polarization (Cianferoni & Spergel, 2014; Weidinger & Novak, 2016). Its expression is correlated with AD severity scoring and measures of epidermal barrier dysfunction, such as transepidermal water loss (Sano et al., 2013). Luo, Zhou, Zhao, Tang, and Lu (2014) demonstrated that the promoter of TSLP is hypomethylated and overexpressed in AD lesional skin compared to healthy controls. Application of a DNMT inhibitor increased TSLP expression, suggesting that demethylation events contribute to TSLP overexpression (Luo et al., 2014). Genetic polymorphisms of the *FCER1* gene, which encode specific subunits of the IgE receptor, have also been implicated in AD since Th2-mediated IgE signaling is an essential component of allergic sensitization (Liang et al., 2016). Luo et al. (2014) reported demethylation and overexpression of the *FCER1G* promoter in monocytes of AD participants compared to healthy controls. Later studies attributed this demethylation event to TSLP-activated pSTAT5 recruitment of a DNA demethylase named TET2 (Liang et al., 2019).

Histone deacetylation is another epigenetic mechanism that can enhance Th2 polarization. The application of HDAC inhibitors in AD murine models showed improvement in skin lesion severity and reduction of IL4 production in CD4+ T cells, and promoted the generation of Tregs in draining lymph nodes (Kim et al., 2010). Whether this finding translates in humans will be of crucial importance given the nonspecific nature and controversy about the etiology of psoriasiform skin lesions observed in mice. Current research suggests that none of the frequently used murine models for the study of AD or psoriasis accurately recapitulate these human skin diseases but rather represent another inflammatory skin disease entity such as allergic or irritant contact dermatitis. Nevertheless, the clinical availability and use of HDAC inhibitors for the treatment of human disease in patients with both AD and CTCL will offer interesting "experiments in nature" and lead to relevant hypothesis-generating observations.

Th17 signaling and psoriasiform epidermal changes in chronic AD may act through epigenetic mechanisms

Th17 population skewing via IL17 production and STAT3 activation has been shown to induce epidermal hyperplasia (Guttman-Yassky & Krueger, 2017), a key feature of both psoriasiform and chronic eczematous lesions (Oyoshi, He, Kumar, Yoon, & Geha, 2009). The pathogenic role of IL17 signaling in chronic AD lesional skin (or specific population subtypes) is just now starting to be elucidated. Aside from its role in T-lymphocyte cell proliferation, miR-155 promotes a shift toward the Th17 axis. Ma, Xue, Wang, Shu, and Zhang (2015) correlated miR-155 overexpression with increased Th17 cell populations, as well as RORγt and IL17 expression in plasma, lesional skin, and perilesional skin obtained from AD participants. Adding a miR-155 mimic to AD-cultured keratinocytes increased the percentage of Th17 cells, whereas the addition of a miR-155 inhibitor decreased the overall percentage of Th17 cells. Further analysis implicated suppressor of cytokine signaling 1 (SOCS1) as the link between miR-155 and Th17 axis skewing since SOCS1 expression negatively correlated with Th17 markers.

miR-10a-5p, best known for its antiproliferative properties in many cancers (Jia et al., 2014; Khan et al., 2015), may also acts as a protective cellular signal for limiting epidermal hyperplasia. miR-10a-5p has been shown to be overexpressed in AD lesional skin (Rebane et al., 2014) and targets genes involved in cell cycle progression and proliferation (Vaher et al., 2019). One such target is hyaluronan synthase 3 (HAS3), an enzyme involved in hyaluronic acid synthesis that is induced by proinflammatory cytokines such as IL4, IL13, and IFN-γ (Sayo et al., 2002). This suggests that miR-10a-5p plays a regulatory role in AD by limiting keratinocyte proliferation and keratinocyte-driven inflammation. This is further supported by evidence that downregulation of miR-10a-5p is also associated with delayed wound healing (Madhyastha, Madhyastha, Nakajima, Omura, & Maruyama, 2012; Simoes et al., 2019). However, miR-10a-5p is insufficient alone to suppress keratinocyte proliferation in AD as shown by persistent elevations in Ki-67 and HAS3 (another miR-10a-5p target) despite significant overexpression of miR-10a-5p (Ohtani et al., 2009; Vaher et al., 2019). This suggests that miR-10a-5p may act in coordination with other miRNAs and/or other cellular signals such as IL19 and IL22, which promote epidermal hyperplasia in AD skin. Selective targeting of miRNAs for the treatment of a chronic disease like AD may therefore be beneficial when used in combination with other primary therapies.

Diagnostic epigenetic biomarkers of AD

As discussed, environmental factors play a focal role in AD and have an impact on DNA methylation patterns in AD-associated genes. DNA methylation is a complex phenomenon that may vary between cell type, age of participants, skin site, and chronicity of disease state. Though many studies have correlated DNA methylation patterns with gene expression and AD risk, establishment of causation is lacking. The lack of causation is particularly evident in studies that did not validate observations with DNA methylase inhibitors or follow specific methylation changes over time. Given recent technologic advances in translational genetics that have allowed for large-scale screening of methylation patterns, the longitudinal study of DNA methylation patterns in a given cell type or tissue over time in the same patient cohort may yield important insights into the onset or progression of disease activity and serve as a useful noninvasive biomarker of disease. Therefore additional studies evaluating DNA methylation are needed to establish the impact of these epigenetic modifications on AD pathogenesis at a molecular level. The ability to screen large numbers of miRNAs and predict putative miRNA targets will lead to more informed decisions as to which miRNA-gene target pairs to further study and evaluate for particular patient cohorts or disease states. Isolating miRNAs and collecting epigenetic data from serum or plasma samples via exosomes as opposed to biopsies of skin lesions offers an even less invasive approach to studying epigenetic modifications as potential disease biomarkers.

Epigenetics as a potential therapeutic approach in AD

DNMT inhibitors and TET inhibitors are actively being studied for the treatment of myelodysplastic and hematologic malignancies (Gros et al., 2012; Guan et al., 2018). There are no human studies on therapeutic modulation of methylation-modifying enzymes in AD. However, since TET2 demethylation directly impacts expression of proinflammatory genes strongly associated with AD, it may be a desirable therapeutic target for future study. miRNA antagonists or agonists offer another therapeutic potential for further study in human disease and AD. The transfection of keratinocytes with these synthetic miRNAs could be used to restore normal expression for dysregulated genes associated with AD and offer personalized therapeutic options in the future (Specjalski & Jassem, 2019).

Histone deacetylase inhibitors (HDACi) are also the subject of study in inflammatory diseases due to their ability to lower levels of proinflammatory cytokines and inhibit angiogenesis. Vorinostat, the first US Food and Drug Administration-approved HDACi, is the focus of study in preclinical and clinical trials of many cancers (Hull, Montgomery, & Leyva, 2016). The effectiveness of HDACi in AD and other allergic diseases has yet to be studied in humans. The impact on Th2 cytokines has, however, been

TABLE 17.3	Biologic effects of histone deacetylase inhibitors (HDACi) in various preclinical models of allergic disease	
Disease	**Model system**	**Effects of HDACi on disease phenotype**
Asthma	Mouse	Reduction in interleukin-4 (IL4) and IL5 levels in bronchoalveolar fluid; improvement in subepithelial fibrosis and goblet cell metaplasia
AR	Mouse	Reduction of IL4, IL5, and IL13 levels in bronchoalveolar fluid; attenuation of bronchial hyperreactivity
	Nasal epithelial cells	Increased expression of tight junction genes (*TJP1, OCLN, CLDN4, CLDN7*)
AD	Mouse	Reduction in CD4+ T cell IL4 production; amelioration of inflammatory skin lesions

AD, atopic dermatitis; *AR*, allergic rhinitis.

studied in a number of preclinical models of allergic disease (Table 17.3) suggesting their potential benefit for the treatment of atopic disease in humans. The principal concern with the use of HDACi or other medications that alter epigenetic modifications and the expression of multiple genes is serious adverse events or unwanted biologic effects during treatment. Vorinostat, for example, is associated with ventricular arrhythmias (Suraweera, O'Byrne, & Richard, 2018) possibly due to changes in the expression of cardiac ion channels (Lugenbiel et al., 2018). This is perhaps the reason why use is limited to advanced, treatment-resistant cancers and will likely limit the widespread use of this drug class unless more specific HDACi with a more favorable side effect profile are developed. Additional studies elucidating the specific mechanisms of regulating these epigenetic modifications may also lead to improved, more targeted therapies that will allow for their use in dermatology in the future.

Summary

Our understanding of AD and its pathogenesis has increased tremendously over the last decade. Nevertheless, significant research gaps still exist in our understanding of this chronic skin condition. Epigenetic studies have integrated DNA methylation changes, miRNA, and histone modifications into the pathogenic model of AD and created a framework by which these modifications may promote immune dysregulation and epidermal barrier dysfunction. Current research supports the role of epigenetics modifications on the regulation of specific T-lymphocyte populations in the skin, bacterial colonization, and known disease-modifying environmental factors such as tobacco exposure and vitamin D deficiency. The potential for DNA methylation status and miRNA signatures to serve as noninvasive biomarkers of disease activity or endotyping disease subtypes is promising. With the rapid translational revolution happening in the field of translational genetics, we are likely to see the advancement and testing of small molecules that target and modify pathogenic epigenetic modifications in AD and other dermatologic conditions. This represents an exciting opportunity to uncover novel mechanisms of disease that exist beyond exons and commonly known susceptibility loci found in patients with AD.

Acknowledgments

JWF is supported in part by the Rockefeller University CTSA award grant UL1TR001866 and KL2TR001865 from the National Center for Advancing Translational Sciences (NCATS), National Institutes of Health (NIH) Clinical and Translational Science Award (CTSA) program.

Further readings

Czarnowicki, T., He, H., Krueger, J. G., & Guttman-Yassky, E. (2019). Atopic dermatitis endotypes and implications for targeted therapeutics. *The Journal of Allergy and Clinical Immunology, 143*(1), 1–11. https://doi.org/10.1016/j.jaci.2018.10.032. https://www.ncbi.nlm.nih.gov/pubmed/30612663.

Potaczek, D. P., Harb, H., Michel, S., Alhamwe, B. A., Renz, H., & Tost, J. (2017). Epigenetics and allergy: From basic mechanisms to clinical applications. *Epigenomics, 9*(4), 539–571. https://doi.org/10.2217/epi-2016-0162. https://www.ncbi.nlm.nih.gov/pubmed/28322581.

Weidinger, S., & Novak, N. (2016). Atopic dermatitis. *Lancet, 387* (10023), 1109–1122. https://doi.org/10.1016/S0140-6736(15)00149-X. https://www.ncbi.nlm.nih.gov/pubmed/26377142.

References

Abeck, D., & Mempel, M. (1998). *Staphylococcus aureus* colonization in atopic dermatitis and its therapeutic implications. *The British Journal of Dermatology, 139*(Suppl 53), 13–16. https://doi.org/10.1046/j.1365-2133.1998.1390s3013.x. https://www.ncbi.nlm.nih.gov/pubmed/9990408.

Alaskhar Alhamwe, B., Khalaila, R., Wolf, J., von Bulow, V., Harb, H., Alhamdan, F., et al. (2018). Histone modifications and their role in epigenetics of atopy and allergic diseases. *Allergy Asthma and Clinical Immunology, 14*, 39. https://doi.org/10.1186/s13223-018-0259-4. https://www.ncbi.nlm.nih.gov/pubmed/29796022.

Bin, L., & Leung, D. Y. (2016). Genetic and epigenetic studies of atopic dermatitis. *Allergy Asthma and Clinical Immunology, 12*, 52. https://doi.org/10.1186/s13223-016-0158-5. https://www.ncbi.nlm.nih.gov/pubmed/27777593.

Bradbury, J. (2003). Human epigenome project—Up and running. *PLoS Biology, 1*(3), E82. https://doi.org/10.1371/journal.pbio.0000082. https://www.ncbi.nlm.nih.gov/pubmed/14691553.

Chen, X. F., Zhang, L. J., Zhang, J., Dou, X., Shao, Y., Jia, X. J., et al. (2018). MiR-151a is involved in the pathogenesis of atopic dermatitis by regulating interleukin-12 receptor β2. *Experimental Dermatology, 27*(4), 427–432. https://doi.org/10.1111/exd.13276. https://www.ncbi.nlm.nih.gov/pubmed/27992076.

Cho, H. J., Sheen, Y. H., Kang, M. J., Lee, S. H., Lee, S. Y., Yoon, J., et al. (2019). Prenatal 25-hydroxyvitamin D deficiency affects development of atopic dermatitis via DNA methylation. *The Journal of Allergy and Clinical Immunology, 143*(3), 1215–1218. https://doi.org/10.1016/j.jaci.2018.10.010. https://www.ncbi.nlm.nih.gov/pubmed/30352202.

Cianferoni, A., & Spergel, J. (2014). The importance of TSLP in allergic disease and its role as a potential therapeutic target. *Expert Review of Clinical Immunology, 10*(11), 1463–1474. https://doi.org/10.1586/1744666X.2014.967684. https://www.ncbi.nlm.nih.gov/pubmed/25340427.

Clausen, M. L., Slotved, H. C., Krogfelt, K. A., Andersen, P. S., & Agner, T. (2016). In vivo expression of antimicrobial peptides in atopic dermatitis. *Experimental Dermatology, 25*(1), 3–9. https://doi.org/10.1111/exd.12831. https://www.ncbi.nlm.nih.gov/pubmed/26269388.

Cui, J., Chen, Y., Wang, H. Y., & Wang, R. F. (2014). Mechanisms and pathways of innate immune activation and regulation in health and cancer. *Human Vaccines & Immunotherapeutics, 10*(11), 3270–3285. https://doi.org/10.4161/21645515.2014.979640. https://www.ncbi.nlm.nih.gov/pubmed/25625930.

Czarnowicki, T., He, H., Krueger, J. G., & Guttman-Yassky, E. (2019). Atopic dermatitis endotypes and implications for targeted therapeutics. *The Journal of Allergy and Clinical Immunology, 143*(1), 1–11. https://doi.org/10.1016/j.jaci.2018.10.032. https://www.ncbi.nlm.nih.gov/pubmed/30612663.

De Benedetto, A., Agnihothri, R., McGirt, L. Y., Bankova, L. G., & Beck, L. A. (2009). Atopic dermatitis: A disease caused by innate immune defects? *Journal of Investigative Dermatology, 129*(1), 14–30. https://doi.org/10.1038/jid.2008.259. https://www.ncbi.nlm.nih.gov/pubmed/19078985.

De Benedetto, A., Rafaels, N. M., McGirt, L. Y., Ivanov, A. I., Georas, S. N., Cheadle, C., et al. (2011). Tight junction defects in patients with atopic dermatitis. *The Journal of Allergy and Clinical Immunology, 127*(3), 773–786.e1-7. https://doi.org/10.1016/j.jaci.2010.10.018. https://www.ncbi.nlm.nih.gov/pubmed/21163515.

Faura Tellez, G., Nawijn, M. C., & Koppelman, G. H. (2014). Protocadherin-1: Epithelial barrier dysfunction in asthma and eczema. *The European Respiratory Journal, 43*(3), 671–674. https://doi.org/10.1183/09031936.00179713. https://www.ncbi.nlm.nih.gov/pubmed/24585862.

Ferreira, M. A., Vonk, J. M., Baurecht, H., Marenholz, I., Tian, C., Hoffman, J. D., et al. (2017). Shared genetic origin of asthma, hay fever and eczema elucidates allergic disease biology. *Nature Genetics, 49*(12), 1752–1757. https://doi.org/10.1038/ng.3985. https://www.ncbi.nlm.nih.gov/pubmed/29083406.

Fishman, M. A., & Perelson, A. S. (1994). Th1/Th2 cross regulation. *Journal of Theoretical Biology, 170*(1), 25–56. https://doi.org/10.1006/jtbi.1994.1166. https://www.ncbi.nlm.nih.gov/pubmed/7967633.

Gambichler, T., Skrygan, M., Tomi, N. S., Altmeyer, P., & Kreuter, A. (2006). Changes of antimicrobial peptide mRNA expression in atopic eczema following phototherapy. *The British Journal of Dermatology, 155*(6), 1275–1278. https://doi.org/10.1111/j.1365-2133.2006.07481.x. https://www.ncbi.nlm.nih.gov/pubmed/17107401.

Gambichler, T., Skrygan, M., Tomi, N. S., Othlinghaus, N., Brockmeyer, N. H., Altmeyer, P., & Kreuter, A. (2008). Differential mRNA expression of antimicrobial peptides and proteins in atopic dermatitis as compared to psoriasis vulgaris and healthy skin. *International Archives of Allergy and Immunology, 147*(1), 17–24. https://doi.org/10.1159/000128582. https://www.ncbi.nlm.nih.gov/pubmed/18446049.

Gros, C., Fahy, J., Halby, L., Dufau, I., Erdmann, A., Gregoire, J. M., et al. (2012). DNA methylation inhibitors in cancer: Recent and future approaches. *Biochimie, 94*(11), 2280–2296. https://doi.org/10.1016/j.biochi.2012.07.025. https://www.ncbi.nlm.nih.gov/pubmed/22967704.

Guan, Y., Tiwari, A. D., Hasipek, M., Grabowski, D., Parker, Y., Hirsch, C. M., et al. (2018). Lessons from nature: A novel class of TET inhibitors for TET2 mutant associated diseases. *Blood, 132*(Suppl 1), 4345–4345. https://doi.org/10.1182/blood-2018-99-117186.

Guttman-Yassky, E., & Krueger, J. G. (2017). Atopic dermatitis and psoriasis: Two different immune diseases or one spectrum? *Current Opinion in Immunology, 48*, 68–73. https://doi.org/10.1016/j.coi.2017.08.008. https://www.ncbi.nlm.nih.gov/pubmed/28869867.

Hawkes, J. E., Nguyen, G. H., Fujita, M., Florell, S. R., Callis Duffin, K., Krueger, G. G., & O'Connell, R. M. (2016). microRNAs in psoriasis. *The Journal of Investigative Dermatology, 136*(2), 365–371. https://doi.org/10.1038/JID.2015.409. https://www.ncbi.nlm.nih.gov/pubmed/26802234.

Hellings, P. W., Vandenberghe, P., Kasran, A., Coorevits, L., Overbergh, L., Mathieu, C., & Ceuppens, J. L. (2002). Blockade of CTLA-4 enhances allergic sensitization and eosinophilic airway inflammation in genetically predisposed mice. *European Journal of Immunology, 32*(2), 585–594. https://onlinelibrary.wiley.com/doi/10.1002/1521-4141(200202)32:2%3C585::AID-IMMU585%3E3.0.CO;2-U. https://www.ncbi.nlm.nih.gov/pubmed/11828376.

Hinz, D., Bauer, M., Roder, S., Olek, S., Huehn, J., Sack, U., et al. (2012). Cord blood Tregs with stable FOXP3 expression are influenced by prenatal environment and associated with atopic dermatitis at the age of one year. *Allergy, 67*(3), 380–389. https://doi.org/10.1111/j.1398-9995.2011.02767.x. https://www.ncbi.nlm.nih.gov/pubmed/22187950.

Howell, M. D., Fairchild, H. R., Kim, B. E., Bin, L., Boguniewicz, M., Redzic, J. S., et al. (2008). Th2 cytokines act on S100/A11 to downregulate keratinocyte differentiation. *The Journal of Investigative Dermatology, 128*(9), 2248–2258. https://doi.org/10.1038/jid.2008.74. https://www.ncbi.nlm.nih.gov/pubmed/18385759.

Hull, E. E., Montgomery, M. R., & Leyva, K. J. (2016). HDAC inhibitors as epigenetic regulators of the immune system: Impacts on cancer therapy and inflammatory diseases. *BioMed Research International, 2016*, 8797206. https://doi.org/10.1155/2016/8797206. https://www.ncbi.nlm.nih.gov/pubmed/27556043.

Irvine, A. D., McLean, W. H., & Leung, D. Y. (2011). Filaggrin mutations associated with skin and allergic diseases. *The New England Journal of Medicine, 365*(14), 1315–1327. https://doi.org/10.1056/NEJMra1011040. https://www.ncbi.nlm.nih.gov/pubmed/21991953.

Jia, H., Zhang, Z., Zou, D., Wang, B., Yan, Y., Luo, M., et al. (2014). MicroRNA-10a is down-regulated by DNA methylation and functions as a tumor suppressor in gastric cancer cells. *PLoS One, 9*(1), e88057. https://doi.org/10.1371/journal.pone.0088057. https://www.ncbi.nlm.nih.gov/pubmed/24498243.

Jjingo, D., Conley, A. B., Yi, S. V., Lunyak, V. V., & Jordan, I. K. (2012). On the presence and role of human gene-body DNA methylation. *Oncotarget, 3*(4), 462–474. https://doi.org/

10.18632/oncotarget.497. https://www.ncbi.nlm.nih.gov/pubmed/22577155.

Kantor, R., Kim, A., Thyssen, J. P., & Silverberg, J. I. (2016). Association of atopic dermatitis with smoking: A systematic review and meta-analysis. *Journal of the American Academy of Dermatology*, *75*(6), 1119–1125e1. https://doi.org/10.1016/j.jaad.2016.07.017. https://www.ncbi.nlm.nih.gov/pubmed/27542586.

Khan, S., Wall, D., Curran, C., Newell, J., Kerin, M. J., & Dwyer, R. M. (2015). MicroRNA-10a is reduced in breast cancer and regulated in part through retinoic acid. *BMC Cancer*, *15*, 345. https://doi.org/10.1186/s12885-015-1374-y. https://www.ncbi.nlm.nih.gov/pubmed/25934412.

Kim, B. E., Leung, D. Y., Boguniewicz, M., & Howell, M. D. (2008). Loricrin and involucrin expression is down-regulated by Th2 cytokines through STAT-6. *Clinical Immunology*, *126*(3), 332–337. https://doi.org/10.1016/j.clim.2007.11.006. https://www.ncbi.nlm.nih.gov/pubmed/18166499.

Kim, M. J., Kim, S. N., Lee, Y. W., Choe, Y. B., & Ahn, K. J. (2016). Vitamin D status and efficacy of vitamin D supplementation in atopic dermatitis: A systematic review and meta-analysis. *Nutrients*, *8*(12). https://doi.org/10.3390/nu8120789. https://www.ncbi.nlm.nih.gov/pubmed/27918470.

Kim, T. H., Jung, J. A., Kim, G. D., Jang, A. H., Cho, J. J., Park, Y. S., & Park, C. S. (2010). The histone deacetylase inhibitor, trichostatin A, inhibits the development of 2, 4-dinitrofluorobenzene-induced dermatitis in NC/Nga mice. *International Immunopharmacology*, *10*(10), 1310–1315. https://doi.org/10.1016/j.intimp.2010.08.004. https://www.ncbi.nlm.nih.gov/pubmed/20728595.

Kumar, D., Puan, K. J., Andiappan, A. K., Lee, B., Westerlaken, G. H., Haase, D., et al. (2017). A functional SNP associated with atopic dermatitis controls cell type-specific methylation of the VSTM1 gene locus. *Genome Medicine*, *9*(1), 18. https://doi.org/10.1186/s13073-017-0404-6. https://www.ncbi.nlm.nih.gov/pubmed/28219444.

Liang, Y., Chang, C., & Lu, Q. (2016). The genetics and epigenetics of atopic dermatitis-filaggrin and other polymorphisms. *Clinical Reviews in Allergy & Immunology*, *51*(3), 315–328. https://doi.org/10.1007/s12016-015-8508-5. https://www.ncbi.nlm.nih.gov/pubmed/26385242.

Liang, Y., Yu, B., Chen, J., Wu, H., Xu, Y., Yang, B., & Lu, Q. (2019). Thymic stromal lymphopoietin epigenetically upregulates Fc receptor gamma subunit-related receptors on antigen-presenting cells and induces TH2/TH17 polarization through dectin-2. *The Journal of Allergy and Clinical Immunology*, *144*(4), 1025–1035 e7. https://doi.org/10.1016/j.jaci.2019.06.011. https://www.ncbi.nlm.nih.gov/pubmed/31251950.

Lu, Q. (2013). The critical importance of epigenetics in autoimmunity. *Journal of Autoimmunity*, *41*, 1–5. https://doi.org/10.1016/j.jaut.2013.01.010. https://www.ncbi.nlm.nih.gov/pubmed/23375849.

Lugenbiel, P., Govorov, K., Rahm, A. K., Wieder, T., Gramlich, D., Syren, P., et al. (2018). Inhibition of histone deacetylases induces K+ channel remodeling and action potential prolongation in HL-1 atrial cardiomyocytes. *Cellular Physiology and Biochemistry*, *49*(1), 65–77. https://doi.org/10.1159/000492840. https://www.ncbi.nlm.nih.gov/pubmed/30134221.

Luo, Y., Zhou, B., Zhao, M., Tang, J., & Lu, Q. (2014). Promoter demethylation contributes to TSLP overexpression in skin lesions of patients with atopic dermatitis. *Clinical and Experimental Dermatology*, *39*(1), 48–53. https://doi.org/10.1111/ced.12206. https://www.ncbi.nlm.nih.gov/pubmed/24341479.

Ma, L., Xue, H. B., Wang, F., Shu, C. M., & Zhang, J. H. (2015). MicroRNA-155 may be involved in the pathogenesis of atopic dermatitis by modulating the differentiation and function of T helper type 17 (Th17) cells. *Clinical and Experimental Immunology*, *181*(1), 142–149. https://doi.org/10.1111/cei.12624. https://www.ncbi.nlm.nih.gov/pubmed/25761610.

Madhyastha, R., Madhyastha, H., Nakajima, Y., Omura, S., & Maruyama, M. (2012). MicroRNA signature in diabetic wound healing: Promotive role of miR-21 in fibroblast migration. *International Wound Journal*, *9*(4), 355–361. https://doi.org/10.1111/j.1742-481X.2011.00890.x. https://www.ncbi.nlm.nih.gov/pubmed/22067035.

Nakamura, T., Sekigawa, I., Ogasawara, H., Mitsuishi, K., Hira, K., Ikeda, S., & Ogawa, H. (2006). Expression of DNMT-1 in patients with atopic dermatitis. *Archives for Dermatological Research*, *298*(5), 253–256. https://doi.org/10.1007/s00403-006-0682-0. https://www.ncbi.nlm.nih.gov/pubmed/16897079.

Noh, Y. H., Lee, J., Seo, S. J., & Myung, S. C. (2018). Promoter DNA methylation contributes to human β-defensin-1 deficiency in atopic dermatitis. *Animal Cells and Systems*, *22*(3), 172–177. https://doi.org/10.1080/19768354.2018.1458652. https://www.ncbi.nlm.nih.gov/pubmed/30460095.

Ohtani, T., Memezawa, A., Okuyama, R., Sayo, T., Sugiyama, Y., Inoue, S., & Aiba, S. (2009). Increased hyaluronan production and decreased E-cadherin expression by cytokine-stimulated keratinocytes lead to spongiosis formation. *The Journal of Investigative Dermatology*, *129*(6), 1412–1420. https://doi.org/10.1038/jid.2008.394. https://www.ncbi.nlm.nih.gov/pubmed/19122650.

Oyoshi, M. K., He, R., Kumar, L., Yoon, J., & Geha, R. S. (2009). Cellular and molecular mechanisms in atopic dermatitis. *Advances in Immunology*, *102*, 135–226. https://doi.org/10.1016/S0065-2776(09)01203-6. https://www.ncbi.nlm.nih.gov/pubmed/19477321.

Pope, S. M., Brandt, E. B., Mishra, A., Hogan, S. P., Zimmermann, N., Matthaei, K. I., et al. (2001). IL-13 induces eosinophil recruitment into the lung by an IL-5- and eotaxin-dependent mechanism. *The Journal of Allergy and Clinical Immunology*, *108*(4), 594–601. https://doi.org/10.1067/mai.2001.118600. https://www.ncbi.nlm.nih.gov/pubmed/11590387.

Potaczek, D. P., Harb, H., Michel, S., Alhamwe, B. A., Renz, H., & Tost, J. (2017). Epigenetics and allergy: From basic mechanisms to clinical applications. *Epigenomics*, *9*(4), 539–571. https://doi.org/10.2217/epi-2016-0162. https://www.ncbi.nlm.nih.gov/pubmed/28322581.

Quinn, S. R., Mangan, N. E., Caffrey, B. E., Gantier, M. P., Williams, B. R., Hertzog, P. J., et al. (2014). The role of Ets2 transcription factor in the induction of microRNA-155 (miR-155) by lipopolysaccharide and its targeting by interleukin-10. *The Journal of Biological Chemistry*, *289*(7), 4316–4325. https://doi.org/10.1074/jbc.M113.522730. https://www.ncbi.nlm.nih.gov/pubmed/24362029.

Quraishi, B. M., Zhang, H., Everson, T. M., Ray, M., Lockett, G. A., Holloway, J. W., et al. (2015). Identifying CpG sites associated with eczema via random forest screening of epigenome-scale DNA methylation. *Clinical Epigenetics*, *7*, 68. https://doi.org/10.1186/s13148-015-0108-y. https://www.ncbi.nlm.nih.gov/pubmed/26199674.

Rebane, A., & Akdis, C. A. (2013). MicroRNAs: Essential players in the regulation of inflammation. *The Journal of Allergy and Clinical Immunology*, *132*(1), 15–26. https://doi.org/10.1016/j.jaci.2013.04.011. https://www.ncbi.nlm.nih.gov/pubmed/23726263.

Rebane, A., Runnel, T., Aab, A., Maslovskaja, J., Ruckert, B., Zimmermann, M., et al. (2014). MicroRNA-146a alleviates chronic skin inflammation in atopic dermatitis through suppression of innate immune responses in keratinocytes. *The Journal of Allergy and Clinical Immunology, 134*(4), 836-847 e11. https://doi.org/10.1016/j.jaci.2014.05.022.   https://www.ncbi.nlm.nih.gov/pubmed/24996260.

Renert-Yuval, Y., & Guttman-Yassky, E. (2019). What's new in atopic dermatitis. *Dermatologic Clinics, 37*(2), 205–213.   https://doi.org/10.1016/j.det.2018.12.007.   https://www.ncbi.nlm.nih.gov/pubmed/30850043.

Rodriguez, E., Baurecht, H., Wahn, A. F., Kretschmer, A., Hotze, M., Zeilinger, S., et al. (2014). An integrated epigenetic and transcriptomic analysis reveals distinct tissue-specific patterns of DNA methylation associated with atopic dermatitis. *The Journal of Investigative Dermatology, 134*(7), 1873–1883. https://doi.org/10.1038/jid.2014.87.   https://www.ncbi.nlm.nih.gov/pubmed/24739813.

Sano, Y., Masuda, K., Tamagawa-Mineoka, R., Matsunaka, H., Murakami, Y., Yamashita, R., et al. (2013). Thymic stromal lymphopoietin expression is increased in the horny layer of patients with atopic dermatitis. *Clinical and Experimental Immunology, 171*(3), 330–337.   https://doi.org/10.1111/cei.12021. https://www.ncbi.nlm.nih.gov/pubmed/23379440.

Sayo, T., Sugiyama, Y., Takahashi, Y., Ozawa, N., Sakai, S., Ishikawa, O., et al. (2002). Hyaluronan synthase 3 regulates hyaluronan synthesis in cultured human keratinocytes. *The Journal of Investigative Dermatology, 118*(1), 43–48. https://doi.org/10.1046/j.0022-202x.2001.01613.x.   https://www.ncbi.nih.gov/pubmed/11851874.

Simoes, A., Chen, L., Chen, Z., Zhao, Y., Gao, S., Marucha, P. T., et al. (2019). Differential microRNA profile underlies the divergent healing responses in skin and oral mucosal wounds. *Scientific Reports, 9*(1),   7160.   https://doi.org/10.1038/s41598-019-43682-w. https://www.ncbi.nlm.nih.gov/pubmed/31073224.

Simpson, M. R., Brede, G., Johansen, J., Johnsen, R., Storro, O., Saetrom, P., & Oien, T. (2015). Human breast milk miRNA, maternal probiotic supplementation and atopic dermatitis in offspring. *PLoS One, 10*(12), e0143496. https://doi.org/10.1371/journal.pone.0143496.   https://www.ncbi.nlm.nih.gov/pubmed/26657066.

Sonkoly, E., Janson, P., Majuri, M. L., Savinko, T., Fyhrquist, N., Eidsmo, L., et al. (2010). MiR-155 is overexpressed in patients with atopic dermatitis and modulates T-cell proliferative responses by targeting cytotoxic T lymphocyte-associated antigen 4. *The Journal of Allergy and Clinical Immunology, 126*(3), 581–589. e1-20. https://doi.org/10.1016/j.jaci.2010.05.045. https://www.ncbi.nlm.nih.gov/pubmed/20673989.

Specjalski, K., & Jassem, E. (2019). MicroRNAs: Potential biomarkers and targets of therapy in allergic diseases? *Archivum Immunologiae et Therapiae Experimentalis, 67*(4), 213–223. https://doi.org/10.1007/s00005-019-00547-4. https://www.ncbi.nlm.nih.gov/pubmed/31139837.

Stevens, M. L., Zhang, Z., Johansson, E., Jagpal, A., Ruff, B. P., He, H., et al. (2019). Disease-associated—KIF3A—genetic variants alter gene methylation and expression resulting in skin barrier dysfunction and increased risk for atopic dermatitis. *The Journal of Allergy and Clinical Immunology, 143*(2), AB90. https://doi.org/10.1016/j.jaci.2018.12.276.   https://doi.org/10.1016/j.jaci.2018.12.276.

Suraweera, A., O'Byrne, K. J., & Richard, D. J. (2018). Combination therapy with histone deacetylase inhibitors (HDACi) for the treatment of cancer: Achieving the full therapeutic potential of HDACi. *Frontiers in Oncology, 8*, 92. https://doi.org/10.3389/fonc.2018.00092.   https://www.ncbi.nlm.nih.gov/pubmed/29651407.

Tan, H. T., Ellis, J. A., Koplin, J. J., Martino, D., Dang, T. D., Suaini, N., et al. (2014). Methylation of the filaggrin gene promoter does not affect gene expression and allergy. *Pediatric Allergy and Immunology, 25*(6), 608–610.   https://doi.org/10.1111/pai.12245. https://www.ncbi.nlm.nih.gov/pubmed/24912553.

Terman, J. R., Mao, T., Pasterkamp, R. J., Yu, H. H., & Kolodkin, A. L. (2002). MICALs, a family of conserved flavoprotein oxidoreductases, function in plexin-mediated axonal repulsion. *Cell, 109*(7), 887–900. https://doi.org/10.1016/s0092-8674(02)00794-8. https://www.ncbi.nlm.nih.gov/pubmed/12110185.

Thurmann, L., Grutzmann, K., Klos, M., Bieg, M., Winter, M., Polte, T., et al. (2018). Early-onset childhood atopic dermatitis is related to NLRP2 repression. *The Journal of Allergy and Clinical Immunology, 141*(4), 1482–1485.e16. https://doi.org/10.1016/j.jaci.2017.11.018. https://www.ncbi.nlm.nih.gov/pubmed/29233739.

Vaher, H., Runnel, T., Urgard, E., Aab, A., Carreras Badosa, G., Maslovskaja, J., et al. (2019). miR-10a-5p is increased in atopic dermatitis and has capacity to inhibit keratinocyte proliferation. *Allergy* https://doi.org/10.1111/all.13849. https://www.ncbi.nlm.nih.gov/pubmed/31049964.

Weidinger, S., & Novak, N. (2016). Atopic dermatitis. *Lancet, 387* (10023), 1109–1122. https://doi.org/10.1016/S0140-6736(15)00149-X. https://www.ncbi.nlm.nih.gov/pubmed/26377142.

Xiao, M., Li, J., Li, W., Wang, Y., Wu, F., Xi, Y., et al. (2017). MicroRNAs activate gene transcription epigenetically as an enhancer trigger. *RNA Biology, 14*(10), 1326–1334. https://doi.org/10.1080/15476286.2015.1112487.   https://www.ncbi.nlm.nih.gov/pubmed/26853707.

Yoshikawa, Y., Sasahara, Y., Takeuchi, K., Tsujimoto, Y., Hashida-Okado, T., Kitano, Y., & Hashimoto-Tamaoki, T. (2013). Transcriptional analysis of hair follicle-derived keratinocytes from donors with atopic dermatitis reveals enhanced induction of IL32 Gene by IFN-γ. *International Journal of Molecular Sciences, 14*(2), 3215–3227.   https://doi.org/10.3390/ijms14023215. https://www.ncbi.nlm.nih.gov/pubmed/23385231.

Zeng, Y. P., Nguyen, G. H., & Jin, H. Z. (2016). MicroRNA-143 inhibits IL-13-induced dysregulation of the epidermal barrier-related proteins in skin keratinocytes via targeting to IL-13Ralpha1. *Molecular and Cellular Biochemistry, 416*(1-2), 63–70. https://doi.org/10.1007/s11010-016-2696-z. https://www.ncbi.nlm.nih.gov/pubmed/27048505.

Ziyab, A. H., Karmaus, W., Holloway, J. W., Zhang, H., Ewart, S., & Arshad, S. H. (2013). DNA methylation of the filaggrin gene adds to the risk of eczema associated with loss-of-function variants. *Journal of the European Academy of Dermatology and Venereology, 27*(3), e420–e423.   https://doi.org/10.1111/jdv.12000. https://www.ncbi.nlm.nih.gov/pubmed/23003573.

Zou, J., Presky, D. H., Wu, C. Y., & Gubler, U. (1997). Differential associations between the cytoplasmic regions of the interleukin-12 receptor subunits β1 and β2 and JAK kinases. *The Journal of Biological Chemistry, 272*(9), 6073–6077. https://doi.org/10.1074/jbc.272.9.6073.   https://www.ncbi.nlm.nih.gov/pubmed/9038232.

18

Clinical Evidence: Internal Factors

LAWRENCE S. CHAN

KEY POINTS

- Less than 50% of patients affected with atopic dermatitis have a genetic mutation of the skin barrier protein, filaggrin. Thus additional contributing factors, barrier defects, and beyond could account for disease triggering of the other 50% of patients with atopic dermatitis but without filaggrin mutation.
- Patients affected with ichthyosis vulgaris and genetic defect of skin barrier protein filaggrin do not all develop atopic dermatitis. Thus skin barrier defect-enabled external triggers are not the only factors contributing to the atopic dermatitis development.
- Patients with atopic dermatitis have an abnormal "resting" internal immune milieu during disease remission, suggesting an abnormal internal immune milieu as a contributing factor. Additionally, patients with atopic dermatitis have other co-morbidities suggesting an underlying immune abnormality. Moreover, the atopic march phenomenon may indicate an internal immune milieu that allows such "atopic expansion."
- Patients with a history atopic dermatitis can suffer eczema vaccinatum, a life-threatening, widespread vaccinia virus with systemic illness when exposed to smallpox vaccine, even at a time of clinical inactivity of atopic dermatitis, providing further support of an internal triggering factor.
- Patients with atopic dermatitis history can suffer eczema herpeticum, a widespread herpetic infection when exposed to herpes simplex virus, even at a time of clinical inactivity of atopic dermatitis, again supporting an abnormal internal milieu.

Introduction

With delineated evidence gathered from laboratory studies at the immunologic and molecular levels to implicate external contributing factors of atopic dermatitis (see Chapters 11–17), we now examine the internal factors from the perspective of clinical evidence. Although clinical evidence is not as robust as that collected through the immunologic or molecular level of investigation, it nevertheless provides a supporting documentation from a unique angle. Clinical evidence provides a sense of reality, a sense of living proof, so to speak. In fact, any medical theory or purely laboratory-based research result unsupported by clinical evidence will be deemed invalid for the actual disease.

The Oxford Living Dictionaries defines the term *clinical* (2019b) as "relating to the observation and treatment of actual patients rather than theoretical or laboratory studies... (of a disease or condition) causing observable and recognizable symptoms." The term is defined in Merriam-Webster (Clinical, 2019a) as "of, relating to, or conducted in or as if in a clinic: such as a: involving direct observation of the patient or b: based on or characterized by observable and diagnosable symptoms." Clinical evidence therefore is data gathered from the clinical observations or clinical studies.

To collect clinical evidence, we gather all the data relating to the symptoms and signs of what we can observe, obtain, and measure about and from actual patient encounters, rather than by theoretic consideration, speculation, or purely laboratory investigation. Nevertheless, laboratory data are also part of the supporting evaluation of clinical data and of documenting clinical evidence. One simple example is the clinical evaluation of early clinical failure of treatment of a gram-negative bacteria sepsis (bloodstream infection). To collect clinical evidence accurately and correctly, the clinical investigators must first establish that all these patients indeed have bloodstream infection by gram-negative bacteria documented by results of blood culture, a laboratory method. In addition, the clinical researchers must measure many parameters to develop a set of criteria for determining the predictors for early clinical failure. These parameters would include "purely clinical data" such as blood pressure, respiratory rate, altered mental status, but they would also include "laboratory data" such as white blood cell count. Together, these data provide the valuable predictors for early clinical failure on treatment for gram-negative sepsis (Rac et al., 2020). Similarly, to collect clinical data and to document clinical evidence in relation to development of atopic dermatitis, some laboratory-generated information, such as serum level of immunoglobulin E (IgE), bacterial culture results, skin histopathology report, genetic mutation information in skin barrier protein, immunologic status, and other clinically supportive laboratory data, is also included. The following discussions delineate some reasons to suggest that internal factors play a significant role in atopic dermatitis development.

Skin barrier defect is not synonymous with atopic dermatitis

One of the reasonable arguments against external factor as the sole contributor for atopic dermatitis goes like this: If the cause of atopic dermatitis is exclusively external, then it should naturally follow that in those patients with skin barrier defect, the resulting easy entry of the offending substance (pathogens or allergens) into the skin should, eventually, lead to development of chronic immune reactions in all patients. Therefore we should find that all patients with skin barrier defect should eventually develop atopic dermatitis when they reach adulthood. Is this conclusion supported by clinical evidence? The answer is a definite no. Outside-in dysregulation leads to atopic dermatitis, but apparently not in all cases.

Not all patients with filaggrin gene mutation develop atopic dermatitis

Filaggrin, one of the major skin barrier proteins that form a protective layer at the stratum corneum level of the skin, is now well documented to be defective, due to genetic mutation, in patients affected by an ichthyosis condition termed ichthyosis vulgaris, with a documented reduction in thickness of granular layer of the epidermis under electron microscopy (Erickson & Kahn, 1970; Smith et al., 2006). In addition, filaggrin mutation in ichthyosis vulgaris causes various abnormal structure organization in the epidermis, including perinuclear retraction of keratin filaments, impaired loading of lamellar body contents, nonuniform extracellular distribution of secreted organelle contents, and abnormal lamellar bilayer architecture. These structural abnormalities predictably link to the functional defect, such as increased transepidermal water loss, an objective indicator of defective skin barrier function (Gruber et al., 2011). If an external factor is the only component needed to induce atopic dermatitis, one would expect that sooner or later all patients affected by ichthyosis vulgaris will develop atopic dermatitis, as our reason goes. However, this does not seem to be the clinical finding. First, it is now clear that not all patients affected with ichthyosis vulgaris develop atopic dermatitis, and this fact is well documented by reports published in different parts of the world (Blunder et al., 2018; Li et al., 2013; Oji et al., 2009; Sekiya et al., 2017). A study showed that even with compound heterozygosity (biallelic filaggrin null mutation), some patients affected by ichthyosis vulgaris do not develop the atopic dermatitis disease (Sekiya et al., 2017). In a study report published in 2009, there is a significantly higher number of antigen presenting cells (CD1a+ Langerhans cells) present in the nonlesional epidermis of ichthyosis vulgaris patients affected with atopic dermatitis than those patients unaffected with atopic dermatitis. Thus the finding of this study suggests that an immunologic factor other than or in addition to epidermal barrier defect may account for the atopic dermatitis development (Oji et al., 2009).

Another recently reported finding of enhanced expression of genes related to xenobiotic metabolism occurred only in the nonlesional skin of patients with atopic dermatitis, not in those patients with ichthyosis vulgaris, which also supports the notion that factors other than skin barrier defect of filaggrin may be involved in the development of atopic dermatitis. Specifically, investigators found that the genes involved in the processing of pollutants, endocrine disruptors, and xenobiotics, particularly glucuronidation, were substantially upregulated in the skin of atopic dermatitis patients but not in that of ichthyosis vulgaris patients. Glucuronidation is a chemical process that converts the less biologically active form of glucuronides to reactive metabolite acylglucuronides (Fujiwara, Yoda, & Tukey, 2018). In other words, detoxification genes are highly activated in atopic dermatitis. Importantly, these enhancements exhibited in the skin of patients affected with atopic dermatitis, with or without filaggrin gene mutation, further reduce the importance of filaggrin gene mutation as a sole triggering factor for atopic dermatitis. These investigators suggested that an inflammatory triggering of local metabolism of noxious molecules might be the key factor that could transform a subinflammatory skin to an overt inflamed skin observed in atopic dermatitis (Blunder et al., 2018).

Not all atopic dermatitis patients have an identifiable filaggrin gene mutation

Conversely, we can ask the question from the opposite direction: Do all patients affected by atopic dermatitis have the mutation of major skin barrier protein filaggrin? The answer is, again, no (Blunder et al., 2018; Chen et al., 2011; Hoppe et al., 2015; Martin et al., 2020; Nomura et al., 2009; Park, Park, Seok, Li, & Seo, 2016; Polcari, Becker, Stein, Smith, & Paller, 2014; Zhang, Guo, Wang, Shi et al., 2011). An early study based in Japan indicates that only a little over 20% of atopic dermatitis patients carry some form of filaggrin gene mutations (Nomura et al., 2008). A subsequent study in Japanese atopic dermatitis patients reveals that just 25% of patients carry one or more filaggrin mutations (Nomura et al., 2009), significantly lower than the high percentage (near 50%) of mutation present in European atopic dermatitis patients (Barker et al., 2007; Sandilands et al., 2007). Similarly, in a study of Singaporean patients with atopic dermatitis, only 20% carry one or more filaggrin gene mutations (Chen et al., 2011). Further, filaggrin mutations occur in Han Chinese atopic dermatitis patients with an overall rate of 31% (Zhang, Guo, Wang, Shi et al., 2011; Zhang, Guo, Wang, Yu et al., 2011). Among African patients affected by both atopic dermatitis and ichthyosis vulgaris, a study documents that only 22% of these patients carry heterozygous filaggrin mutation (Polcari et al., 2014). In a study of Korean patients with atopic dermatitis, the investigators discovered that only 68 among the 1110 atopic dermatitis patients have filaggrin mutations (6.1%): 18 patients have the heterozygous 3321 delA mutations, 49 patients have the heterozygous, and 1 patient has the homozygous p.K4022X mutations (Park et al., 2016). Another study of Korean atopic dermatitis showed that four filaggrin null mutations (3321 delA, K4022X, S3296X, and S2889X) were detected in only 16% of the 70 tested patients (On et al., 2017).

Not surprisingly, patients with filaggrin mutations tend to have poorer skin hydration, earlier disease onset, and more severe atopic dermatitis (Park et al., 2016). Overall, approximately 10% to 50% of patients in different cohorts affected by atopic dermatitis harbor mutations at different regions of the filaggrin gene (Osawa, Akiyama, & Shimizu, 2011; Park et al., 2016). The next logical question to ask is: Do those atopic dermatitis patients who have no filaggrin gene mutation have genetic mutations of other skin barrier proteins such as loricrin or involucrin? Barrier dysfunctions due to yet-to-be-discovered mutations of those nonfilaggrin barrier proteins, if existed, may account for the external triggering factor in atopic dermatitis. At the present time, however, we do not have the answer, and there is no literature report as of June 2020. This question is important to answer as it would help decipher whether atopic dermatitis is a pure inside-out or outside-in process, or a combination of both. The following paragraphs will examine the internal immune milieu of patients affected by atopic dermatitis.

Th2 immune type correlates with inside-out dysregulation in atopic dermatitis

The internal "resting" immune milieu is skewed toward Th2 in atopic dermatitis patients

Another reasoning argues against external factor as the sole contributor for atopic dermatitis is as follows: If the cause of atopic dermatitis is exclusively external, then the immunologic status of the patients affected by atopic dermatitis should remain normal when the patient is lesion free and would become activated only when it is in a lesional condition. The best way to answer this question is to examine the immune milieu of these patients when their skin disease is inactive. The data obtained during inactive disease stage are essential for determining the internal immune milieu because once the disease is active the immune data may simply reflect a reactive immune state rather than a resting immune state. Study results, although somewhat limited thus far, point to an abnormal resting immune system in atopic dermatitis patients (Howell, Richard, et al., 2006; Howell, Wollenberg, et al., 2006; Howell et al., 2011; Reed, Scott, & Bray, 2012; Turner, Bauer, & Nimmo-Smith, 1962).

Abnormal upregulation of Th2-type cytokines

The Th2-type immune milieu is essential for the development of any allergic diseases. IL4, a key Th2 cytokine, is critical for IgE production and is the driver for Th2 lymphocyte development and atopic diseases (Abbas, Kenneth, & Sher, 1996; Kuhn, Rajewsky, & Muller, 1991; Murphy & Steven, 2002; Ricci, Matucci, & Rossi, 1997). IL13 is a Th2 cytokine with its gene located close to IL4 gene on the same chromosome, 5q31, and its protein shares the same cellular receptor (IL4 receptor-α) with IL4. Both IL4 and IL13 are known for their stimulatory role in allergic diseases (Shirakawa et al., 2000; Wilis-Karp, 2000). Studies have also shown a higher level of IL13 than IL4 in atopic dermatitis skin lesions (Bieber, 2020). Besides IL4 and IL13, evidence shows that IL10 plays a significant role in allergic diseases (Ricci et al., 1997).

Animal models further support the role of the Th2 immune milieu in atopic dermatitis. Epidermally expressed IL4 by transgenesis in mice induces a chronic, pruritic, inflammatory skin disease that fulfills the clinical diagnosis of human atopic dermatitis. Before the disease onset, there are already upregulations of Th2-type cytokines (IL4, IL5, IL6, IL13) detected in the "normal appearing" skin of these IL4-transgenic mice, and the Th2 cytokine upregulation went higher still after the onset of skin lesions (Chan, Robinson, & Xu, 2001; Chen et al., 2004). Epidermal expression of IL4 in BALB/c mice, a strain with principal internal Th2 immune milieu, induces a much earlier disease onset and a more severe skin inflammation than IL4 expressing in C57BL/6 mice, a strain with predominant internal Th1 immune milieu (Chan et al., 2001; Reichle, Chen, Shao-xia, & Chan, 2011).

Patients with atopic dermatitis have an immune dysregulation and a predominant Th2-type cytokine milieu (Bos, Wierenga, Smitt, van der Heijden, & Kapsenberg, 1992). The Th2 immune milieu is also suppressive to immune defense against certain infectious microorganisms. One of the best clinical examples is observed in the disease of leprosy, a chronic bacterial infection caused by *Mycobacterium leprae*. Patients with a milder/resistant form of tuberculous leprosy have strong skin mRNA expressions for IFN-γ and IL2, the Th1-type cytokines; patients with a severe/multibacillary form of lepromatous leprosy, however, have skin cytokine mRNAs predominant for IL4, IL5, and IL10, the Th2 types (Yamamura et al., 1991). Human allergen-specific CD4+ T-cell clones obtained from atopic patients produce Th2 cytokines IL4, and not Th1 cytokine IFN-γ, when stimulated in the presence of autologous antigen presenting cells, regardless if the antigen presenting cells are derived from active or inactive disease state. By contrast, T-cell clones obtained from nonatopic donors exposed to the same allergen produce Th1 cytokine IFN-γ under the identical stimulating condition, further supporting the Th2-skewed immune milieu in the resting state of atopic dermatitis (Wierenga et al., 1990).

Peripheral blood mononuclear cells derived from atopic dermatitis patients have a greater tendency for spontaneous release of IL4 and IL10, suggesting T cells of atopic dermatitis are skewed toward a Th2 response (Ohmen et al., 1995; Tang & Kemp, 1994). Secretion of IL4 induces expression and secretion of the pruritus-inducing cytokine IL31 from helper T cells and mast cells, further amplifying Th2 cytokine effects in atopic diseases (McLeod, Baker, & Ryan, 2015), and leads to constant itch-scratch cycles exacerbating the chronic skin inflammation (Stott et al., 2013).

In the absence of a comprehensive study on the nonlesional skin cytokine milieu or skin cytokine milieu during the inactive disease stage of atopic patients, one can still learn some useful insights by comparing the cytokine milieu between two common inflammatory skin diseases, atopic dermatitis and psoriasis. In contrast to the prominent Th2 immune milieu in atopic dermatitis skin, psoriasis skin is marked with a strong Th1 immune response. Evidence obtained from lesional skin of atopic dermatitis patients shows an inability to produce sufficient amounts of human defensins and inflammatory cytokines tumor necrosis factor-α (TNF-α) and IFN-γ (Nomura et al., 2003). Moreover, Th2 cytokines, IL13 and IL4, inhibit TNF-α- and IFN-γ-induced human β-defensin production (Albanesi et al., 2007). These findings help define the cytokine patterns that drive immune deviation toward a Th2 immune response in atopic dermatitis, in contrast to that of psoriasis.

Atopic dermatitis patients have immune-mediated comorbidities

Besides the documented Th2 immune deviations, some patients affected by atopic dermatitis also have comorbidities related to underlying immunologic conditions. These include autoimmune diseases such as alopecia areata, gastrointestinal immune-mediated disorders, and cardiovascular diseases (Paller et al., 2018; Silverberg, 2019). The occurrence of these comorbidities suggests an underlying immune deviation in patients affected by atopic dermatitis. However, it is not completely clear if these comorbidities exist before atopic dermatitis develops or they occur as a sequela of atopic dermatitis development.

Th2 immune response cytokines suppress expressions of skin barrier proteins

While we would like to highlight the distinct properties of outside-in and inside-out dysregulation in atopic dermatitis, the two are intimately connected. Study results show that the major Th2 cytokines, IL4 and IL13, alone or in combination could suppress the expression of three critical stratum corneum–located primary skin barrier proteins: filaggrin, involucrin, and loricrin (Bao et al., 2017; Bao, Jamie, Huayi, Kui, & Lawrence, 2016; Di et al., 2016). In addition, the combination of three Th2 cytokines (IL4, IL13, and IL31) suppresses the expression of claudin-1, a tight junction protein important for skin barrier function (Gruber et al., 2015). These data show that internal immune derangements observed in atopic dermatitis could induce skin barrier defects even in the absence of genetic mutations. Thus internal immune deviation (an inside-out dysregulation) could lead to external contributing factors: skin barrier weakness–related penetration of pathogens and allergens (an outside-in dysregulation), provoking the development of atopic dermatitis. More details on this aspect are discussed in Chapter 11.

Atopic March

One of the well-known clinical phenomena in relationship to atopic dermatitis is atopic march, which documents the occurrence of extracutaneous atopic diseases such as asthma, food allergy, and allergic rhinitis after patients developed cutaneous atopic dermatitis in early childhood (Davidson et al., 2019). While the pathomechanism of atopic march is not completely understood and is being pursued by physicians and scientists in the field, there is some evidence pointing to an internal immune dysregulation. For example, the majority of IgE detected from patients with asthma is not accounted for by known allergens in patients with highest total IgE levels, supporting a notion of internal IgE dysregulation. A history of infant-onset atopic dermatitis together with a parental family history of atopy increased the risk of subsequent upper or lower airway allergic manifestations, suggesting a genetic link of atopy. Accordingly, field experts support recommendations to examine if early immune interventions utilizing systemic Th2 inhibition could prevent atopic march in high-risk children with atopic dermatitis (Davidson et al., 2019).

Increased risk of atopic dermatitis–associated viral infections

Observations of increased viral-related skin infections in patients of atopic dermatitis include eczema vaccinatum, eczema herpeticum, eczema coxsackium, and a higher occurrence of human papillomavirus infections. The details of these viral infections are delineated next.

Eczema vaccinatum

The most dramatic clinical evidence illustrating an abnormal immune milieu in atopic dermatitis is none other than the rare occurrence of eczema vaccinatum. In such event, patients with atopic dermatitis develop systemic illness and widespread smallpox lesions after being exposed to people recently vaccinated against smallpox. Eczema vaccinatum can be fatal and can occur in patients with or without active dermatitis lesions, even in patients who have had no active skin disease for years. Results of early and recent studies suggest this phenomenon occurs because of altered immune defense against the smallpox viruses (Copeman & Wallace, 1964; Lane & Goldstein, 2003; Reed et al., 2012; Turner et al., 1962; Waddington, Bray, Evans, & Richards, 1964).

Investigators have demonstrated an enhanced vaccinia virus replication in skin samples from nonlesional skin of atopic dermatitis patients, compared to skin samples from psoriasis patients and healthy individuals in an ex vivo experiment and linked to LL-37. LL-37 is an antimicrobial peptide known to suppress vaccinia virus replication in a dose-dependent manner. In nonlesional skin of atopic dermatitis patients, vaccinia viruses fail to induce expression of LL-37, in contrast to LL-37 induction observed in nonlesional skin from psoriasis patients and normal individuals. Furthermore, the combination of Th2 cytokines IL4 and IL13 enhances the vaccinia virus replication and suppresses expression of LL-37 by the vaccinia virus–stimulated keratinocytes (Howell et al., 2006). In the clinical situation, increased levels of IL4 and IL13 in atopic dermatitis would likely suppress LL-37 expression, thereby contributing to unchecked replication of vaccinia viruses as observed in eczema vaccinatum.

Additional evidence pointing to pathomechanism of eczema vaccinatum is from the study of macrophage inflammatory protein 3 alpha (MIP-3α), a C-C chemokine that plays an important role in innate and adaptive immune response and has documented antimicrobial activities against the vaccinia virus. Investigators have demonstrated that the skin lesions from atopic dermatitis patients exhibited only 50% of the MIP-3α expressed by that of psoriasis patients. Furthermore, preincubation with IL4 and IL13 significantly suppresses the induced expression of this chemokine in keratinocytes when stimulated with the vaccinia virus (Kim et al., 2007).

Eczema herpeticum

Another excellent clinical evidence to support an altered resting immune milieu in patients affected by atopic dermatitis is the clinical disease of eczema herpeticum. Eczema herpeticum, also termed Kaposi varicelliform eruption, occurs when atopic dermatitis patients develop widespread herpetic blistering eruptions secondary to exposure to herpes simplex viruses (Wollenberg & Eliszbeth, 2007; Wollenberg, Helen-Caroline, & Jurgen, 2011). Eczema herpeticum manifests with fever, viremia, skin erosion, lymphadenopathy, keratoconjunctivitis, and (in severe cases) meningitis. The fact that it occurs in patients with or without active skin disease further supports the notion of an altered resting immune milieu in atopic dermatitis patients (Sun & Peck, 2017).

In addition, these atopic dermatitis patients have a significantly higher level of total serum IgE (Beck et al., 2009; Hata et al., 2010; Peng et al., 2007), and there is an inverse correlation between IgE level and LL-37 expression in the skin (Howell, Wollenberg et al., 2006). Patients with a history of eczema herpeticum have a defect in their skin's ability to induce expressions of HBD-2, HBD-3, and cathelicidin (LL-37), the three important epidermis-produced antimicrobial peptides. They also have a higher level of Th2 cytokine IL13 in nonlesional skin, compared to those atopic dermatitis patients with no history of eczema herpeticum. This high level of IL13 may predispose these patients for eczema herpeticum development (Hata et al., 2010; Howell, Wollenberg et al., 2006).

The tendency to develop eczema herpeticum has been linked with STAT6 single nucleotide polymorphisms (SNPs), particularly at a 2-SNP (CT) haplotype (Howell et al., 2011). Resting peripheral blood CD8+ T cells obtained from atopic dermatitis patients with a history of eczema herpeticum have defective interferon-gamma (IFN-γ) production in response to stimulation with herpes simplex virus in vitro, and these patients have an HLA-B7 genotype (Mathias et al., 2013). Moreover, IFN-α and IL29 mRNAs and proteins are significantly reduced in the atopic dermatitis patients with a history of eczema herpeticum, compared to those patients without the history of eczema herpeticum, when their resting peripheral blood mononuclear cells are stimulated with herpes virus in culture. Further studies

document a significant inhibition of upstream regulators IRF3, IRF7, and IRF9 in atopic patients with the history of eczema herpeticum. IRFs are important transcription factors involving in a good deal of viral recognition signaling pathways, and some examples are toll-like receptors, cytoplasmic DNA sensors, and cytoplasmic RNA sensor RIG1 (Bin et al., 2014). Subsequently, atopic dermatitis patients with the history of eczema herpeticum have shown functional defect in genetic variants of the interferon-pathway gene encoding interferon-gamma receptor 1 (IFNGR1) (Gao et al., 2015).

Eczema coxsackium

Atopic dermatitis patients have also developed eczema coxsackium, extensive skin blistering, when exposed to *Coxsackie* viruses, and it can occur in the absence of active atopic dermatitis skin lesions. In contrast to the limited skin involvement observed in the typical *Coxsackie* viral infection (i.e., hand, foot, and mouth disease), eczema coxsackium manifests with fever and widespread lesions of papules, blisters, and erosions, a clinical morphology similar to that of eczema herpeticum (Horsten, Fisker, & Bygum, 2016; Mathes et al., 2013). Although the pathophysiology of eczema coxsackium is not fully understood, an altered internal immune response may play an important role, as documented in the study results on eczema herpeticum and eczema vaccinatum (Bin et al., 2014; Howell, Richard, et al., 2006; Howell, Wollenberg et al., 2006; Kim et al., 2007).

High-risk cervical human papillomavirus infection

Clinical evidence demonstrates an association between increased infections of high-risk cervical human papillomavirus and female atopic dermatitis patients (Morgan et al., 2015). Atopic dermatitis is significantly more commonly identified in patients affected with high-risk human papillomavirus infection (8.3%) than in patients with negative infection ($P = .007$). Since high-risk human papillomavirus infection is more likely to persist in immunosuppressed women, the data seem to suggest that atopic dermatitis is associated with a level of immunosuppression or an altered immune response as discussed earlier.

Summary

We have examined available clinical evidence in relation to the development of atopic dermatitis to pursue an answer whether internal or external contributing factors are triggers for atopic dermatitis development. From the data showing that not all patients with ichthyosis vulgaris and skin barrier protein filaggrin mutation developed atopic dermatitis, that not all patients affected by atopic dermatitis have identified filaggrin mutation, that some internal immune milieu of Th2 deviations existed in patients with atopic dermatitis, that Th2 cytokines can suppress skin barrier protein expression in the absence of gene mutation, and that widespread

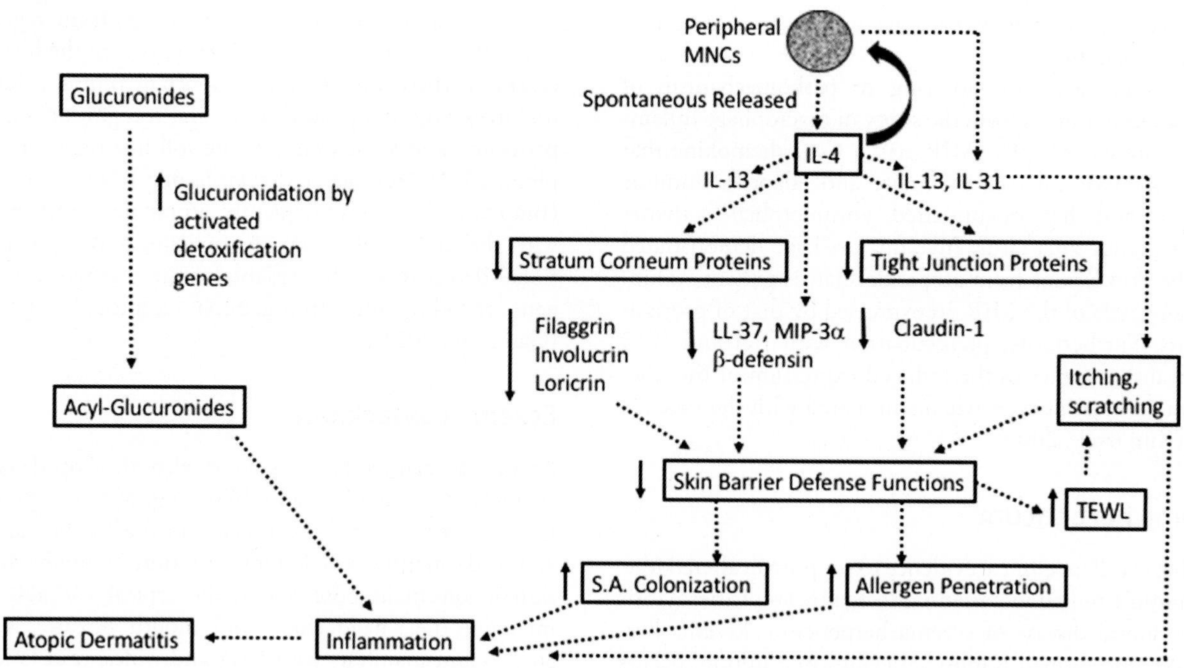

• **Fig. 18.1** Schematic depiction of a proposed mechanism in which abnormal internal immune milieu would trigger the development of atopic dermatitis. *Curve arrow* indicates an autocrine stimulation loop. *Dotted arrows* indicate directions of influence. *Up and down solid arrows* indicate up- and downregulations, respectively. *LL-37,* A cathelicidin-type of antimicrobial peptide; *MIP-3α,* macrophage inflammatory protein-3α; *MNCs,* mononuclear cells; *S.A., Staphylococcus aureus; TEWL,* transepidermal water loss.

viral infection (such as eczema vaccinatum, eczema herpeticum, and eczema coxsackium) can occur in patients with a history of atopic dermatitis but no active skin disease, the hypothesis that all cases of atopic dermatitis can be developed without an altered internal immune milieu cannot be supported. Fig. 18.1 depicts a proposed mechanism in which internal immune deviation toward Th2 milieu would trigger the type of inflammation observed in atopic dermatitis.

Further readings

Boguniewicz, M. (2017). Biologic therapy for atopic dermatitis: Moving beyond the practice parameter and guidelines. *Journal of Allergy and Clinical Immunology Practice, 5*(6), 1477–1487. https://doi.org/10.1016/j.jaip.2017.08.031.

Hofmann, M. A., Kiecker, F., & Zuberbier, T. (2016). A systematic review of the role of interleukin-17 and the interleukin-20 family in inflammatory allergic skin diseases. *Current Opinions in Allergy and Clinical Immunology, 16*(5), 451–457. https://doi.org/10.1097/ACI.0000000000000310.

Paller, A. S., Kabashima, K., & Bieber, T. (2017). Therapeutic pipeline for atopic dermatitis: End of the drought? *Journal of Allergy and Clinical Immunology, 140*(3), 633–643. https://doi.org/10.1016/j.jaci.2017.07.006.

References

Abbas, A. K., Murphy, K. M., & Sher, A. (1996). Functional diversity of helper T lymphocytes. *Nature, 383*(6603), 787–793. https://doi.org/10.1038/383787a0.

Albanesi, C., Fairchild, H. R., Madonna, S., Scarponi, C., De Pita, O., Leung, D. Y. M., & Howell, M. D. (2007). IL-4 and IL-13 negatively regulate TNF-α and IFN-γ-induced β-defensin expression through STAT-6, suppressor of cytokine signaling (SOCS)-1 and SOCS-3. *The Journal of Immunology, 179*(2), 984–992. https://doi.org/10.4049/jimmunol.179.2.984.

Bao, L., Alexander, J. B., Zhang, H., Shen, K., & Chan, L. S. (2016). Interleukin-4 downregulation of involucrin expression in human epidermal keratinocytes involves Stat6 sequestration of the coactivator CREB-binding protein. *Journal of Interferon & Cytokine Research, 36*(6), 374–381. https://doi.org/10.1089/jir.2015.0056.

Bao, L., Mohan, G. C., Alexander, J. B., Doo, C., Shen, K., Bao, J., & Chan, L. S. (2017). A molecular mechanism for IL-4 suppression of loricrin transcription in epidermal keratinocytes: Implication for atopic dermatitis pathogenesis. *Innate Immunity, 23*(8), 641–647. https://doi.org/10.1177/1753425917732823.

Barker, J. N. W. N., Palmer, C. N. A., Zhao, Y., Liao, H., Hull, P. R., Lee, S. P., Allen, M. H., et al. (2007). Null mutations in the filaggrin gene (FLG) determine major susceptibility to early-onset atopic dermatitis that persists into adulthood. *Journal of Investigative Dermatology, 127*(3), 564–567. https://doi.org/10.1038/sj.jid.5700587.

Beck, L. A., Boguniewicz, M., Hata, T., Schneider, L. C., Hanifin, J., Gallo, R., Paller, A. S., et al. (2009). Phenotype of atopic dermatitis subjects with a history of eczema herpeticum. *Journal of Allergy and Clinical Immunology, 124*(2), 260–269. https://doi.org/10.1016/j.jaci.2009.05.020.

Bieber, T. (2020). Interleukin-13: Targeting an underestimated cytokine in atopic dermatitis. *Allergy 75,* 54–62. https://doi.org/10.1111/all.13954.

Bin, L., Edwards, M. G., Heiser, R., Streib, J., Richers, B., Hall, C., & Leung, D. Y. M. (2014). Identification of novel gene signatures in atopic dermatitis complicated by eczema herpeticum. *Journal of Allergy and Clinical Immunology, 13*(4), 848–855. https://doi.org/10.1016/j.jaci.2014.07.018.

Blunder, S., Koks, S., Koks, G., Reimann, E., Hackl, H., Gruber, R., Moosbrugger-Martinz, V., Schmuth, M., & Dubrac, S. (2018). Enhanced expression of genes related to xenobiotic metabolism in the skin of patients with atopic dermatitis but not with ichthyosis vulgaris. *Journal of Investigative Dermatology*, *138*, 98–108. https://doi.org/10.1016/j.jid.2017.08.036.

Bos, J. D., Wierenga, E. A., Smitt, J. H. S., van der Heijden, F. L., & Kapsenberg, M. L. (1992). Immune dysregulation in atopic dermatitis. *Archives of Dermatology*, *128*(11), 1509–1512. https://doi.org/10.1001/archderm.1992.01680210087014.

Chan, L. S., Robinson, N., & Xu, L. (2001). Expression of interleukin-4 in the epidermis of transgenic mice results in a pruritic inflammatory skin disease: An experimental animal model to study atopic dermatitis. *Journal of Investigative Dermatology*, *117*(4), 977–983.

Chen, H., Common, J. E. A., Haines, R. L., Balakrishnan, A., Brown, S. J., Goh, C. S. M., Cordell, H. J., et al. (2011). Wide spectrum of filaggrin-null mutations in atopic dermatitis highlights differences between Singaporean Chinese and European populations. *British Journal of Dermatology*, *165*(1), 106–114. https://doi.org/10.1111/j.1365-2133.2011.10331.x.

Chen, L., Martinez, O., Overbergh, L., Mathieu, C., Prabhakar, B. S., & Chan, L. S. (2004). Early up-regulation of Th2 cytokines and late surge of Th1 cytokines in an atopic dermatitis model. *Clinical & Experimental Allergy*, *138*(3), 375–387. https://doi.org/10.1111/j.1365-2249.2004.02649.x.

Clinical. (2019a). *Merriam Webster online*. https://merriam-webster.com/dictionary/clinical. Accessed 05.06.2019.

Clinical. (2019b). *Oxford Living Dictionaries*. https://en.oxforddictionaries.com/definition/clinical. Accessed 05.06.2019.

Copeman, P. W., & Wallace, H. J. (1964). Eczema vaccinatum. *British Medical Journal*, *2*, 906–908.

Davidson, W. F., Leung, D. Y. M., Beck, L. A., Berin, C. M., Boguniewicz, M., Busse, W. W., et al. (2019). Report from the National Institute of Allergy and Infectious Diseases workshop on 'atopic dermatitis and the atopic march: mechanisms and interventions'. *Journal of Allergy and Clinical Immunology*, *143*(3), 894–913. https://doi.org/10.1016/j.jaci.2019.01.003.

Di, Z.-H., Ma, L., Qi, R.-Q., Sun, X.-D., Huo, W., Zhang, L., et al. (2016). T helper 1 and T help 2 cytokines differentially modulate expression of filaggrin and its processing proteases in human keratinocytes. *Chinese Medical Journal*, *129*(3), 295–303. https://doi.org/10.4103/0366-6999.174489.

Erickson, L., & Kahn, G. (1970). The granular layer thickness in atopy and ichthyosis vulgaris. *Journal of Investigative Dermatology*, *54*(1), 11–12.

Fujiwara, R., Yoda, E., & Tukey, R. H. (2018). Species differences in drug glucuronidation: Humanized UDP-glucuronosyltransferase 1 mice and their application for predicting drug glucuronidation and drug-induced toxicity in humans. *Drug Metabolism and Pharmacokinetics*, *33*(1), 9–16. https://doi.org/10.1016/j.dmpk.2017.10.002.

Gao, L., Bin, L., Rafaels, N. M., Huang, L., Potee, J., Ruczinski, I., et al. (2015). Targeted deep sequencing identifies rare loss-of-function variants in IFNGR1 for risk of atopic dermatitis complicated by eczema herpeticum. *Journal of Allergy and Clinical Immunology*, *136*(6), 1591–1600. https://doi.org/10.1016/j.jaci.2015.06.047.

Gruber, R., Bornchen, C., Rose, K., Daubmann, A., Volksdorf, T., Wladykowski, E., et al. (2015). Diverse regulation of claudin-1 and claudin-4 in atopic dermatitis. *The American Journal of Pathology*, *185*(10), 2777–2789. https://doi.org/10.1016/j.ajpath.2015.06.021.

Gruber, R., Elias, P. M., Crumrine, D., Lin, T.-K., Brandner, J. M., Hachem, J.-P., et al. (2011). Filaggrin genotype in ichthyosis vulgaris predicts abnormalities in epidermal structure and function. *The American Journal of Pathology*, *178*(5), 2252–2263. https://doi.org/10.1016/j.ajpath.2011.01.053.

Hata, T. R., Kotol, P., Boguniewicz, M., Taylor, P., Paik, A., Jackson, J., Nguyen, M., et al. (2010). History of eczema herpeticum is associated with the inability to induce human β-defensin (HBD)-2, HBD-3 and cathelicidin in the skin of patients with atopic dermatitis. *British Journal of Dermatology*, *163*(3), 659–661. https://doi.org/10.1111/j.1365-2133.2010.09892.x.

Hoppe, T., Winge, M. C. G., Bradley, M., Nordenskjold, M., Vahlquist, A., Torma, H., & Berne, B. (2015). Moisturizing treatment of patients with atopic dermatitis and ichthyosis vulgaris improves dtry skin, but has a modest effect on gene expression regardless of FLG genotype. *Journal of the European Academy of Dermatology and Venereology*, *29*(1), 174–177. https://doi.org/10.1111/jdv.12333.

Horsten, H.-H., Fisker, N., & Bygum, A. (2016). Eczema coxsackium caused by coxsackievirus A6. *Pediatric Dermatology*, *33*(3), e230–e231. https://doi.org/10.1111/pde.12874.

Howell, M. D., Richard, L. G., Boguniewicz, M., Jones, J. F., Wong, C., Strieb, J. E., & Leung, D. Y. M. (2006). Cytokine milieu of atopic dermatitis skin subverts the innate immune response to vaccinia virus. *Immunity*, *24*(3), 341–348. https://doi.org/10.1016/j.immuni.2006.02.006.

Howell, M. D., Wollenberg, A., Gallo, R. L., Flaig, M., Streib, J. E., Wong, C., et al. (2006). Cathelicidin deficiency predisposes to eczema herpeticum. *Journal of Allergy and Clinical Immunology*, *117*(4), 836–841. https://doi.org/10.1016/j.jaci.2005.12.1345.

Howell, M. D., Gao, P., Kim B, E., Lesley, L. J., Streib, J. E., Taylor, P. A., et al. (2011). The signal transducer and activator of transcription 6 gene (STAT6) increases the propensity of patients with atopic dermatitis toward disseminated viral skin infections. *Journal of Allergy and Clinical Immunology*, *128*(5), 1006–1014. https://doi.org/10.1016/j.jaci.2011.06.003.

Kim, B. E., Donald, Y. M. L., Streib, J. E., Boguniewicz, M., Hamid, Q. A., & Michael, D. H. (2007). Macrophage inflammatory protein 3 alpha (MIP-3a) deficiency in AD skin and role in innate immune response to vaccinia virus. *Journal of Allergy and Clinical Immunology*, *119*(2), 457–463. https://doi.org/10.1016/j.jaci.2006.10.005.

Kuhn, R., Rajewsky, K., & Muller, W. (1991). Generation and analysis of interleukin-4 deficient mice. *Science*, *254*(5032), 707–710.

Lane, J. M., & Goldstein, J. (2003). Adverse events occurring after smallpox vaccination. *Seminars in Pediatric Infectious Diseases*, *14*(3), 189–195. https://doi.org/10.1016/S1045-1870(03)00032-3.

Li, M., Cheng, R., Shi, M., Liu, J., Zhang, G., Liu, Q., Yu, H., & Yao, Z. (2013). Analyses of FLG mutation frequency and filaggrin expression in isolated ichthyosis vulgaris (IV) and atopic dermatitis-associated IV. *British Journal of Dermatology*, *168*(6), 1335–1338. https://doi.org/10.1111/bjd.12206.

Martin, M. J., Estravis, M., Garcia-Sanchez, A., Davila, I., Isidoro-Garcia, M., & Sanz, C. (2020). Genetics and epigenetics of atopic dermatitis: An updated systematic review. *Genes*, *11*, 442. https://doi.org/10.3390/genes11040442.

Mathes, E. F., Oza, V., Frieden, I. J., Cordoro, K. M., Yagi, S., Howard, R., et al. (2013). Eczema coxsackium' and unusual cutaneous findings in an enterovirus outbreak. *Pediatrics*, *132*(1), e149–e157. https://doi.org/10.1542/peds.2012-3175.

Mathias, R. A., Weinberg, A., Boguniewicz, M., Zaccaro, D. J., Armstrong, B., Schneider, L. C., et al. (2013). Atopic dermatitis complicated by eczema herpeticum is associated with HLA B7 and reduced interferon-g-producing CD8+ T cells. *British Journal of Dermatology, 169*(3), 700–703. https://doi.org/10.1111/bjd.12382.

McLeod, J. J. A., Baker, B. N., & Ryan, J. J. (2015). Mast cell production and responses to IL-4 and IL-13. *Cytokine, 75*(1), 57–61. https://doi.org/10.1016/j.cyto.2015.05.019.

Morgan, T. K., Hanifin, J., Mahmood, M., Larson, B., Baig-Lewis, S., Long, T., et al. (2015). Atopic dermatitis is associated with cervical high risk human papillomavirus infection. *Journal of Lower Genital Tract Disease, 19*(4), 345–349. https://doi.org/10.1097/LGT.0000000000000147.

Murphy, K. M., & Reiner, S. L. (2002). The lineage decisions of helper T cells. *Nature Reviews Immunology, 2*(12), 933–944. https://doi.org/10.1038/nri954.

Nomura, I., Goleva, E., Howell, M. D., Hamid, Q. A., Ong, P. Y., Hall, C. F., et al. (2003). Cytokine milieu of atopic dermatitis, as compared to psoriasis, skin prevents induction of innate immune response genes. *The Journal of Immunology, 171*(6), 3262–3269. https://doi.org/10.4049/jimmunol.171.6.3262.

Nomura, T., Akiyama, M., Sandilands, A., Nemoto-Hasebe, I., Sakai, K., Nagasaki, A., et al. (2008). Specific filaggrin mutations cause ichthyosis vulgaris and are significantly associated with atopic dermatitis in Japan. *Journal of Investigative Dermatology, 128*(6), 1436–1441. https://doi.org/10.1038/sj.jid.5701205.

Nomura, T., Akiyama, M., Sandilands, A., Nemoto-Hasebe, I., Sakai, K., Nagasaki, A., et al. (2009). Prevalent and rare mutations in the gene encoding filaggrin in Japanese patients with ichthyosis vulgaris and atopic dermatitis. *Journal of Investigative Dermatology, 129*(5), 1302–1305. https://doi.org/10.1038/jid.2008.372.

Ohmen, J. D., Hanifin, J. M., Nickoloff, B. J., Rea, T. H., Wyzykowski, R., Kim, J., et al. (1995). Overexpression of IL-10 in atopic dermatitis: Contrasting cytokine patterns with delayed-type hypersensitivity reactions. *The Journal of Immunology, 154*(4), 1956–1963.

Oji, V., Seller, N., Sandilands, A., Gruber, R., Gerss, J., Huffmeier, U., et al. (2009). Ichthyosis vulgaris: Novel FLG mutations in the German population and high presence of CD1a+ cells in the epidermis of the atopic subgroup. *British Journal of Dermatology, 160*(4), 771–781. https://doi.org/10/1111/j.1365-2133.2008.08999.x.

On, H. R., Lee, S. E., Kim, S.-E., Hong, W. J., Kim, H. J., Nomura, T., et al. (2017). Filaggrin mutation in Korean patients with atopic dermatitis. *Medical Journal, 58*(2), 395–400. https://doi.org/10.3349/ymj.2017.58.2.395.

Osawa, R., Akiyama, M., & Shimizu, H. (2011). Filaggrin gene defects and the risk of developing allergic disorders. *Allergology International, 60*(1), 1–9. https://doi.org/10.2332/allergolint.10-RAI-0270.

Paller, A., Jaworski, J. C., Simpson, E. L., Boguniewicz, M., Russell, J. J., Block, J. K., et al. (2018). Major comorbidities of atopic dermatitis: Beyond allergic disorders. *American Journal of Clinical Dermatology, 19*(6), 821–838. https://doi.org/10.1007/s40257-018-0383-4.

Park, K. Y., Park, M. K., Seok, J., Li, K., & Seo, S. J. (2016). Clinical characteristics of Korean patients with filaggrin-related atopic dermatitis. *Clinical and Experimental Dermatology, 41*(6), 595–600. https://doi.org/10.1111/ced.12854.

Peng, W. M., Jenneck, C., Bussmann, C., Bogdanow, M., Hart, J., Leung, D. Y. M., et al. (2007). Risk factors of atopic dermatitis patients for eczema herpeticum. *Journal of Investigative Dermatology, 127*(5), 1261–1263. https://doi.org/10.1038/sj.jid.5700657.

Polcari, I., Becker, L., Stein, S. L., Smith, M. S., & Paller, A. (2014). Filaggrin gene mutations in Africans with both ichthyosis vulgaris

and atopic dermatitis. *Pediatric Dermatology, 31*(4), 489–492. https://doi.org/10.1111/pde.12355.

Rac, H., Gould, A. P., Bookstaver, P. B., Justo, J., Kohn, J. A., & Al-Hasan, M. N. (2020). Evaluation of early clinical failure criteria for gram-negative bloodstream infections. *Clinical Microbiology and Infection, 26*, 73–77. https://doi.org/10.1016/j.cmi.2019.05.017.

Reed, J. L., Scott, D. E., & Bray, M. (2012). Eczema vaccinatum. *Clinical Infectious Diseases, 54*(6), 832–840. https://doi.org/10.1093/cid/cir952.

Reichle, M. E., Chen, L., Lin, S.-X., & Chan, L. S. (2011). The Th2 system immune milieu enhances cutaneous inflammation in the K14-IL-4-transgenic atopic dermatitis model. *Journal of Investigative Dermatology, 131*(3), 791–794. https://doi.org/10.1038/jid.2010.382.

Ricci, M., Matucci, A., & Rossi, O. (1997). IL-4 as a key factor influencing the development of allergen-specific Th2-like cells in atopic dermatitis. *Journal of Investigational Allergology and Clinical Immunology, 7*(3), 144–150.

Sandilands, A., Terron-Kwiatkowski, A., Hull, P. R., O'Regan, G. M., Clayton, T. H., Watson, R. M., et al. (2007). Comprehensive analysis of the gene encoding filaggrin uncovers prevalent and rare mutations in ichthyosis vulgaris and atopic dermatitis. *Nature Genetics, 39*(5), 650–654. https://doi.org/10.1038/ng2020.

Sekiya, A., Kono, M., Tsujiuchi, H., Kobayashi, T., Nomura, T., Kitakawa, M., et al. (2017). Compound heterozygotes for filaggrin gene mutations do not always show severe atopic dermatitis. *Journal of the European Academy of Dermatology and Venereology, 31*(1), 158–162. https://doi.org/10.1111/jdv.13871.

Shirakawa, T., Deichmann, K. A., Izuhara, K., Mao, X.-Q., Adra, C. N., & Hopkin, J. M. (2000). Atopy and asthma: genetic variants of IL-4 and IL-13 signaling. *Immunology Today, 21*(2), 60–64. https://doi.org/10.1016/S0167-5699(99)01492-9.

Silverberg, J. I. (2019). Comorbidities and the impact of atopic dermatitis. *The Annals of Allergy, Asthma, & Immunology, 123*(2), 144–151. https://doi.org/10.1016/j.anai.2019.04.020.

Smith, F. J. D., Irvine, A. D., Terron-Kwiakowski, A., Sandilands, A., Campbell, L. E., Zhao, Y., et al. (2006). Loss-of-function mutations in the gene encoding filaggrin cause ichthyosis vulgaris. *Nature Genetics, 38*(3), 337–342. https://doi.org/10.1038/ng1743.

Stott, B., Lavender, P., Lahmann, S., Pennino, D., Durham, S., & Schmidt-Weber., C. B. (2013). Human IL-31 is induced by IL-4 and promotes Th2-driven inflammation. *Journal of Allergy and Clinical Immunology, 132*(2), 446–454. https://doi.org/10.1016/j.jaci.2013.03.050.

Sun, D., & Peck, Y. O. (2017). Infectious complications in atopic dermatitis. *Immunology and Allergy Clinics of North America, 37*(1), 75–93. https://doi.org/10.1016/j.iac.2016.08.015.

Tang, M. L., & Kemp, A. S. (1994). Spontaneous expression of IL-4 mRNA in lymphocytes from children with atopic dermatitis. *Clinical & Experimental Allergy, 97*(3), 491–498. https://doi.org/10.1111/j.1365-2249.1994.tb06115.x.

Turner, W., Bauer, D. J., & Nimmo-Smith, R. H. (1962). Eczema vaccinatum treated with n-methylisatin beta-thiosemicarbazone. *British Medical Journal, 12*(5288), 1317–1319. https://doi.org/10.1136/bmj.1.5288.1317.

Waddington, E., Bray, P. T., Evans, A. D., & Richards, I. D. (1964). Cutaneous complications of mass vaccination against smallpox in South Wales. *Transactions of the St. John's Hospital Dermatological Society, 50*, 22–42.

Wierenga, E. A., Snoek, M., de Groot, C., Chretien, I., Bos, J. D., Jansen, H. M., & Kapsenberg, M. L. (1990). Evidence for compartmentalization of functional subsets of CD2+ T lymphocytes in atopic patient. *The Journal of Immunology, 144*(12), 4651–4656.

Wilis-Karp, M. (2000). The gene encoding interleukin-13: A susceptibility locus for asthma and related traits. *Respiratory Research, 1*(1), 19–23. https://doi.org/10.1186/rr7.

Wollenberg, A., & Klein, E. (2007). Current aspects of innate and adaptive immunity in atopic dermatitis. *Clinical Reviews in Allergy & Immunology, 33*(1-2), 35–44. https://doi.org/10.1007/s12016-007-0032-9.

Wollenberg, A., Rawer, H.-C., & Schauber, J. (2011). Innate immunity in atopic dermatitis. *Clinical Reviews in Allergy & Immunology, 41*(3), 272–281. https://doi.org/10.1007/s12016-010-8227-x.

Yamamura, M., Uyemura, K., Deans, R. J., Weinberg, K., Rea, T. H., Bloom, B. R., & Modlin., R. L. (1991). Defining protective responses to pathogens: Cytokine profiles in leprosy lesions. *Science, 254*(5029), 277–279.

Zhang, H., Guo, Y., Wang, W., Shi, M., Chen, X., & Yao, Z. (2011). Mutations in the filaggrin gene in Han Chinese patients with atopic dermatitis. *Allergy, 66*(3), 420–427. https://doi.org/10.1111/j.1398-9995.2010.02493.x.

Zhang, H., Guo, Y., Wang, W., Yu, X., & Yao, Z. (2011). Association of FLG mutations between ichthyosis vulgaris and atopic dermatitis in Han Chinese. *Allergy, 66*(9), 1252–1254. https://doi.org/10.1111/j.1398-9995.2011.02597.x.

19

Therapeutic Guideline Overview

SAFIYYAH BHATTI, ALEXIS TRACY, AND LAWRENCE F. EICHENFIELD

KEY POINTS

- Multiple clinical guidelines, consensus statements, and expert management recommendations have been published for atopic dermatitis.
- Most prominent guidelines are from the American Academy of Dermatology and the College of Allergy, Asthma & Immunology Joint Task published in 2014 and 2012, respectively.
- Guidelines discuss diagnostic and grading severity criteria, which are generally used in clinical trials rather than clinical practice.
- There is a commonality among most guideline documents in terms of recommendations of standard interventions with moisturization, topical corticosteroids, topical calcineurin inhibitors, and phosphodiesterase-4 inhibitors.
- Systemic therapy recommendations are actively changing with introduction of new systemic immunomodulatory agents and other emerging therapies.

Introduction

Treatments for atopic dermatitis (AD) have evolved over the years. As our understanding of the underlying pathophysiology grows, treatment options broaden and treatment strategies are refined. This chapter provides a bird's-eye view on the general therapeutic guideline, taking into account the recently published consensus. Following this chapter, the section Clinician's Corner will then be divided into discussions of therapeutics from the perspectives of encountering the external factors (see Chapters 20, 21, and 22), the internal factors (see Chapter 23), and the combined approaches (see Chapters 24, 25, 26, and 27).

Overview of recently published guidelines

This chapter serves to provide a unified, consolidated overview of recently published therapeutic guidelines for the management of AD. Guidelines and similar documents, including consensus statements and expert management recommendations, are pursued and published to assist in the clinical care and management of AD patients. Many

of these are produced through professional organizations that relate to specialty societies, including dermatology and allergy organizations, as well as pediatric and other primary care health care professional groups. Guidelines may vary by region, country, and continent; others are international initiatives. This chapter aims to review and emphasize the most essential current guidelines related to caring for patients with AD across the age groups, conscious that it can only relate a selection of them with cursory sampling of the actual recommendations.

This chapter will draw most of its focus from the American Academy of Allergy, Asthma & Immunology/ American College of Allergy, Asthma & Immunology Joint Task Force 2012 AD Practice Parameter (JTF) and the 2014 American Academy of Dermatology (AAD) guidelines. The JTF Practice Parameter is an update of the 2004 parameter on AD; it is a single document with an executive summary, followed by evidence-based summary statements and an annotated flowchart of the diagnosis and management of AD. The AAD guidelines are organized into four separate publications. The AAD work group and JTF ranked their recommendations in similar manners, AAD from "A" to "C" and JTF from "A" to "D." Both of these are based on the grade of evidence available for these clinical practices.

Diagnostic and severity grading criteria for atopic dermatitis

The diagnosis of AD is clinically based. In making this diagnosis, physicians should consider patient history, lesion morphology and distribution, and associated clinical signs. Various groups have created formal guidelines to aid in making a correct and reliable diagnosis of AD, though guideline criteria vary in sensitivity, specificity, and applicability to epidemiologic or clinical studies versus utility in clinical practice.

The 1980 Hanifin and Rajka criteria is one of the earliest and most recognized sets of diagnostic criteria for AD. The diagnosis of AD requires that one must meet 3 of 4 major criteria and 3 of 23 minor criteria (Table 19.1). Though comprehensive and commonly used in clinical trials, the

TABLE 19.1 Clinical diagnostic criteria for atopic dermatitis

Major criteria (3 of 4 must be present)	Minor criteria (≥3 must be present)
Typical morphology and distribution of skin lesions: flexural involvement in adults, facial and extensor involvement in infants Pruritus Chronic or relapsing disease Personal and/or family history of atopy (asthma, allergic rhinoconjunctivitis, atopic dermatitis)	Early age of onset Xerosis Ichthyosis Facial pallor and/or erythema Pityriasis alba Orbital darkening Dennie-Morgan infraorbital folds Anterior neck folds Subcapsular cataract Keratoconus Recurrent conjunctivitis Immediate (type 1) skin-test reactivity Increased serum total immunoglobulin E concentration Hyperlinear palms Keratosis pilaris Cheilitis Nonspecific hand and foot eczema Areolar eczema Pruritus upon sweating Wind intolerance White dermatographism Perifollicular accentuation Susceptibility to bacterial and viral infections (particularly *Staphylococcus aureus* and herpes simplex) or impaired cell-mediated immunity Triggers: foods, environmental factors, emotional stressors, and skin irritants

Derived from Hanifin, J. M., & Rajka, G. (1980). Diagnostic features of atopic dermatitis. *Acta Dermato-Venereologica (Stockholm), 92*, S44–S47.

criteria can be difficult to incorporate into clinical practice—additionally, several of the minor criteria are nonspecific or uncommon (Eichenfield et al., 2014a, 2014b). Several international groups have proposed modifications to address these limitations (e.g., Kang and Tian criteria, International Study of Asthma and Allergies in Childhood [ISAAC] criteria) (Eichenfield et al., 2014a, 2014b). A systematically distilled version of the Hanifin and Rajka criteria created by the UK Working Party is often utilized for epidemiologic studies. The core set consists of one mandatory and five major criteria, all of which do not require laboratory testing. Both the Hanifin and Rajka and the UK Working Party diagnostic schemes have been validated in studies and tested in several different populations. The original UK criteria cannot be applied to very young children, although revisions to include infants have since been proposed (Eichenfield et al., 2014a, 2014b).

A 2003 consensus conference directed by the American Academy of Dermatology suggested diagnostic schemes based on revised Hanifin and Rajka criteria that are simplified and applicable to the wide age range that can be affected by this disease (Table 19.2) (Eichenfield et al., 2014a, 2014b). This version has been formally validated in children, but not adults (Udkoff et al., 2017); however, it has been accepted by many for use in clinical trials, as well as considered a pragmatic approach for the clinical setting.

The JTF and AAD guidelines both define AD as a chronic pruritic inflammatory disease that more commonly affects the pediatric population and is a diagnosis that is clinically based on patient's history, characteristic clinical findings, and exclusion of other dermatoses. Both of these guidelines agree that the disease can be familial; however, the AAD guidelines associate AD with history of type 1 allergies, allergic rhinitis, and asthma (Eichenfield et al., 2014a, 2014b). The JTF guidelines assert the necessity of an atopic history, whereas the AAD guidelines only distinguish atopy as an important feature. The JTF guidelines outline the typical appearance according to the chronicity of AD lesions as pruritic, erythematous papulovesicular lesions associated with excoriation and serous exudate in the acute setting, whereas findings of lichenification, papules, and excoriations can be seen in patients with chronic AD. In contrast, AAD guidelines focus more on the standardized criteria based on the revised Hanifin and Rajka diagnostic schemes discussed earlier (see Table 19.1) (Eichenfield et al., 2017).

Multiple guideline's criteria discuss the differential diagnosis and suggest judicial use of skin biopsy specimens or other tests (such as serum immunoglobulin E [IgE], potassium hydroxide preparation, contact allergy patch testing, and/or genetic testing), which may be helpful to rule out other or associated skin conditions. The AAD guidelines mandate the exclusion of other common cutaneous

TABLE 19.2	Features in the diagnosis of atopic dermatitis

Features to be considered in the diagnosis of patients with atopic dermatitis (AD)
Essential features (these must be present)
- Pruritus
- Eczema
- Typical morphology and age-specific patterns (as specified below)
- Chronic or relapsing history

Patterns include:
- Facial and extensor involvement in infants and children
- Current or history of flexural lesions in any age group
- Lack of involvement of groin and axillary regions

Important features (these support the diagnosis and are present in the majority of cases)
- Early age of onset
- Atopy
- Personal and/or family history
- Immunoglobulin E reactivity
- Xerosis

Associated features (these are nonspecific and cannot be used to define the diagnosis of AD for research and epidemiologic studies; however, they can suggest the diagnosis of AD)
- Facial pallor, white dermographism, delayed blanch response
- Perifollicular accentuation/lichenification/prurigo lesions
- Keratosis pilaris/pityriasis alba/hyperlinear palms/ichthyosis

Exclusionary conditions
- Psoriasis
- Photosensitivity dermatoses
- Scabies
- Contact dermatitis
- Ichthyoses
- Seborrheic dermatitis
- Cutaneous T-cell lymphoma
- Immune deficiency diseases
- Erythroderma of other causes

disorders before the diagnosis of AD; however, the JTF guidelines suggest this through thorough reevaluation. Other considerations discussed by the AAD work group include the lack of a requirement for specific biomarkers for a diagnosis or severity assessment and recommend against routine IgE levels (Eichenfield et al., 2017).

Severity grading criteria

There are a myriad of disease severity scales, the most common being the Eczema Area and Severity Index (EASI), Scoring Atopic Dermatitis (SCORAD), Investigator's Global Assessment (IGA), and the Six Area, Six Sign Atopic Dermatitis (SASSAD) severity score.

As there are currently more than 20 different named instruments to measure the severity of AD, all of which assess different aspects of AD in different ways, a major obstacle exists in advancing evidence-based treatment.

Because of this, the global Harmonising Outcome Measures for Eczema (HOME) initiative was created with the aim to standardize and validate a core set of outcome measurements for AD. As outlined on the HOME for eczema group webpage, the HOME outcome domains are divided into four categories: clinical signs measured by using a physician-assessed instrument, symptoms measured by using a patient-assessed instrument, health-related quality of life, and long-term control of flares (Schmitt et al., 2014).

The EASI score evaluates the AD involvement based on the extent of dermatitis and the degree of erythema, papulation, excoriation, and lichenification by body regions. The SCORAD takes into consideration both the physician's objectives on extent and severity as well as the subjective patient assessment of itch and sleeplessness. The Patient-Oriented Eczema Measure (POEM) is a short questionnaire solely based on the patient's perspective in relation to symptoms and frequency. The Three Item Severity Scale (TISS) is another simplified scale that shows promise for future use in clinical practice, although it needs further testing.

The available literature suggests that the SCORAD index, the EASI score, and POEM severity scale have been adequately tested and validated, and therefore their use can be considered when practical (Eichenfield et al., 2014a, 2014b). For clinical studies, the HOME group states that all trials should measure the core domains (as referenced earlier) as this will enable trials to be compared and combined in meta-analyses. Worldwide consensus was reached that these core outcome domains should be used in all future AD trials. However, the inclusion of core outcomes does not preclude the use of any additional domains, scales, or instruments. The HOME group recommends the use of EASI score for the clinical signs core outcome, and POEM for patient reported symptoms core outcome. For the quality of life core outcome, they recommend the Dermatology Life Quality Index (DLQI) for adults, Children's Dermatology Life Quality Index (CDLQI) for children, and the Infants' Dermatitis Quality of Life Index (IDQoL) for infants. The RECAP (Recap of Eczema Control for Atopic Eczema) and the ADCT (Atopic Dermatitis Control Tool) are recommended as the long-term control outcome measures (Harmonizing Outcome Measures for Eczema [HOME], 2020; Schmitt et al., 2014).

These scales are primarily used in clinical trials and only rarely in clinical practice. IGA, as its name reflects, uses investigational global assessments (IGAs) in its studies. Many different IGAs have been utilized, and recently a validated IGA has been developed and recommended for use by the International Eczema Council (2014; Simpson et al., 2020).

Body surface area (BSA) is a standard assessment in clinical studies and may be a useful measure in clinical practice.

The AAD guidelines state that for the general management of patients with AD, available disease severity measurement scales are not recommended for routine clinical practice because they were not designed for this purpose. Additionally, they recommend that clinicians ask general questions about itch, sleep, impact on daily activity, and persistence of disease, and currently available scales should be used mainly when practical (Eichenfield et al., 2014a, 2014b).

Nonpharmaceutic agents: moisturization, wet wrap therapy, and bleach baths

Topical therapies are the mainstay of AD treatment and are commonly used with other interventions to combat different components of this complex disease. In this section we focus on the current guidelines with reference to the JTF and AAD recommendations on these common nonpharmaceutic therapies: moisturizers, wet wrap therapy, and bleach baths.

Moisturization

Xerosis is one of the cardinal clinical features of AD. Dryness, essentially ubiquitous in AD patients, is secondary to a dysfunctional epidermal barrier and transepidermal water loss—factors that moisturizers help alleviate to some degree. Moisturizers may include emollients (i.e., glycol, soy sterols), occlusive agents (i.e., petrolatum, dimethicone, mineral oil), and humectants (i.e., glycerol, lactic acid, urea).

Moisturizers help to hydrate the skin—this has been supported both subjectively by patients and objectively by means of microscopy to assess changes in the skin's capacitance/conductance. A number of clinical trials have shown that moisturizers lessen the symptoms and signs of AD, including pruritus, erythema, fissuring, and lichenification. Additionally, multiple randomized clinical trials have demonstrated that moisturizer use decreases the amount of prescription antiinflammatory treatments needed for disease control.

Most all guideline documents state that regardless of severity, moisturizers should be incorporated in all AD patient regimens and continued as part of a maintenance plan for prevention of flares due to strong evidence that it can reduce disease severity and the need for pharmacologic intervention. The JTF and AAD guidelines concur that moisturizers increase skin hydration by improving skin barrier function and reducing transepidermal water loss. Both agree that moisturizers are a main primary treatment for mild disease and an important adjunctive therapy in moderate and severe disease (Eichenfield et al., 2017).

It is expert consensus that moisturizers should be applied soon after bathing to improve skin hydration, though there is not an optimal amount or frequency of application defined by systematic studies. In the JTF and AAD guidelines, liberal and frequent application is suggested. The AAD and JTF guidelines acknowledge that most ointments carry the advantage of being preservative and fragrance free; however, no specific recommendations regarding vehicle systems and types of moisturizers have been made (Eichenfield et al., 2017).

Prescription emollient devices (PEDs) are generally agents with distinct ratios of lipids that mimic normal skin.

They are designed and proposed to target defects in skin barrier function seen in AD patients. They have not been shown to be superior to other moisturizing products, and therefore AAD guidelines do not recommend their use (Eichenfield et al., 2017).

Among the few trials that have been conducted to compare and contrast specific moisturizing products, a specific moisturizer has not been deemed superior—this includes the PEDs. Choice of moisturizer is largely based on patient and provider preference, though ideally the chosen agent is effective and free of additives, fragrances, and other sensitizing agents. Despite the lack of specifics, both the JTF and AAD guidelines recommend incorporating moisturizers as part of the AD patient regimen in times of active disease, maintenance, and flare prevention.

Wet wrap therapy

AAD guidelines recommend that the use of wet wrap therapy with or without a topical corticosteroid (TCS) can be advised for patients with moderate to severe AD to decrease disease severity and water loss during flares (Eichenfield et al., 2017).

Both the JTF and AAD guidelines recommend wet wrap therapy with use of TCS in the setting of significant flares/refractory disease. This method tends to involve applying TCS followed by wet gauze and a second layer of dry gauze to seal in the medication. Some experts utilize two layers of clothing over TCS as an alternative. Wet wraps help to occlude and increase penetration of the therapeutic agent; additionally, it decreases water loss and provides a barrier against scratching. It should be mentioned that caution should be taken when using mid- to high-potency steroids as there is an increased chance of systemic side effects particularly if used widely on skin, though only the JTF guidelines recommend against overuse of wet wrap therapy (Eichenfield et al., 2017).

Bleach baths

In patients with moderate to severe AD and clinical signs of secondary bacterial infections, antimicrobial bleach baths may be recommended to reduce disease severity. For the population of AD patients that have frequent, recurrent bacterial infections both the JTF and AAD guidelines support the consideration of incorporating bleach baths in both active and maintenance periods. The effect of bleach baths on microbial colonization has been challenged by some experts (Eichenfield et al., 2017).

As an aside, there are no standards regarding frequency or duration of bathing appropriate for patients with AD, though both JTF and AAD guidelines recommend bathing with warm water and applying moisturizer shortly after bathing (Eichenfield et al., 2017). Studies have supported the utility of more frequent bathing with moisturization to follow versus infrequent bathing (Cardona et al., 2019). Limited use of nonsoap cleansers that are neutral to low pH, hypoallergenic, and fragrance free is recommended. There is not sufficient evidence to support adding oils or emollients to bath water; that being said, JTF supports additives such as baking soda or oatmeal for symptomatic relief while the AAD advises against such additives with the exception being bleach for reasons discussed earlier (Eichenfield et al., 2017).

Topical modalities: corticosteroids, calcineurin inhibitors, and phosphodiesterase-4 inhibitors

This section will focus on topical antiinflammatory therapies used in the treatment of AD. We focus on the current guidelines with reference to the JTF and AAD recommendations on pharmaceutic therapies, including TCS, topical calcineurin inhibitors (TCI), and phosphodiesterase-4 (PDE4) inhibitors. The choice of which topical therapy to use as maintenance therapy will depend on patient/caregiver and provider preference, access to medications (including formulary status and cost of medication), lesion location (TCS use in sensitive skin areas such as the face and eyes should be limited), and the effectiveness and tolerability observed with a particular agent (Eichenfield et al., 2015).

Topical corticosteroids

TCS products are used in the management of AD in both adults and children and are the mainstay of antiinflammatory therapy when nonpharmacologic interventions have failed (Eichenfield et al., 2014a, 2014b). According to both AAD and JTF guidelines, low-potency TCS are generally suggested for maintenance therapy, whereas intermediate and high-potency TCS are recommended for the acute control of AD. Twice-daily application of TCS is commonly recommended for the treatment of acute AD (Eichenfield et al., 2017), while some studies state that daily TCS may be as effective (Williams, 2007).

Once healing is achieved (regression of eczema and improvement or resolution of itching), the goal of therapy should be long-term disease control, extending the relapse-free time for as long as possible and minimizing signs and symptoms. The use of moisturizers alone as maintenance therapy without a topical antiinflammatory may be sufficient for mild AD. For this purpose, emollients can be effective, but patients or family members should be educated to reapply topical antiinflammatory therapies with signs of relapse.

Proactive therapy with TCS may be started after eczema heals (Eichenfield et al., 2015). For proactive maintenance therapy, the AAD suggests once- to twice-weekly application of TCS in commonly flaring areas to prevent relapses, whereas the JTF discusses long-term control with twice-weekly TCS. Although no optimal quantity of TCS has been definitively recommended, AAD guidelines highlight

the fingertip unit method applied over an area equivalent to 2 palms in addition to the use of charts that propose quantities that are age and area based (Eichenfield et al., 2017). Providers may also find it helpful to prescribe specific amounts of a topical agent to be used over the course of 1 week or month to ensure proper use of TCS, TCI, and/or moisturizers (Eichenfield et al., 2015). Both AAD and JTF guidelines caution use of TCS on areas of thin skin, such as the face, neck, and skin folds, because adverse effects are directly related to the surface area of affected skin, skin thickness, use of occlusive dressing, and potency and duration of TCS administered (Eichenfield et al., 2017).

Topical calcineurin inhibitors

TCI, including tacrolimus and pimecrolimus, are a distinct class of steroid-sparing, antiinflammatory agents that have been shown to be efficacious in acute flares and maintenance therapy of AD in both adults and children 2 years and older (Eichenfield et al., 2017). Tacrolimus ointment (0.03%) and pimecrolimus cream (1%) are approved as short-term and noncontinuous chronic treatments of AD in the United States, Canada, and Europe for children 2 years of age and older with mild to moderate AD. In addition, 0.1% tacrolimus ointment is approved for treatment of moderate to severe AD in children 16 years of age and older. The AAD and JTF guidelines agree that use of TCI at sites of sensitive or thin skin offers an advantage over use of TCS (Eichenfield et al., 2017). TCI are usually offered as a second-line therapy for acute and chronic treatment of AD in patients who have not responded adequately to other topical treatments or when those treatments are not recommended (Eichenfield et al., 2014a, 2014b).

Twice-daily application of either tacrolimus ointment or pimecrolimus cream is efficacious in treating inflamed AD lesions and improving or resolving pruritus. Proactive or maintenance therapy for AD that includes intermittent application of TCI twice daily or two to three times weekly to recurrent sites of involvement has been shown to reduce relapse and is recommended per AAD and JTF guidelines although not per US Food and Drug Administration (FDA) guidelines. Both AAD and JTF guidelines emphasize the importance of counseling patients on potential side effects to prevent premature discontinuation of treatment. Although not discussed in the JTF practice parameter, the AAD guidelines recommend the preceding use of TCI with TCS, where appropriate, to lessen the severity of local skin reactions with recommendation to initially use TCS to control a flare, whereas TCI can be applied as maintenance therapy to prevent relapse. In addition to informing patients about immediate site reactions with TCI, both guidelines advocate for proactive guidance regarding the FDA's boxed warning for potential risk of malignancy (Eichenfield et al., 2017).

According to the European guidelines, although TCS remain the mainstay of therapy, tacrolimus and pimecrolimus are preferred in sensitive skin areas and for long-term use. Per European guidelines for children with AD, twice-weekly treatment with tacrolimus 0.03% ointment is recommended as it has been observed to reduce the number of flares and to prolong flare-free intervals and may be cost saving in children with moderate or severe AD (Wollenberg et al., 2018a, 2018b).

Topical phosphodiesterase-4 inhibitors

Crisaborole 2% topical ointment is a nonsteroidal anti-inflammatory PDE4 inhibitor approved in 2016 by the FDA in the United States to treat mild to moderate AD in patients 2 years or older. As crisaborole was introduced after their publication, there are no current AAD or JTF guidelines available on this particular drug. When considering step-up therapy in mild to moderate AD when symptoms are not well controlled with a low to medium potency TCS, either TCS dose or potency can be increased, or a TCI or crisaborole can be added. Based on safety and efficacy profiles, it has been suggested that TCS be used to treat symptom exacerbations, followed by long-term maintenance therapy with a lower dose of a TCS and/or a TCI or crisaborole. Crisaborole can be used as a first-line agent in patients based on their established adverse event profiles with TCS or TCI use with the goal to proactively prevent relapses (Boguniewicz et al., 2018).

Phototherapy

The AAD and JTF guidelines both recommend phototherapy as a treatment for AD refractory to topical treatments. Consideration of availability, cost, patient skin type, skin cancer history, and patient use of photosensitizing medications might help with the selection of phototherapy. Although AAD guidelines outline the multiple forms of light therapy without a definitive recommendation of a particular therapy, the JTF guidelines consider narrow-band ultraviolet B (UVB) as the most effective phototherapy option, given its low-risk profile, relative efficacy, availability, and provider comfort level. JTF guidelines additionally suggest using UVA1 for acute exacerbations, UVB modalities for chronic AD, and photochemotherapy with psoralen and UVA only for patients with severe widespread AD. AAD guidelines state that phototherapy can be used as maintenance therapy in patients with chronic disease. Dosing and frequency of phototherapy are dependent on minimal erythema dose, Fitzpatrick skin type, or both (Eichenfield et al., 2017).

Systemic therapies

Adults with severe recalcitrant AD that is not well controlled by intensive topical treatment or phototherapy and those for whom phototherapy is not a viable option may be offered systemic therapies. The choice of a systemic treatment will depend upon severity of AD, impact on the patient's quality of life, the patient's age and sex, family planning issues, presence of comorbidities, adverse effects, the patient's preferences, and costs. This section will focus on current immunomodulating agents, systemic steroids, the biologic dupilumab, and emerging therapies.

Systemic immunomodulatory agents

Systemic immunomodulatory agents are indicated for the subset of adult and pediatric patients in whom optimized topical regimens and/or phototherapy do not adequately control the signs and symptoms of disease (Sidbury et al., 2014). Both AAD and JTF guidelines recommend immunomodulatory agents in a subset of patients with severe AD refractory to topical regimens and phototherapy or when quality of life is severely affected (Eichenfield et al., 2017).

Physicians should optimize topical therapy before considering systemic medications for AD. Patients who have inadequate response should be evaluated for exacerbating factors such as cutaneous infection and for alternative diagnoses such as allergic contact dermatitis. Adequate education needs to be delivered to improve adherence to topical therapy. The general approach should be an intensive clearance period with a TCS followed by a safe and individualized regimen of intermittent TCS, TCI, or emollients to prevent flares. Phototherapy should be considered before the use of other systemic therapy if accessible and practical.

The International Eczema Council (2014) recommends a systematic approach (Fig. 19.1) to assess patients with severe signs and/or symptoms of AD and/or impact on quality of life before starting systemic therapy. One approach for identifying a candidate for systemic therapy is to utilize a disease severity score. The two most extensively validated disease severity scores are SCORAD, which incorporates the intensity of disease signs and extent along with the patient-reported sleep loss and itch, and EASI. Documentation of severe, extensive disease and/or QoL impairment at several time points with adequate topical therapy enables a holistic rationale for moving to systemic therapy (Simpson et al., 2017).

Several systemic therapies are used both on- and off-label for the treatment of moderate to severe pediatric and adult AD refractory to topical therapy and/or phototherapy. These include methotrexate, cyclosporine A, azathioprine, mycophenolate mofetil, prednisone, and biologics, which currently only include dupilumab. Although both guidelines agree that there is a paucity of data indicating the relative efficacy of each systemic agent, the AAD guidelines suggest that cyclosporine, methotrexate, mycophenolate mofetil, and azathioprine are widely used and more efficacious in treating AD when compared with interferon-gamma (IFN-γ) and oral calcineurin inhibitors.

Although the AAD tabulates dosages, monitoring, adverse effects, interactions, and contraindications of systemic immunomodulants, the JTF emphasizes potential serious adverse effects. Therefore the agent used is based on provider and patient preferences for injection versus tablets,

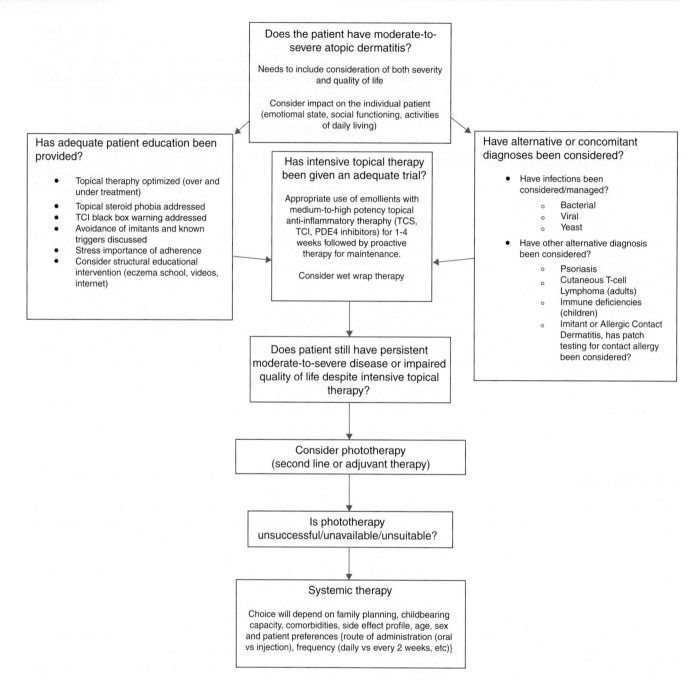

Does the patient have moderate-to-severe atopic dermatitis?

Needs to include consideration of both severity and quality of life

Consider impact on the individual patient (emotional state, social functioning, activities of daily living)

Has adequate patient education been provided?

- Topical therapy optimized (over and under treatment)
- Topical steroid phobia addressed
- TCI black box warning addressed
- Avoidance of imitants and known triggers discussed
- Stress importance of adherence
- Consider structural educational intervention (eczema school, videos, internet)

Has intensive topical therapy been given an adequate trial?

Appropriate use of emollients with medium-to-high potency topical anti-inflammatory therapy (TCS, TCI, PDE4 inhibitors) for 1-4 weeks followed by proactive therapy for maintenance.

Consider wet wrap therapy

Have alternative or concomitant diagnoses been considered?

- Have infections been considered/managed?
  - Bacterial
  - Viral
  - Yeast
- Have other alternative diagnosis been considered?
  - Psoriasis
  - Cutaneous T-cell Lymphoma (adults)
  - Immune deficiencies (children)
  - Imitant or Allergic Contact Dermatitis, has patch testing for contact allergy been considered?

Does patient still have persistent moderate-to-severe disease or impaired quality of life despite intensive topical therapy?

Consider phototherapy (second line or adjuvant therapy)

Is phototherapy unsuccessful/unavailable/unsuitable?

Systemic therapy

Choice will depend on family planning, childbearing capacity, comorbidities, side effect profile, age, sex and patient preferences {route of administration (oral vs injection), frequency (daily vs every 2 weeks, etc)}

• **Fig. 19.1** Algorithm to determine when to initiate systemic immunomodulatory therapy in patients with atopic dermatitis. (Adapted from the International Eczema Council.) Abbreviations: Topical corticosteroid (TCS), Topical Calcineurin inhibitors (TCI), phosphodiesterase 4 (PDE4).

cost, childbearing capacity, age, comorbidities, and side effect profile (Eichenfield et al., 2017).

Systemic steroids

Systemic steroids are approved by the FDA for patients with moderate to severe AD, owing to their broad label for inflammatory skin disease in both adult and pediatric populations; however, there is minimal safety and efficacy data for their use in AD, and they are not recommended by the

AAD (Boguniewicz et al., 2017). The European guidelines similarly emphasize that "well known side-effects limit their use especially for long-term treatment" and that they have a largely unfavorable risk:benefit ratio (Wollenberg et al., 2018a, 2018b).

Dupilumab

Dupilumab is a biologic agent indicated for moderate to severe AD in patients age 6 years and older at the time of this publication. Given the timing of introduction of this biologic agent, many guideline documents have not included dupilumab in recommendations. The European guidelines recommend dupilumab as a disease-modifying drug for patients with moderate to severe AD, in whom topical treatment is not sufficient and other systemic treatment is not advisable (Wollenberg et al., 2018a, 2018b). Dupilumab was the first systemic biologic indicated in the United States for the treatment of pediatric AD in children age 12 years and older and may be considered first-line for this age group when AD cannot be adequately controlled with topical agents (steroids, calcineurin inhibitors, or PDE inhibitors) supplanting methotrexate, cyclosporine, azathioprine, or mycophenolate mofetil. Comparative trials for methotrexate, cyclosporine, azathioprine, or mycophenolate mofetil have not been performed in pediatric AD. Neither AAD or JTF guidelines include a discussion of newer biologics or small-molecule agents such as dupilumab (Eichenfield et al., 2017).

Emerging therapies

Several targeted therapies, both small molecules and biologics, are under investigation for the treatment of moderate to severe AD. Due to guideline documents and consensus statements requiring time to assess newly introduced medications, there are limited discussions of newer biologics or small-molecule agents such as Janus kinase (JAK) inhibitors in most of the publications to date. Novel targeted therapies are being studied in children and adolescents with moderate to severe AD, including both topical and systemic JAK inhibitors as well as other systemic biologics. Baricitinib has been studied for AD in adults, and abrocitinib and upadacitinib, both JAK inhibitors, have completed phase 3 clinical trials for adolescent AD (age 12–17 years) and adults. Tralokinumab and lebrikizumab, both interleukin-13 (IL13) inhibitors, have phase 3 trials underway for patients aged 12 to 17 years as well as adult trials. Risankizumab, an IL23 inhibitor, has a phase 2 trial for patients aged 12 to 17 years. Two other small molecules, ODC-9101 and fevipiprant, which target the chemoattractant receptor-homologous molecule expressed on T helper (Th2) cells, are in phase 2 trials for adults with moderate to severe AD. Other agents in development for adults with moderate to severe AD include two agents that target IL31, nemolizumab and BMS-981164 (Boguniewicz et al., 2017). Again, neither AAD or JTF guidelines include a discussion of newer biologics or small-molecule agents such as JAK inhibitors.

Antihistamines

Topical and oral antihistamines have little evidence to support their use. The AAD advises against general use of systemic sedating and nonsedating antihistamines; however, both JTF and AAD guidelines suggest sedating antihistamines for short-term sporadic use in patients with disturbed sleep caused by pruritus (Eichenfield et al., 2017).

Food allergy guidelines

The AAD and JTF guidelines encourage active assessment for clinical signs of food allergy during AD office visits. Both groups oppose allergy testing independent of clinical assessment. The JTF encourages initial diagnostic use of food-specific IgE antibody testing in patients with AD with clinical presentation suspicious for food allergy. In this subset of patients, oral food challenge is subsequently recommended if IgE test results are negative. Both groups strongly recommend against food elimination based on allergy tests alone, citing the low specificity of such testing and the potential for nutritional deficiencies. The AAD also recommends against elimination diets based on the presence of AD or a suspicious history alone. The National Institute of Allergy and Infectious Diseases (NIAID) Food and Allergy Expert Panel guidelines suggest the consideration of limited food allergy testing in patients less than 5 years of age with refractory AD despite optimal therapeutic management and/or a clinical history of an allergic reaction immediately after specific food exposure (Eichenfield et al., 2017).

Peanut allergy guidelines

Based on data generated in the Learning Early About Peanut Allergy (LEAP) trial and existing guidelines from the American Academy of Allergy, Asthma & Immunology and the American Academy of Pediatrics, health care providers should recommend introducing peanut-containing products into the diets of "high-risk" infants early on in life (between 4 and 11 months of age) in countries where peanut allergy is prevalent because delaying the introduction of peanut can be associated with an increased risk of peanut allergy. Infants with early-onset atopic disease, such as severe eczema, or egg allergy in the first 4 to 6 months of life, might benefit from evaluation by an allergist or physician trained in management of allergic diseases in this age group to diagnose any food allergy and assist in implementing these suggestions regarding the appropriateness of early peanut introduction (Fleischer et al., 2015).

Summary

In conclusion, we reviewed current guidelines as well as consensus statements and expert management recommendations for AD. This included the diagnostic and grading severity criteria created and assessed by multiple organizations, and recommendations for standard treatment interventions both nonpharmacologic and pharmacologic with focus on guidelines as put forth by *Journal of the American Academy of Dermatology* and Asthma & Immunology Joint Task Force 2012 AD Practice Parameter. Overall, there is commonality among most guidelines with minor variations in general recommendations regarding moisturization, TCS, TCI, and PDE4 inhibitors. Systemic therapy recommendations are actively changing as this field continues to expand with new and exciting therapies such as systemic immunomodulatory agents. As novel and emerging therapies continue to be researched and introduced, we hope that this gives patients and providers a better understanding of this disease, more treatment options, and significant improvement in patient quality of life.

Further reading

National Eczema Association. https://nationaleczema.org/.

American Academy of Dermatology: Eczema types: Atopic dermatitis overview. https://www.aad.org/public/diseases/eczema/types/atopic-dermatitis.

Paller, A., & Mancini, A. (2020). Hurwitz Clinical Pediatric Dermatology: A Textbook of Skin. *Disorders of Childhood and Adolescence.* New York: Elsevier.

References

Boguniewicz, M., Andrew, F., Lisa, A. B., Block, J., Eichenfield, L. F., Fonacier, L., et al. (2017). Expert perspectives on management of moderate-to-severe atopic dermatitis: A multidisciplinary consensus addressing current and emerging therapies. *The Journal of Allergy and Clinical Immunology: In Practice,* 5(6), 1519–1531. https://doi.org/10.1016/j.jaip.2017.08.005.

Boguniewicz, M., Fonacier, L., Guttman-Yassky, E., Ong, P. Y., Silverberg, J., & Farrar, J. R. (2018). Atopic dermatitis yardstick: Practical recommendations for an evolving therapeutic landscape. *Annals of Allergy, Asthma & Immunology,* 120(1), 10–22. https://doi.org/10.1016/j.anai.2017.10.039.

Cardona, I. D., Kempe, E. E., Lary, C., Ginder, J. H., & Jain, N. (2019). Frequent versus infrequent bathing in pediatric atopic dermatitis: A randomized clinical trial. *The Journal of Allergy and Clinical Immunology: In Practice,* 8(3), 1014–1021. https://doi.org/10.1016/j.jaip.2019.10.042.

Eichenfield, L. F., Ahluwalia, J., Waldman, A., Borok, J., Udkoff, J., & Boguniewicz., M. (2017). Current guidelines for the evaluation and management of atopic dermatitis: A comparison of the Joint Task Force Practice Parameter and American Academy of Dermatology guidelines. *The Journal of Allergy and Clinical Immunology,* 139(4), S49–S57. https://doi.org/10.1016/j.jaci.2017.01.009.

Eichenfield, L. F., Mark, B., Eric, L. S., John, J. R., Block, J. K., Feldman, S. R., et al. (2015). Translating atopic dermatitis management guidelines into practice for primary care providers. *Pediatrics,* 136(3), 554–565. https://doi.org/10.1542/peds.2014-3678.

Eichenfield, L. F., Wynnis, L. T., Berger, T. G., Krol, A., Paller, A. S., Schwarzenberger, K., et al. (2014a). Guidelines of care for the management of atopic dermatitis. Section 1. Diagnosis and assessment of atopic dermatitis. *Journal of the American Academy of Dermatology,* 70(2), 338–351. https://doi.org/10.1016/j.jaad.2013.10.010.

Eichenfield, L. F., Wynnis, L. T., Berger, T. G., MD, Krol, A., Paller, A. S., Schwarzenberger, K., et al. (2014b). Guidelines of care for the management of atopic dermatitis. Section 2. Management and treatment of atopic dermatitis with topical therapies. *Journal of the American Academy of Dermatology,* 71(1), 116–132. https://doi.org/10.1016/j.jaad.2014.03.023.

Fleischer, D. M., Sicherer, S., Greenhawt, M., Campbell, D., Chan, E., Muraro, A., et al. (2015). Consensus communication on early peanut introduction and the prevention of peanut allergy in high-risk infants. *Annals of Allergy, Asthma & Immunology,* 115(2), 87–90. https://doi.org/10.1016/j.anai.2015.06.001.

Hanifin, J. M., & Rajka, G. (1980). Diagnostic features of atopic dermatitis. *Acta Dermato-Venereologica (Stockholm),* 92(suppl), 44–47.

Harmonizing Outcome Measures for Eczema (HOME). n.d. Harmonizing Outcome Measures for Eczema (HOME). http://www.homeforeczema.org/. Accessed 26.07.2020.

International Eczema Council. 2014. International Eczema Council". Accessed January 31, 2020. http://www.eczemacouncil.org/.

Schmitt, J., Spuls, P. I., Thomas, K. S., Simpson, E., Furue, M., Deckert, S., et al. (2014). The harmonising outcome measures for eczema (HOME) statement to assess clinical signs of atopic eczema in trials. *The Journal of Allergy and Clinical Immunology,* 134(4), 800–807. https://doi.org/10.1016/j.jaci.2014.07.043.

Sidbury, R., Davis, D. M., Cohen, D. E., Cordoro, K. M., Berger, T. G., Bergman, J. N., et al. (2014). Guidelines of care for the management of atopic dermatitis: Section 3. Management and treatment with phototherapy and systemic agents. *Journal of the American Academy of Dermatology,* 71(2), 327–349. https://doi.org/10.1016/j.jaad.2014.03.030.

Simpson, E. L., Bruin-Weller, M., Flohr, C., Ardern-Jones, M. R., Barbarot, S., Deleuran, M., et al. (2017). When does atopic dermatitis warrant systemic therapy? Recommendations from an expert panel of the International Eczema Council. *Journal of the American Academy of Dermatology,* 77(4), 623–633. https://doi.org/10.1016/j.jaad.2017.06.042.

Simpson, E., Bissonnette, R., Eichenfield, L., Guttman-Yassky, E., King, B., Silverberg, J. I., et al. (2020). The Validated Investigator Global Assessment for Atopic Dermatitis (vIGA-AD): The development and reliability testing of a novel clinical outcome measurement instrument for the severity of atopic dermatitis. *Journal of the American Academy of Dermatology,* 83(3), 839–846. https://doi.org/10.1016/j.jaad.2020.04.104.

Udkoff, J., Eichenfield, L. F., Matiz, C., Friedlander, S., Dohil, M., Tom, W., et al. (2017). Validation of the American Academy of Dermatology Diagnostic Criteria for Atopic Dermatitis and Modification into a Checkbox Form. Chicago, Illinois: Presentation; World Congress of Pediatric Dermatology.

Williams, H. C. (2007). Established corticosteroid creams should be applied only once daily in patients with atopic eczema. *British Medical Journal,* 334(7606), 1272. https://doi.org/10.1136/bmj.39195.636319.80.

Wollenberg, A., Barbarot, S., Bieber, T., Christen-Zaech, S., Deleuran, M., Fink-Wagner, A., et al. (2018a). Consensus-based European guidelines for treatment of atopic eczema (atopic dermatitis) in adults and children: Part I. *Journal of the European Academy of Dermatology and Venerology,* 32(5), 657–682. https://doi.org/10.1111/jdv.14891.

Wollenberg, A., Barbarot, S., Bieber, T., Christen-Zaech, S., Deleuran, M., Fink-Wagner, A., et al. (2018b). Consensus-based European guidelines for treatment of atopic eczema (atopic dermatitis) in adults and children: Part II. *Journal of the European Academy of Dermatology and Venerology,* 32(6), 850–878. https://doi.org/10.1111/jdv.14888.

20
Topical Therapies

JOSEPH M. YARDMAN-FRANK, MARY E. LOGUE, AND AIMEE C. SMIDT

KEY POINTS

- Optimal bathing practices can improve atopic dermatitis (AD) symptoms and limit disease flares. Best practices include daily bathing for less than 10 minutes in lukewarm water, utilizing neutral to mildly acidic nonsoap cleansers, and the immediate application of postbath emollients.
- Topical corticosteroids represent the standard of care for acute AD flares. However, their prolonged use should be avoided, and their strength, vehicle, and frequency of application should be customized to each patient.
- Topical calcineurin inhibitors represent a second-line therapy for AD in those patients who have either failed topical cortical steroid treatment, require long-term antiinflammatory treatment, or require treatment to sensitive areas such as the eyelids, face, and genitalia. Phosphodiesterase-4 inhibitors are a newer class of topical antiinflammatory medication, which represents an alternative to topical steroids and topical calcineurin inhibitors.
- Topical antimicrobials are not recommended for the routine management of AD; we also discuss the role of dilute bleach as a bath additive and other such practices.

Introduction

Topical management for atopic dermatitis (AD) includes specific guidance on bathing, topical antiinflammatory medications, and antimicrobial approaches. This chapter summarizes the evidence behind and provides recommendations for optimal bathing practices, including frequency, duration, use of cleansers, and additives, and discusses the role of dilute bleach baths. The role of topical antiinflammatory medications is also reviewed, including topical corticosteroid utilization, and gives guidance on how to optimize acute flare management. Second-line therapies, including topical calcineurin inhibitors and phosphodiesterase-4 inhibitors, are similarly discussed, and recommendations are made for the role of these medications in AD. Lastly, the history behind the use of topical antimicrobial treatments and the importance of limiting their utilization is discussed. In sum, this chapter aims to provide an overview of the topical approach to AD, providing recommendations to optimize maintenance and flare-free intervals as well as guidance on the management of acute flares and refractory situations.

Bathing

Bathing represents a crucial component in the management of AD for epithelial hydration. It is also a salient factor of skin hygiene and can remove allergens, irritants, scale, and crust (Eichenfield et al., 2014; Prezzano & Beck, 2017). However, due to accompanying evaporation, overbathing or improper bathing can also lead to epithelial dryness and decreased epithelial barrier function driven by transepidermal water loss and the drying of the stratum corneum (Eichenfield et al., 2014; LePoidevin, Lee, & Shi, 2019). In practice, patients are often subject to conflicting recommendations from providers. Here, the aim is to present evidence supporting frequency and duration of bathing, the use of specific cleansers and/or soaps, dilute bleach baths, bath additives, and other less-studied bathing practices that may be observed in clinical practice.

Frequency of bathing

It is essential to note that all bathing recommendations discussed here are accompanied by the additional directive for application of a moisturizer or emollient ideally within 3 minutes of bathing. The time window is ideal at sealing in hydration and preventing the negative aspects of evaporation. Baths should be taken in lukewarm to warm water that is comfortable to the patient's skin; excessively hot or cold water temperatures should be avoided. Further, no literature to date directly compares baths versus showers in AD patients, and as such, all recommendations in this chapter should be applied to both bathing methods.

The American management of AD guidelines recommends daily bathing, whereas the European guidelines do not explicitly comment on frequency (Eichenfield et al., 2014; Wollenberg et al., 2018a). Regardless, patients often receive conflicting recommendations. Historically, primary care physicians tend to recommend infrequent bathing; conversely, allergists, immunologists, and dermatologists have recommended frequent bathing (Cardona, Stillman, & Jain, 2016). These conflicting messages have been driven by the fact that some physicians have viewed bathing as drying to the skin, and specialists have viewed it as hydrating. Multiple survey studies have confirmed this trend (Cardona, Kempe, Hatzenbeuhler,

Antaya, Cohen, & Jain, 2015; Kempe, Jain, & Cardona, 2013). Up to 75% of patients/families have reported confusion in how frequently to bathe, and 45.6% have reported receiving conflicting advice (Cardona et al., 2016; Kempe et al., 2013). The primary benefit of bathing most likely stems from its hydrating qualities rather than its cleansing properties (Koutroulis, Petrova, Kratimenos, & Gaughan, 2014).

Type of bathing and duration

Similar to the frequency of bathing, recommendations for duration historically lack consensus. The American Academy of Dermatology (US) guidelines recommend 5- to 10-minute baths, followed by the immediate application of emollients (Eichenfield et al., 2014). European guidelines recommend shorter (5-minute) baths, with the addition of bath oils in the final 2 minutes, followed by patting dry, and the immediate application of emollients (Wollenberg et al., 2018a). Retrospective cohort studies have not shown a statistical significance between short bathing (<5 minutes) versus medium length bathing (5–10 minutes); extended baths (10–30 minutes) are associated with more severe AD (Koutroulis, Pyle, Kopylov, Little, Gaughan, & Kratimenos, 2016). This association of severity with longer duration of bathing may be confounding as those with more severe AD may bathe longer (Koutroulis et al., 2016). Those with severe AD and those with frequent infections are often recommended to take "soak and smear" baths, which consist of bathing for approximately 10 minutes, followed by the immediate application of antiinflammatory medications (Cardona et al., 2016; Eichenfield et al., 2014; LePoidevin et al., 2019). The US guidelines explicitly recommend such baths for patients with frequent exacerbations (Eichenfield et al., 2014).

Cleansers, soaps, and bathing practices

An essential component of bathing is the appropriate use of cleansers and soaps. The epidermis has a mildly acidic pH ranging between 4 and 5.5 (Eichenfield et al., 2014; Prezzano & Beck, 2017). This acid mantle is crucial for skin's innate antimicrobial action and maintenance of the skin barrier (Ali & Yosipovitch, 2013). Most soaps are alkaline due to the process of saponification. Exposure of the skin to this alkalinity can disrupt the epithelium's acid mantle and be directly damaging to the stratum corneum leading to increased water loss and causing rigidity of the lipid components (Kulthanan, Maneeprasopchoke, Varothai, & Nuchkull, 2014; Prezzano & Beck, 2017). Soaps also remove physiologically normal oils and contain detergents and surfactants that can damage the epithelium leading to irritation and dry skin (Ananthapadmanabhan, Moore, Kumar, Misra, & Meyer, 2004; White, Jenkinson, & Lloyd, 1987).

Patients are presented with an abundance of options when choosing bathing products, including soaps, cleansers, and synthetic detergents (syndets). Soaps are made of long-chain fatty acid alkali salts created from the process of saponification; cleansers are mixtures of water and some form of active compound, including soaps, emulsifiers, surfactants, and detergents (Mukhopadhyay, 2011). Syndets are nonsoap synthetic surfactants. One study examined the pH of all commercially available soaps and cleansers and found that all bars of soap had a pH between 9.9 and 10.7 except for syndet bars, which had a pH of 7 (Kulthanan et al., 2014). In the same study, most liquid cleansers were found to be less alkaline, but many still had a pH between 7.5 and 9.6; again, liquid syndets had a pH of 7 (Kulthanan et al., 2014). Based on the harmful effects of soaps and alkalinity, patients with AD are usually advised to use nonsoap hypoallergenic cleansers containing a neutral or mildly acidic pH (Eichenfield et al., 2014; Prezzano & Beck, 2017). Guidelines from Korea, Italy, and the United States directly recommend the use of syndets (LePoidevin et al., 2019). Notably, one study found that for patients with AD, the daily use of mildly acidic syndets significantly reduced clinical severity and symptomology in patients compliant with the regimen compared to those who were not (Kim et al., 2012). Further, some data have shown that there may be no significant difference in eczematous symptoms when the use of soap is compared with bathing with water alone (Stoughton, Lew, Clendenning, Fisher, & Kress, 1960). Thus daily cleanser use is not needed in AD patients, especially prepubertal children, as their potentially sensitive skin may be at high risk of experiencing irritating effects, and the sebum content of their skin is relatively lower (compared to adolescents and/or adults). In sum, the usage of neutral to mildly acidic cleansers should be recommended to patients, and they should also be counseled on the harmful effects of alkalinity.

Patients should also be directed to avoid damaging the epithelial barrier when using cleansers and take active steps to minimize friction when applying or removing soaps. They should be counseled to gently apply cleansers with the hands or soft microfiber cloths only, and to avoid the use of rougher texture wash cloths, loofahs, firm sponges, and/or scrubbing, as there is a risk of direct physical irritation. Cleansers should be quickly and gently rinsed off.

One unique aspect of bathing to be stressed with patients is the appropriate application of emollients. In 2009, a crossover study compared bathing without any application of emollients, bathing with immediate application, bathing with delayed 30-minute application, and emollient application without bathing effects on epithelial hydration (Chiang & Eichenfield, 2009). This study found that patients who did not apply an emollient postbathing had decreased epithelial hydration in comparison to the emollient treatment arms (Chiang & Eichenfield, 2009). Thus patients should be counseled that bathing without any application of an emollient may have directly negative impacts on epithelial hydration and be instructed to always use a postbath emollient.

Dilute bleach baths

In the past decade, dilute bleach baths have been increasingly recommended as an adjunct therapy for AD, especially for those patients who experience frequent infections as a trigger for flares. Bleach bath use was initially prompted by subjective parental reports of children's symptoms lessening in summer months when they were often swimming in chlorinated pools (Kusari, Allison, Schairer, & Eichenfield, 2019). The active component of bleach is sodium hypochlorite, which reacts with water to form hypochlorous acid. Hypochlorous acid then further dissociates, forming hypochlorite and superoxide radicals. These superoxide radicals are cytotoxic to bacteria and other microbes, including *Staphylococcal aureus* (Chong & Fonacier, 2016). It was initially thought that dilute bleach baths provided an antimicrobial method free of concerns for resistance, which could both prevent infection and address *S. aureus* colonization (Chong & Fonacier, 2016; Maarouf, Hendricks, & Shi, 2019).

To perform a dilute bleach bath, 0.25 cup of household bleach (typically 6% sodium hypochlorite) is added to a regular-sized bathtub half-full of warm water in which the patient bathes for 5 to 10 minutes. With these instructions, the bleach concentration ends up being approximately 0.005% (Eriksson, van der Plas, Mörgelin, & Sonesson, 2017). Some recommend a capful to a smaller bath for infants/toddlers and more (0.5 cup to full tub) for older children, teens, and adults. It is recommended to include the term *dilute* so that patients are not fearful of exposure to full concentration and its potentially harmful effects.

Further studies now demonstrate the benefit of bleach baths to be antiinflammatory and antipruritic most likely due to microbiome modulation (Fukuyama et al., 2018). Hypochlorite's antiinflammatory properties are multifactorial and include the inhibition of nuclear factor kappa B (NFκB), decreased mitogen-activated protein kinase (MAPK) activation, reduction of immunoglobulin E (IgE), reduction of proinflammatory cytokines, and decreased levels of interleukin-12 (IL12), which drives the conversion from a T helper 2 (Th2) to a T helper 1 (Th1) inflammatory response (Fukuyama et al., 2018; Leung et al., 2013). Hypochlorite's antipruritic properties are currently hypothesized to be due to reduced peripheral nerve stimulation (Fukuyama et al., 2018). Interestingly, in vitro studies have found that bleach is cytotoxic and can eradicate biofilms but not at doses below 0.01% (Eriksson et al., 2017). Importantly, the use of dilute bleach baths has not been found to be harmful to the epithelial barrier function, nor does it seem to affect epithelial hydration any differently than water, although the data are based on a one-time only exposure (Shi et al., 2016).

The initial study that investigated the use of dilute bleach baths was conducted in 2009. Patients with moderate to severe AD were treated with 2 weeks of oral cephalexin and then randomized to receive either intranasal mupirocin and dilute bleach baths or a placebo for 3 months (Huang, Abrams, Tlougan, Rademaker, & Paller, 2009). This study found significant improvement in AD severity and affected area for the treatment group (Huang et al., 2009). In the past decade, multiple studies, including three randomized controlled trials (RCTs), have failed to replicate these findings (Chopra, Paras, Sacotte, & Jonathan, 2017; Hon et al., 2016; Kusari et al., 2019). Multiple systemic reviews, via pooled data analysis, have also failed to show any statistically significant benefit of dilute bleach baths over regular baths (Chopra et al., 2017; Kusari

et al., 2019). Yet, each of these reviews has shown that both methods of bathing decrease the severity of AD (Chopra et al., 2017; Kusari et al., 2019). The lack of replicable benefit of dilute bleach baths versus regular water baths could indicate that its primary benefit may be via epithelial hydration or that it could be a product of small poorly designed studies. Interestingly, dilute bleach baths side effect profile is not significantly different from regular baths, thus they are frequently recommended as a safe and effective adjunctive strategy (Asch, Vork, Joseph, Major-Elechi, & Tollefson, 2019; Chopra et al., 2017).

The Canadian, Italian, and Taiwanese guidelines recommend dilute bleach baths for patients with frequent infections (Chu et al., 2015; Galli et al., 2016; Weinstein et al., 2017). Considering the cumulative evidence, dilute bleach baths provide a low-cost adjunctive treatment that may provide relief to patients with severe, frequently exacerbated AD and should be recommended for those patients. A few limited studies have investigated the potential use of bleach wipes or body wash containing bleach for those of whom submergent bathing is not feasible (Ryan, Richard, Cockerell, Hand, & Ghali, 2013). Although early results are promising, they are not readily available as part of clinical practice. In the meantime, these patients may choose to make their own dilute bleach solution and use a soaked gauze to apply to active skin lesions. A 0.005% sodium hypochlorite solution can be made by adding 4.15 mL (~1 tsp) of 6% household bleach to 500 mL of water, and this may be used as a spray-on body wash. Other patients may choose to swim in chlorinated pools; it should be suggested to limit the amount of times going into and out of the pool to curb transepithelial water loss and drying effect. Lastly, patients should be counseled that following sodium hypochlorite exposure, they may briefly rinse the skin with tap water to prevent residual bleach from potentially causing epithelial irritation.

Bath additives

Bath additives most commonly include oils or emollients. Conventional oils are balmandol, paraffin, soybean, mineral, and olive oil surfactant (Maarouf et al., 2019). The primary theory behind their use is that oils leave a film on the skin that can promote hydration as well as functioning as a humectant (retaining moisture) (Santer et al., 2018). However, investigational studies have not shown any significant benefit to their use (Eichenfield et al., 2014; Santer et al., 2018). It is also essential to note that although commonly suggested, olive oil has been shown to negatively impact the epithelial barrier in AD patients (Danby et al., 2013). While bath additives are mentioned in a few international guidelines, they cannot be explicitly recommended as a component of care. Patients should be counseled that they can make bath surfaces slippery and can pose a safety hazard in this way.

Other bathing practices

Additional practices worth mentioning include the use of acetic acid (vinegar) baths, the influence of water hardness, home therapies such as addition of oatmeal or rice bran, and balneotherapy. Acetic acid has anti–*S. aureus* properties, and it has historically been used in the inpatient setting, similar to dilute bleach baths, for patients with AD flares (Asch et al., 2019). Although it has decades of historical use, it has not been formally investigated and therefore cannot receive a specific recommendation.

Water hardness also has been thought to be associated with triggering AD. It has been hypothesized that the high concentrations of calcium and magnesium in water could irritate the skin, that hard water contains individual irritants, and that hard water leads to more aggressive soap use that in turn could damage the epithelium (Font-Ribera et al., 2015; Maarouf et al., 2019). Large-scale epidemiologic studies have failed to identify an association with water hardness and AD (Font-Ribera et al., 2015). The addition of water softeners also has not been proven to be beneficial (Eichenfield et al., 2014).

Oatmeal and rice bran are commonly used home remedies that may be encountered in clinical practice. As oatmeal contains hydrophilic carbohydrates, it is thought to help with epithelial hydration (Kurtz & Wallo, 2007). It also contains vitamin E and saponin, which can be cleansing and antioxidative (Saeed, Butt, McDonald-Gibson, & Collier, 1981). Rice bran contains inositol and γ-oryzanol, which can be antiinflammatory by inhibiting NFκB and other acids that are thought to benefit epithelial health (Fujiwaki & Furusho, 1992; Islam et al., 2009). However, robust clinical evidence is lacking for these modalities, and their use cannot be directly recommended.

Balneotherapy involves bathing in mineral springs. This practice is centuries old, and the three most studied geographic areas are the Dead Sea, La Roche-Posay Thermal Center in France, and the Blue Lagoon in Iceland. Each location has different mineral properties, but for AD, they all claim to decrease inflammation and improve skin hydration (Huang, Seité, & Adar, 2018). Although a few small trials have shown clinical benefit of balneotherapy in AD, there are no robust controlled trials to date. Therefore balneotherapy is likely unfeasible for the majority of patients. Lastly, similar to balneotherapy, families may express interest in the utilization of magnesium (Epsom) salts ($MgSO_4$) and potassium permanganate as Epsom salts are theoretically hydrating and potassium permanganate is an antiseptic. No robust clinical evidence supports their use in AD and therefore they cannot be specifically recommended.

Recommendations

In conclusion, taking into consideration the entirety of the existing evidence around bathing, our recommendations are in concordance with the American Academy of Dermatology and European guidelines as follows:
- Daily bathing is recommended.
- Baths/showers with lukewarm water should be less than 10 minutes, followed by the immediate application of emollients.
- Appropriate cleansers are nonsoap based and neutral to mildly acidic.

- Cleansers should be applied gently with hands, rinsed off with water, and patted dry.
- Aggressive physical manipulation and scrubbing, including the use of sponges, wash cloths, and loofahs, should be avoided.
- Dilute bleach baths can be considered for patients with frequent AD exacerbations or infections as triggers.
- Bath additives or home remedies should not be explicitly recommended but do not need to be discouraged.

Topical management with antiinflammatories

Topical corticosteroids (TCS), topical calcineurin inhibitors (TCI), and/or phosphodiesterase-4 (PDE4) inhibitors should be considered in patients who fail to respond to gentle skin care and emollient therapy regimens alone. Topical antimicrobials should also be considered as adjunct treatment in appropriate patients. Topical medications contain both active ingredients and vehicles. Table 20.1 depicts the various vehicle contents and their appropriate application conditions.

Topical corticosteroids

TCS were introduced in the 1950s and subsequently found to be effective for a number of skin diseases. Today there are several preparations and strengths with hundreds of RCTs

TABLE 20.1 Vehicles of topical medications and their appropriate application conditions

Vehicle type	Purpose	Example/use
Powder	Drying	Aesthetically acceptable; hygiene, body folds
Gel, shake suspension	Drying, cooling	Lightweight, less comedogenic
Liquid (lotion, solution, foam)	Drying to neutral	Diffuse or hair-bearing surfaces
Oil	Neutral to emollient	Diffuse surfaces
Cream (water in oil or oil in water)	Neutral to emollient	Patient preference, elegance, may sting if applied to eroded surfaces
Ointment-paste	Barrier/occlusion	Protective; diaper, body folds, erosions
Ointment	Emollient/occlusion	Infants and young children, maximal absorption but greasy, less elegant

supporting their efficacy and safety (Hoare, Li Wan Po, & Williams, 2000). TCS are considered standard treatment for AD owing to their effective antiinflammatory properties. TCS downregulate T lymphocytes, monocytes, macrophages, and dendritic cells resulting in impaired antigen processing and suppression of proinflammatory cytokine production. As such, TCS are an effective way to treat and/or prevent the pruritus and inflammation associated with AD (Schadt & Jackson, 2018).

TCS are divided into seven classes based on vasoconstriction properties (Table 20.2). Class VII is the lowest potency; class I is the highest. Patient age, anatomic site of application, and the severity of dermatitis are all important considerations when deciding which class of TCS is appropriate. Additionally, insurance coverage may vary between options within the same class, affecting cost to the patient. Older children and adults may have preferences for TCS vehicle. Petroleum-based products (ointments) may not be realistic during a school day or sports activities as compared to cream formulations that readily absorb, while ointments are preferred for their potency and tolerability in infants who are not affected by the choice of vehicle. Vehicles that contain water or alcohol for consistent emulsification (lotions, foams, and some creams) may be more elegant to use but can also sting on contact, especially to open or eroded skin. Lotions, solutions, gels, and foams are less commonly used for patients with AD compared with other inflammatory skin conditions, but their use may be helpful to consider for scalp and other hair bearing areas. Involving the patient/family in choice of vehicle may improve compliance, as consistency with application when used is integral to therapeutic success. Ensuring families are provided with sufficient quantity of medication and adequate refills is important.

Application frequency is generally recommended at twice daily. According to more recent data, once-daily application of certain TCS may be sufficient. Duration and frequency of therapy vary based on clinical picture and clinician/patient preferences. For example, for severe flares, short-burst high-potency TCS followed by a quick taper in potency and/or frequency of application can be an effective regimen (Thomas et al., 2002).

TABLE 20.2 Topical corticosteroid classification

Class	Potency	Examples
VII	Low	Hydrocortisone acetate cream, ointment, gel, lotion, and solution 0.5%–2.5%
VI	Low	Alclometasone dipropionate cream and ointment 0.05% Betamethasone valerate lotion 0.05% Desonide cream, gel, ointment, lotion, and foam 0.05% Fluocinolone acetonide cream and solution 0.01% Triamcinolone acetonide cream and lotion 0.025%
V	Medium	Betamethasone valerate cream and lotion 0.1% Clocortolone pivalate cream 0.1% Fluocinolone acetonide cream 0.025% or oil and shampoo 0.01% Fluticasone propionate cream and lotion 0.05% Flurandrenolide cream and lotion 0.05% Hydrocortisone butyrate cream, ointment, lotion, and solution 0.1% Hydrocortisone valerate cream 0.2% Triamcinolone acetonide ointment 0.025% or lotion 0.1%
IV	Medium	Betamethasone valerate foam 0.12% Desoximetasone cream 0.05% Fluocinolone acetonide ointment 0.025% Flurandrenolide ointment 0.05% Mometasone furoate cream and lotion 0.1% Triamcinolone acetonide cream and ointment 0.1%
III	High	Betamethasone dipropionate cream and lotion 0.05% Betamethasone valerate ointment 0.1% and foam 0.12% Fluticasone propionate ointment 0.005% Triamcinolone acetonide ointment 0.1% or cream 0.5%
II	High	Betamethasone dipropionate cream and lotion 0.05% Desoximetasone cream and ointment 0.25% or gel 0.05% Fluocinonide cream, ointment, gel, and solution 0.05% Mometasone furoate ointment 0.1% Triamcinolone acetonide ointment 0.5%
I	Ultrahigh	Betamethasone dipropionate ointment 0.05% Clobetasol propionate gel, ointment, cream, lotion, foam, and solution 0.05% Fluocinonide cream 0.1% Flurandrenolide tape 4 mcg/cm^2 Halobetasol propionate ointment and cream 0.05%

In our practice, we often employ the analogy of briefly using such medication as a "fire extinguisher." Alternatively, for more mild to moderate flares in chronic low-level AD, an alternative approach can be to use the lowest potency TCS and increase potency based on a failure to respond. TCS also safely and effectively can be used as preventive therapy (i.e., application once to twice weekly to sites of recurrent dermatitis as a form of prophylaxis, but families must be counseled not to overuse. It is important to teach patients and families how to recognize flares and remissions so topical therapy can be tapered or escalated appropriately (Brown, Nicole, Liang, Stockwell, & Friedman, 2018; Shi, Nanda, Lee, Armstrong, & Lio, 2013). The Eczema Action Plan was developed as a more formalized approach to this recommendation. It is a written plan organized into a color-coded (e.g., green, yellow, red) stepwise approach to address mild, moderate, and severe flares. Each step includes a description of each type of flare followed by respective emollient therapy and/or TCS application recommendations (Sauder, McEvoy, & Louise Ramien, 2016). These plans can be tailored and reviewed between providers and patients/families.

In general, patients should be counseled that in order to be effective, TCS may take several days but should not be used for more than approximately 2 weeks to the same site to prevent complications, and the treatment may need to be changed if it is not effective in this time frame.

There is not yet a universal standardized measure for topical application quantity. Proposed methods have included fingertip units (FTUs), which equates to the amount of product that fits on a fingertip, and the rule of 9s, which divides anatomic areas to approximate 9% body surface (Fox, Helfrich, & Kang, 2018). These methods can be difficult to realistically apply in clinical practice, especially within the pediatric population. In our practice, we typically recommend parents use a "thin layer" to the affected area only, avoiding contact with unaffected skin. Children have a high body surface area (BSA) to weight ratio, which translates to higher absorption compared to adults for a given amount of medication. For these reasons, it is important to use the lowest effective potency TCS in the long-term management and reserve mid- to high-potency or superhigh-potency TCS for intermittent, short courses for flares. Face, neck, genitalia, and skin folds also require lower potency TCS as thinner and/or occluded skin allows for greater absorption and potential for complications (Eichenfield et al., 2014). Although not precise, FTU is commonly used to estimate the quantity of topical medication and utilized as a guide for age-appropriate quantity for topical medications (Tables 20.3 and 20.4).

The most worrisome consequence of inappropriate or overuse of TCS is systemic absorption, leading to hypothalamic-pituitary-adrenal (HPA) axis suppression. The risk of HPA axis suppression is low and usually attributed to prolonged, daily or extensive use of potent TCS, particularly with concurrent use of oral, intranasal, and inhaled corticosteroids, or in areas under occlusion (such as the diaper area of an infant). Other worrisome side effects of prolonged, daily use of TCS include the potential for skin atrophy, telangiectasia, purpura, hypertrichosis, and striae formation. Steroid-induced glaucoma is an ophthalmologic site-specific side effect. Such side effects generally resolve over the subsequent months following discontinuation, though

TABLE 20.3	Estimated quantity of topical medication by fingertip unit (FTU)	
Approximate FTUs for 1 application	Weight of ointment for 1 application	Tube size for once-daily application x 10 days
Face and neck: 2.5	1.25 g	15 g
Trunk, front or back: 7	3.5 g	45 g
One arm: 3	1.5 g	15 g
One hand, both sides: 1	0.5 g	15 g
One leg: 6	3 g	45 g
One foot: 2	1 g	15 g

TABLE 20.4	Estimated application of topical medication by age factor				
Age	Face and neck (FTUs)	Arm and hand (FTUs)	Leg and foot (FTUs)	Trunk (front) (FTUs)	Trunk (back) and buttocks (FTUs)
6–10 years	2	2.5	4.5	3.5	5
3–5 years	1.5	2	3	3	3.5
1–2 years	1.5	1.5	2	2	3
3–11 months	1	1	1.5	1	1.5

FTUs, Fingertip units.

striae do tend to be irreversible once formed. TCS can also induce dermatoses of the face, including rosacea, acne, and perioral dermatitis (Schadt & Jackson, 2018). Another side effect of which clinicians should be aware is topical steroid withdrawal (TSW; red skin syndrome). It is hypothesized that sudden withdrawal of TCS leads to a rebound effect secondary to increased nitric oxide levels resulting in vasodilation of the cutaneous blood vessels. It can present as burning, erythema, and edema or as papules, pustules, and nodules (Hajar et al., 2015; Sheary, 2018, 2019). These presentations can be confused for a flare of the underlying disease and vice versa. As a result, therapy may be escalated or tapered inappropriately. TSW should be highly considered if a patient presents with a primary complaint of burning, confluent erythema days to weeks after TCS discontinuation, and/or a history of prolonged use of TCS on the face or genitals. Although the incidence of cutaneous TCS side effects is also low, it is important to discuss with families and monitor for these changes clinically. Clinicians should also be aware of the potential for patients to develop allergic contact dermatitis to the TCS and/or vehicle. Consider patch testing if dermatitis fails to improve or worsen with TCS therapy. In summary, it is important to emphasize the importance of avoiding continuous, daily application of TCS for long periods of time and promoting an as-needed approach. Of note, the aforementioned maintenance therapy regimen of low-potency TCS has not been associated with cutaneous side effects or HPA axis suppression.

Steroid phobia refers to the phenomenon not infrequently encountered in clinical practice in which families/parents or patients are unwilling to use TCS because of fear of their side effects or other concerns. This is not uncommon and typically results in inappropriate and/or ineffective use and may confuse the clinical picture if the provider is not attuned to the possibility. Therefore families should be counseled consistently regarding the safety of TCS when used appropriately and intermittently (Beattie & Lewis-Jones, 2003; Capozza & Schwartz, 2019; Charman, Morris, & Williams, 2000). It may also be helpful to remember that because TCS were primarily developed in the 1950s, there is sparse US Food and Drug Administration (FDA) approval in this category for older drugs, but hundreds of RCTs have shown safety and efficacy for this use. It can also be reassuring for some families to be educated on the natural role of steroids in normal human physiology. Additionally, clinicians should be aware that pharmacy package inserts included with TCS on dispensation address all potential side effects associated with the entire class and may be a source of unnecessary concern/anxiety to parents.

Topical calcineurin inhibitors

TCI were introduced in the 2000s with FDA approval for the treatment of AD. They inhibit calcineurin-dependent T-cell activation preventing production of proinflammatory cytokines and mediators.

There are currently two agents, tacrolimus ointment (0.03% and 0.1%) and pimecrolimus cream (1%).

Tacrolimus is approved for moderate to severe AD and found to be as effective as a midpotency TCS. Pimecrolimus is approved for mild to moderate AD. TCI are approved as a second-line therapy, and as such, insurance denials and the need for prior authorizations are common. TCI approval often requires failure to respond to TCS and/or application to anatomically sensitive locations (i.e., thin skin at eyelids, face, or genitalia) to avoid the potential side effects associated with TCS. TCI should be considered for patients who are failing to adequately respond to TCS regimens, need application to sensitive areas such as the face and skin folds, have a history of steroid-induced atrophy, or require long-term uninterrupted use of medication. There are also age-approved variations in TCI. Tacrolimus 0.03% ointment and pimecrolimus 0.1% cream are approved for use in patients 2 years and older. Tacrolimus 0.01% ointment is currently approved only in patients 15 years and older. Of note, clinical trials have shown tacrolimus 0.03% and pimecrolimus to be safe and effective in children under 2 years of age, including infants (Martins et al., 2015). Application frequency is optimal at twice-daily application. They are also safely and effectively used as maintenance therapy (i.e., application two to three times weekly to sites of recurrent dermatitis as a form of prophylaxis).

The most common adverse side effect of TCI is an initial stinging or burning sensation at the site of application often in direct proportion to disease severity. These sensations tend to decrease in severity after the first several applications and can be mitigated by pretreatment with TCS (Martins et al., 2015). In our practice we have found this to be more common with the cream vehicle than with the ointment. There have also been six reports of patients, five with AD and one with cheilitis, developing pigmented macules at the site of TCI application (Hickey, Robson, Barker, & Smith, 2005; Shi, Joo, & Sharon, 2014; Zattra, Albertin, & Belloni Fortina, 2010). There are also two case reports of lentigines developing in areas of resolved chronic AD in the absence of TCI use (Shayegan & Lauren, 2019).

It is important to note that TCI come with a black box warning for lymphoma, based on rare cases of lymphoma reports in patients using TCI, as well as theoretic increased risks extrapolated from high-dose oral calcineurin-inhibitor therapy in posttransplant patients and animal studies. A causal relationship has never been established, and the current 10-year surveillance studies have not found any evidence of increased malignancy rates to date (Koo et al., 2005; Tennis, Gelfand, & Rothman, 2011). Overall, TCI have an excellent safety profile, and there is no evidence to suggest routine blood monitoring. They have shown little to no systemic absorption, unless there is a severe barrier defect such as in Nethertons syndrome.

Other topical antiinflammatories

The newest topical agent FDA approved in 2016 for mild to moderate AD is crisaborole 2% topical ointment. It is a PDE4 inhibitor that results in a downstream decrease in the production of proinflammatory cytokines. Twice-daily topical application demonstrated rapid and sustainable reduction in both inflammation and pruritus associated with AD. It has low systemic absorption and is rapidly metabolized. Initial studies showed low incidence of pain (including stinging/burning) at application site; in our practice we have noted this to be more common. PDE4 inhibitors therefore represent another safe and efficacious topical alternative to TCS and TCI. More specific recommendations regarding the use of PDE4 inhibitors is pending future research (Paller et al., 2016).

Recommendations

In conclusion, taking into consideration the entirety of the existing evidence around topical therapeutics, our strong recommendation is in concordance with the American Academy of Dermatology and European guidelines and is as follows:

- TCS are recommended for AD patients who have failed gentle skin care and regular bland-emollient therapy alone.
- Twice-daily application of TCS is considered safe and effective for acute flares and twice-weekly application to stubborn areas to prevent flares.
- Providers should thoroughly address patient questions and concerns, particularly regarding steroid phobia.
- TCI are an effective, steroid-sparing alternative for acute and chronic AD, and when used as maintenance therapy.
- TCI have particular utility for sensitive areas, long-term use, and patient's with steroid recalcitrance or atrophy.
- Providers should counsel patients regarding the burning/stinging sensation associated with initial TCI application.
- PDE4 inhibitors are a newer, safe, and effective steroid sparing alternative to TCI that has been shown effective with twice-daily application.

Topical antimicrobials

The history of utilizing topical antimicrobials for the management of AD has primarily been driven by the recognition of high *S. aureus* colonization rates among patients (see earlier). Although wide variation exists, it has been documented that between 30% and nearly 100% of patients with AD are colonized with *S. aureus* (Totté et al., 2016). In pooled data analysis via a high-quality systematic review, *S. aureus* colonization is found on 39% of nonlesional skin and 70% of lesional skin (Totté et al., 2016). It is also recognized that bacterial density is associated with severity of disease and that exacerbations are significantly associated with *S. aureus* colonization (Hashim, Chen, Hebert, & Kircik, 2019; Wollenberg et al., 2018b). In contrast, approximately 30% of the general population demonstrated colonization, promoting the use of topical antimicrobials as adjunct therapy for the management of AD (Ryu et al., 2014).

Patients with AD are known to have decreased epithelial barrier function along with chronic Th2-driven inflammatory dysfunction, which makes them especially prone to infection. *S. aureus* also independently activates numerous immunologic inflammatory pathways and produces superantigens and protease inhibitors that possibly contribute to chronic inflammation (Eichenfield et al., 2014). *S. aureus* is a known biofilm-producing organism, further complicating the disease process as biofilm may block the epithelial glands contributing to chronic inflammation and itching (Di Domenico et al., 2019).

Although addressing *S. aureus* colonization via topical antimicrobials (either alone or in combination with TCS) in the management of AD may seem logical, review of current evidence does not support routine use. A 2008 Cochrane review on the topic (Birnie et al., 2008), including the use of topical antibiotics alone, topical antibiotics plus topical steroids, and topical antibiotics plus topical steroids and topical antifungals, demonstrated that although these combinations reduce *S. aureus* colonization, this does not result in any significant clinical improvement when compared to sole TCS use (Birnie et al., 2008). Over the past decade, this finding has been replicated across multiple RCTs and updated systematic reviews (Harris & Cooper, 2017; Nankervis et al., 2017).

In addition, there is growing concern about resistance to antibiotics more broadly and therefore a need to limit unnecessary exposure to antimicrobials. Although geographic and regional differences exist, skin samples have demonstrated *S. aureus* resistance rates as high as 100% to bacitracin, 50% to macrolides, 42.6% to neomycin, 33.9% to mupirocin, 33.5% to methicillin, 14.7% to gentamycin, 6% to clindamycin, and 5.5% to tetracycline (Bessa et al., 2016; Biedenbach, Samuel, Johnson, Hoban, & Hackel, 2014; Weitz et al., 2016). These rates of resistance coupled with the risk resistance potentiation, the absence of clinical significance in addressing *S. aureus* colonization, and the lack of long-term clinical benefits should prompt the questioning of the routine use of topical antibiotics in this patient population. Considering this, the most recent AD guidelines from Asia, Australia, Europe, and North America have all recommended against the routine use of topical antibiotics or have elected to exclude topical antibiotics completely (Chu et al., 2015; Eichenfield et al., 2014; Rubel et al., 2013; Weinstein et al., 2017; Wollenberg et al., 2018b).

Current recommendations include obtaining surface bacterial cultures with sensitivities to help guide specific therapy and the tracking of resistance (Chong & Fonacier, 2016; Weitz et al., 2016). Investigational studies have found that primary care providers with exposure to dermatology education/clinical exposure are much more likely to culture acutely infected lesions and avoid topical antibiotics than those without. In some cases of superinfected AD, a short course of topical mupirocin can be added as an adjunct to TCS and/or oral antistaphylococcal antibiotics but should be done judiciously (Silverberg & Durán-McKinster, 2017). In our experience, in many cases simply using appropriate TCS is sufficient to repair the damaged skin barrier, and oral antibiotics can be avoided if the patient is markedly better once culture results are known. However, if infection is strongly suspected and/or culture demonstrates heavy growth of bacteria, a 7- to 10-day course of oral antistaphylococcal antibiotics is given. Clinical infection in AD may sometimes represent eczema herpeticum (herpes simplex virus), which requires antiviral coverage but is often also complicated by secondary bacterial infection.

Other antimicrobial approaches include dilute bleach baths as referenced earlier, silver-impregnated dressings, and antimicrobial clothing (Birnie et al., 2008; Friedman & Goldman, 2011; LePoidevin et al., 2019; Wollenberg et al., 2018b). Although there is a logical role for antimicrobial textiles and clothing, their evidence is sparse with mixed results (Friedman & Goldman, 2011; Wollenberg et al., 2018b).

Recommendations for topical treatments

- TCS are recommended for AD patients who have failed gentle skin care and regular bland-emollient therapy alone. Twice-daily application of TCS is considered safe and effective for acute flares.
- TCI are an effective, steroid-sparing alternative for acute and chronic AD, and when used as maintenance therapy. TCI have particular utility for sensitive areas, long-term use, and patient's with steroid recalcitrance or atrophy.
- PDE4 inhibitors are a newer, safe, and effective steroid sparing alternative to TCI that has been shown effective with twice daily application.
- Topical antimicrobials are not recommended for the routine management of AD.
- Areas that appear infected clinically should be cultured and have sensitivities performed.
- Patients with signs of infection while on TCS should receive a 7- to 10-day course of an oral antistaphylococcal agent guided by resulting sensitivities.

Summary

Topical treatments for AD commonly include bathing, antiinflammatories, and antimicrobials. These treatments could work together to generate a defense mechanism against allergens and invading microorganisms and to dial down inflammation, thus helping to improve the skin conditions of patients affected by the disease.

Further readings

Ring, J. (2016). *Atopic dermatitis: Eczema.* Springer.

Silverberg, J. I., & Silverberg, N. B. (Eds.), (2017). *Dermatologic clinics: Atopic dermatitis.* Elsevier.

References

Ali, S. M., & Yosipovitch, G. (2013). Skin pH: From basic science to basic skin care. *Acta Dermato-Venereologica, 93*(3), 261–267. https://doi.org/10.2340/00015555-1531.

Ananthapadmanabhan, K. P., Moore, D. J., Kumar, S., Misra, M., & Meyer, F. (2004). Cleansing without compromise: The impact of cleansers on the skin barrier and the technology of mild cleansing. *Dermatologic Therapy, 17*(1), 16–25. https://doi.org/10.1111/j.1396-0296.2004.04s1002.x.

Asch, S., Vork, D. L., Joseph, J., Major-Elechi, B., & Tollefson, M. M. (2019). Comparison of bleach, acetic acid, and other topical anti-infective treatments in pediatric atopic dermatitis: A retrospective cohort study on antibiotic exposure. *Pediatric Dermatology, 36*(1), 115–120. https://doi.org/10.1111/pde.13663.

Beattie, P. E., & Lewis-Jones, M. S. (2003). Parental knowledge of topical therapies in the treatment of childhood atopic dermatitis. *Clinical and Experimental Dermatology, 28*(5), 549–553. https://doi.org/10.1046/j.1365-2230.2003.01357.x.

Bessa, G. R., Vanessa, P. Q., Daiane, C. M., Caroline, L., Magda, B. W., Renan, R. B., & D'Azevedo, P. A. (2016). *Staphylococcus aureus* resistance to topical antimicrobials in atopic dermatitis. *Anais Brasileiros De Dermatologia, 91*(5), 604–610. https://doi.org/10.1590/abd1806-4841.20164860.

Biedenbach, D. J., Samuel, K. B., Johnson, S. A., Hoban, D. J., & Hackel, M. (2014). Susceptibility of *Staphylococcus aureus* to topical agents in the United States: A sentinel study. *Clinical Therapeutics, 36*(6), 953–960. https://doi.org/10.1016/j.clinthera.2014.04.003.

Birnie, A. J., Bath-Hextall, F. J., Ravenscroft, J. C., & Williams, H. C. (2008). Interventions to reduce *Staphylococcus aureus* in the management of atopic eczema. *The Cochrane Database of Systematic Reviews, 3,* CD003871. https://doi.org/10.1002/14651858.CD003871.pub2.

Brown, J., Nicole, W. W., Liang, A., Stockwell, M. S., & Friedman, S. (2018). Does an eczema action plan improve atopic dermatitis? A single-site randomized controlled trial. *Clinical Pediatrics, 57*(14), 1624–1629. https://doi.org/10.1177/0009922818795906.

Capozza, K., & Schwartz, A. (2019). Does it work and is it safe? Parents' perspectives on adherence to medication for atopic dermatitis. *Pediatric Dermatology, 37*(1), 58–61. https://doi.org/10.1111/pde.13991. Accessed 01.09.2019.

Cardona, I. D., Kempe, E., Hatzenbeuhler, J. R., Antaya, R. J., Cohen, B., & Jain, N. (2015). Bathing frequency recommendations for children with atopic dermatitis: Results of three observational pilot surveys. *Pediatric Dermatology, 32*(4), e194–e196. https://doi.org/10.1111/pde.12618.

Cardona, I. D., Stillman, L., & Jain, N. (2016). Does bathing frequency matter in pediatric atopic dermatitis? *Annals of Allergy, Asthma & Immunology, 117*(1), 9–13. https://doi.org/10.1016/j.anai.2016.05.014.

Charman, C. R., Morris, A. D., & Williams, H. C. (2000). Topical corticosteroid phobia in patients with atopic eczema. *British Journal of Dermatology, 142*(5), 931–936. https://doi.org/10.1046/j.1365-2133.2000.03473.x.

Chiang, C., & Eichenfield, L. F. (2009). Quantitative assessment of combination bathing and moisturizing regimens on skin hydration in atopic dermatitis. *Pediatric Dermatology, 26*(3), 273–278. https://doi.org/10.1111/j.1525-1470.2009.00911.x.

Chong, M., & Fonacier, L. (2016). Treatment of eczema: Corticosteroids and beyond. *Clinical Reviews in Allergy & Immunology, 51*(3), 249–262. https://doi.org/10.1007/s12016-015-8486-7.

Chopra, R., Paras, P. V., Sacotte, R., & Jonathan, I. S. (2017). Efficacy of bleach baths in reducing severity of atopic dermatitis: A systematic review and meta-analysis. *Annals of Allergy, Asthma & Immunology, 119*(5), 435–440. https://doi.org/10.1016/j.anai.2017.08.289.

Chu, C.-Y., Lee, C.-H., Shih, I.-H., Chen, H.-C., Huang, P.-H., Yang, C.-Y., et al. (2015). Taiwanese dermatological association consensus for the management of atopic dermatitis. *Dermatologica Sinica, 33*(4), 220–230. https://doi.org/10.1016/j.dsi.2015.06.004.

Danby, S. G., AlEnezi, T., Sultan, A., Lavender, T., Chittock, J., Brown, K., & Cork, M. J. (2013). Effect of olive and sunflower seed oil on the adult skin barrier: Implications for neonatal skin care. *Pediatric Dermatology, 30*(1), 42–50. https://doi.org/10.1111/j.1525-1470.2012.01865.x.

Di Domenico, E. G., Cavallo, I., Capitanio., B., Ascenzioni, F., Pimpinelli, F., Morrone, A., & Ensoli, F. (2019). *Staphylococcus aureus* and the cutaneous microbiota biofilms in the pathogenesis of atopic dermatitis. *Microorganisms, 7*(9), 301: 1–22. https://doi.org/10.3390/microorganisms7090301. 301.

Eichenfield, L. F., Wynnis, L. T., Berger, T. G., Krol, A., Paller, A. S., Schwarzenberger, K., et al. (2014). Guidelines of care for the management of atopic dermatitis: Section 2. Management and treatment of atopic dermatitis with topical therapies. *Journal of the American Academy of Dermatology, 71*(1), 116–132. https://doi.org/10.1016/j.jaad.2014.03.023.

Eriksson, S., van der Plas, M. J. A., Mörgelin, M., & Sonesson, A. (2017). Antibacterial and antibiofilm effects of sodium hypochlorite against *Staphylococcus aureus* isolates derived from patients with atopic dermatitis. *British Journal of Dermatology, 177*(2), 513–521. https://doi.org/10.1111/bjd.15410.

Fleischer, D. M., Udkoff, J., Borok, J., Friedman, A., Nicol, N., Bienstock, J., et al. (2017). Atopic dermatitis: Skin care and topical therapies. *Seminars in Cutaneous Medicine and Surgery, 36*(3), 104–110. https://doi.org/10.12788/j.sder.2017.035.

Font-Ribera, L., Gracia-Lavedan, E., Esplugues, A., Ballester, F., Jiménez Zabala, A., Santa Marina, L., et al. (2015). Water hardness and eczema at 1 and 4 y of age in the INMA birth cohort. *Environmental Research, 142*(October), 579–585. https://doi.org/10.1016/j.envres.2015.07.013.

Fox, M., Helfrich, Y., & Kang, S. (2018). Other Topical Medications. In *Dermatology*, (4th ed., pp. 2263–77). Philadelphia, PA: Elsevier. http://www.clinicalkey.com/#!/content/book/3-s2.0-B9780702066275900129X?scrollTo=%23hl0001116.

Friedman, B.-C., & Goldman, R. D. (2011). Anti-staphylococcal treatment in dermatitis. *Canadian Family Physician Medecin De Famille Canadien, 57*(6), 669–671.

Fujiwaki, T., & Furusho, K. (1992). The effects of rice bran broth bathing in patients with atopic dermatitis. *Acta Paediatrica Japonica: Overseas Edition, 34*(5), 505–510. https://doi.org/10.1111/j.1442-200x.1992.tb00997.x.

Fukuyama, T., Martel, B. C., Linder, K. E., Ehling, S., Ganchingco, J. R., & Bäumer, W. (2018). Hypochlorous acid is antipruritic and anti-inflammatory in a mouse model of atopic dermatitis. *Clinical and Experimental Allergy, 48*(1), 78–88. https://doi.org/10.1111/cea.13045.

Galli, E., Neri, I., Ricci, G., Baldo, E., Barone, M., Fortina, A. B., et al. (2016). Consensus conference on clinical management of pediatric atopic dermatitis. *Italian Journal of Pediatrics, 42*, 26. https://doi.org/10.1186/s13052-016-0229-8.

Glines, K. R., Katherine, M. S., Freeze, M., Cline, A., Strowd, L. C., & Feldman, S. R. (2019). An update on the topical and oral therapy options for treating pediatric atopic dermatitis. *Expert Opinion on Pharmacotherapy, 20*(5), 621–629. https://doi.org/10.1080/14656566.2018.1561868.

Hajar, T., Yael, A. L., Hanifin, J. M., Nedorost, S. T., Lio, P. A., Paller, A. S., et al. (2015). A systematic review of topical corticosteroid withdrawal ('steroid addiction') in patients with atopic dermatitis and other dermatoses and (the National Eczema Association Task Force). *Journal of the American Academy of Dermatology, 72*(3), 541–549. https://doi.org/10.1016/j.jaad.2014.11.024.

Harris, V. R., & Cooper, A. J. (2017). Atopic dermatitis: The new frontier. *The Medical Journal of Australia, 207*(8), 351–356.

Hashim, P. W., Chen, T., Hebert, A. A., & Kircik, L. H. (2019). Topical treatment for the management of atopic dermatitis. *Journal of Drugs in Dermatology, 18*(s2), s112–s116.

Hengge, U. R., Ruzicka, T., Schwartz, R. A., & Cork, M. J. (2006). Adverse effects of topical glucocorticosteroids. *Journal of the American Academy of Dermatology, 54*(1), 1–15. https://doi.org/10.1016/j.jaad.2005.01.010.

Hickey, J. R., Robson, A., Barker, J. N. W. N., & Smith, C. H. (2005). Does topical tacrolimus induce lentigines in children with atopic dermatitis? A report of three cases. *British Journal of Dermatology, 152*(1), 152–154. https://doi.org/10.1111/j.1365-2133.2004.06280.x.

Hoare, C., Li Wan Po, A., & Williams, H. (2000). Systematic review of treatments for atopic eczema. *Health Technology Assessment (Winchester, England), 4*(37), 1–191.

Hon, K. L., Tsang, Y. C. K., Lee, V. W. Y., Pong, N. H., Ha, G., Lee, S. T., et al. (2016). Efficacy of sodium hypochlorite (bleach) baths to reduce *Staphylococcus aureus* colonization in childhood onset moderate-to-severe eczema: A randomized, placebo-controlled cross-over trial. *Journal of Dermatological Treatment, 27*(2), 156–162. https://doi.org/10.3109/09546634.2015.1067669.

Huang, A., Seité, S., & Adar, T. (2018). The use of balneotherapy in dermatology. *Clinics in Dermatology, 36*(3), 363–368. https://doi.org/10.1016/j.clindermatol.2018.03.010.

Huang, J. T., Abrams, M., Tlougan, B., Rademaker, A., & Paller, A. S. (2009). Treatment of *Staphylococcus aureus* colonization in atopic dermatitis decreases disease severity. *Pediatrics, 123*(5), e808–e814. https://doi.org/10.1542/peds.2008-2217.

Islam, M. S., Yoshida, H., Matsuki, N., Ono, K., Nagasaka, R., Ushio, H., et al. (2009). Antioxidant, free radical-scavenging, and NF-kappaB-inhibitory activities of phytosteryl ferulates: Structure-activity studies. *Journal of Pharmacological Sciences, 111*(4), 328–337. https://doi.org/10.1254/jphs.09146fp.

Koo, J. Y. M., Fleischer, A. B., Abramovits, W., Pariser, D. M., McCall, C. O., Horn, T. D., et al. (2005). Tacrolimus ointment is safe and effective in the treatment of atopic dermatitis: Results in 8000 patients. *Journal of the American Academy of Dermatology, 53*(2 Suppl 2), S195–S205. https://doi.org/10.1016/j.jaad.2005.04.063.

Kempe, E., Jain, N., & Cardona, I. (2013). Bathing frequency recommendations for pediatric atopic dermatitis: Are we adding to parental frustration? *Annals of Allergy, Asthma & Immunology, 111*(4), 298–299. https://doi.org/10.1016/j.anai.2013.07.016.

Kim, H., Ban, J., Park, M.-R., Kim, D.-S., Kim, H.-Y., Han, Y., et al. (2012). Effect of bathing on atopic dermatitis during the summer season. *Asia Pacific Allergy, 2*(4), 269–274. https://doi.org/10.5415/apallergy.2012.2.4.269.

Koutroulis, I., Petrova, K., Kratimenos, P., & Gaughan, J. (2014). Frequency of bathing in the management of atopic dermatitis: To bathe or not to bathe? *Clinical Pediatrics, 53*(7), 677–681. https://doi.org/10.1177/0009922814526980.

Koutroulis, I., Pyle, T., Kopylov, D., Little, A., Gaughan, J., & Kratimenos, P. (2016). The association between bathing habits and severity of atopic dermatitis in children. *Clinical Pediatrics, 55*(2), 176–181. https://doi.org/10.1177/0009922815594346.

Kulthanan, K., Maneeprasopchoke, P., Varothai, S., & Nuchkull, P. (2014). The ph of antiseptic cleansers. *Asia Pacific Allergy, 4*(1), 32–36. https://doi.org/10.5415/apallergy.2014.4.1.32.

Kurtz, E. S., & Wallo, W. (2007). Colloidal oatmeal: History, chemistry and clinical properties. *Journal of Drugs in Dermatology, 6*(2), 167–170.

Kusari, A., Allison, M. H., Schairer, D., & Eichenfield, L. F. (2019). Atopic dermatitis: New developments. *Dermatologic Clinics, 37*(1), 11–20. https://doi.org/10.1016/j.det.2018.07.003.

LePoidevin, L. M., Lee, D. E., & Shi, V. Y. (2019). A comparison of international management guidelines for atopic dermatitis. *Pediatric Dermatology, 36*(1), 36–65. https://doi.org/10.1111/pde.13678.

Leung, T. H., Zhang, L. F., Wang, J., Ning, S., Knox, S. J., & Kim, S. K. (2013). Topical hypochlorite ameliorates NF-KB–mediated skin diseases in mice. *The Journal of Clinical Investigation, 123*(12), 5361–5370. https://doi.org/10.1172/JCI70895.

Maarouf, M., Hendricks, A. J., & Shi, V. Y. (2019). Bathing additives for atopic dermatitis - A systematic review. *Dermatitis: Contact, Atopic, Occupational, Drug, 30*(3), 191–197. https://doi.org/10.1097/DER.0000000000000459.

Martins, J. C., Martins, C., Aoki, V., Gois, A. F. T., Ishii, H. A., & da Silva, E. M. K. (2015). Topical tacrolimus for atopic dermatitis. *Cochrane Database of Systematic Reviews, 7*(7), 1–35. https://doi.org/10.1002/14651858.CD009864.pub2.

Mukhopadhyay, P. (2011). Cleansers and their role in various dermatological disorders. *Indian Journal of Dermatology, 56*(1), 2–6. https://doi.org/10.4103/0019-5154.77542.

Nankervis, H., Thomas, K. S., Delamere, F. M., Barbarot, S., Smith, S., Rogers, N. K., & Williams, H. C. (2017). What is the evidence base for atopic eczema treatments? A summary of published randomized controlled trials. *British Journal of Dermatology, 176*(4), 910–927. https://doi.org/10.1111/bjd.14999.

Ohtsuki, M., Morimoto, H., & Nakagawa, H. (2018). Tacrolimus ointment for the treatment of adult and pediatric atopic derma-titis: Review on safety and benefits. *The Journal of Dermatology, 45*(8), 936–942. https://doi.org/10.1111/1346-8138.14501.

Paller, A. S., Wynnis, L. T., Lebwohl, M. G., Blumenthal, R. L., Boguniewicz, M., Call, R. S., et al. (2016). Efficacy and safety of crisaborole ointment, a novel, nonsteroidal phosphodiesterase 4 (PDE4) inhibitor for the topical treatment of atopic dermatitis (AD) in children and adults. *Journal of the American Academy of Dermatology, 75*(3), 494–503. E6. https://doi.org/10.1016/j.jaad.2016.05.046.

Prezzano, J. C., & Beck, L. A. (2017). Long-term treatment of atopic dermatitis. *Dermatologic Clinics, 35*(3), 335–349. https://doi.org/10.1016/j.det.2017.02.007.

Rubel, D., Thirumoorthy, T., Soebaryo, R. W., Weng, S. C. K., Gabriel, T. M., Villafuerte, L. L., et al. (2013). Consensus guidelines for the management of atopic dermatitis: An Asia–Pacific perspective. *The Journal of Dermatology, 40*(3), 160–171. https://doi.org/10.1111/1346-8138.12065.

Ryan, C., Richard, E. S., Cockerell, C. J., Hand, S., & Ghali, F. E. (2013). Novel sodium hypochlorite cleanser shows clinical response and excellent acceptability in the treatment of atopic dermatitis. *Pediatric Dermatology, 30*(3), 308–315. https://doi.org/10.1111/pde.12150.

Ryu, S., Peter, I. S., Ho Seo, C., Cheong, H., & Park, Y. (2014). Colonization and infection of the skin by S. Aureus: Immune system evasion and the response to cationic antimicrobial peptides. *International Journal of Molecular Sciences, 15*(5), 8753–8772. https://doi.org/10.3390/ijms15058753.

Saeed, S. A., Butt, N. M., McDonald-Gibson, W. J., & Collier, H. O. J. (1981). Inhibitor(s) of prostaglandin biosynthesis in extracts of oat (*Avena sativa*) seeds. *Biochemical Society Transactions, 9*(5), 444. https://doi.org/10.1042/bst0090444.

Santer, M., Matthew, J. R., Francis, N. A., Stuart, B., Rumsby, K., Chorozoglou, M., et al. (2018). Emollient bath additives for the treatment of childhood eczema (BATHE): Multicentre pragmatic parallel group randomised controlled trial of clinical and cost effectiveness. *BMJ (Clinical Research Ed.), 361*, k1332. https://doi.org/10.1136/bmj.k1332.

Sauder, M. B., McEvoy, A., & Louise Ramien, M. (2016). Prescribing success: Developing an integrated prescription and eczema action plan for atopic dermatitis. *Journal of the American Academy of Dermatology, 75*(6), 1281–1283. https://doi.org/10.1016/j.jaad.2016.08.029.

Schadt, C. R., & Jackson, S. M., 2018. Glucocorticoids. In *Dermatology*, (4th ed., pp. 2186–99). Philadelphia, PA: Elsevier. http://www.clinicalkey.com/#!/content/book/3-s2.0-B9780702062759001252.

Shayegan, L. H., & Lauren, C. T. (2019). The itch that… freckles? Development of lentigines in areas of resolved chronic atopic dermatitis. *Pediatric Dermatology, 36*(6), 970–972. https://doi.org/10.1111/pde.13996.

Sheary, B. (2018). Steroid withdrawal effects following long-term topical corticosteroid use. *Dermatitis: Contact, Atopic, Occupational, Drug, 29*(4), 213–218. https://doi.org/10.1097/DER.0000000000000387.

Sheary, B. (2019). Topical steroid withdrawal: A case series of 10 children. *Acta Dermato-Venereologica, 99*(6), 551–556. https://doi.org/10.2340/00015555-3144.

Shi, V. Y., Foolad, N., Ornelas, J. N., Hassoun, L. A., Monico, G., Takeda, N., et al. (2016). Comparing the effect of bleach and water baths on skin barrier function in atopic dermatitis: A split-body randomized controlled trial. *British Journal of Dermatology, 175*(1), 212–214. https://doi.org/10.1111/bjd.14483.

Shi, V. Y., Joo, J. S., & Sharon, V. R. (2014). Multiple labial melanotic macules occurring after topical application of calcineurin inhibitors. *Dermatology Online Journal, 20*(8), 12.

Shi, V. Y., Nanda, S., Lee, K., Armstrong, A. W., & Lio, P. A. (2013). Improving patient education with an eczema action plan: A randomized controlled trial. *JAMA Dermatology, 149*(4), 481–483. https://doi.org/10.1001/jamadermatol.2013.2143.

Silverberg, N. B., & Durán-McKinster, C. (2017). Special considerations for therapy of pediatric atopic dermatitis. *Dermatologic Clinics, 35*(3), 351–363. https://doi.org/10.1016/j.det.2017.02.008.

Stoughton, R. B., Lew, W. P., Clendenning, W., Fisher, S., & Kress, M. (1960). Management of patients with eczematous diseases: use of soap versus no soap. *The Journal of the American Medical Association, 173*(11), 1196–1198. https://doi.org/10.1001/jama.1960.03020290022004.

Tennis, P., Gelfand, J. M., & Rothman, K. J. (2011). Evaluation of cancer risk related to atopic dermatitis and use of topical calcineurin inhibitors. *The British Journal of Dermatology, 165*(3), 465–473. https://doi.org/10.1111/j.1365-2133.2011.10363.x.

Totté, J. E. E., van der Feltz, W. T., Hennekam, M., van Belkum, A., van Zuuren, E. J., & Pasmans, S. G. M. A. (2016). Prevalence and odds of *Staphylococcus aureus* carriage in atopic dermatitis: A systematic review and meta-analysis. *The British Journal of Dermatology, 175*(4), 687–695. https://doi.org/10.1111/bjd.14566.

Weinstein, M., Bergman, J., Drucker, A. M., Lynde, C., Marcoux, D., Rehmus, W., & Cresswell-Melville, A. (2017). Atopic dermatitis: A practical guide to management. *Atopic Dermatitis, 12*(3), 6–10.

Weitz, N. A., Brody, E., Lauren, C. T., Morel, K. D., Paladine, H., Garzon, M. C., & Krause, M. C. (2016). Management of infectious aspects of atopic dermatitis in primary care: A resident survey. *Clinical Pediatrics, 55*(14), 1295–1299. https://doi.org/10.1177/0009922815627347.

White, M. I., Jenkinson, D. M., & Lloyd, D. H. (1987). The effect of washing on the thickness of the stratum corneum in normal and atopic individuals. *British Journal of Dermatology, 116*(4), 525–530. https://doi.org/10.1111/j.1365-2133.1987.tb05873.x.

Wollenberg, A., Barbarot, S., Bieber, T., Christen-Zaech, S., Deleuran, M., Fink-Wagner, A., et al. (2018a). Consensus-based european guidelines for treatment of atopic eczema (atopic dermatitis) in adults and children: Part I. *Journal of the European Academy of Dermatology and Venereology, 32*(5), 657–682. https://doi.org/10.1111/jdv.14891.

Wollenberg, A., Barbarot, S., Bieber, T., Christen-Zaech, S., Deleuran, M., Fink-Wagner, A., et al. (2018b). Consensus-based european guidelines for treatment of atopic eczema (atopic dermatitis) in adults and children: Part II. *Journal of the European Academy of Dermatology and Venereology, 32*(6), 850–878. https://doi.org/10.1111/jdv.14888.

Zattra, E., Albertin, C., & Belloni Fortina, A. (2010). Labial melanotic macule after application of topical tacrolimus: Two case reports. *Acta Dermato-Venereologica, 90*(5), 527. https://doi.org/10.2340/00015555-0878.

21

Wound Care

PENELOPE HIRT, DIVYA J. AICKARA, DANIELA SANCHEZ, AND HADAR LEV-TOV

KEY POINTS

- Issues with wound healing in patients with atopic dermatitis (AD) relate to innate inability to repair the barrier, defective angiogenesis, abnormal microbial colonization, and a prolonged inflammatory phase.
- Patients with AD are at a higher risk for hypersensitivity reactions such as allergic contact dermatitis to various dressings and topical medications.
- General measures that may help in the treatment of both AD and wound include moisturizing to restore barrier, hypochlorous acid, and adequate nutrition.
- Complementary and alternative treatments emerge as promising tools to treat wounds in AD patients.

Introduction

A critical function of the skin, a protein layer, is to provide a physiologic and protective barrier to the external environment. It represents the primary interface between the body and the environment. In addition to preventing loss of moisture and electrolytes from the inside, the skin is a key element in the host defense system preventing the penetration of harmful stimuli—microbial organisms, chemical irritants, toxins, as well as solar and ionizing radiation—from the outside (Bangert, Brunner, & Stingl, 2011). This physiologic barrier function is primarily carried out by two structures in the epidermis: the stratum corneum (SC) and intercellulalr tight junctions (TJs).

As a barrier organ, the skin encounters a variety of antigens and environmental insults on a daily basis. When immune surveillance responds inappropriately to an otherwise harmless antigen and passes this information on to the adaptive system, various pathologic conditions can develop, such as autoimmunity, allergy, chronic inflammation, and delayed wound healing (Clark & Kupper, 2005; Kupper & Fuhlbrigge, 2004).

Many inflammatory skin diseases, including atopic dermatitis (AD), are perpetuated by inappropriate and/or hyperactive immune responses under the circumstances of genetic predisposition, exposure to internal or external triggers, and disruption of barrier integrity—and their interactions. In this chapter we aim to delineate the pathophysiology of skin

barrier disruption in AD and discuss methods of management to repair this defect.

Atopic dermatitis pathobiology: Relationship to wound care

Previously, our understanding of the pathobiology of AD consisted of three main schools of thought: skin barrier abnormalities (outside-in hypothesis), defects in immune response (inside-out hypothesis), and altered skin resident microbiota (Boguniewicz & Leung, 2011; Brunner, Leung, & Guttman-Yassky, 2018; Kuo, Yoshida, De Benedetto, & Beck, 2013). Increased transepidermal water loss has been detected in AD patients at birth (Kelleher et al., 2015), and loss-of-function mutations in filaggrin—which encodes a protein indispensable for barrier formation and function—were found in over 40% of AD patients (Blunder et al., 2017; Palmer et al., 2006). However, recent findings showed that abnormal immunity can also lead to a loss of barrier function through downregulation of filaggrin in patients without the filaggrin gene mutation (Howell et al., 2009).

From an immunologic perspective, AD begins with an acute phase with excessive T-helper type 2 (Th2), Th22, and Th17 cell activation (Brandt & Sivaprasad, 2011; Gittler et al., 2012). Transition to the chronic phase is marked by the onset of Th1 cell activation and the continued presence of Th2 and Th22 cells (Brandt & Sivaprasad, 2011; Gittler et al., 2012; Guttman-Yassky, Krueger, & Lebwohl, 2017). Allergens and microbes such as *Staphylococcus aureus* and *Malassezia* spp. have been reported to trigger AD by inducing Th2 cytokine production (Bieber, 2008; Glatz et al., 2015; Hon et al., 2016; Kobayashi et al., 2015; Soumelis, 2017; Totte et al., 2016; Travers, 2014). Moreover, Th2 cytokine responses can be induced by keratinocytes that produce thymic stromal lymphopoietin (TSLP), which translates to Th2 polarization and production of interleukin-4 (IL4) and IL13 (Guttman-Yassky et al., 2017). Their effectors—IL25 and IL33—synergize with to further promote Th2 cytokine responses (Wang & Liu, 2009).

All of these processes result in two AD hallmarks: reduction in barrier proteins such as loricrin and filaggrin, and reduction in lipids (free fatty acids and ceramides) (Danso et al., 2014; Guttman-Yassky et al., 2017; Nygaard et al., 2017), translating into a defective epidermal permeability barrier. IL22 also promotes hyperplasia, downregulates terminal differentiation, synergizes with IL17 to induce the S100 genes, and induces keratinocyte production of type 2 cytokines (Guttman-Yassky et al., 2017; Lou et al., 2017; Souwer, Szegedi, Kapsenberg, & de Jong, 2010). Whether skin inflammation in AD is initiated by skin barrier dysfunction or by immune deregulation is still in debate. Additionally, innate lymphoid cells 2 (ILC-2) were recently implicated in AD through the production of IL4, IL5, IL13, and IL6 (Konya & Mjosberg, 2016; Mjosberg & Eidsmo, 2014; Roediger, Kyle, Le Gros, & Weninger, 2014). The subject of skin barrier is further discussed in Chapters 5 and 11.

Wound healing biology

Wound healing is an intricate process regulated by sequential and overlapping phases, including hemostasis, inflammation, proliferation, and remodeling. Under physiologic conditions this process is highly efficient; however, under pathologic conditions chronic wounds may develop (Lindley, Stojadinovic, Pastar, & Tomic-Canic, 2016).

Upon injury, hemostasis initiates fibrin clot formation, which serves as a scaffold and a source of growth factors and chemokines that recruit inflammatory cells to migrate into the wound bed (Singer & Clark, 1999). These inflammatory cells release growth factors and IL1, IL6, tumor necrosis factor-α (TNF-α), platelet-derived growth factor (PDGF), and fibroblast growth factor-2 (FGF-2) (Eming, Martin, & Tomic-Canic, 2014; Lindley et al., 2016).

Fibroblasts proliferate and produce provisional matrix over which keratinocytes migrate from the wound margins (Eming et al., 2014). Additionally, rearrangement of integrins and cytoskeletal components takes place and there is expression of proteases such as matrix metalloproteinase (MMP), which allows keratinocyte migration (Eming et al., 2014). This process is then followed by keratinocyte proliferation. Aberrant execution of any of these steps results in healing impairment and development of chronic wounds. Notably, this model is predominantly studied in wounds that feature both epidermal and at least partial dermal injuries.

Biologic underpinning for wound healing impairment in atopic dermatitis

The wound healing process in AD patients is characterized by a prolonged inflammatory phase. This leads to epidermal hyperplasia and tissue remodeling, resulting in the development of spongiosis (Levin, Friedlander, & Del Rosso, 2013). A proposed mechanism underlying the impaired wound healing in AD is depicted in Fig. 21.1.

EGF epidermal growth factor; hCAP18 human cathelicidin protein 18; IL-4 interleukin -4; MIF macrophage migration inhibitory factor; PPAR-α peroxisome proliferator-activator receptor α; TSLP Thymic stromal lymphopoietin; VEGF vascular endothelial growth factor

Wounds in AD are caused mostly by epidermal injury and disruption, rather than dermal alterations. The wound healing process in AD can rarely cause issues such as postsurgical complications. Issues with AD wound healing in general relate to innate inability to repair the barrier, defective angiogenesis, and abnormal microbial colonization, among others. These challenges are subtle but may further impact the patients' quality of life. Therefore clinicians should pay attention to wound and exudate care in patients with AD.

Various genes and molecules may delay wound healing in AD leading to the phenotypic changes noted earlier. In this section preclinical evidence is presented in support of the role of the following elements in the potential healing impairment in AD: IL4, caspases, hyperforin, TSLP, histamine, epidermal growth factor (EGF), various chemokines, vascular endothelial growth factor (VEGF), human cathelicidin protein 18 (hCAP18)/LL-37, peroxisome proliferator-activator receptor α (PPAR-α), tenascin-C, and altered microbiome environment.

Interleukin-4

IL4 is a Th2 cytokine secreted by activated T lymphocytes and innate immune cells that affects keratinocyte differentiation (Howell et al., 2006; Kagami et al., 2005). IL4 reduces keratinocyte expression of epidermal differentiation complex genes, decreases the expression of defensins, alters the expression of keratins, and increases the production of the chemokine CCL26 (eotaxin 3) (Albanesi et al., 2007; Omori-Miyake, Yamashita, Tsunemi, Kawashima, & Yagi, 2014; Owczarek et al., 2010).

Importantly, IL4 is a therapuetic target in patients with AD. In clinical trials of subjects with moderate to severe AD, disease scores improved after anti-IL4Rα human antagonist antibody treatment (Lewkowich et al., 2008).

In an IL4 transgenic (Tg) mouse model that presents an AD-like phenotype (Zhao, Bao, Chan, DiPietro, & Chen, 2016), IL4 Tg mice had delayed wound closure and reepithelialization. Additionally, the wounds showed an increased expression of proinflammatory cytokines/chemokines, elevated infiltration of neutrophils, macrophages, CD3+ lymphocytes and epidermal dendritic T lymphocytes, and larger amounts of granulation tissue (Zhao et al., 2016).

Serezani et al. (2017) found that IL4 represses the expression of fibronectin by keratinocytes, leading to a delay in wound repair. Moreover, IL4 modulated fibronectin in an in vivo model, improving wound repair (Serezani et al., 2017). Importantly, acute IL4 stimulation resulted in modulating expression of genes involved in cell growth and survival and diminished the expression of genes involved in cell adhesion. Chronic stimulation with IL4 resulted in increased expression of genes involved in cell projection and adhesion and decreased expression of genes participating in response to wounding and defense. Taken together, IL4 appears to stimulate a disorganized epithelial structure and contribute to an

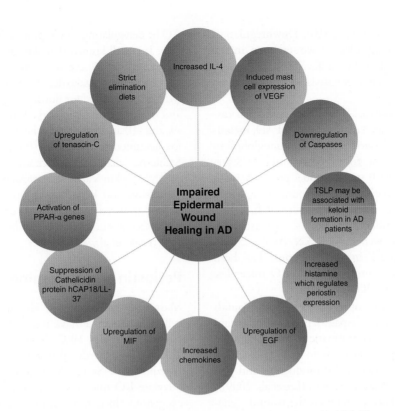

• **Fig. 21.1** Proposed mechanisms underlying the impaired wound healing process in atopic dermatitis *(AD)*. Elements involved in a compromised wound healing environment in AD include increased interleukin-4 *(IL4)*, induced mast cell expression of vascular endothelial growth factor *(VEGF)*, downregulation of caspases, thymic stromal lymphopoietin *(TSLP)* associated with keloid formation, histamine regulating periostin expression and mediating tissue remodeling, upregulation of epidermal growth factor *(EGF)*, increased various chemokines, upregulation of macrophage migration inhibitory factor *(MIF)*, suppression of human cathelicidin protein 18 *(hCAP18)/LL-37*, activation of peroxisome proliferator-activator receptor α *(PPAR-α)* and tenascin-C, as well as strict elimination diets.

increased susceptibility to microorganism invasion, which are also characteristics of AD lesions (Serezani et al., 2017).

Vascular endothelial growth factors/angiogenesis

Angiogenesis is the growth of new blood vessels from preexisting vessels and occurs physiologically in wound healing. Lymphangiogenesis can be activated in inflammation and tumor metastasis (Varricchi, Granata, Loffredo, Genovese, & Marone, 2015). AD as well as other inflammatory skin disorders, including psoriasis, are characterized by altered angiogenesis, lymphangiogenesis, or both (Genovese et al., 2012). Mast cells in AD lesions may stimulate angiogenesis via the release of proangiogenic factors (Detoraki et al., 2009, 2010; Kawakami, Ando, Kimura, Wilson, & Kawakami, 2009). It has been established that plasma and skin concentrations of VEGF are increased in AD (Brockow et al., 2002; Zhang, Matsuo, & Morita, 2006). A possible association between polymorphisms of the VEGF/VEGFR genes and AD has been established (Namkung et al., 2013; Zablotna et al., 2010). Moreover, IL9/IL9 receptor genes are overexpressed in AD, and IL9 induces VEGF secretion from mast cells (Sismanopoulos et al., 2012).

Interestingly, mast cells express corticotropin-releasing hormone receptors, which leads to the secretion of VEGF

(Cao et al., 2005). It is well known that stress worsens AD, and stress stimulates the release of corticotropin-releasing hormone and corticotropin-releasing hormone-induced mast cell-derived VEGF (Cao et al., 2005).

Semaphorins are a large family of secreted and membrane-associated proteins associated with axon guidance. They have been associated with angiogenesis (Bussolino, Giraudo, & Serini, 2014). Semaphorin IIIA was shown to improve skin lesions in the NC/Nga model of AD through the modulation of angiogenesis (Jung et al., 2010; Yamaguchi et al., 2008). Skin microcirculation in AD is further discussed in Chapter 12.

Caspases 1 and 8

Caspases (cysteine-aspartic proteases, cysteine aspartases, or cysteine-dependent aspartate-directed proteases) are protease enzymes playing essential roles in programmed cell death. Caspase-1, also known as IL1-converting enzyme, proteolytically cleaves the precursors of IL1β and IL18 and forms part of inflammasome. Caspase-8 is involved in the programmed cell death induced by Fas and various apoptotic stimuli.

Caspases play important roles in both chronic wound healing response and the pathogenesis of AD, therefore better understanding of caspases' function may ellucidate the wound response in AD (Li et al., 2010). Downregulation of epidermal caspase-8 recapitulates a wound even in the absence of trauma to the skin (Lee et al., 2009). Moreover, in humans, systemic deficiency of caspase-8 causes eczema (Chun et al., 2002).

Christopher et al. found that deletion of epidermal caspase-8 in a mouse model shared many features of AD, including acanthosis, scaling, elevated serum immunoglobulins, mast cell infiltration, and spongiosis (Scharschmidt & Segre, 2008). A C8 knockout (KO) mouse model presented with maximal levels of Th2 markers relative in young mice, which waned as the animal aged. These genes included IL4, IL5, IL9, and IL13 and chemokine receptor 4 (Scharschmidt & Segre, 2008; Schmidt-Weber, Akdis, & Akdis, 2007). Overexpression of caspase-1 in the epidermis has been reported to phenotypically mimic caspase-8 KO mice (Lee et al., 2009; Yamanaka et al., 2000).

Caspase-1 was found to be upregulated in both wounds and the caspase-8 KO mouse. Caspase-1 plays an important role in the inflammasome conformation and inflammatory response stimulating epithelial stem cell proliferation and tissue remodeling (through TSLP production and p38 mitogen-activated protein kinase activation) (Lee et al., 2009).

There are various similarities between the wound signature in AD and the wound healing response seen in caspase-8 deficiency. Caspase-8 KO mouse models have many features of AD, including acanthosis, scaling, elevated serum immunoglobulins, mast cell infiltration, and spongiosis (Li et al., 2010). Li et al. (2010) concluded that an unknown factor that normally would induce the expression of epidermal caspase-8 following wound closure may be impaired in AD, resulting in the sustained repression of caspase-8.

Thymic stromal lymphopoietin

TSLP is a Th2 cytokine that recently has been described in the pathogenesis of fibrosis. TSLP roles in systemic sclerosis (Christmann et al., 2013; Usategui et al., 2013), idiopathic pulmonary fibroblasts (Datta et al., 2013), and IL13-induced AD (Oh et al., 2011) have been described.

Subcutaneous injection of TSLP-induced skin fibrosis in a murine model (Jessup et al., 2008) and in the transgenic IL13 AD mouse model, the neutralization of TSLP, reduced collagen deposition and the inflammatory response (Oh et al., 2011). Shin et al. (2016) proposed that TSLP is an inducer of extracellular matrix synthesis and activator of the CXCR4/SDF-1 axis in skin fibrosis, especially in keloid pathogenesis. Although keloids in AD patients are rare, the data suggest that its formation in those patients is mediated through TSLP; however, more research needs to be done to establish a relationship in human pathobiology.

Role of the microbiome

Brauweiler, Goleva, Hall, and Leung (2015) proposed that Th2 cytokines, as well as staphylococcal lipoteichoic acid (LTA), may contribute to delayed wound healing and pathology of

AD by deregulating MMP production and altering cell migration. It is well known that skin of AD patients is chronically colonized with *S. aureus* (Travers et al., 2010; Zabielinski, McLeod, Aber, Izakovic, & Schachner, 2013). Moreover, MMPs are required for normal migration and wound closure, and overexpression is observed in chronic wounds. MMP-1, -9, and -10 are expressed at the wound edges and are required for keratinocyte migration (Inoue, Kratz, Haegerstrand, & Stahle-Backdahl, 1995; Rechardt et al., 2000).

Th2 cytokines are overexpressed in AD, and inhibit MMP expression and keratinocyte migration. Overexpression of MMPs induced by LTA may contribute to skin disease as well. Recent studies have described MMP expression in AD skin (Esaki et al., 2015).

Periostin and histamine

Mast cells contribute to the healing process and mast cell–deficient mice have impaired wound healing (Hebda, Collins, & Tharp, 1993; Noli & Miolo, 2001; Trautmann, Toksoy, Engelhardt, Brocker, & Gillitzer, 2000; Weller, Foitzik, Paus, Syska, & Maurer, 2006). Histidine decarboxylase KO mice resulted in delayed would healing, and exogenous histamine administration restored the normal healing process (Numata et al., 2006). Interestingly, H_1R antagonists (but not H_2R antagonists) were found to reduce wound closure in mice (Weller et al., 2006), and H_1R antagonist inhibits the synthesis of collagen 1 by dermal fibroblasts (Murota, Bae, Hamasaki, Maruyama, & Katayama, 2008). Moreover, there is an increase in mast cell number in fibrotic tissues, including scleroderma skin and keloids (Atkins & Clark, 1987; Hawkins, Claman, Clark, & Steigerwald, 1985). Yang et al. (2014) cultured dermal fibroblasts derived from wild type (WT) or periostin KO (PN[-/-]) mice and stimulated them with histamine. They found increased expression of colagen 1 mRNA after 48 hours of coincubation with histamine and concluded that histamine-mediated tissue remodeling may require the expression of periostin as a second messenger to elicit tissue remodeling (Yang et al., 2014). Taniguchi et al. (2014) studied how periostin regulates the proliferation and differentiation of keratinocytes. Fibroblasts secrete periostin, which stimulated IL1α-induced IL6 production and activated IL6 production through the nuclear factor (NF)–κB pathway (Taniguchi et al., 2014). Histamine is a major proinflammatory mediator that is increased in AD patients, therefore understanding the histamine-periostin pathway may explain the wound healing physiology in these patients.

Epidermal growth factor

The EGF pathway is essential for keratinocyte proliferation and differentiation and for proper wound healing (Berlanga-Acosta et al., 2009; Repertinger et al., 2004). Upregulation of this pathway has been found in chronic inflammatory skin disorders, including psoriasis and AD (Pastore, Mascia, Mariani, & Girolomoni, 2008).

Zhang, Xiao, Gibson, Bass, and Khurana Hershey (2014) described that EGF treatment in human keratinocytes and HaCat keratinocytes resulted in a decrease of IL17A and IL6 expression in the skin. In vivo, EGF may attenuate IL6 production in the skin and reduce local Th17 response. This suggests a protective role for EGF in AD and a new role for EGF in modulating IL17 responses in the skin.

Chemokines

Fibrogenic and fibrosis-associated cytokines (TGF-β1, IL11, and IL17) as well as the chemokine superfamily have been shown to regulate atopic skin inflammation (Gombert et al., 2005; Homey et al., 2002; Pivarcsi et al., 2004). CCL11, CCL17, CCL22, CCL26, CCL27, and CX$_3$CL1 interactions are directly correlated with disease activity and severity (Homey, Meller, Savinko, Alenius, & Lauerma, 2007).

Gaspar et al. (2013) identified chemokine-mediated pathways regulating tissue remodeling in AD. They analyzed the chemokine receptor expression of human dermal fibroblasts and showed that among the CCR3 ligands, the chemokine CCL26 is the most highly expressed in AD, and that the keratinocytes were the predominant source (Gaspar et al., 2013).

Macrophage migration inhibitory factor

Macrophage migration inhibitory factor (MIF) is a lymphokine involved in cell-mediated immunity, immunoregulation, and inflammation and plays a role in the regulation of macrophage function in host defense through the suppression of antiinflammatory effects of glucocorticoids. MIF has been identified as a key effector of estrogen effetcs on wound repair (Gilliver, Emmerson, Bernhagen, & Hardman, 2011). Moreover, endothelial MIF expression is upregulated in AD (Gomez, Diepgen, Neumann, & Sorg, 1990; Hizawa, Yamaguchi, Takahashi, Nishihira, & Nishimura, 2004). Therefore this cytokine may play a role in the healing process of AD skin.

Cathelicidin protein hCAP18/LL-37

hCAP18/LL-37 is an endogenous antimicrobial peptide (AMP) that plays a crucial role in barrier protection. Wounding of the skin induces hCAP18/LL-37 expression in normal skin (Dorschner et al., 2001). In AD lesions, the expression of hCAP18 mRNA was suppressed following wounding. It is hypothesized that the abundant inflammatory response in AD neutralizes the expected induction of hCAP18 (Mallbris et al., 2010). Inability to upregulate hCAP18 in eczema following injury is likely to affect antimicrobial protection and tissue repair in AD.

Peroxisome proliferator-activated receptors

PPARs are ligand-activated transcription factors that belong to the nuclear receptor superfamily. The PPAR family genes are activated by various fatty acid metabolites produced during inflammatory responses and regulate other signaling pathways, including NFκB, through ligand-dependent transrepression (Lefebvre, Chinetti, Fruchart, & Staels, 2006; Ricote & Glass, 2007). Skin injury was found to stimulate PPAR-α reexpression in keratinocytes during the healing process, and PPAR-α$^{-/-}$ mice have a transient delay in initial wound healing (Michalik et al., 2001; Tan et al., 2001). Interesntingly, PPAR-α–deficient mice display many features similar to AD, including increased epidermal thickening, dermal inflammatory cell infiltrate, and other atopic features such as lung inflammation and hyperactivity (Staumont-Salle et al., 2008). Understanding the PPAR-α pathway and its regulators may help scientist to better discern the healing process in AD patients.

Tenascin-C

Tenascin-C is part of the tenascins family, which are expressed in human tissues during organogenesis as well as embryogenesis and wound healing (Chiquet-Ehrismann & Chiquet, 2003). Upregulation of the tenascin-C expression was found to be specific to AD lesions, and tenascin-C was markedly upregulated by IL4 and IL13, and moderately upregulated by interferón-gamma (Ogawa et al., 2005). Human keratinocytes are a major source of tenascin-C, especially during the early phase of wound healing (Latijnhouwers et al., 1997). The high expression of tenascin-C in the skin lesion of AD patients might reflect the process for remodeling or overrepairing the inflammatory lesion by keratinocytes. Taken together, these pathways that may be dysregulated in AD may help to understand some of the phenotypical observations that have been made pertaining to wound healing impairment in AD. However, better translational evidence is needed to provide a comprehensive model for wound healing impairment in AD.

Surgical complications in atopic dermatitis

AD management is often complicated by colonization of *S. aureus* (Fukunaga et al., 2012). Colonization with this bacterium is a risk factor for certain infections such as skin cellulitis and osteomyelitis. Thus atopic patients are at increased risk of infection when facing surgical procedures that break the protective skin barrier (Fukunaga et al., 2012).

Among patients undergoing cardiac surgery, 70% to 80% of wounds in those with mediastinitis following conventional median sternotomy have positive cultures for *S. aureus* (Fukunaga et al., 2012). Thus it has been suggested that AD patients undergoing sternotomy are at an increased risk of mediastinitis given the *S. aureus* burden associated with AD and the infectious risk this poses postoperatively (Fukunaga et al., 2012). Of note, no postoperative mediastinitis has been observed in AD patients who underwent thoracotomy, suggesting that may be a more favorable surgical approach in patients with AD requiring cardiac intervention (Fukunaga et al., 2012).

AD has additionally been found to be an independent risk factor for surgical site infection following anterior cruciate ligament reconstruction (ACLR) (Kawata et al., 2018). This is thought to be due to the aforementioned susceptibility of *S. aureus* colonization of atopic skin lesions (Kawata et al., 2018). Rates of surgical site infection following ACLR are low, ranging from 0.14% to approximately 2.32%. Nonetheless, this rare complication has the potential to cause significant repercussions, as it may require further surgical intervention or even graft removal (Kawata et al., 2018).

Wound care in atopic dermatitis

General measures for patients with wounds and atopic dermatitis

An impaired barrier predisposes to skin injuries, which can progress to nonhealing wounds. The pillar of wound prevention is barrier repair through moisturization. Moisturizers have broad utility within dermatology, especially for AD, since they help alleviate symptoms and improve barrier function (Kim & Leung, 2018; Simpson et al., 2014). Therefore moisturizers represent a pillar in wound prevention.

Microorganisms colonize human skin and resultant wounds as well as the mouth, digestive, and reproductive tracts. As a result, the number of bacteria colonizing the human body far exceeds the number of our own cells (Mancl, Kirsner, & Ajdic, 2013). Moreover, it is well known that AD patients are chronically colonized with *S. aureus* (Travers et al., 2010; Zabielinski et al., 2013), and the presence of *S. aureus* is correlated with flares. Failure to heal of wounds has been associated with biofilms, as they have been shown to prevent wound contracture and epithelialization, disrupt the host immune response, and induce chronic inflammation (Miller et al., 2014).

Hypochlorous acid (HOCl) exhibits antiinflammatory effects through blockade of NFκB signaling in keratinocytes (Leung et al., 2013) and decreases sensory nerve transmission by inhibiting intracellular calcium signaling, reducing pain and itch symptoms (Fukuyama et al., 2018). HOCl also reduces serum levels of IL1β, IL6, and TNF-α (Fukuyama et al., 2018) proinflammatory cytokines elevated in skin and serum (Smith, Nicholson, Parks-Miller, & Hamzavi, 2017). Moreover, HOCl decreases sensory nerve transmission by inhibiting intracellular calcium signaling, thus reducing pain and itch symptoms (Fukuyama et al., 2018). Sakarya, Gunay, Karakulak, Ozturk, and Ertugrul (2014) found that stabilized HOCl solution had dose-dependent favorable effects on fibroblast and keratinocyte migration. Due to the antiinflammatory properties, HCOl is a useful solution to be used in patients with AD and chronic wounds.

Drug delivery vehicles

Various drug delivery systems may be utilized to treat chronic wounds. In patients with AD and wounds, clinicians have an opportunity to leverage the vehicles to benefit patients with AD. The most common examples are ointments and hydrogels, which can improve the impaired barrier for these patients.

In general, the barrier function of the skin poses a drug delivery challenge. Optimal drug delivery systems should feature nontoxicity, good biocompatibility and biodegradability, drug stability, and optimized drug absorption and bioavailability (Yun, Lee, & Park, 2015). Relative to other drug delivery vehicles commonly used in AD such as ointments, hydrogels have demonstrated bioequivalence, higher ease of use, and patient satisfaction; this may prove to be a useful tool in wound management in AD. Hydrogels are composed of a network of three-dimensional hydrophilic polymers that can withstand swelling without losing their structural integrity. They can be used as drug delivery systems given their biocompatibility, flexibility, and ability to hold high water content (Harrison & Spada, 2018).

A hydrogel formulation containing desonide has been found easy to use, quick to disappear, comfortable, soothing, nondrying, and not greasy or shiny on the skin by AD patients. Desonide hydrogel 0.05% was found to be equally effective to desonide ointment 0.05% at reducing AD symptoms. However, when compared to desonide ointment, desonide hydrogel has higher rates of patient satisfaction for absorbability and lack of greasiness. This hydrogel preparation has consistently been rated higher by patients than other vehicles, has higher rates of patient adherence, and has been found to be efficacious in a shorter time frame than other vehicles. Furthermore, hydrogel formulations improved skin hydration when compared to a moisturizing lotion (Harrison & Spada, 2018).

Dressings and textiles

The treatment of chronic wounds typically involves the application of various dressings, and often these products contain active medications. Additionally, people with AD may exhibit increased percutaneous drug absorption due to their skin's impaired barrier function. Therefore patients with AD are at a higher risk for hypersensitivity reactions such as allergic contact dermatitis.

Many dressings when in contact with fluids, including wound exudate, change their composition into hydrogels. This property can help hydrate and improve the defective barrier seen in patients with AD.

Wound care regime in AD may include wet wrap therapy, which helps to rehydrate and soothe the skin. Fabric wraps are to be soaked in warm water and applied to the affected areas of the skin. A dry layer is then applied over the wet one, such as pajamas, which can be worn as a top layer to maintain the wet dressings undisturbed. This process is best done after the patient has bathed and moisturized the skin. The wet wraps can be left on overnight (Nicol, Boguniewicz, Strand, & Klinnert, 2014).

Hydrocolloid dressings containing ceramides may have a positive therapeutic effect in AD. The SC functions as a watertight protective barrier from external insults, partially via composition of various lipids. Ceramide, a sphingolipid, is a major component of the lipid bilayer, accounting for almost half of the lipids in the SC by weight. This sphingolipid is intimately involved with the skin's barrier function (Tsuchiya et al., 2013). Low levels of ceramides in the SC are associated with the dry skin and barrier-disruption exhibited in AD. Furthermore, insufficient levels of ceramides can lead to increased susceptibility to infection, increased transepidermal water loss (TEWL), and skin inflammation. These deleterious processes may eventually trigger erosions following excoriations and other minor trauma, which would subsequently be difficult to heal given the skin's disrupted barrier function (Tsuchiya et al., 2013).

Topical ceramide can be utilized to improve skin barrier function (Tsuchiya et al., 2013). More recently it was found to accelerate wound healing as well (Tsuchiya et al., 2013). Hydrocolloid dressings containing 0.3% ceramide-2 showed reduction in wound size and greater regeneration of epidermal and dermal layers in mice models relative to control (thickness of regenerated epidermis/dermis was 3.27 times thicker, on average, for ceramide group compared to control group). Ceramide dressings also helped reduce the wound-related increase in TEWL, suggesting they may be of use in the management of wounds in AD (Tsuchiya et al., 2013). Dressings and textiles specially coated with zinc may also have beneficial effects on the management of AD. Textiles that capitalize on zinc's intrinsic antibacterial and antioxidative properties, such as Benevit Zink+, have demonstrated rapid improvement of AD symptom severity with regard to pruritus and sleep quality when utilized overnight (Reed et al., 2016).

Cutaneous superinfection of atopic lesions with *S. aureus* plays a significant role in inflammation and exacerbations seen in AD. In fact, AD severity can be correlated with cutaneous *S. aureus* colonization (Haug et al., 2006). Therefore treatment of AD and AD-associated wounds includes antimicrobial components in an effort to reduce the *S. aureus* burden, leading to a positive effect on the disease overall (Haug et al., 2006).

Silver products have historically been used as antimicrobial wound dressings, given silver's antiseptic properties and the relatively low drug resistance associated with it (Haug et al., 2006). Newer developments show these antimicrobial effects are exhibited by silver-coated textiles as well, such as Padycare textiles (micromesh with 20% woven silver filaments). In vitro studies of these textiles demonstrate their ability to significantly reduce the bioburden of *S. aureus*, *Pseudomonas aeruginosa*, and *Candida albicans* (Haug et al., 2006). Importantly, the antimicrobial efficacy of silver-impregnated textiles is reduced with repetitive washing (from >99% reduction in *Escherichia coli* growth to 81.6% [deionized water only] to 75.1% [deionized water and detergent] reduction in *E. coli* growth) (Reed et al., 2016).

Chitosan functionalized textiles have similar antibacterial properties, particularly against *S. aureus*, Methicillin-resistant *S. aureus* (MRSA), and vancomycin-resistant *S. aureus* (VRSA), making it a prime candidate for possible management of wounds in AD (Costa, Silva, Veiga, Tavaria, & Pintado, 2018). Chitosan is a cationic biopolymer with unique biologic properties that is found widely in nature, composed of fungi and the exoskeletons of insects as well as marine invertebrates. As a free molecule, chitosan inhibits bacterial growth and adhesion. Chitosan appears to bypass the antibiotic resistance mechanisms typical to the *Staphylococcus* spp., allowing it to have significant bactericidal activity on MRSA and VRSA. In vivo studies with AD patients demonstrated that cotton-based clothing with a chitosan antimicrobial finish aided in modulating the cutaneous bacterial profile by reducing *S. aureus* counts and increasing coagulase-negative *Staphylococci*. Therefore chitosan functionalized textiles may be a viable alternative to traditional antibiotic regimes in AD wound management (Costa et al., 2018).

Other textiles have been implemented in AD management, including silk. Silk inherently reduces irritation in AD given its unique smooth texture (Haug et al., 2006). Additionally, products such as Dermasilk combine the smoothness of silk with an antimicrobial coating, making it an optimal textile for AD patients with wounds at risk for infection (Haug et al., 2006). Nonetheless, it is important to consider costs when recommending such specialty dressings and textiles, as they may be high.

The role of nutrition in wound care

The role of nutrition in wound healing of eczematous patients is a concept that has not been studied directly. However, with the current knowledge of the role of nutrition in the pathogenesis of AD and to promote wound healing, clinicians should consider educating patients about the importance of (1) adequate nutrition and clarifying the common misconceptions about food allergies, and (2) the role of micronutrients, polyunsaturated fatty acid (PUFA), and healthy microbiome to attenuate inflammation and to promote wound healing in AD.

Adequate nutrition

Evaluating AD patients' nutritional status and ensuring sufficient calories from a balanced diet of carbohydrates, fats, and protein, and supplementing protein, fluid, and vitamins A and C, is needed for adequate wound healing. Strict elimination diets are more likely to lead to nutritional deficiencies (Liu et al., 2001) and delayed wound healing (Stechmiller, 2010). Therefore, to prevent nutritional deficiency and the subsequent delayed wound healing in AD patients, it is important to clarify the common misconceptions associated with food allergies. Nutrition is further discussed in Chapter 8.

Vitamins and minerals

While various vitamin and mineral deficiencies have been shown to play a role in the pathogenesis of AD and wound healing, the evidence for their use in the treatment or prevention of AD in pediatric and adult patients has been unconvincing (Bath-Hextall, Delamere, & Williams, 2009).

Zinc is an essential cofactor for metalloenzymes involved in cellular function. Deficiency of zinc has been correlated with impaired wound healing (Gil & Rueda, 2002; Stechmiller, 2010), but there is no proven benefit of oral zinc supplementation in AD treatment. Zinc deficiency disturbs all phases of wound healing. In the inflammatory phase, there is reduced immunity and augmented susceptibility to infections. In the proliferative phase, there is decreased collagen synthesis and tensile strength. Finally, in the remodeling phase, there is a diminishing of fibroblast proliferation, collagen synthesis, and epithelialization (Gil & Rueda, 2002; Stechmiller, 2010).

Oxidative stress has been proposed as another pathophysiologic factor contributing to AD, therefore suppression of oxidative stress via the supplementation of antioxidants may be an effective treatment strategy. Selenium is strongly involved in antioxidant functions; however, its direct wounding healing role in still unclear (Stechmiller, 2010).

Several vitamins, including A, C, and E, are known to protect cells against free radical damage and have been hypothesized to play a possible role in the prevention and management of AD (Foolad, Brezinski, Chase, & Armstrong, 2013). Various mechanisms of the role of vitamin D in AD have been proposed, including immunomodulation, reduced cell proliferation, and improved epidermal barrier function (Amestejani et al., 2012; Galli et al., 2015; Kim, Kim, Lee, Choe, & Ahn, 2016; Norizoe et al., 2014; Zhang, Wu, & Sun, 2013). Cathelicidin is an AMP induced by vitamin D that promotes wound healing. Vitamin D and its receptor signaling control structural integrity of epithelial barriers with implications for wound healing (Zhang et al., 2013).

While recommendations for micronutrient supplementation are unknown in the treatment of AD and the specific roles micronutrients play in wound healing, dermatologists should remind their patients that maintaining a healthy, wholesome diet with less processed foods has been shown to benefit patients with AD.

Polyunsaturated fatty acids

For wound healing in AD patients, adequate PUFA dietary intake may help to rebuild the structural integrity of the damaged skin barrier and support synthesis of signaling molecules, which influence the inflammatory response in the skin (Kiecolt-Glaser, Glaser, & Christian, 2014).

There are a multitude of ceramide species found in both the dermis and the epidermis. Biochemically, n-3 and n-6 are essential fatty acids that are particularly significant in maintaining a healthy skin barrier as they contribute to the formation of ceramides (Elias et al., 2014). However, a deficiency is difficult to produce unless a fat-free diet is maintained.

Immune dysregulation plays an important role in the pathogenesis of AD and is needed for proper wound

healing regulation of the immune system and attenuation of inflammation. There are diverse advantageous effects on the immune response that have been attributed to the long-chain n-3 fatty acids eicosapentaenoic acid (EPA) and docosahexaenoic acid (DHA) (Calder, Kremmyda, Vlachava, Noakes, & Miles, 2010). Through different mechanisms, these n-3 fatty acids have an inhibitory or regulatory effect on the immune response. One example is the regulatory effect of these n-3 fatty acids on antigen presentation and adhesion molecule expression, as part of the Th1 and Th2 response, as well as on proinflammatory cytokine and eicosanoid production (Calder et al., 2010; Harbige, 2003). Protectins and resolvins are n-3 PUFA-derived molecules, which play an important role in switching from initiation to the resolution phase of inflammation.

The biochemical effects of PUFAs are known to benefit the integrity of skin barrier by optimizing skin lipid biology and are known to attenuate multiple inflammatory cascades within the immune system.

Probiotics

Gut probiotics and commensals may moderate skin wound healing through effects on systemic immunity and enhanced nutrient absorption. The differences in gut microbiota between those with atopic diseases and controls have been described. AD patients have higher proportion of *Clostridia, Clostridium difficile, E. coli*, and *S. aureus* and decreased *Bifidobacteria, Bacteroidetes*, and *Bacteroides* in the gut microbiome than in healthy controls (Abrahamsson et al., 2012; Kirjavainen, Arvola, Salminen, & Isolauri, 2002; Lee et al., 2016; Nylund et al., 2015; Penders et al., 2006).

Certain bacterial strains have the potential to attenuate skin inflammation when administered systemically by changing the composition of gut microbiome. For example, a study found *Lactobacillus paracasei* modifies the composition of intestinal microbiota by increasing *Bifidobacteria* and *Lactobacilli* microbiota and also reinforces skin barrier and decreases skin sensitivity while significantly increasing Th1 cell-dependent immune responses (Benyacoub et al., 2014). Also, it was found that supplementation of probiotics such as *Lactobacillus reuteri* encourages an upregulation of antiinflammatory IL10, which induces Foxp3+ Treg lymphocytes to minimize tissue damage at the wound edge (Erdman & Poutahidis, 2014).

Aside from manipulating the immune system, the gut microbiota and orally introduced probiotics may achieve improved absorption of nutrients essential for skin wound healing, especially vitamins, minerals, and cofactors for enzymes involved in tissue repair (Askelson, Campasino, Lee, & Duong, 2014; Kaplan, Gonul, Dincer, Dincer Kaya, & Babul, 2004; Rutherfurd, Chung, Thomas, Zou, & Moughan, 2012). Additionally, several *Lactobacilli* spp., including *Lactobacillus coryniformis* and *Lactobacillus rossiae*, have been shown to produce vitamin B_{12}, which is valuable for wound healing (De Angelis et al., 2014). *L. reuteri* and *Lactobacillus acidophilus* were shown to increase absorption of dietary vitamin D and E, known to be important for wound healing (Degirolamo, Rainaldi, Bovenga, Murzilli, & Moschetta, 2014; Jones, Martoni, & Prakash, 2013; Oda, Tu, Menendez, Nguyen, & Bikle, 2016; Roager et al., 2014). Though a therapeutic potential of probiotic bacteria for wound healing in disorders exists, more definitive studies are needed to explore the benefit of probiotics in wound healing for AD patients. The microbiome and probiotics are further discussed in Chapters 6 and 24.

Complementary and alternative medicine in wound care

Complementary and alternative medicine (CAM) is commonly practiced throughout the world. In China, CAM represent up to 40% of all health care practice (WHO, 2002). Up to 80% of populations in Asia and Africa utilize CAM as their primary form of medicine. Despite CAM-prevalent utilization around the world, there is a need of clinical research to elucidate mechanisms of action and validate its use.

Due to the worldwide prevalence of chronic wounds and their notorious difficulty in treatment, CAM regimens have been clinically evaluated for their efficacy. Moreover, there are an increasing number of trials studying CAM to treat patients with AD. Interestingly there is a growing interest in CAM as a primary, maintenance, or simultaneous treatment for AD (Lu et al., 2018). Patients with AD and their family members may choose CAM as their primary approach to relieve their illness or at least to improve the duration and quality of symptomatic relief.

Standard treatment for chronic wounds and AD can be expensive, painful, and frustrating; moreover, it may be associated with various adverse effects. Among other widely practiced alternative wound healing methods and AD treatments, the topical application of honey, vitamins, and herbs as well as dietary modifications are some examples of CAM therapies with some evidence supporting their use in clinical studies. Additional CAM treatments are discussed in Chapters 26 and 27.

Curcumin

Turmeric *(Curcuma longa)* is a popular bright yellow spice used worldwide in traditional medicine and for cooking and dye. Curcumin is the active constituent of turmeric. The use of curcumin in medicine has been heavily studied, particularly with regard to its role in modulating inflammation (He et al., 2015; Kocaadam & Sanlier, 2017). In some Eastern countries, curcumin's antiinflammatory effects are exploited as a part of AD management (Vollono et al., 2019).

Curcumin's role in AD has also been described. Curcumin modulates protein kinase C-θ pathway in vitro, leading to the inhibition of T-cell activation (Lee et al., 2012). In mice, it was also found to ameliorate ovalbumin-induced AD pathology through inhibition of TSLP, IL33, IL4, IL5, L13, IL31 and reduced STAT-6 phosphorylation (Sharma, Sethi, & Naura, 2019).

In mice, oral administration reduced the production of proinflammatory cytokines by keratinocytes, improving cutaneous signs of AD such as inflammation and dermoepidermal thickening (Heng, Song, Harker, & Heng, 2000). Importantly, in humans, daily applications of a combination herbal extract cream (Herbavate) that contains *C. longa* was found to alleviate AD symtoms (Rawal, Shah, Jayaraaman, & Jaiswal, 2009).

Curcumin has been studied in wound healing. Animal model studies have demonstrated topical application of curcumin accelerates wound healing and reepithelialization rates when compared to controls (Vollono et al., 2019). Topical application of curcumin was found to have a more robust effect on wound healing when compared to oral administration. This is likely due to the higher availability of curcumin at the wound site when applied topically (Vollono et al., 2019). However, topical application may lead to yellowish or brown discoloration, and patients should be warned in advance about this potential side effect.

Curcumin is thought to play an active role in wound healing, particularly during the inflammatory and proliferative phases (Vollono et al., 2019). Curcumin has been observed to reduce inflammation through the suppression of TNF-α, an inflammatory mediator involved in the inflammatory phase of wound healing (see Introduction). In the proliferative phase, studies have shown that curcumin may increase hydroxyproline and collagen synthesis, accelerate the maturation of collagen fibers, and reduce the number of MMPs. Curcumin has also been shown to promote the differentiation of fibroblasts into myofibroblasts, thus aiding in wound contraction and resulting in a shorter epithelization period (Vollono et al., 2019).

Although promising for the treatment of both AD and wounds, curcumin has been associated with allergic contact dermatitis and has emerged as a contact allergen (Chaudhari, Tam, & Barr, 2015; Fischer & Agner, 2004; Ghasemi, Saxtrup, Al-Khafagi, Thorup, & Sommerlund, 2018; Hata et al., 1997; Kiec-Swierczynska & Krecisz, 1998; Liddle, Hull, Liu, & Powell, 2006; Lopez-Villafuerte & Clores, 2016; Thompson & Tan, 2006). Historically, it was thought that patients with AD were less likely to develop contact dermatitis; however, more recent evidence has shown that patients with AD have similar if not higher rates of positive patch test results to common contact allergens (Aquino & Fonacier, 2014; Lugovic & Lipozencic, 1997; Simonsen, Johansen, Deleuran, Mortz, & Sommerlund, 2017). Therefore caution needs to be taken when using topical curcumin for wounds in patients with AD due to possible increased risk of contact allergic dermatitis.

Glycerol

Glycerol is a trihydroxy alcohol widely used in dermatologic preparations. Topical glycerol application aids in increasing epidermal hydration, which is of utmost importance in the management of skin diseases characterized by xerosis and impaired epidermal barrier function, such as AD (Fluhr,

Darlenski, & Surber, 2008). Glycerol additionally promotes the process of wound healing (Hara, Ma, & Verkman, 2002; Hara-Chikuma & Verkman, 2008) and has antiirritant and antimicrobial properties, among other functions. Gram-negative bacteria in particular appear to be more susceptible to glycerol than gram-positive bacteria (Fluhr et al., 2008). Glycerol's wound healing properties combined with its antiirritant, antimicrobial, and hydrating qualities suggest this topical agent may be of potential use in treating wounds in AD.

Hyperforin

Hyperforin is a major active constituent of St. John wort (*Hypericum perforatum* L.) extract, a traditional herbal medicine with wound healing properties (Samadi et al., 2010; Suntar et al., 2011) and potential antiinflammatory properties in AD (Schempp, Windeck, Hezel, & Simon, 2003). Takada, Yonekawa, Matsumoto, Furuya, and Sokabe (2017) proposed that hyperforin/2-hydroxylpropyl-beta-cyclodextrin (HPβCD) is a potent targeted therapeutic agent that can be used to promote epidermal wound healing and treat AD. They measured the stretch-induced Ca^{2+} responses ex vivo in atopic skin and found that the Ca^{2+} response was impaired in AD. The effect was recovered after the application of hyperforin/HPβCD, suggesting the therapeutic properties and potential to promote epidermal wound healing and treat AD (Takada et al., 2017).

Summary

The wound healing process in AD patients is overall altered. Various genes and molecules have been described in atopic skin that may be involved in the delayed healing process. Issues with healing may relate to innate inability to repair the barrier, defective angiogenesis, and abnormal microbial colonization, among others. In general, these challenges are subtle but impact patients' quality of life. Wound healing in AD can rarely cause issues such as postsurgical complications.

Special drug delivery vehicles commonly used in AD such as ointments and hydrogels prove to be useful tools in wound management in AD. Caution needs to be taken when considering special dressings and textiles in patients with AD due to the increased risk of development of allergic contact dermatitis.

Also, adequate nutrition is needed to address both AD and enhancement of skin healing properties. PUFA, healthy microbiome, and wholesome diet are needed to attenuate inflammation and to maintain a healthy SC. CAM interventions are receiving increased attention among physicians and researchers, and its role is being investigated for both wound healing and AD.

Further readings

Choi, F. D., Sung, C. T., Juhasz, M. L., & Mesinkovsk, N. A. (2019). Oral collagen supplementation: A systematic review of dermatological applications. *Journal of Drugs in Dermatology, 18*(1), 9–16.

Donovan, M., Ambach, A., Thomas-Collignon, A., Prado, C., Bernard, D., Jammayrac, O., et al. (2013). Calmodulin-like skin protein level increases in the differentiated epidermal layers in atopic dermatitis. *Experimental Dermatology, 22*(12), 836–837. https://doi.org/10.1111/exd.12274.

Fenner, J., & Silverberg, N. B. (2018). Oral supplements in atopic dermatitis. *Clinical Dermatology, 36*(5), 653–658. https://doi.org/10.1016/j.clindermatol.2018.05.010.

Guo, L., Chen, H., Li, Y., Zhou, Q., & Sui, Y. (2013). An aquaporin 3-notch1 axis in keratinocyte differentiation and inflammation. *PLoS One, 8*(11), e80179. https://doi.org/10.1371/journal.pone.0080179.

Kramer, A., Guggenbichler, P., Heldt, P., Junger, M., Ladwig, A., Thierbach, H., et al. (2006). Hygienic relevance and risk assessment of antimicrobial-impregnated textiles. *Current Problems in Dermatology, 33*, 78–109. https://doi.org/10.1159/000093938.

Li, W., Sandhoff, R., Kono, M., Zerfas, P., Hoffmann, V., Ding, B. C., et al. (2007). Depletion of ceramides with very long chain fatty acids causes defective skin permeability barrier function, and neonatal lethality in ELOVL4 deficient mice. *International Journal of Biological Sciences, 3*(2), 120–128. https://doi.org/10.7150/ijbs.3.120.

Miles, E. A., & Calder, P. C. (2017). Can early omega-3 fatty acid exposure reduce risk of childhood allergic disease? *Nutrients, 9*(7), 784. https://doi.org/10.3390/nu9070784.

Park, J. Y., Shin, M. S., Hwang, G. S., Yamabe, N., Yoo, J. E., Kang, K. S., et al. (2018). Beneficial effects of deoxyshikonin on delayed wound healing in diabetic mice. *International Journal of Molecular Science, 19*(11), 3660. https://doi.org/10.3390/ijms19113660.

Park, K. S., & Park, D. H. (2019). The effect of Korean red ginseng on full-thickness skin wound healing in rats. *Journal of Ginseng Research, 43*(2), 226–235. https://doi.org/10.1016/j.jgr.2017.12.006.

Slattery, J., MacFabe, D. F., & Frye, R. E. (2016). The significance of the enteric microbiome on the development of childhood disease: A review of prebiotic and probiotic therapies in disorders of childhood. *Clinical Medicine Insights: Pediatrics, 10*, 91–107. https://doi.org/10.4137/CMPed.S38338.

Song, H. J., Grant, I., Rotondo, D., Mohede, I., Sattar, N., Heys, S. D., & Wahle, K. W. (2005). Effect of CLA supplementation on immune function in young healthy volunteers. *European Journal of Clinical Nutrition, 59*(4), 508–517. https://doi.org/10.1038/sj.ejcn.1602102.

Varricchi, G., Granata, F., Loffredo, S., Genovese, A., & Marone, G. (2015). Angiogenesis and lymphangiogenesis in inflammatory skin disorders. *Journal of the American Academy of Dermatology, 73*(1), 144–153. https://doi.org/10.1016/j.jaad.2015.03.041.

References

Abrahamsson, T. R., Jakobsson, H. E., Andersson, A. F., Bjorksten, B., Engstrand, L., & Jenmalm, M. C. (2012). Low diversity of the gut microbiota in infants with atopic eczema. *The Journal of Allergy and Clinical Immunology, 129*(2), 434–440. https://doi.org/10.1016/j.jaci.2011.10.025. 440.e1-2.

Albanesi, C., Fairchild, H. R., Madonna, S., Scarponi, C., De Pita, O., Leung, D. Y., & Howell, M. D. (2007). IL-4 and IL-13 negatively regulate TNF-alpha- and IFN-gamma-induced beta-defensin expression through STAT-6, suppressor of cytokine signaling (SOCS)-1, and SOCS-3. *Journal of Immunology, 179*(2), 984–992. https://doi.org/10.4049/jimmunol.179.2.984.

Amestejani, M., Salehi, B. S., Vasigh, M., Sobhkhiz, A., Karami, M., Alinia, H., et al. (2012). Vitamin D supplementation in the treatment of atopic dermatitis: A clinical trial study. *Journal of Drugs in Dermatology*, 11(3), 327–330.

Aquino, M., & Fonacier, L. (2014). The role of contact dermatitis in patients with atopic dermatitis. *The Journal of Allergy and Clinical Immunology: In Practice*, 2(4), 382–387. https://doi.org/10.1016/j.jaip.2014.05.004.

Askelson, T. E., Campasino, A., Lee, J. T., & Duong, T. (2014). Evaluation of phytate-degrading *Lactobacillus* culture administration to broiler chickens. *Applied and Environmental Microbiology*, 80(3), 943–950. https://doi.org/10.1128/AEM.03155-13.

Atkins, F. M., & Clark, R. A. (1987). Mast cells and fibrosis. *Archives of Dermatology*, 123(2), 191–193.

Bangert, C., Brunner, P. M., & Stingl, G. (2011). Immune functions of the skin. *Clinics in Dermatology*, 29(4), 360–376. https://doi.org/10.1016/j.clindermatol.2011.01.006.

Bath-Hextall, F., Delamere, F. M., & Williams, H. C. (2009). Dietary exclusions for improving established atopic eczema in adults and children: Systematic review. *Allergy*, 64(2), 258–264. https://doi.org/10.1111/j.1398-9995.2008.01917.x.

Benyacoub, J., Bosco, N., Blanchard, C., Demont, A., Philippe, D., Castiel-Higounenc, I., & Gueniche, A. (2014). Immune modulation property of *Lactobacillus paracasei* NCC2461 (ST11) strain and impact on skin defences. *Beneficial Microbes*, 5(2), 129–136. https://doi.org/10.3920/BM2013.0014.

Berlanga-Acosta, J., Gavilondo-Cowley, J., Lopez-Saura, P., Gonzalez-Lopez, T., Castro-Santana, M. D., Lopez-Mola, E., et al. (2009). Epidermal growth factor in clinical practice—A review of its biological actions, clinical indications and safety implications. *International Wound Journal*, 6(5), 331–346. https://doi.org/10.1111/j.1742-481X.2009.00622.x.

Bieber, T. (2008). Atopic dermatitis. *The New England Journal of Medicine*, 358(14), 1483–1494. https://doi.org/10.1056/NEJMra074081.

Blunder, S., Ruhl, R., Moosbrugger-Martinz, V., Krimmel, C., Geisler, A., Zhu, H., et al. (2017). Alterations in epidermal eicosanoid metabolism contribute to inflammation and impaired late differentiation in FLG-mutated atopic dermatitis. *The Journal of Investigative Dermatology*, 137(3), 706–715. https://doi.org/10.1016/j.jid.2016.09.034.

Boguniewicz, M., & Leung, D. Y. (2011). Atopic dermatitis: A disease of altered skin barrier and immune dysregulation. *Immunological Reviews*, 242(1), 233–246. https://doi.org/10.1111/j.1600-065X.2011.01027.x.

Brandt, E. B., & Sivaprasad, U. (2011). Th2 cytokines and atopic dermatitis. *Journal of Clinical & Cellular Immunology*, 2(3). https://doi.org/10.4172/2155-9899.1000110.

Brauweiler, A. M., Goleva, E., Hall, C. F., & Leung, D. Y. M. (2015). Th2 cytokines suppress lipoteichoic acid-induced matrix metalloproteinase expression and keratinocyte migration in response to wounding. *The Journal of Investigative Dermatology*, 135(10), 2550–2553. https://doi.org/10.1038/jid.2015.181.

Brockow, K., Akin, C., Huber, M., Scott, L. M., Schwartz, L. B., & Metcalfe, D. D. (2002). Levels of mast-cell growth factors in plasma and in suction skin blister fluid in adults with mastocytosis: Correlation with dermal mast-cell numbers and mast-cell tryptase. *The Journal of Allergy and Clinical Immunology*, 109(1), 82–88. https://doi.org/10.1067/mai.2002.120524.

Brunner, P. M., Leung, D. Y. M., & Guttman-Yassky, E. (2018). Immunologic, microbial, and epithelial interactions in atopic dermatitis. *Annals of Allergy, Asthma and Immunology*, 120(1), 34–41. https://doi.org/10.1016/j.anai.2017.09.055.

Bussolino, F., Giraudo, E., & Serini, G. (2014). Class 3 semaphorin in angiogenesis and lymphangiogenesis. *Chemical Immunology and Allergy*, 99, 71–88. https://doi.org/10.1159/000353315.

Calder, P. C., Kremmyda, L. S., Vlachava, M., Noakes, P. S., & Miles, E. A. (2010). Is there a role for fatty acids in early life programming of the immune system?". *The Proceedings of the Nutrition Society*, 69(3), 373–380. https://doi.org/10.1017/S0029665110001552.

Cao, J., Papadopoulou, N., Kempuraj, D., Boucher, W. S., Sugimoto, K., Cetrulo, C. L., & Theoharides, T. C. (2005). Human mast cells express corticotropin-releasing hormone (CRH) receptors and CRH leads to selective secretion of vascular endothelial growth factor. *Journal of Immunology*, 174(12), 7665–7675. https://doi.org/10.4049/jimmunol.174.12.7665.

Chaudhari, S. P., Tam, A. Y., & Barr, J. A. (2015). Curcumin: A contact allergen. *The Journal of Clinical and Aesthetic Dermatology*, 8(11), 43–48.

Chiquet-Ehrismann, R., & Chiquet, M. (2003). Tenascins: Regulation and putative functions during pathological stress. *The Journal of Pathology*, 200(4), 488–499. https://doi.org/10.1002/path.1415.

Christmann, R. B., Mathes, A., Affandi, A. J., Padilla, C., Nazari, B., Bujor, A. M., et al. (2013). Thymic stromal lymphopoietin is up-regulated in the skin of patients with systemic sclerosis and induces profibrotic genes and intracellular signaling that overlap with those induced by interleukin-13 and transforming growth factor beta. *Arthritis and Rheumatism*, 65(5), 1335–1346. https://doi.org/10.1002/art.37859.

Chun, H. J., Zheng, L., Ahmad, M., Wang, J., Speirs, C. K., Siegel, R. M., et al. (2002). Pleiotropic defects in lymphocyte activation caused by caspase-8 mutations lead to human immunodeficiency. *Nature*, 419(6905), 395–399. https://doi.org/10.1038/nature01063.

Clark, R., & Kupper, T. (2005). Old meets new: The interaction between innate and adaptive immunity. *The Journal of Investigative Dermatology*, 125(4), 629–637. https://doi.org/10.1111/j.0022-202X.2005.23856.x.

Costa, E. M., Silva, S., Veiga, M., Tavaria, F. K., & Pintado, M. M. (2018). Chitosan's biological activity upon skin-related microorganisms and its potential textile applications. *World Journal of Microbiology and Biotechnology*, 34(7), 93. https://doi.org/10.1007/s11274-018-2471-2.

Danso, M. O., van Drongelen, V., Mulder, A., van Esch, J., Scott, H., van Smeden, J., et al. (2014). TNF-alpha and Th2 cytokines induce atopic dermatitis-like features on epidermal differentiation proteins and stratum corneum lipids in human skin equivalents. *The Journal of Investigative Dermatology*, 134(7), 1941–1950. https://doi.org/10.1038/jid.2014.83.

Datta, A., Alexander, R., Sulikowski, M. G., Nicholson, A. G., Maher, T. M., Scotton, C. J., & Chambers, R. C. (2013). Evidence for a functional thymic stromal lymphopoietin signaling axis in fibrotic lung disease. *Journal of Immunology*, 191(9), 4867–4879. https://doi.org/10.4049/jimmunol.1300588.

De Angelis, M., Bottacini, F., Fosso, B., Kelleher, P., Calasso, M., Di Cagno, R., et al. (2014). *Lactobacillus rossiae*, a vitamin B12 producer, represents a metabolically versatile species within the Genus *Lactobacillus*. *PLoS One*, 9(9), e107232. https://doi.org/10.1371/journal.pone.0107232.

Degirolamo, C., Rainaldi, S., Bovenga, F., Murzilli, S., & Moschetta, A. (2014). Microbiota modification with probiotics induces hepatic bile acid synthesis via downregulation of the Fxr-Fgf15 axis in mice. *Cell Reports*, 7(1), 12–18. https://doi.org/10.1016/j.celrep.2014.02.032.

Detoraki, A., Granata, F., Staibano, S., Rossi, F. W., Marone, G., & Genovese, A. (2010). Angiogenesis and lymphangiogenesis in bronchial asthma. *Allergy, 65*(8), 946–958. https://doi.org/10.1111/j.1398-9995.2010.02372.x.

Detoraki, A., Staiano, R. I., Granata, F., Giannattasio, G., Prevete, N., de Paulis, A., et al. (2009). Vascular endothelial growth factors synthesized by human lung mast cells exert angiogenic effects. *The Journal of Allergy and Clinical Immunology, 123*(5), 1142–1149. https://doi.org/10.1016/j.jaci.2009.01.044. 1149.e1-5.

Dorschner, R. A., Pestonjamasp, V. K., Tamakuwala, S., Ohtake, T., Rudisill, J., Nizet, V., et al. (2001). Cutaneous injury induces the release of cathelicidin anti-microbial peptides active against group A *Streptococcus*. *The Journal of Investigative Dermatology, 117*(1), 91–97. https://doi.org/10.1046/j.1523-1747.2001.01340.x.

Elias, P. M., Gruber, R., Crumrine, D., Menon, G., Williams, M. L., Wakefield, J. S., et al. (2014). Formation and functions of the corneocyte lipid envelope (CLE). *Biochimica et Biophysica Acta, 1841*(3), 314–318. https://doi.org/10.1016/j.bbalip.2013.09.011.

Eming, S. A., Martin, P., & Tomic-Canic, M. (2014). Wound repair and regeneration: Mechanisms, signaling, and translation. *Science Translational Medicine, 6*(265). https://doi.org/10.1126/scitranslmed.3009337. 265sr6.

Erdman, S. E., & Poutahidis, T. (2014). Probiotic 'glow of health': It's more than skin deep. *Beneficial Microbes, 5*(2), 109–119. https://doi.org/10.3920/BM2013.0042.

Esaki, H., Ewald, D. A., Ungar, B., Rozenblit, M., Zheng, X., Xu, H., et al. (2015). Identification of novel immune and barrier genes in atopic dermatitis by means of laser capture microdissection. *The Journal of Allergy and Clinical Immunology, 135*(1), 153–163. https://doi.org/10.1016/j.jaci.2014.10.037.

Fischer, L. A., & Agner, T. (2004). Curcumin allergy in relation to yellow chlorhexidine solution used for skin disinfection prior to surgery. *Contact Dermatitis, 51*(1), 39–40. https://doi.org/10.1111/j.0105-1873.2004.0378f.x.

Fluhr, J. W., Darlenski, R., & Surber, C. (2008). Glycerol and the skin: Holistic approach to its origin and functions. *The British Journal of Dermatology, 159*(1), 23–34. https://doi.org/10.1111/j.1365-2133.2008.08643.x.

Foolad, N., Brezinski, E. A., Chase, E. P., & Armstrong, A. W. (2013). Effect of nutrient supplementation on atopic dermatitis in children: A systematic review of probiotics, prebiotics, formula, and fatty acids. *JAMA Dermatology, 149*(3), 350–355.

Fukunaga, N., Yuzaki, M., Shomura, Y., Fujiwara, H., Nasu, M., & Okada, Y. (2012). Clinical outcomes of open heart surgery in patients with atopic dermatitis. *Asian cardiovascular & thoracic annals, 20*(2), 137–140. https://doi.org/10.1177/0218492311433311.

Fukuyama, T., Martel, B. C., Linder, K. E., Ehling, S., Ganchingco, J. R., & Baumer, W. (2018). Hypochlorous acid is antipruritic and anti-inflammatory in a mouse model of atopic dermatitis. *Clinical and Experimental Allergy, 48*(1), 78–88. https://doi.org/10.1111/cea.13045.

Galli, E., Rocchi, L., Carello, R., Giampietro, P. G., Panei, P., & Meglio, P. (2015). Serum vitamin D levels and vitamin D supplementation do not correlate with the severity of chronic eczema in children. *European Annals of Allergy and Clinical Immunology, 47*(2), 41–47.

Gaspar, K., Kukova, G., Bunemann, E., Buhren, B. A., Sonkoly, E., Szollosi, A. G., et al. (2013). The chemokine receptor CCR3 participates in tissue remodeling during atopic skin inflammation. *Journal of Dermatological Science, 71*(1), 12–21. https://doi.org/10.1016/j.jdermsci.2013.04.011.

Genovese, A., Detoraki, A., Granata, F., Galdiero, M. R., Spadaro, G., & Marone, G. (2012). Angiogenesis, lymphangiogenesis and atopic dermatitis. *Chemical Immunology and Allergy, 96*, 50–60. https://doi.org/10.1159/000331883.

Ghasemi, H., Saxtrup, K., Al-Khafagi, A. A. M., Thorup, B., & Sommerlund, M. (2018). [Allergic contact dermatitis caused by curcumin-containing chlorhexidine]. *Ugeskrift for Laeger, 180*(42).

Gil, A., & Rueda, R. (2002). Interaction of early diet and the development of the immune system. *Nutrition Research Reviews, 15*(2), 263–292. https://doi.org/10.1079/NRR200248.

Gilliver, S. C., Emmerson, E., Bernhagen, J., & Hardman, M. J. (2011). MIF: A key player in cutaneous biology and wound healing. *Experimental Dermatology, 20*(1), 1–6. https://doi.org/10.1111/j.1600-0625.2010.01194.x.

Gittler, J. K., Shemer, A., Suarez-Farinas, M., Fuentes-Duculan, J., Gulewicz, K. J., Wang, C. Q., et al. (2012). Progressive activation of T(H)2/T(H)22 cytokines and selective epidermal proteins characterizes acute and chronic atopic dermatitis. *The Journal of Allergy and Clinical Immunology, 130*(6), 1344–1354. https://doi.org/10.1016/j.jaci.2012.07.012.

Glatz, M., Buchner, M., von Bartenwerffer, W., Schmid-Grendelmeier, P., Worm, M., Hedderich, J., & Folster-Holst, R. (2015). *Malassezia* spp.-specific immunoglobulin E level is a marker for severity of atopic dermatitis in adults. *Acta Dermato-Venereologica, 95*(2), 191–196. https://doi.org/10.2340/00015555-1864.

Gombert, M., Dieu-Nosjean, M. C., Winterberg, F., Bunemann, E., Kubitza, R. C., Da Cunha, L., et al. (2005). CCL1-CCR8 interactions: An axis mediating the recruitment of T cells and Langerhans-type dendritic cells to sites of atopic skin inflammation. *Journal of Immunology, 174*(8), 5082–5091. https://doi.org/10.4049/jimmunol.174.8.5082.

Gomez, R. S., Diepgen, T. L., Neumann, C., & Sorg, C. (1990). Detection of migration inhibitory factor (MIF) by a monoclonal antibody in the microvasculature of inflamed skin. *Archives of Dermatological Research, 282*(6), 374–378. https://doi.org/10.1007/bf00372087.

Guttman-Yassky, E., Krueger, J. G., & Lebwohl, M. G. (2017). Systemic immune mechanisms in atopic dermatitis and psoriasis with implications for treatment. *Experimental Dermatology* https://doi.org/10.1111/exd.13336.

Hara, M., Ma, T., & Verkman, A. S. (2002). Selectively reduced glycerol in skin of aquaporin-3-deficient mice may account for impaired skin hydration, elasticity, and barrier recovery. *The Journal of Biological Chemistry, 277*(48), 46616–46621. https://doi.org/10.1074/jbc.M209003200.

Hara-Chikuma, M., & Verkman, A. S. (2008). Aquaporin-3 facilitates epidermal cell migration and proliferation during wound healing. *Journal of Molecular Medicine, 86*(2), 221–231. https://doi.org/10.1007/s00109-007-0272-4.

Harbige, L. S. (2003). Fatty acids, the immune response, and autoimmunity: A question of n-6 essentiality and the balance between n-6 and n-3. *Lipids, 38*(4), 323–341.

Harrison, I. P., & Spada, F. (2018). Hydrogels for atopic dermatitis and wound management: A superior drug delivery vehicle. *Pharmaceutics, 10*(2). https://doi.org/10.3390/pharmaceutics10020071.

Hata, M., Sasaki, E., Ota, M., Fujimoto, K., Yajima, J., Shichida, T., & Honda, M. (1997). Allergic contact dermatitis from curcumin (turmeric). *Contact Dermatitis, 36*(2), 107–108. https://doi.org/10.1111/j.1600-0536.1997.tb00426.x.

Haug, S., Roll, A., Schmid-Grendelmeier, P., Johansen, P., Wuthrich, B., Kundig, T. M., & Senti, G. (2006). Coated textiles in the treatment of atopic dermatitis. *Current Problems in Dermatology, 33*, 144–151. https://doi.org/10.1159/000093941.

Hawkins, R. A., Claman, H. N., Clark, R. A., & Steigerwald, J. C. (1985). Increased dermal mast cell populations in progressive systemic sclerosis: a link in chronic fibrosis? *Annals of Internal Medicine, 102*(2), 182–186. https://doi.org/10.7326/0003-4819-102-2-182.

He, Y., Yue, Y., Zheng, X., Zhang, K., Chen, S., & Du, Z. (2015). Curcumin, inflammation, and chronic diseases: How are they linked? *Molecules, 20*(5), 9183–9213. https://doi.org/10.3390/molecules20059183.

Hebda, P. A., Collins, M. A., & Tharp, M. D. (1993). Mast cell and myofibroblast in wound healing. *Dermatologic Clinics, 11*(4), 685–696.

Heng, M. C., Song, M. K., Harker, J., & Heng, M. K. (2000). Drug-induced suppression of phosphorylase kinase activity correlates with resolution of psoriasis as assessed by clinical, histological and immunohistochemical parameters. *The British Journal of Dermatology, 143*(5), 937–949. https://doi.org/10.1046/j.1365-2133.2000.03767.x.

Hizawa, N., Yamaguchi, E., Takahashi, D., Nishihira, J., & Nishimura, M. (2004). Functional polymorphisms in the promoter region of macrophage migration inhibitory factor and atopy. *American Journal of Respiratory and Critical Care Medicine, 169*(9), 1014–1018. https://doi.org/10.1164/rccm.200307-933OC.

Homey, B., Alenius, H., Muller, A., Soto, H., Bowman, E. P., Yuan, W., et al. (2002). CCL27-CCR10 interactions regulate T cell-mediated skin inflammation. *Nature Medicine, 8*(2), 157–165. https://doi.org/10.1038/nm0202-157.

Homey, B., Meller, S., Savinko, T., Alenius, H., & Lauerma, A. (2007). Modulation of chemokines by staphylococcal superantigen in atopic dermatitis. *Chemical Immunology and Allergy, 93,* 181–194. https://doi.org/10.1159/000100895.

Hon, K. L., Tsang, Y. C., Pong, N. H., Ng, C., Ip, M., & Leung, T. F. (2016). Clinical features and *Staphylococcus aureus* colonization/infection in childhood atopic dermatitis. *The Journal of Dermatological Treatment, 27*(3), 235–240. https://doi.org/10.3109/09546634.2015.1093586.

Howell, M. D., Gallo, R. L., Boguniewicz, M., Jones, J. F., Wong, C., Streib, J. E., & Leung, D. Y. (2006). Cytokine milieu of atopic dermatitis skin subverts the innate immune response to vaccinia virus. *Immunity, 24*(3), 341–348. https://doi.org/10.1016/j.immuni.2006.02.006.

Howell, M. D., Kim, B. E., Gao, P., Grant, A. V., Boguniewicz, M., DeBenedetto, A., et al. (2009). Cytokine modulation of atopic dermatitis filaggrin skin expression. *The Journal of Allergy and Clinical Immunology, 124*(3 Suppl 2), R7–R12. https://doi.org/10.1016/j.jaci.2009.07.012.

Inoue, M., Kratz, G., Haegerstrand, A., & Stahle-Backdahl, M. (1995). Collagenase expression is rapidly induced in wound-edge keratinocytes after acute injury in human skin, persists during healing, and stops at re-epithelialization. *The Journal of Investigative Dermatology, 104*(4), 479–483. https://doi.org/10.1111/1523-1747.ep12605917.

Jessup, H. K., Brewer, A. W., Omori, M., Rickel, E. A., Budelsky, A. L., Yoon, B. R., et al. (2008). Intradermal administration of thymic stromal lymphopoietin induces a T cell- and eosinophil-dependent systemic Th2 inflammatory response. *Journal of Immunology, 181*(6), 4311–4319. https://doi.org/10.4049/jimmunol.181.6.4311.

Jones, M. L., Martoni, C. J., & Prakash, S. (2013). Oral supplementation with probiotic *L. reuteri* NCIMB 30242 increases mean circulating 25-hydroxyvitamin D: A post hoc analysis of a randomized controlled trial. *The Journal of Clinical Endocrinology and Metabolism, 98*(7), 2944–2951. https://doi.org/10.1210/jc.2012-4262.

Jung, M. K., Hur, D. Y., Song, S. B., Park, Y., Kim, T. S., Bang, S. I., et al. (2010). Tannic acid and quercetin display a therapeutic effect in atopic dermatitis via suppression of angiogenesis and TARC expression in Nc/Nga mice. *The Journal of Investigative Dermatology, 130*(5), 1459–1463. https://doi.org/10.1038/jid.2009.401.

Kagami, S., Saeki, H., Komine, M., Kakinuma, T., Tsunemi, Y., Nakamura, K., et al. (2005). Interleukin-4 and interleukin-13 enhance CCL26 production in a human keratinocyte cell line, HaCaT cells. *Clinical and Experimental Immunology, 141*(3), 459–466. https://doi.org/10.1111/j.1365-2249.2005.02875.x.

Kaplan, B., Gonul, B., Dincer, S., Dincer Kaya, F. N., & Babul, A. (2004). Relationships between tensile strength, ascorbic acid, hydroxyproline, and zinc levels of rabbit full-thickness incision wound healing. *Surgery Today, 34*(9), 747–751. https://doi.org/10.1007/s00595-004-2827-0.

Kawakami, T., Ando, T., Kimura, M., Wilson, B. S., & Kawakami, Y. (2009). Mast cells in atopic dermatitis. *Current Opinion in Immunology, 21*(6), 666–678. https://doi.org/10.1016/j.coi.2009.09.006.

Kawata, M., Sasabuchi, Y., Taketomi, S., Inui, H., Matsui, H., Fushimi, K., et al. (2018). Atopic dermatitis is a novel demographic risk factor for surgical site infection after anterior cruciate ligament reconstruction. *Knee Surgery, Sports Traumatology, Arthroscopy, 26*(12), 3699–3705. https://doi.org/10.1007/s00167-018-4958-7.

Kelleher, M., Dunn-Galvin, A., Hourihane, J. O., Murray, D., Campbell, L. E., McLean, W. H., & Irvine, A. D. (2015). Skin barrier dysfunction measured by transepidermal water loss at 2 days and 2 months predates and predicts atopic dermatitis at 1 year. *The Journal of Allergy and Clinical Immunology, 135*(4), 930–935. https://doi.org/10.1016/j.jaci.2014.12.013. e1.

Kiecolt-Glaser, J. K., Glaser, R., & Christian, L. M. (2014). Omega-3 fatty acids and stress-induced immune dysregulation: Implications for wound healing. *Military Medicine, 179*(11 Suppl), 129–133. https://doi.org/10.7205/MILMED-D-14-00167.

Kiec-Swierczynska, M., & Krecisz, B. (1998). Occupational allergic contact dermatitis due to curcumin food colour in a pasta factory worker. *Contact Dermatitis, 39*(1), 30–31. https://doi.org/10.1111/j.1600-0536.1998.tb05809.x.

Kim, B. E., & Leung, D. Y. M. (2018). Significance of skin barrier dysfunction in atopic dermatitis. *Allergy, Asthma & Immunology Research, 10*(3), 207–215. https://doi.org/10.4168/aair.2018.10.3.207.

Kim, M. J., Kim, S. N., Lee, Y. W., Choe, Y. B., & Ahn, K. J. (2016). Vitamin D status and efficacy of vitamin D supplementation in atopic dermatitis: A systematic review and meta-analysis. *Nutrients, 8*(12). https://doi.org/10.3390/nu8120789.

Kirjavainen, P. V., Arvola, T., Salminen, S. J., & Isolauri, E. (2002). Aberrant composition of gut microbiota of allergic infants: A target of bifidobacterial therapy at weaning? *Gut, 51*(1), 51–55.

Kobayashi, T., Glatz, M., Horiuchi, K., Kawasaki, H., Akiyama, H., Kaplan, D. H., et al. (2015). Dysbiosis and *Staphylococcus aureus* colonization drives inflammation in atopic dermatitis. *Immunity, 42*(4), 756–766. https://doi.org/10.1016/j.immuni.2015.03.014.

Kocaadam, B., & Sanlier, N. (2017). Curcumin, an active component of turmeric (*Curcuma longa*), and its effects on health. *Critical Reviews in Food Science and Nutrition, 57*(13), 2889–2895. https://doi.org/10.1080/10408398.2015.1077195.

Konya, V., & Mjosberg, J. (2016). Lipid mediators as regulators of human ILC2 function in allergic diseases. *Immunology Letters*, *179*, 36–42. https://doi.org/10.1016/j.imlet.2016.07.006.

Kuo, I. H., Yoshida, T., De Benedetto, A., & Beck, L. A. (2013). The cutaneous innate immune response in patients with atopic dermatitis. *The Journal of Allergy and Clinical Immunology*, *131*(2), 266–278. https://doi.org/10.1016/j.jaci.2012.12.1563.

Kupper, T. S., & Fuhlbrigge, R. C. (2004). Immune surveillance in the skin: Mechanisms and clinical consequences. *Nature Reviews Immunology*, *4*(3), 211–222. https://doi.org/10.1038/nri1310.

Latijnhouwers, M., Bergers, M., Ponec, M., Dijkman, H., Andriessen, M., & Schalkwijk, J. (1997). Human epidermal keratinocytes are a source of tenascin-C during wound healing. *The Journal of Investigative Dermatology*, *108*(5), 776–783. https://doi.org/10.1111/1523-1747.ep12292170.

Lee, E., Lee, S. Y., Kang, M. J., Kim, K., Won, S., Kim, B. J., et al. (2016). Clostridia in the gut and onset of atopic dermatitis via eosinophilic inflammation. *Annals of Allergy, Asthma and Immunology*, *117*(1), 91–92. https://doi.org/10.1016/j.anai.2016.04.019. e1.

Lee, H. S., Kim, Y. D., Na, B. R., Kim, H. R., Choi, E. J., Han, W. C., et al. (2012). Phytocomponent p-Hydroxycinnamic acid inhibits T-cell activation by modulation of protein kinase C-theta-dependent pathway. *International Immunopharmacology*, *12*(1), 131–138. https://doi.org/10.1016/j.intimp.2011.11.001.

Lee, P., Lee, D. J., Chan, C., Chen, S. W., Ch'en, I., & Jamora, C. (2009). Dynamic expression of epidermal caspase 8 simulates a wound healing response. *Nature*, *458*(7237), 519–523. https://doi.org/10.1038/nature07687.

Lefebvre, P., Chinetti, G., Fruchart, J. C., & Staels, B. (2006). Sorting out the roles of PPAR alpha in energy metabolism and vascular homeostasis. *The Journal of Clinical Investigation*, *116*(3), 571–580. https://doi.org/10.1172/jci27989.

Leung, T. H., Zhang, L. F., Wang, J., Ning, S., Knox, S. J., & Kim, S. K. (2013). Topical hypochlorite ameliorates NF-kappaB-mediated skin diseases in mice. *The Journal of Clinical Investigation*, *123*(12), 5361–5370. https://doi.org/10.1172/jci70895.

Levin, J., Friedlander, S. F., & Del Rosso, J. Q. (2013). Atopic dermatitis and the stratum corneum: Part 3: The immune system in atopic dermatitis. *The Journal of Clinical and Aesthetic Dermatology*, *6*(12), 37–44.

Lewkowich, I. P., Lajoie, S., Clark, J. R., Herman, N. S., Sproles, A. A., & Wills-Karp, M. (2008). Allergen uptake, activation, and IL-23 production by pulmonary myeloid DCs drives airway hyperresponsiveness in asthma-susceptible mice. *PLoS One*, *3*(12), e3879. https://doi.org/10.1371/journal.pone.0003879.

Li, C., Lasse, S., Lee, P., Nakasaki, M., Chen, S. W., Yamasaki, K., et al. (2010). Development of atopic dermatitis-like skin disease from the chronic loss of epidermal caspase-8. *Proceedings of the National Academy of Sciences of the United States of America*, *107*(51), 22249–22254. https://doi.org/10.1073/pnas.1009751108.

Liddle, M., Hull, C., Liu, C., & Powell, D. (2006). Contact urticaria from curcumin. *Dermatitis: Contact, Atopic, Occupational, Drug*, *17*(4), 196–197. https://doi.org/10.2310/6620.2006.06004.

Lindley, L. E., Stojadinovic, O., Pastar, I., & Tomic-Canic, M. (2016). Biology and biomarkers for wound healing. *Plastic and Reconstructive Surgery*, *138*(3 Suppl), 18s–28s. https://doi.org/10.1097/prs.0000000000002682.

Liu, T., Howard, R. M., Mancini, A. J., Weston, W. L., Paller, A. S., Drolet, B. A., et al. (2001). Kwashiorkor in the United States: Fad diets, perceived and true milk allergy, and nutritional ignorance. *Archives of Dermatology*, *137*(5), 630–636.

Lopez-Villafuerte, L., & Clores, K. H. (2016). Contact dermatitis caused by turmeric in a massage oil. *Contact Dermatitis*, *75*(1), 52–53. https://doi.org/10.1111/cod.12549.

Lou, H., Lu, J., Choi, E. B., Oh, M. H., Jeong, M., Barmettler, S., et al. (2017). Expression of IL-22 in the skin causes Th2-biased immunity, epidermal barrier dysfunction, and pruritus via stimulating epithelial Th2 cytokines and the GRP pathway. *Journal of Immunology*, *198*(7), 2543–2555. https://doi.org/10.4049/jimmunol.1600126.

Lu, C. L., Liu, X. H., Stub, T., Kristoffersen, A. E., Liang, S. B., Wang, X., et al. (2018). Complementary and alternative medicine for treatment of atopic eczema in children under 14 years old: A systematic review and meta-analysis of randomized controlled trials. *BMC Complementary and Alternative Medicine*, *18*(1), 260. https://doi.org/10.1186/s12906-018-2306-6.

Lugovic, L., & Lipozencic, J. (1997). Contact hypersensitivity in atopic dermatitis. *Arhiv za Higijenu Rada i Toksikologiju*, *48*(3), 287–296.

Mallbris, L., Carlen, L., Wei, T., Heilborn, J., Nilsson, M. F., Granath, F., & Stahle, M. (2010). Injury downregulates the expression of the human cathelicidin protein hCAP18/LL-37 in atopic dermatitis. *Experimental Dermatology*, *19*(5), 442–449. https://doi.org/10.1111/j.1600-0625.2009.00918.x.

Mancl, K. A., Kirsner, R. S., & Ajdic, D. (2013). Wound biofilms: Lessons learned from oral biofilms. *Wound Repair and Regeneration*, *21*(3), 352–362. https://doi.org/10.1111/wrr.12034.

Michalik, L., Desvergne, B., Tan, N. S., Basu-Modak, S., Escher, P., Rieusset, J., et al. (2001). Impaired skin wound healing in peroxisome proliferator-activated receptor (PPAR)alpha and PPARbeta mutant mice. *The Journal of Cell Biology*, *154*(4), 799–814. https://doi.org/10.1083/jcb.200011148.

Miller, K. G., Tran, P. L., Haley, C. L., Kruzek, C., Colmer-Hamood, J. A., Myntti, M., & Hamood, A. N. (2014). Next science wound gel technology, a novel agent that inhibits biofilm development by gram-positive and gram-negative wound pathogens. *Antimicrobial Agents and Chemotherapy*, *58*(6), 3060–3072. https://doi.org/10.1128/AAC.00108-14.

Mjosberg, J., & Eidsmo, L. (2014). Update on innate lymphoid cells in atopic and non-atopic inflammation in the airways and skin. *Clinical and Experimental Allergy*, *44*(8), 1033–1043. https://doi.org/10.1111/cea.12353.

Murota, H., Bae, S., Hamasaki, Y., Maruyama, R., & Katayama, I. (2008). Emedastine difumarate inhibits histamine-induced collagen synthesis in dermal fibroblasts. *Journal of Investigational Allergology & Clinical Immunology*, *18*(4), 245–252.

Namkung, J. H., Lee, J. E., Kim, E., Huh, I. S., Park, T., Shin, E. S., et al. (2013). Single nucleotide polymorphism in the FLT4 gene is associated with atopic dermatitis in Koreans. *Cytokine*, *62*(1), 110–114. https://doi.org/10.1016/j.cyto.2013.02.006.

Nicol, N. H., Boguniewicz, M., Strand, M., & Klinnert, M. D. (2014). Wet wrap therapy in children with moderate to severe atopic dermatitis in a multidisciplinary treatment program. *The Journal of Allergy and Clinical Immunology: In Practice*, *2*(4), 400–406. https://doi.org/10.1016/j.jaip.2014.04.009.

Noli, C., & Miolo, A. (2001). The mast cell in wound healing. *Veterinary Dermatology*, *12*(6), 303–313. https://doi.org/10.1046/j.0959-4493.2001.00272.x.

Norizoe, C., Akiyama, N., Segawa, T., Tachimoto, H., Mezawa, H., Ida, H., & Urashima, M. (2014). Increased food allergy and vitamin D: Randomized, double-blind, placebo-controlled trial. *Pediatrics International*, *56*(1), 6–12. https://doi.org/10.1111/ped.12207.

Numata, Y., Terui, T., Okuyama, R., Hirasawa, N., Sugiura, Y., Miyoshi, I., et al. (2006). The accelerating effect of histamine on the cutaneous wound-healing process through the action of basic fibroblast growth factor. *The Journal of Investigative Dermatology, 126*(6), 1403–1409. https://doi.org/10.1038/sj.jid.5700253.

Nygaard, U., van den Bogaard, E. H., Niehues, H., Hvid, M., Deleuran, M., Johansen, C., & Vestergaard, C. (2017). The "alarmins" HMBG1 and IL-33 downregulate structural skin barrier proteins and impair epidermal growth. *Acta Dermato-Venereologica, 97*(3), 305–312. https://doi.org/10.2340/00015555-2552.

Nylund, L., Nermes, M., Isolauri, E., Salminen, S., de Vos, W. M., & Satokari, R. (2015). Severity of atopic disease inversely correlates with intestinal microbiota diversity and butyrate-producing bacteria. *Allergy, 70*(2), 241–244. https://doi.org/10.1111/all.12549.

Oda, Y., Tu, C. L., Menendez, A., Nguyen, T., & Bikle, D. D. (2016). Vitamin D and calcium regulation of epidermal wound healing. *The Journal of Steroid Biochemistry and Molecular Biology, 164*, 379–385. https://doi.org/10.1016/j.jsbmb.2015.08.011.

Ogawa, K., Ito, M., Takeuchi, K., Nakada, A., Heishi, M., Suto, H., et al. (2005). Tenascin-C is upregulated in the skin lesions of patients with atopic dermatitis. *Journal of Dermatological Science, 40*(1), 35–41. https://doi.org/10.1016/j.jdermsci.2005.06.001.

Oh, M. H., Oh, S. Y., Yu, J., Myers, A. C., Leonard, W. J., Liu, Y. J., et al. (2011). IL-13 induces skin fibrosis in atopic dermatitis by thymic stromal lymphopoietin. *Journal of Immunology, 186*(12), 7232–7242. https://doi.org/10.4049/jimmunol.1100504.

Omori-Miyake, M., Yamashita, M., Tsunemi, Y., Kawashima, M., & Yagi, J. (2014). In vitro assessment of IL-4- or IL-13-mediated changes in the structural components of keratinocytes in mice and humans. *The Journal of Investigative Dermatology, 134*(5), 1342–1350. https://doi.org/10.1038/jid.2013.503.

Owczarek, W., Paplinska, M., Targowski, T., Jahnz-Rozyk, K., Paluchowska, E., Kucharczyk, A., & Kasztalewicz, B. (2010). Analysis of eotaxin 1/CCL11, eotaxin 2/CCL24 and eotaxin 3/CCL26 expression in lesional and non-lesional skin of patients with atopic dermatitis. *Cytokine, 50*(2), 181–185. https://doi.org/10.1016/j.cyto.2010.02.016.

Palmer, C. N., Irvine, A. D., Terron-Kwiatkowski, A., Zhao, Y., Liao, H., Lee, S. P., et al. (2006). Common loss-of-function variants of the epidermal barrier protein filaggrin are a major predisposing factor for atopic dermatitis. *Nature Genetics, 38*(4), 441–446. https://doi.org/10.1038/ng1767.

Pastore, S., Mascia, F., Mariani, V., & Girolomoni, G. (2008). The epidermal growth factor receptor system in skin repair and inflammation. *The Journal of Investigative Dermatology, 128*(6), 1365–1374. https://doi.org/10.1038/sj.jid.5701184.

Penders, J., Stobberingh, E. E., Thijs, C., Adams, H., Vink, C., van Ree, R., & van den Brandt, P. A. (2006). Molecular fingerprinting of the intestinal microbiota of infants in whom atopic eczema was or was not developing. *Clinical and Experimental Allergy, 36*(12), 1602–1608. https://doi.org/10.1111/j.1365-2222.2006.02599.x.

Pivarcsi, A., Gombert, M., Dieu-Nosjean, M. C., Lauerma, A., Kubitza, R., Meller, S., et al. (2004). CC chemokine ligand 18, an atopic dermatitis-associated and dendritic cell-derived chemokine, is regulated by staphylococcal products and allergen exposure. *Journal of Immunology, 173*(9), 5810–5817. https://doi.org/10.4049/jimmunol.173.9.5810.

Rawal, R. C., Shah, B. J., Jayaraaman, A. M., & Jaiswal, V. (2009). Clinical evaluation of an Indian polyherbal topical formulation in the management of eczema. *Journal of Alternative and Complementary Medicine, 15*(6), 669–672. https://doi.org/10.1089/acm.2008.0508.

Rechardt, O., Elomaa, O., Vaalamo, M., Paakkonen, K., Jahkola, T., Hook-Nikanne, J., et al. (2000). Stromelysin-2 is upregulated during normal wound repair and is induced by cytokines. *The Journal of Investigative Dermatology, 115*(5), 778–787. https://doi.org/10.1046/j.1523-1747.2000.00135.x.

Reed, R. B., Zaikova, T., Barber, A., Simonich, M., Lankone, R., Marco, M., et al. (2016). Potential environmental impacts and antimicrobial efficacy of silver- and nanosilver-containing textiles. *Environmental Science & Technology, 50*(7), 4018–4026. https://doi.org/10.1021/acs.est.5b06043.

Repertinger, S. K., Campagnaro, E., Fuhrman, J., El-Abaseri, T., Yuspa, S. H., & Hansen, L. A. (2004). EGFR enhances early healing after cutaneous incisional wounding. *The Journal of Investigative Dermatology, 123*(5), 982–989. https://doi.org/10.1111/j.0022-202X.2004.23478.x.

Ricote, M., & Glass, C. K. (2007). PPARs and molecular mechanisms of transrepression. *Biochimica et Biophysica Acta, 1771*(8), 926–935. https://doi.org/10.1016/j.bbalip.2007.02.013.

Roager, H. M., Sulek, K., Skov, K., Frandsen, H. L., Smedsgaard, J., Wilcks, A., et al. (2014). *Lactobacillus acidophilus* NCFM affects vitamin E acetate metabolism and intestinal bile acid signature in monocolonized mice. *Gut Microbes, 5*(3), 296–303. https://doi.org/10.4161/gmic.28806.

Roediger, B., Kyle, R., Le Gros, G., & Weninger, W. (2014). Dermal group 2 innate lymphoid cells in atopic dermatitis and allergy. *Current Opinion in Immunology, 31*, 108–114. https://doi.org/10.1016/j.coi.2014.10.008.

Rutherfurd, S. M., Chung, T. K., Thomas, D. V., Zou, M. L., & Moughan, P. J. (2012). Effect of a novel phytase on growth performance, apparent metabolizable energy, and the availability of minerals and amino acids in a low-phosphorus corn-soybean meal diet for broilers. *Poultry Science, 91*(5), 1118–1127. https://doi.org/10.3382/ps.2011-01702.

Sakarya, S., Gunay, N., Karakulak, M., Ozturk, B., & Ertugrul, B. (2014). Hypochlorous Acid: An ideal wound care agent with powerful microbicidal, antibiofilm, and wound healing potency. *Wounds, 26*(12), 342–350.

Samadi, S., Khadivzadeh, T., Emami, A., Moosavi, N. S., Tafaghodi, M., & Behnam, H. R. (2010). The effect of *Hypericum perforatum* on the wound healing and scar of cesarean. *Journal of Alternative and Complementary Medicine, 16*(1), 113–117. https://doi.org/10.1089/acm.2009.0317.

Scharschmidt, T. C., & Segre, J. A. (2008). Modeling atopic dermatitis with increasingly complex mouse models. *The Journal of Investigative Dermatology, 128*(5), 1061–1064. https://doi.org/10.1038/sj.jid.5701201.

Schempp, C. M., Windeck, T., Hezel, S., & Simon, J. C. (2003). Topical treatment of atopic dermatitis with St. John's wort cream—A randomized, placebo controlled, double blind half-side comparison. *Phytomedicine, 10*(Suppl 4), 31–37. https://doi.org/10.1078/1433-187x-00306.

Schmidt-Weber, C. B., Akdis, M., & Akdis, C. A. (2007). TH17 cells in the big picture of immunology. *The Journal of Allergy and Clinical Immunology, 120*(2), 247–254. https://doi.org/10.1016/j.jaci.2007.06.039.

Serezani, A. P. M., Bozdogan, G., Sehra, S., Walsh, D., Krishnamurthy, P., Sierra Potchanant, E. A., et al. (2017). IL-4 impairs wound healing potential in the skin by repressing fibronectin expression. *The Journal of Allergy and Clinical Immunology, 139*(1), 142–151.e5 https://doi.org/10.1016/j.jaci.2016.07.012. e5.

Sharma, S., Sethi, G. S., & Naura, A. S. (2019). Curcumin ameliorates ovalbumin-induced atopic dermatitis and blocks the progression of atopic march in mice. *Inflammation, 43,* 358–369. https://doi.org/10.1007/s10753-019-01126-7.

Shin, J. U., Kim, S. H., Kim, H., Noh, J. Y., Jin, S., Park, C. O., et al. (2016). TSLP is a potential initiator of collagen synthesis and an activator of CXCR4/SDF-1 axis in keloid pathogenesis. *The Journal of Investigative Dermatology, 136*(2), 507–515. https://doi.org/10.1016/j.jid.2015.11.008.

Simonsen, A. B., Johansen, J. D., Deleuran, M., Mortz, C. G., & Sommerlund, M. (2017). Contact allergy in children with atopic dermatitis: A systematic review. *The British Journal of Dermatology, 177*(2), 395–405. https://doi.org/10.1111/bjd.15628.

Simpson, E. L., Chalmers, J. R., Hanifin, J. M., Thomas, K. S., Cork, M. J., McLean, W. H., et al. (2014). Emollient enhancement of the skin barrier from birth offers effective atopic dermatitis prevention. *The Journal of Allergy and Clinical Immunology, 134*(4), 818–823. https://doi.org/10.1016/j.jaci.2014.08.005.

Singer, A. J., & Clark, R. A. (1999). Cutaneous wound healing. *The New England Journal of Medicine, 341*(10), 738–746. https://doi.org/10.1056/nejm199909023411006.

Sismanopoulos, N., Delivanis, D. A., Alysandratos, K. D., Angelidou, A., Vasiadi, M., Therianou, A., & Theoharides, T. C. (2012). IL-9 induces VEGF secretion from human mast cells and IL-9/IL-9 receptor genes are overexpressed in atopic dermatitis. *PLoS One, 7*(3), e33271. https://doi.org/10.1371/journal.pone.0033271.

Smith, M. K., Nicholson, C. L., Parks-Miller, A., & Hamzavi, I. H. (2017). Hidradenitis suppurativa: An update on connecting the tracts. *F1000Research, 6,* 1272. https://doi.org/10.12688/f1000research.11337.1.

Soumelis, V. (2017). Molecular and cellular discoveries in inflammatory dermatoses. *Journal of the European Academy of Dermatology and Venereology, 31*(Suppl 5), 3–7. https://doi.org/10.1111/jdv.14373.

Souwer, Y., Szegedi, K., Kapsenberg, M. L., & de Jong, E. C. (2010). IL-17 and IL-22 in atopic allergic disease. *Current Opinion in Immunology, 22*(6), 821–826. https://doi.org/10.1016/j.coi.2010.10.013.

Staumont-Salle, D., Abboud, G., Brenuchon, C., Kanda, A., Roumier, T., Lavogiez, C., et al. (2008). Peroxisome proliferator-activated receptor alpha regulates skin inflammation and humoral response in atopic dermatitis. *The Journal of Allergy and Clinical Immunology, 121*(4), 962–968.e6 https://doi.org/10.1016/j.jaci.2007.12.1165. e6.

Stechmiller, J. K. (2010). Understanding the role of nutrition and wound healing. *Nutrition in Clinical Practice, 25*(1), 61–68. https://doi.org/10.1177/0884533609358997.

Suntar, I., Akkol, E. K., Keles, H., Oktem, A., Baser, K. H., & Yesilada, E. (2011). A novel wound healing ointment: A formulation of *Hypericum perforatum* oil and sage and oregano essential oils based on traditional Turkish knowledge. *Journal of Ethnopharmacology, 134*(1), 89–96. https://doi.org/10.1016/j.jep.2010.11.061.

Takada, H., Yonekawa, J., Matsumoto, M., Furuya, K., & Sokabe, M. (2017). Hyperforin/HP-beta-cyclodextrin enhances mechanosensitive Ca(2+) signaling in HaCaT keratinocytes and in atopic skin ex vivo which accelerates wound healing. *BioMed Research International, 2017,* 8701801. https://doi.org/10.1155/2017/8701801.

Tan, N. S., Michalik, L., Noy, N., Yasmin, R., Pacot, C., Heim, M., et al. (2001). Critical roles of PPAR beta/delta in keratinocyte response to inflammation. *Genes & Development, 15*(24), 3263–3277. https://doi.org/10.1101/gad.207501.

Taniguchi, K., Arima, K., Masuoka, M., Ohta, S., Shiraishi, H., Ontsuka, K., et al. (2014). Periostin controls keratinocyte proliferation and differentiation by interacting with the paracrine IL-1alpha/IL-6 loop. *The Journal of Investigative Dermatology, 134*(5), 1295–1304. https://doi.org/10.1038/jid.2013.500.

Thompson, D. A., & Tan, B. B. (2006). Tetrahydracurcumin-related allergic contact dermatitis. *Contact Dermatitis, 55*(4), 254–255. https://doi.org/10.1111/j.1600-0536.2006.00857.x.

Totte, J. E., van der Feltz, W. T., Hennekam, M., van Belkum, A., van Zuuren, E. J., & Pasmans, S. G. (2016). Prevalence and odds of *Staphylococcus aureus* carriage in atopic dermatitis: A systematic review and meta-analysis. *The British Journal of Dermatology, 175*(4), 687–695. https://doi.org/10.1111/bjd.14566.

Trautmann, A., Toksoy, A., Engelhardt, E., Brocker, E. B., & Gillitzer, R. (2000). Mast cell involvement in normal human skin wound healing: Expression of monocyte chemoattractant protein-1 is correlated with recruitment of mast cells which synthesize interleukin-4 in vivo. *The Journal of Pathology, 190*(1), 100–106. https://europepmc.org/article/MED/10640999. https://pubmed.ncbi.nlm.nih.gov/10640999/.

Travers, J. B. (2014). Toxic interaction between Th2 cytokines and *Staphylococcus aureus* in atopic dermatitis. *The Journal of Investigative Dermatology, 134*(8), 2069–2071. https://doi.org/10.1038/jid.2014.122.

Travers, J. B., Kozman, A., Mousdicas, N., Saha, C., Landis, M., Al-Hassani, M., et al. (2010). Infected atopic dermatitis lesions contain pharmacologic amounts of lipoteichoic acid. *The Journal of Allergy and Clinical Immunology, 125*(1), 146–152. https://doi.org/10.1016/j.jaci.2009.09.052. e1-2.

Tsuchiya, S., Ichioka, S., Sekiya, N., Tajima, S., Iwasaki, T., & Numata, S. (2013). The effect of a hydrocolloid dressing containing ceramide-2 on split-thickness wounds in a laser-induced erosion model. *Advances in Skin & Wound Care, 26*(5), 224–229. https://doi.org/10.1097/01.asw.0000428952.00149.77.

Usategui, A., Criado, G., Izquierdo, E., Del Rey, M. J., Carreira, P. E., Ortiz, P., et al. (2013). A profibrotic role for thymic stromal lymphopoietin in systemic sclerosis. *Annals of the Rheumatic Diseases, 72*(12), 2018–2023. https://doi.org/10.1136/annrheumdis-2012-202279.

Varricchi, G., Granata, F., Loffredo, S., Genovese, A., & Marone, G. (2015). Angiogenesis and lymphangiogenesis in inflammatory skin disorders. *Journal of the American Academy of Dermatology, 73*(1), 144–153. https://doi.org/10.1016/j.jaad.2015.03.041.

Vollono, L., Falconi, M., Gaziano, R., Iacovelli, F., Dika, E., Terracciano, C., et al. (2019). Potential of curcumin in skin disorders. *Nutrients, 11*(9). https://doi.org/10.3390/nu11092169.

Wang, Y. H., & Liu, Y. J. (2009). Thymic stromal lymphopoietin, OX40-ligand, and interleukin-25 in allergic responses. *Clinical and Experimental Allergy, 39*(6), 798–806. https://doi.org/10.1111/j.1365-2222.2009.03241.x.

Weller, K., Foitzik, K., Paus, R., Syska, W., & Maurer, M. (2006). Mast cells are required for normal healing of skin wounds in mice. *The FASEB Journal, 20*(13), 2366–2368. https://doi.org/10.1096/fj.06-5837fje.

WHO. (2002). *Traditional medicine strategy 2002–2005.* World Health Organization.

Yamaguchi, J., Nakamura, F., Aihara, M., Yamashita, N., Usui, H., Hida, T., et al. (2008). Semaphorin3A alleviates skin lesions and scratching behavior in NC/Nga mice, an atopic dermatitis model. *The Journal of Investigative Dermatology, 128*(12), 2842–2849. https://doi.org/10.1038/jid.2008.150.

Yamanaka, K., Tanaka, M., Tsutsui, H., Kupper, T. S., Asahi, K., Okamura, H., et al. (2000). Skin-specific caspase-1-transgenic mice show cutaneous apoptosis and pre-endotoxin shock condition with a high serum level of IL-18. *Journal of Immunology, 165*(2), 997–1003. https://doi.org/10.4049/jimmunol.165.2.997.

Yang, L., Murota, H., Serada, S., Fujimoto, M., Kudo, A., Naka, T., & Katayama, I. (2014). Histamine contributes to tissue remodeling via periostin expression. *The Journal of Investigative Dermatology*, *134*(8), 2105–2113. https://doi.org/10.1038/jid.2014.120.

Yun, Y. H., Lee, B. K., & Park, K. (2015). Controlled drug delivery: Historical perspective for the next generation. *Journal of Controlled Release*, *219*, 2–7. https://doi.org/10.1016/j.jconrel.2015.10.005.

Zabielinski, M., McLeod, M. P., Aber, C., Izakovic, J., & Schachner, L. A. (2013). Trends and antibiotic susceptibility patterns of methicillin-resistant and methicillin-sensitive *Staphylococcus aureus* in an outpatient dermatology facility. *JAMA Dermatology*, *149*(4), 427–432. https://doi.org/10.1001/jamadermatol.2013.2424.

Zablotna, M., Sobjanek, M., Glen, J., Niedoszytko, M., Wilkowska, A., Roszkiewicz, J., & Nedoszytko, B. (2010). Association between the -1154 G/A promoter polymorphism of the vascular endothelial growth factor gene and atopic dermatitis. *Journal of the European Academy of Dermatology and Venereology*, *24*(1), 91–92. https://doi.org/10.1111/j.1468-3083.2009.03307.x.

Zhang, Y., Matsuo, H., & Morita, E. (2006). Increased production of vascular endothelial growth factor in the lesions of atopic dermatitis. *Archives of Dermatological Research*, *297*(9), 425–429. https://doi.org/10.1007/s00403-006-0641-9.

Zhang, Y. G., Wu, S., & Sun, J. (2013). Vitamin D, vitamin D receptor, and tissue barriers. *Tissue Barriers*, *1*(1). https://doi.org/10.4161/tisb.23118.

Zhang, Z., Xiao, C., Gibson, A. M., Bass, S. A., & Khurana Hershey, G. K. (2014). EGFR signaling blunts allergen-induced IL-6 production and Th17 responses in the skin and attenuates development and relapse of atopic dermatitis. *Journal of Immunology*, *192*(3), 859–866. https://doi.org/10.4049/jimmunol.1301062.

Zhao, Y., Bao, L., Chan, L. S., DiPietro, L. A., & Chen, L. (2016). Aberrant wound healing in an epidermal interleukin-4 transgenic mouse model of atopic dermatitis. *PLoS One*, *11*(1), e0146451. https://doi.org/10.1371/journal.pone.0146451.

22

Skin Barrier Repair

MICHELLE V. Y., JENNIFER ORNELAS, AND SMITA AWASTHI

KEY POINTS

- Moisturizers help with skin barrier repair and continue to be the mainstay of maintenance treatment and prevention of flares in atopic dermatitis (AD).
- Though greasier moisturizer delivery systems such as ointments and creams are most effective, patient compliance should be weighed in selection of an appropriate delivery system.
- Though a tremendous variety of moisturizers at difference price points exist on the market, studies do not show that one moisturizer or moisturizer ingredient is significantly better than another in patients with AD.
- Natural moisturizers such as sunflower seed oil and virgin coconut oil show promise in AD, whereas olive oil may increase skin penetration and promote inflammation.
- Proactive use of moisturizers during infancy may have a protective effect on the incidence of AD.

Introduction

Moisturizers are the key to skin barrier regulation and repair and the mainstay of treatment for atopic dermatitis (AD) along with topical medications (Leung, Hon, & Robson, 2007). Moisturizers have been shown to reduce transepidermal water loss and improve barrier function, preventing flares and the need for topical corticosteroid use in patients with AD (Lodén et al., 2002). Daily use of moisturizer improves xerosis, resolves pruritus quicker, and lengthens the time to flare compared to no treatment (Agrawal & Woodfolk, 2014). Thus daily use of moisturizers to preserve barrier function is fundamental to preventing flares and maintaining quiescent periods in AD.

The skin barrier

Skin is the largest organ of the body and functions as an interface between the internal and external environment. The skin is an essential factor to human survival as a physical barrier against harmful external agents and in protecting against dehydration. The stratum corneum is a major component of the skin barrier, which plays a key role in these important functions. In the stratum corneum, keratinocytes terminally differentiate into corneocytes, which are embedded into a lipid-rich extracellular matrix (Flohr & Mann, 2014). Corneocytes are characterized by cornified envelopes that contain densely packed keratin filaments cemented by several proteins, particularly filaggrin molecules. Filaggrin degradation produces natural moisturizing factor, which is responsible for hydration of the stratum corneum, as well as regulation of its pH (Tsakok, Woolf, Smith, Weidinger, & Flohr, 2019). As a result, acidification by filaggrin metabolites helps to retain the skin barrier (Elias, 2015; Flohr & Mann, 2014; Flohr et al., 2010; Kezic et al., 2008). The filaggrin metabolites, which make up natural moisturizing factor, include amino acids, lactic acids, salts, and urea (Schwartz & Friedman, 2016). Natural moisturizing factors in the extracellular matrix attract and bind water to maintain moisturization and lipids. The lipids are made from breakdown products of keratinocytes and corneocyte membranes, called lamellar granules (Schwartz & Friedman, 2016). Lamellar lipids are composed of cholesterol, free fatty acids, ceramides, and other sphingolipids (Schwartz & Friedman, 2016). Disruptions and disorders of these biochemical pathways can impair the skin barrier and increase its vulnerability to environmental insults and transepidermal water loss (Leung & Hon, 2015; Leung et al., 2007). Additional details of the skin barrier are discussed in Chapters 5, 11, and 15.

AD is a common chronic inflammatory skin disease attributed to both epidermal barrier dysfunction and chronic T helper type 2 (Th2) inflammation (Lin, Zhong, & Santiago, 2018). The impaired barrier function in AD impacts allergic sensitization to protein antigens and microbes, including staphylococcal superantigens, which further exacerbates barrier dysfunction due to altered epidermal differentiation from underlying epidermal inflammation (Lin et al., 2018). Th2-related cytokines, such as interleukin-4 (IL4), further intensify skin barrier impairment by altering keratinocyte differentiation and lipid synthesis in the stratum corneum (Elias, 2014; Hatano et al., 2013). Elevated transepidermal water loss correlates with AD severity. Thus, for patients with AD, restoring hydration and reducing transepidermal water loss with appropriate use of moisturizers plays a key role in repairing epidermal barrier dysfunction (Elias & Wakefield, 2011; Patzelt et al., 2012).

Moisturizers

While there is no consensus regarding the definition of *moisturizer*, the term was initially coined by marketers to promote its function to moisten the skin (Purnamawati, Indrastuti, Danarti, & Saefudin, 2017). Moisturizers address the epidermal repair dysfunction by acting as an occlusive barrier, slowing transepidermal water loss, retaining hydration, and protecting the skin from external irritants (Giam et al., 2016; Szczepanowska, Reich, & Szepietowski, 2008). The terms *moisturizer* and *emollient* are often used interchangeably; however, moisturizers encompass emollients, occlusives, and humectants. Emollient is more specific to a moisturizer that is mostly made up of lipids and their components (Purnamawati et al., 2017). Emollients fill in the space between desquamating corneocytes to create a smooth surface and are used to soften, hydrate, and smooth the skin (Eichenfield et al., 2014; Purnamawati et al., 2017). Examples of emollients include soy sterols, collagen, elastin, shea butter, glycol, and glyceryl stearate (Eichenfield et al., 2014; Hon et al., 2015). Occlusive topical agents are mostly oil based and are similar to intercellular matrix lipids like ceramide, cholesterol, and free fatty acids (Giam et al., 2016; Hon, Leung, & Barankin, 2013; Hon, Pong, et al., 2013). Occlusives form a thin hydrophobic film on the stratum corneum to slow the transepidermal water loss and thus prevent drying (Hon, Leung, et al., 2013; Hon, Pong, et al., 2013; Szczepanowska et al., 2008). Examples of occlusive agents include petrolatum, dimethicone, mineral oil, silicone, olive oil, and lanolins (Eichenfield et al., 2014; Hon, Leung, et al., 2013; Hon, Pong, et al., 2013). Lastly, humectants are agents that attract and hold water from the dermis and the environment to moisturize the skin (Eichenfield et al., 2014; Giam et al., 2016). Humectants include glycerin, sorbitol, and α-hydroxyl acids (Eichenfield et al., 2014). The efficacy of moisturizers depends not only on the ingredients of the moisturizer but also on the proper delivery system to encourage adherence.

Moisturizer delivery systems

Choosing an ideal delivery system for a patient is critical to delivering the most efficacious treatment while also encouraging adherence to treatment. Various delivery systems include ointments, creams, lotions, gels, and oils. A summary of these moisturizer vehicles can be found in Table 22.1.

Ointments

Ointments are made of an emulsion of semisolid containing less than 20% water and volatiles and more than 50% hydrocarbons, waxes, or polyethylene glycols (Mayba & Gooderham, 2018). They contain a greasy base, which often forms an occlusive layer over the skin to prevent dehydration and transepidermal water loss (Mayba & Gooderham, 2018). Ointments are translucent, greasy, do not evaporate, and are the least spreadable compared to the other delivery systems (Buhse et al., 2005; Tan, Feldman, Chang, & Balkrishnan, 2012). They are the most effective and tolerable in drier areas such as the trunk, nonhair-bearing regions, and extremities, including the palms and soles (Del Rosso & Friedlander, 2005). The greasy nature may limit patient adherence, especially on hair-bearing skin (Tan et al., 2012).

Creams

Creams are made of an emulsion of semisolid containing more than 20% water and less than 50% hydrocarbons, waxes, or polyethylene glycols (Buhse et al., 2005). Creams are opaque, viscous, range from nongreasy to mildly greasy,

TABLE 22.1 Moisturizer delivery systems

Vehicle name	Composition	Notes
Ointments	Emulsion of <20% water and volatiles >50% hydrocarbons, waxes, or polyethylene glycols	Most greasy, least spreadable; prevent dehydration and transepidermal water loss (TEWL); do not evaporate
Creams	Emulsion of >20% water and volatiles <50% hydrocarbons, waxes, or polyethylene glycols. Emulsion of either water in oil or oil in water	Less greasy, more spreadable than ointments; evaporate and/or absorbed
Lotions	Aqueous vehicle and >50% water and volatiles	Nongreasy, spreadable; evaporate rapidly thus poorer at slowing TEWL
Gels	Colloidal dispersion of water, acetone, alcohol or propylene glycol, thickened with cellulose derivative. Oily gel: nonalcoholic, lipophilic gel formulation (oil or organic solvents, gelled with an organogelator)	Liquefy on contact with skin and dry as nonocclusive film; easily removed with water and perspiration (except the oily gel); oily gel could slow TEWL
Oils	Mainly triglycerides; also contain fatty acids, phosphatides, sterols, tocopherols, stanols, waxes, and more	Some oils may have skin barrier benefits, but not all oils are created equally

and are made of an emulsion of either water in oil or oil in water (Mayba & Gooderham, 2018). They are less greasy, less viscous, more spreadable than ointments, and usually evaporate or are absorbed when rubbed onto the skin (Mayba & Gooderham, 2018). Creams are effective all over the body, especially in flexural and genital areas and in those areas with both dry and weepy skin conditions (Mayba & Gooderham, 2018; Rosen, Landriscina, & Friedman, 2014). Creams are preferred when an occlusive effect is not as important (Weiss, 2011). Though creams are less hydrating, patients may be more adherent to creams compared to ointments due to the ease of spread and the less greasy texture (Rosen et al., 2014).

Lotions

Lotions are solutions containing an aqueous vehicle and more than 50% water and volatiles (Weiss, 2011). Lotions are thin, opaque, nongreasy, and evaporate rapidly (Mayba & Gooderham, 2018). Lotions are easier to spread, are beneficial for exudative conditions, and are effective in large hair-bearing areas (Weiss, 2011). Lotions evaporate quickly, which is not as beneficial for slowing transepidermal water loss.

Gels

Gels are transparent lattices of organic macromolecules in a semisolid dosage form containing a gelling agent to provide stiffness to a solution or colloidal dispersion for application to the skin (Mayba & Gooderham, 2018; Weiss, 2011). Gels are formulated as a colloidal dispersion of water, acetone, alcohol, or propylene glycol thickened with a cellulose derivative (Weiss, 2011). Gels are usually clear or translucent in a single phase, but opaque in a two-phase system (Mayba & Gooderham, 2018). They are typically thick and nongreasy, except the oily gel, which is a nonalcoholic, lipophilic gel formulation (Mayba & Gooderham, 2018). Gels liquefy upon contact with the skin and then dry as a nonocclusive film (Weiss, 2011). Gels are advantageous and could promote adherence given their cosmetic advantage and ease of use as they are easy to apply to hair-bearing areas and are nongreasy (Weiss, 2011). However, gels are easily removed with water or perspiration and tend to lack emolliating and skin protective properties (Weiss, 2011). An exception is the oily gel, which is characterized by a nonpolar dispersion medium such as oil or organic solvents, gelled with an organogelator (Mayba & Gooderham, 2018). These oily gels are advantageous and could slow transepidermal water loss as they are resistant to water and perspiration (Mayba & Gooderham, 2018).

Oils

Oils include mineral, almond, jojoba, soybean, avocado, coconut, olive, and cannabinoid oils as well as various other vegetable oils. Oils can act as a protective barrier to the skin via the occlusive effect, allowing moisture retention,

and thus may decrease transepidermal water loss (Ziboh, Miller, & Cho, 2000). Plant oils are classified into essential oils and fixed oils, where the latter is not volatile at room temperature (Ziboh et al., 2000). Fixed plant oils are composed of triglycerides, free fatty acids, squalene tocopherols, sterols, stanols, phospholipids, waxes, and other components (Elias, 2014). Certain oils are enriched in these various components and have been shown to improve barrier function, reduce inflammation via activation of peroxisome proliferator-activated receptors (PPARs), and/or provide nutritional benefits (Ansari, Nicolaides, & Fu, 1970; Lin et al., 2018; Ziboh et al., 2000). Plant oils vary by types of free fatty acids, including straight-chain saturated fatty acids (SFAs) and unsaturated fatty acids (UFAs), which have been shown to have differences in slowing transepidermal water loss and irritant skin response (Patzelt et al., 2012). For example, linoleic acid, a long-chain fatty acid and a major lipid in sunflower seed oil, has been shown to maintain the water permeability barrier of the skin, and its metabolite has antiproliferative properties (Elias, Brown, & Ziboh, 1980; Lin et al., 2018; Ziboh et al., 2000). On the other hand, oleic acid, a short-chain fatty acid, causes barrier disruption and could induce dermatitis under continuous application (Lin et al., 2018). Patients often choose these treatments given perceived lower risk of natural products (Karagounis, Gittler, Rotemberg, & Morel, 2019). Some studies have shown skin barrier benefits with sunflower seed oil and virgin coconut oil (Karagounis et al., 2019). Additional natural oils for skin moisturization and barrier repair are discussed later in Alternative and Natural Moisturizers and in Chapter 26.

Moisturizer ingredients

It is well established that moisturizers are the mainstay of treatment for AD and, as such, a tremendous variety of moisturizers at difference price points exist on the market. Increased understanding of the pathophysiology of AD has also led to newer moisturizers, which claim to replenish ceramides or natural moisturizing factor among other claims, though, for the most part, these claims have not been substantiated. Here we review the evidence behind a few of the primary ingredients in moisturizers. A summary of these moisturizer ingredients can be found in Table 22.2.

Lanolin, a wax derived from the sebaceous glands of sheep, is a common ingredient that is either used as moisturizer alone or as an ingredient in many moisturizers. However, there are surprisingly few trials that have investigated the efficacy of lanolin as an emollient. In one study, 173 preterm infants who were treated with a 30% olive oil and 70% lanolin product twice daily for 4 weeks had improvement in their skin condition compared to a water-in-oil emollient cream (Kiechl-Kohlendorfer, Berger, & Inzinger, 2008). The results of this study support the efficacy of lanolin as a moisturizer in AD. Allergic contact dermatitis to lanolin can occur in patients with AD. Contact allergy to lanolin occurs in approximately 2% to 10% of

TABLE 22.2 Moisturizer ingredients

Ingredient	Mechanism of action in AD	Summary of clinical data	Notes
Lanolin	Blocks transepidermal water loss (TEWL)	Few studies Appears efficacious	Allergic contact dermatitis in patients with AD (2%–10%)
Petrolatum	Blocks TEWL, increases stratum corneum thickness, reduces T-cell infiltrate, and upregulates antimicrobial peptides	Improves overall disease severity and pruritus	Cost-effective moisturizer
Ceramides	Help replace lowered levels of epidermal ceramides found in AD to maintain skin integrity and prevent water loss	Effective steroid-sparing moisturizer Unclear if significantly more beneficial than other moisturizer ingredients	Prescription version, EpiCeram, can be costly
Urea	Absorbs water from the atmosphere to help hydrate the superficial layers of the stratum corneum	Preparations with concentrations of 4%–10% may improve erythema, dryness, induration, and papules in AD	Can cause stinging and irritation
Glycerol	Absorbs water from the atmosphere to help hydrate the superficial layers of the stratum corneum	Improves xerosis, dryness, skin hydration, and scaling compared to vehicle Decreased TEWL	
Glycyrrhetinic acid	Exerts antiinflammatory and antibacterial properties	Improves erythema, edema, pruritus, and overall disease severity	Found in licorice root
PEA, cannabinoids	Exerts antiinflammatory and antipruritic properties by binding cannabinoid receptors in the skin (CB1/CB2)	Improves erythema, pruritus, excoriation, scaling, lichenification dryness, and sleep quality	PEA and cannabinoids tested for treatment of AD have minimal to no psychoactive properties
Sunflower seed oil	Rich in linoleic acid, which helps maintain barrier function in epidermis and modulates inflammation through its conversion to arachidonic acid Improved stratum corneum integrity	Improves dryness, hydration, flaking, lichenification, and overall SCORAD	Good alternative for parents/patients who would like a natural emollient option
Olive oil	Causes reduction in stratum corneum integrity and induces irritation	Increases skin hydration, but shown to cause erythema and irritation	Not recommended as an emollient in AD
Virgin coconut oil	Improves skin barrier Rich in lauric acid, which has antibacterial and antiinflammatory properties	Improves SCORAD, decreases TEWL and lower rates of colonization with *Staphylococcus aureas*	Good alternative for parents/patients who would like a natural emollient option
Almond oil	Antioxidant and antibacterial properties	Improves moisture and lipid content of skin Reduces itch	Can lead to percutaneous sensitization

AD, Atopic dermatitis; *PEA,* palmitoylethanolamide.

patients (Fransen, Overgaard, Johansen, & Thyssen, 2018; Pap, Temesvari, Nemeth, Sardy, & Ponyai, 2018).

Petrolatum is a semisolid hydrocarbon that is also found in many moisturizers and is often used as a moisturizer alone. In one trial, patients with AD were randomized to apply either Aquaphor healing ointment, for which the active ingredient is 41% petrolatum, EpiCeram, or Atopiclair three times daily for 3 weeks. Atopiclair contains

glycyrrhetinic acid, which has antiinflammatory and antibacterial properties likely beneficial in the treatment of AD (Aburjai & Natsheh, 2003; Kapoor & Saraf, 2011). Glycyrrhetinic acid is further discussed in Alternative and Natural Moisturizers, later. EpiCeram is a prescription-only cream rich in ceramides used to treat AD (Madaan, 2008). EpiCeram is discussed in more detail in Prescription Emollients, later. In this study, application of Aquaphor healing ointment showed improvement in itch and disease severity that was comparable to the other moisturizers, leading the authors to not only conclude that the over-the-counter petrolatum-based moisturizer was as effective as the other moisturizers, but also 47 times more cost effective (Miller et al., 2011). In another study, occlusion with petrolatum was compared with occlusion alone for 48 hours in nonlesional skin of 13 patients with AD and 39 healthy patients to investigate changes in the cutaneous molecular makeup and structure of the skin in AD. Skin biopsies of occluded areas obtained after 72 hours demonstrated a significant upregulation in antimicrobial peptides, as well as an increased stratum corneum thickness, and significantly reduced T-cell infiltrates in petrolatum-occluded skin compared to both control and occluded-only skin (Czarnowicki et al., 2016). These results confirm that petrolatum is an effective treatment for AD. Studies also show that petrolatum is a far more cost-effective moisturizer compared to other common moisturizers, further supporting its use in the treatment of AD (Xu et al., 2017).

Ceramides are lipids found in high concentration in cell membranes in the stratum corneum. Ceramides help to maintain the integrity of skin and prevent water loss (Agrawal & Woodfolk, 2014). Individuals with AD have been found to have lower epidermal levels of ceramides and pseudoceramides, thus ceramide precursor containing emollients have been developed to treat AD (Agrawal & Woodfolk, 2014; Hon, Leung, et al., 2013; Hon, Pong, et al., 2013). There have been several studies investigating the efficacy of such moisturizers in treating AD. In one study, investigators compared a 6-week course of twice-daily application of a nonprescription ceramide containing cream, Atobarrier cream, to a control nonceramide-containing cream. Patients also applied beclomethasone dipropionate 0.025% cream throughout the study. Those randomized to ceramide-containing cream used on average less topical steroid cream compared to the group randomized to apply a nonceramide-containing cream. As a result the investigators concluded that the ceramide-containing cream was a more effective steroid-sparing moisturizer (Noh, Jung, Park, Koh, & Lee, 2011).

Urea is another ingredient frequently added to moisturizers. As mentioned earlier, it is a natural moisturizing factor that is produced by the degradation of filaggrin in the skin and absorbs water from the atmosphere to help hydrate the superficial layers of the stratum corneum (Schwartz & Friedman, 2016; Warner et al., 1999). Urea cream is available in different concentrations ranging from 1% to 50%. It acts as a humectant in lower concentrations but can be irritating at higher concentrations (>20%) where it is keratolytic (Marini, Krutmann, & Grether-Beck, 2012). In one study, researchers compared application of a 4% urea cream to a 20% glycerin cream and placebo (the vehicle of the glycerin cream) in patients with AD. Patients were instructed to use their designated cream as often as desired, with a minimum of once daily for 1 month. Investigators found that improvement in dryness was equivalent between the glycerin

and urea cream, though there were no significant differences in the patients' perception of dryness at the end of study between the three creams (Lodén et al., 2002). In another study, subjects preferred a 10% urea-containing cream to a vehicle cream in terms of improvement of erythema, dryness, induration, and papules (Wilhelm, Schölermann, Bohnsack, Wilhelm, & Rippke, 1998). Additionally, 5% urea cream has been shown to prolong the time between AD flares compared to no moisturizer (Wiren et al., 2009). However, it should be noted that in the studies mentioned, each moisturizer contained other ingredients, such as petrolatum in the glycerin cream, paraffinum liquidum in the 4% urea cream, and coconut oil and propylene glycol in the latter study, which confounds whether the results are due to the individual ingredients alone (Wiren et al., 2009).

Glycerol is an ingredient that is added to many moisturizers as a humectant. Consequently, it has been investigated as a treatment for AD. In the same study discussed earlier in which a 4% urea cream, a 20% glycerin cream, and placebo (the vehicle of the glycerin cream) were compared in patients with AD, the glycerin cream was additionally found to cause less smarting (a sharp, localized superficial sensation) on application compared to the urea cream (Lodén et al., 2002). In another study that included children ages 2 to 6 with AD, participants were randomized to apply a cream that contained glycerol and paraffin or the vehicle cream twice daily. At week 4, nonresponders were treated open-label with the emollient (the glycerol-containing cream) until week 12, whereas responders stopped treatment. Those who relapsed after stopping treatment at week 8 were then treated open-label on emollient until week 12. Treatment with the glycerol-containing cream led to a significantly greater improvement in the xerosis score of the SCORAD index, objective SCORAD, visual analogue score, and skin hydration (Boralevi et al., 2014). These findings were further supported by a similar study in which a glycerol-containing cream was compared to placebo (vehicle alone) in individuals with AD in a twice-daily application for 4 weeks. Researchers found that areas treated with the glycerol cream had a greater change in SCORAD index, improvement in transepidermal water loss, and skin capacitance compared to vehicle alone (Breternitz, Kowatzki, Langenauer, Elsner, & Fluhr, 2008).

More often than looking for specific ingredients in moisturizers, parents of children with AD can be more focused on avoiding certain ingredients, the most common of which are parabens and phthalates, which are suspected to have endocrine-disrupting effects. Phthalates and parabens can be added to emollients purposefully or released from plastic containers into emollients unintentionally. In a cross-sectional study of more than 800 Danish children ages 4 to 9 years, researchers found that AD and self-reported frequent application of emollients, defined as daily or several times a week, was associated with increased urinary phthalate metabolite and paraben levels (Overgaard et al., 2017). However, it is unclear whether this increase is the result of an increased exposure to phalates and paraben in children with AD or a result of their compromised skin barrier (Overgaard et al., 2017). Furthermore, the difference in excretion of these ubiquitous environmental chemicals was modest, and any health implications of the increased phthalate and paraben exposure are unclear.

When selecting a moisturizer, consumers should also be cognizant of potential contact allergens commonly found in moisturizers, such as fragrances, synthetic dyes, and preservatives. These are discussed further in Chapters 7 and 10, regarding external factors.

Prescription emollients

EpiCeram is a ceramide-rich cream available by prescription only that was approved by the US Food and Drug Administration (FDA) in 2006 as a nonsteroidal lipid barrier emulsion for burning and itching associated with dry skin conditions, including AD, irritant contact dermatitis, radiation dermatitis, and other dermatoses (Madaan, 2008). In a pilot study, EpiCeram was found to be superior to Eucerin cream after a twice-daily 4-week application of each cream to different sites (Kircik, 2014). However, other studies have failed to show the superiority of EpiCeram compared to other moisturizers. In a trial in which patients with AD were randomized to receive either EpiCeram, Atopiclair, a cream containing glycyrrhetinic acid, or Aquaphor healing ointment, three times daily for 3 weeks, no significant difference was found in the improvement in itch and disease severity, as all groups showed improvement (Miller et al., 2011). Moreover, a trial comparing the application of EpiCeram to a colloidal oatmeal–containing cream twice daily or as needed for 3 weeks in children of African descent with AD showed no significant difference in itch reduction or Eczema Area and Severity Index (EASI) score as both creams led to improvement (Nunez et al., 2013). These studies suggest that the benefit of EpiCeram compared to other nonprescription moisturizers may not outweigh its cost.

Mimyx cream is another moisturizer available by prescription containing palmitoylethanolamide (PEA), a synthetic cannabinoid. It was approved by the FDA in 2005 as a nonsteroidal treatment for AD as well as other skin conditions, including radiation dermatitis and allergic contact dermatitis. In a large observational, noncontrolled prospective cohort study involving 2456 participants, twice-daily application of Mimyx for 4 to 6 weeks led to significant improvement in physician assessment of symptoms (dryness, excoriation, pruritus, and erythema) and patient-reported symptoms (decreased loss of sleep related to itching), as well as decreased topical corticosteroid use (Eberlein, Eicke, Reinhardt, & Ring, 2008). In a head-to-head comparison of Mimyx and Eucerin cream applied twice daily in a split-body trial involving 74 patients with AD, more participants preferred Mimyx cream to Eucerin, and patients had a longer duration until flare at the site of Mimyx cream application compared to Eucerin cream (Laumann et al., 2006). Further studies are needed to determine efficacy of Mimyx compared to other nonprescription moisturizers.

Alternative and natural moisturizers

Many individuals and parents of children with AD seek alternative treatments for their condition (Johnston, Bilbao, & Graham-Brown, 2003). As a result, knowledge of safe alternative moisturizers is essential for providers. A summary of these moisturizers can be found in Table 22.2.

Sunflower seed oil has been proposed as a potential treatment for AD. It is rich in linoleic acid, which is needed to maintain normal barrier function in the epidermis and is thought to contribute to the modulation of inflammation through its conversion to arachidonic acid, a precursor to prostaglandin E2 (Eichenfield, McCollum, & Msika, 2009; Elias et al., 1980). In a study of 218 children with AD, twice-daily application for 30 days of a cream containing 2% sunflower oil distillate resulted in an improvement in dryness and flaking (Piccardi, Piccirilli, Choulot, & Msika, 2001). In another study, Msika et al. (2008) randomized 86 children with AD to receive either daily application for 21 days of desonide 0.05% cream or an every other daily application of desonide 0.05% cream alternating with an every other day application of an emollient containing 2% sunflower seed oil. Both groups had similar improvements in SCORAD, but the group treated with an emollient-containing sunflower seed oil had a greater improvement in lichenification (Msika et al., 2008). These results indicate that sunflower seed oil may have a role as a steroid-sparing agent in AD (Msika et al., 2008). While both were small trials, these results are promising, especially for patients and parents who prefer a natural option for a moisturizer.

Olive oil is produced by pressing olives and has also been studied as a treatment for AD. In a small study of 19 volunteers with and without a history of AD, twice-daily application of sunflower seed oil for 4 weeks preserved the stratum corneum integrity, did not cause erythema, and improved hydration (Danby et al., 2013). In contrast, application of olive oil caused a significant reduction in stratum corneum integrity and induced mild erythema in volunteers with and without a history of AD (Danby et al., 2013). Researchers randomized 115 neonates to receive either no oil, four drops of olive oil, or four drops of sunflower seed oil in a twice-daily application for 4 weeks. While there was no difference observed in transepidermal water loss, those in the olive oil group had significantly lower ordering of lipids in the stratum corneum than the no-oil group. The results of these studies demonstrate that olive oil is not a suitable emollient for the treatment of AD due to its ability to increase skin penetration and promote inflammation (Jiang & Zhou, 2003; Katsuta, Iida, Hasegawa, Inomata, & Denda, 2009).

Virgin coconut oil has been investigated as a potential natural plant-based emollient. It is produced by using a cold press method and retains more of its fatty acids compared to nonvirgin coconut oil, which is produced by boiling coconut meat, then heating and bleaching the oils to remove any impurities and the coconut fragrance (Karagounis et al., 2019; Marina, Man, Nazimah, & Amin, 2009). Researchers compared the use of virgin coconut oil to mineral oil as topical emollients applied twice daily for 8 weeks in a study of 117 patients with AD; while both oils led to the improvement or decrease of SCORAD indices and decreased transepidermal water loss, virgin coconut oil was superior to mineral oil (Evangelista, Abad-Casintahan, & Lopez-Villafuerte, 2014). Moreover, virgin coconut oil has been shown to have antibacterial properties against *Staphylococcus aureus* (Verallo-Rowell, Dillague, & Syah-Tjundawan, 2008). Patients with AD treated with virgin coconut oil have lower rates of cutaneous *S. aureus* colonization (Verallo-Rowell et al., 2008). However, these results were not corroborated in a separate study in which virgin coconut oil failed to demonstrate antibacterial activity against several bacteria, including *S. aureus* (Nguyen, Le, Phan, & Tran, 2017). Regardless, virgin coconut oil can be used safely as an effective moisturizer in individuals with AD.

Almond oil is rich in phenolic acids and flavonoids and has been shown to have antioxidant and antibacterial properties (Ahmad, 2010). As a result, almond oil has been trialed for the treatment of AD. In one study of an emollient-containing almond oil and lactic acid, researchers found that twice-daily application for 14 days in individuals with xerotic skin conditions, including AD, had significant reduction in itch and that skin moisture and lipid content were increased (Simon et al., 2018). However, it should be noted that topical application of almond oil has been shown to lead to the percutaneous sensitization in children, so providers should be cognizant of this potential when selecting an emollient for patients (Guillet & Guillet, 2000).

Glycyrrhetinic acid is an active component of the licorice root that has antiinflammatory and antibacterial properties and a low potential to cause allergic contact dermatitis (Aburjai & Natsheh, 2003; Kapoor & Saraf, 2011; Sasseville, 2011). In an aforementioned study included in the petrolatum section, researchers found that three times daily application for 3 weeks of Atopiclar cream, which contains glycyrrhetinic acid cream, led to improvement in itch and disease severity comparable to the other moisturizers in the study (Miller et al., 2011). In another trial involving 60 individuals with AD, participants were randomized to apply a gel with either 1% or 2% glycyrrhetinic acid three times daily for 2 weeks. While both formulations led to improvement, the 2% gel led to superior improvement in erythema, edema, and pruritus (Saeedi, Morteza-Semnani, & Ghoreishi, 2003).

Cannabinoid (CBD) oils and products have recently been postulated as a potential novel treatment for AD. Cannabinoids are a large group of compounds that are similar in structure and biochemically to the main psychoactive compound found in *Cannabis sativa*, delta(9)-tetrahydrocannabinol (THC) (Sheriff, Lin, Dubin, & Khorasani, 2019). Cannabinoids have antiinflammatory and antipruritic properties by binding to receptors found in the skin, which has led to the investigation of their potential treatment for AD (Gaffal, Cron, Glodde, & Tuting, 2013; Milando & Friedman, 2019; Soliman, Henderson, Danell, & Van Dross, 2016; Soliman & Van Dross, 2016).

It is important to note that cannabinoid compounds trialed for the treatment of AD have minimal to no psychoactive properties (Milando & Friedman, 2019). In a small trial of 20 patients with AD, psoriasis, and scars, investigators found that twice-daily application of a CBD oil–enriched ointment for 3 months led to improvement in AD, including itch severity (Palmieri, Laurino, & Vadalà, 2019). As mentioned, Mimyx cream, a prescription-only cream containing PEA (a synthetic cannabinoid), has been shown to be effective in the treatment of AD, and in a small clinical trial, which included twice-daily application to one side of the body, it was shown to be more effective that Eucerin cream in treating AD (Eberlein et al., 2008; Laumann et al., 2006). In a larger observational study of 2456 participants, twice-daily application of a cream containing PEA (Physiogel A.I. Cream) to affected areas for 4 to 6 weeks led to improvement in eczema with improvement in erythema, pruritus, excoriation, scaling, lichenification dryness, and sleep quality (Eberlein et al., 2008). However, in both studies it is unclear if the results are due to PEA or other ingredients contained in the respective PEA creams as they were not compared to vehicle. Further research is needed before moisturizers that contain CBD oil or cannabinoids can be recommended as effective treatment for AD.

In a more recent trend, patients and parents of children with AD have turned more often to complementary and alternative medicine (CAM) due to fears regarding topical corticosteroid use (Johnston et al., 2003). It is important to note, however, that herbal creams, particularly those obtained abroad, may covertly contain topical corticosteroids (Hughes, Higgins, & Pembroke, 1994; Keane, Munn, Vivier, Higgins, & Taylor, 1999; Niggemann & Grüber, 2003; O'Driscoll, Burden, & Kingston, 1992; Wood & Wishart, 1997). Parents should also be educated that natural ingredients have risks and may not be studied as well as prescribed medications. For instance, tea-tree and lavender oils have only recently been found to cause gynecomastia in prepubescent children (Diaz, Luque, Badar, Kornic, & Danon, 2016; Henley, Lipson, Korach, & Bloch, 2007). Consequently, patients and families should be queried on the use of CAM products and counseled on the potential risk of both CAM and prescription medications.

Role of proactive use of moisturizers in prevention of eczema in infants

Children with filaggrin mutations have an increased transepidermal water loss and an increased risk of developing AD (Horimukai et al., 2014). AD has a significant negative socioeconomic impact as well as adverse effects on quality of life. Primary prevention of AD through barrier repair could significantly reduce its burden. It is well established that daily use of moisturizer can improve xerosis, resolve pruritus quicker, and lengthen time to flare compared to no treatment (Agrawal & Woodfolk, 2014). More recently, several studies have demonstrated that use of emollients early in life could prevent AD (Horimukai et al., 2014). Horimukai et al. (2014) performed a randomized controlled trial showing a significantly reduced risk of AD in infants with daily application of moisturizer during the first 32 weeks of life compared with the control group, who occasionally received a minimum amount of petroleum jelly. Simpson et al. (2014) also showed a statistically significant protective effect of daily emollient on incidence of AD compared to the control group that did not use any emollients.

Among infants who are at high risk for AD based on family history of atopy (first-degree relative with family history of AD, allergic rhinitis, or asthma), those who received once-daily application of a ceramide and amino acid–containing emollient had significantly lower rates of AD diagnosis at 12 and 24 months of age, compared to those who used emollients of their choice on an as-needed basis for dry skin. This study suggests a protective effect of daily emollient with ceramides and amino acids (McClanahan et al., 2019).

Summary

Moisturizers continue to be the mainstay for maintenance treatment of AD and show promise in disease prevention with proactive use. Though a variety of moisturizers exist, studies do not show that one moisturizer or moisturizer ingredient, natural or synthetic, is significantly better that another in patients with AD (Hon, Kung, Ng, & Leung, 2018). The cost effectiveness of moisturizers in reducing physician visits, health care utilization, and overall health care costs is indisputable (Xu et al., 2017). Delivery system and parental desire for natural or alternative options should be key considerations for physicians recommending moisturizers to increase adherence to use.

Further readings

Hebert, A.A., Rippke, F., Weber, T.M. et al. (2020). Efficacy of Nonprescription Moisturizers for Atopic Dermatitis: An Updated Review of Clinical Evidence. *American Journal of Clinical Dermatology*, 21, 641–655. https://doi.org/10.1007/s40257-020-00529-9.

Elias, P. M., & Wakefield, J. S. (2011). Therapeutic implications of a barrier-based pathogenesis of atopic dermatitis. *Clinical Reviews in Allergy and Immunology*, 41(3), 282–295. https://doi.org/10.1007/s12016-010-8231-1.

Hon, K. L., Leung, A. K., & Barankin, B. (2013). Barrier repair therapy in atopic dermatitis: an overview. *American Journal of Clinical Dermatology*, 14(5), 389–399. https://doi.org/10.1007/s40257-013-0033-9.

Xu, S., Immaneni, S., Hazen, G. B., Silverberg, J. I., Paller, A. S., & Lio, P. A. (2017). Cost-effectiveness of prophylactic moisturization for atopic dermatitis. *JAMA Pediatrics, 171*(2). e163909-e163909.

References

Aburjai, T., & Natsheh, F. M. (2003). Plants used in cosmetics. *Phytotherapy Research, 17*(9), 987–1000.

Agrawal, R., & Woodfolk, J. A. (2014). Skin barrier defects in atopic dermatitis. *Current Allergy and Asthma Reports, 14*(5), 433. https://doi.org/10.1007/s11882-014-0433-9.

Ahmad, Z. (2010). The uses and properties of almond oil. *Complementary Therapies in Clinical Practice, 16*(1), 10–12. https://doi.org/10.1016/j.ctcp.2009.06.015.

Ansari, M. N., Nicolaides, N., & Fu, H. C. (1970). Fatty acid composition of the living layer and stratum corneum lipids of human sole skin epidermis. *Lipids, 5*(10), 838–845. https://doi.org/10.1007/bf02531977.

Boralevi, F., Saint Aroman, M., Delarue, A., Raudsepp, H., Kaszuba, A., Bylaite, M., & Tiplica, G. S. (2014). Long-term emollient therapy improves xerosis in children with atopic dermatitis. *Journal of the European Academy of Dermatology and Venereology, 28*(11), 1456–1462.

Breternitz, M., Kowatzki, D., Langenauer, M., Elsner, P., & Fluhr, J. W. (2008). Placebo-controlled, double-blind, randomized, prospective study of a glycerol-based emollient on eczematous skin in atopic dermatitis: Biophysical and clinical evaluation. *Skin Pharmacology and Physiology, 21*(1), 39–45.

Buhse, L., Kolinski, R., Westenberger, B., Wokovich, A., Spencer, J., Chen, C. W., et al. (2005). Topical drug classification. *International Journal of Pharmaceutics, 295*(1–2), 101–112. https://doi.org/10.1016/j.ijpharm.2005.01.032.

Czarnowicki, T., Malajian, D., Khattri, S., da Rosa, J. C., Dutt, R., Finney, R., et al. (2016). Petrolatum: Barrier repair and antimicrobial responses underlying this "inert" moisturizer. *Journal of Allergy and Clinical Immunology, 137*(4), 1091–1102.e7.

Danby, S. G., AlEnezi, T., Sultan, A., Lavender, T., Chittock, J., Brown, K., & Cork, M. J. (2013). Effect of olive and sunflower seed oil on the adult skin barrier: Implications for neonatal skin care. *Pediatric Dermatology, 30*(1), 42–50. https://doi.org/10.1111/j.1525-1470.2012.01865.x.

Del Rosso, J., & Friedlander, S. F. (2005). Corticosteroids: Options in the era of steroid-sparing therapy. *Journal of the American Academy of Dermatology, 53*(1 Suppl 1), S50–S58. https://doi.org/10.1016/j.jaad.2005.04.030.

Diaz, A., Luque, L., Badar, Z., Kornic, S., & Danon, M. (2016). Prepubertal gynecomastia and chronic lavender exposure: Report of three cases. *Journal of Pediatric Endocrinology and Metabolism, 29*(1), 103–107.

Eberlein, B., Eicke, C., Reinhardt, H. W., & Ring, J. (2008). Adjuvant treatment of atopic eczema: Assessment of an emollient containing N-palmitoylethanolamine (ATOPA study). *Journal of the European Academy of Dermatology and Venereology, 22*(1), 73–82. https://doi.org/10.1111/j.1468-3083.2007.02351.x.

Eichenfield, L. F., McCollum, A., & Msika, P. (2009). The benefits of sunflower oleodistillate (SOD) in pediatric dermatology. *Pediatric Dermatology, 26*(6), 669–675. https://doi.org/10.1111/j.1525-1470.2009.01042.x.

Eichenfield, L. F., Tom, W. L., Berger, T. G., Krol, A., Paller, A. S., Schwarzenberger, K. et al. (2014). Guidelines of care for the management of atopic dermatitis: Section 2. Management and treatment of atopic dermatitis with topical therapies. *Journal of the American Academy of Dermatology, 71*(1), 116–132. https://doi.org/10.1016/j.jaad.2014.03.023.

Elias, P. M. (2014). Lipid abnormalities and lipid-based repair strategies in atopic dermatitis. *Biochimica et Biophysica Acta, 1841*(3), 323–330. https://doi.org/10.1016/j.bbalip.2013.10.001.

Elias, P. M. (2015). Stratum corneum acidification: How and why? *Experimental Dermatology, 24*(3), 179–180. https://doi.org/10.1111/exd.12596.

Elias, P. M., Brown, B. E., & Ziboh, V. A. (1980). The permeability barrier in essential fatty acid deficiency: Evidence for a direct role for linoleic acid in barrier function. *The Journal of Investigative Dermatology*, *74*(4), 230–233. https://doi.org/10.1111/1523-1747.ep12541775.

Elias, P. M., & Wakefield, J. S. (2011). Therapeutic implications of a barrier-based pathogenesis of atopic dermatitis. *Clinical Reviews in Allergy and Immunology*, *41*(3), 282–295. https://doi.org/10.1007/s12016-010-8231-1.

Evangelista, M. T., Abad-Casintahan, F., & Lopez-Villafuerte, L. (2014). The effect of topical virgin coconut oil on SCORAD index, transepidermal water loss, and skin capacitance in mild to moderate pediatric atopic dermatitis: A randomized, double-blind, clinical trial. *International Journal of Dermatology*, *53*(1), 100–108. https://doi.org/10.1111/ijd.12339.

Flohr, C., England, K., Radulovic, S., McLean, W. H., Campbel, L. E., Barker, J., et al. (2010). Filaggrin loss-of-function mutations are associated with early-onset eczema, eczema severity and transepidermal water loss at 3 months of age. *British Journal of Dermatology*, *163*(6), 1333–1336. https://doi.org/10.1111/j.1365-2133.2010.10068.x.

Flohr, C., & Mann, J. (2014). New insights into the epidemiology of childhood atopic dermatitis. *Allergy*, *69*(1), 3–16. https://doi.org/10.1111/all.12270.

Fransen, M., Overgaard, L. E. K., Johansen, J. D., & Thyssen, J. P. (2018). Contact allergy to lanolin: Temporal changes in prevalence and association with atopic dermatitis. *Contact Dermatitis*, *78*(1), 70–75. https://doi.org/10.1111/cod.12872.

Gaffal, E., Cron, M., Glodde, N., & Tuting, T. (2013). Anti-inflammatory activity of topical THC in DNFB-mediated mouse allergic contact dermatitis independent of CB1 and CB2 receptors. *Allergy*, *68*(8), 994–1000. https://doi.org/10.1111/all.12183.

Giam, Y. C., Hebert, A. A., Dizon, M. V., Van Bever, H., Tiongco-Recto, M., Kim, K. H., et al. (2016). A review on the role of moisturizers for atopic dermatitis. *Asia Pacific Allergy*, *6*(2), 120–128. https://doi.org/10.5415/apallergy.2016.6.2.120.

Guillet, G., & Guillet, M. H. (2000). Percutaneous sensitization to almond oil in infancy and study of ointments in 27 children with food allergy. *Allergie et Immunologie*, *32*(8), 309–311.

Hatano, Y., Adachi, Y., Elias, P. M., Crumrine, D., Sakai, T., Kurahashi, R., et al. (2013). The Th2 cytokine, interleukin-4, abrogates the cohesion of normal stratum corneum in mice: Implications for pathogenesis of atopic dermatitis. *Experimental Dermatology*, *22*(1), 30–35. https://doi.org/10.1111/exd.12047.

Henley, D. V., Lipson, N., Korach, K. S., & Bloch, C. A. (2007). Prepubertal gynecomastia linked to lavender and tea tree oils. *New England Journal of Medicine*, *356*(5), 479–485.

Hon, K. L., Kung, J. S. C., Ng, W. G. G., & Leung, T. F. (2018). Emollient treatment of atopic dermatitis: Latest evidence and clinical considerations. *Drugs in Context*, *7*, 212530. https://doi.org/10.7573/dic.212530.

Hon, K. L., Leung, A. K., & Barankin, B. (2013). Barrier repair therapy in atopic dermatitis: an overview. *American Journal of Clinical Dermatology*, *14*(5), 389–399. https://doi.org/10.1007/s40257-013-0033-9.

Hon, K. L., Pong, N. H., Wang, S. S., Lee, V. W., Luk, N. M., & Leung, T. F. (2013). Acceptability and efficacy of an emollient containing ceramide-precursor lipids and moisturizing factors for atopic dermatitis in pediatric patients. *Drugs in R&D*, *13*(1), 37–42. https://doi.org/10.1007/s40268-013-0004-x.

Hon, K. L., Tsang, Y. C., Pong, N. H., Lee, V. W., Luk, N. M., Chow, C. M., & Leung, T. F. (2015). Patient acceptability, efficacy, and skin biophysiology of a cream and cleanser containing lipid complex with shea butter extract versus a ceramide product for eczema. *Hong Kong Medical Journal*, *21*(5), 417–425. https://doi.org/10.12809/hkmj144472.

Horimukai, K., Morita, K., Narita, M., Kondo, M., Kitazawa, H., Nozaki, M., et al. (2014). Application of moisturizer to neonates prevents development of atopic dermatitis. *Journal of Allergy and Clinical Immunology*, *134*(4), 824–830. e6.

Hughes, J. R., Higgins, E. M., & Pembroke, A. C. (1994). Oral dexamethasone masquerading as a Chinese herbal remedy. *British Journal of Dermatology*, *130*(2), 261. https://doi.org/10.1111/j.1365-2133.1994.tb02916.x.

Jiang, S. J., & Zhou, X. J. (2003). Examination of the mechanism of oleic acid-induced percutaneous penetration enhancement: An ultrastructural study. *Biological and Pharmaceutical Bulletin*, *26*(1), 66–68. https://doi.org/10.1248/bpb.26.66.

Johnston, G. A., Bilbao, R. M., & Graham-Brown, R. A. (2003). The use of complementary medicine in children with atopic dermatitis in secondary care in Leicester. *British Journal of Dermatology*, *149*(3), 566–571. https://doi.org/10.1046/j.1365-2133.2003.05471.x.

Kapoor, S., & Saraf, S. (2011). Topical herbal therapies an alternative and complementary choice to combat acne. *Journal of Medicinal Plants Research*, *5*(6), 650–659.

Karagounis, T. K., Gittler, J. K., Rotemberg, V., & Morel, K. D. (2019). Use of "natural" oils for moisturization: Review of olive, coconut, and sunflower seed oil. *Pediatric Dermatology*, *36*(1), 9–15. https://doi.org/10.1111/pde.13621.

Katsuta, Y., Iida, T., Hasegawa, K., Inomata, S., & Denda, M. (2009). Function of oleic acid on epidermal barrier and calcium influx into keratinocytes is associated with N-methyl D-aspartate-type glutamate receptors. *British Journal of Dermatology*, *160*(1), 69–74. https://doi.org/10.1111/j.1365-2133.2008.08860.x.

Keane, F. M., Munn, S. E., Vivier, A. W., Higgins, E. M., & Taylor, N. F. (1999). Analysis of Chinese herbal creams prescribed for dermatological conditions. *The Western Journal of Medicine*, *170*(5), 257–259.

Kezic, S., Kemperman, P. M., Koster, E. S., de Jongh, C. M., Thio, H. B., Campbell, L. E., et al. (2008). Loss-of-function mutations in the filaggrin gene lead to reduced level of natural moisturizing factor in the stratum corneum. *The Journal of Investigative Dermatology*, *128*(8), 2117–2119. https://doi.org/10.1038/jid.2008.29.

Kiechl-Kohlendorfer, U., Berger, C., & Inzinger, R. (2008). The effect of daily treatment with an olive oil/lanolin emollient on skin integrity in preterm infants: A randomized controlled trial. *Pediatric Dermatology*, *25*(2), 174–178. https://doi.org/10.1111/j.1525-1470.2008.00627.x.

Kircik, L. H. (2014). Effect of skin barrier emulsion cream vs a conventional moisturizer on transepidermal water loss and corneometry in atopic dermatitis: A pilot study. *Journal of Drugs in Dermatology*, *13*(12), 1482–1484.

Laumann, A., Lai, S., Lucky, A. W., Schlessinger, J., Jarratt, M., Jones, T. M., & Simpson, E. L. (2006). The efficacy and safety of Mimyx cream in reducing the risk of relapse in atopic dermatitis. *Journal of Investigative Dermatology*, *126*, 45.

Leung, A. K., Hon, K. L., & Robson, W. L. (2007). Atopic dermatitis. *Advances in Pediatrics*, *54*, 241–273. https://doi.org/10.1016/j.yapd.2007.03.013.

Leung, T. N., & Hon, K. L. (2015). Eczema therapeutics in children: What do the clinical trials say? *Hong Kong Medical Journal*, *21*(3), 251–260. https://doi.org/10.12809/hkmj144474.

Lin, T.-K., Zhong, L., & Santiago, J. L. (2018). Anti-inflammatory and skin barrier repair effects of topical application of some plant oils. *International Journal of Molecular Sciences*, *19*(1), 70.

Lodén, M., Andersson, A.-C., Anderson, C., Bergbrant, I.-M., Frodin, T., Ohman, H., et al. (2002). A double-blind study comparing the effect of glycerin and urea on dry, eczematous skin in atopic patients. *Acta Dermato-Venereologica*, *82*(1), 45–47.

Madaan, A. (2008). Epiceram for the treatment of atopic dermatitis. *Drugs of Today (Barcelona)*, *44*(10), 751–755. https://doi.org/10.1358/dot.2008.44.10.1276838.

Marina, A. M., Man, Y. B., Nazimah, S. A., & Amin, I. (2009). Antioxidant capacity and phenolic acids of virgin coconut oil. *International Journal of Food Sciences and Nutrition*, *60*(Suppl 2), 114–123. https://doi.org/10.1080/09637480802549127.

Marini, A., Krutmann, J., & Grether-Beck, S. (2012). Urea and skin: A well-known molecule revisited. *Treatment of Dry Skin Syndrome*, 493–501.

Mayba, J. N., & Gooderham, M. J. (2018). A guide to topical vehicle formulations. *Journal of Cutaneous Medicine and Surgery*, *22*(2), 207–212. https://doi.org/10.1177/1203475417743234.

McClanahan, D., Wong, A., Kezic, S., Samrao, A., Hajar, T., Hill, E., & Simpson, E. L. (2019). A randomized controlled trial of an emollient with ceramide and filaggrin-associated amino acids for the primary prevention of atopic dermatitis in high-risk infants. *Journal of the European Academy of Dermatology and Venereology*, *33*(11), 2087–2094.

Milando, R., & Friedman, A. (2019). Cannabinoids: Potential role in inflammatory and neoplastic skin diseases. *American Journal of Clinical Dermatology*, *20*(2), 167–180.

Miller, D. W., Koch, S. B., Yentzer, B. A., Clark, A. R., O'Neill, J. R., Fountain, J., et al. (2011).An over-the-counter moisturizer is as clinically effective as, and more cost-effective than, prescription barrier creams in the treatment of children with mild-to-moderate atopic dermatitis: A randomized, controlled trial. *Journal of Drugs in Dermatology*, *10*(5), 531–537.

Msika, P., De Belilovsky, C., Piccardi, N., Chebassier, N., Baudouin, C., & Chadoutaud, B. (2008). New emollient with topical corticosteroid-sparing effect in treatment of childhood atopic dermatitis: SCORAD and quality of life improvement. *Pediatric Dermatology*, *25*(6), 606–612. https://doi.org/10.1111/j.1525-1470.2008.00783.x.

Nguyen, V. T. A., Le, T. D., Phan, H. N., & Tran, L. B. (2017). Antibacterial activity of free fatty acids from hydrolyzed virgin coconut oil using lipase from. *Candida rugosa Journal of Lipids*, *2017*, 7170162. https://doi.org/10.1155/2017/7170162.

Niggemann, B., & Grüber, C. (2003). Side-effects of complementary and alternative medicine. *Allergy*, *58*(8), 707–716.

Noh, S., Jung, J. Y., Park, W. S., Koh, H. J., & Lee, K. H. (2011). The steroid-sparing effect of an emollient APDDR-0801 in patients with atopic dermatitis. *Korean Journal of Dermatology*, *49*(3), 227–233.

Nunez, C., Hogan, D., Humphrey, M., Zhang, P., Lisante, T. A., & Doshi, U. (2013). A colloidal oatmeal OTC cream is as clinically effective as a prescription barrier repair cream for the management of mild to moderate atopic dermatitis in African American children. *Journal of the American Academy of Dermatology*, *68*(4), Ab73.

O'Driscoll, J., Burden, A. D., & Kingston, T. P. (1992). Potent topical steroid obtained from a Chinese herbalist. *British Journal of Dermatology*, *127*(5), 543–544. https://doi.org/10.1111/j.1365-2133.1992.tb14859.x.

Overgaard, L. E. K., Main, K. M., Frederiksen, H., Stender, S., Szecsi, P. B., Williams, H. C., & Thyssen, J. P. (2017). Children with atopic dermatitis and frequent emollient use have increased urinary levels of low-molecular-weight phthalate metabolites and parabens. *Allergy*, *72*(11), 1768–1777. https://doi.org/10.1111/all.13157.

Palmieri, B., Laurino, C., & Vadalà, M. (2019). A therapeutic effect of cbd-enriched ointment in inflammatory skin diseases and cutaneous scars. *La Clinica Terapeutica*(2), e93–e99.

Pap, E. B., Temesvari, E., Nemeth, I., Sardy, M., & Ponyai, G. (2018). Contact hypersensitivity in adolescents. *Pediatric Dermatology*, *35*(6), 769–773. https://doi.org/10.1111/pde.13609.

Patzelt, A., Lademann, J., Richter, H., Darvin, M. E., Schanzer, S., Thiede, G., et al. (2012). In vivo investigations on the penetration of various oils and their influence on the skin barrier. *Skin Research and Technology*, *18*(3), 364–369. https://doi.org/10.1111/j.1600-0846.2011.00578.x.

Piccardi, N., Piccirilli, A., Choulot, J., & Msika, P. (2001). Sunflower oil oleo distillate for atopy treatment: An in vitro and clinical evaluation. *Journal of Investigative Dermatology*, *117*(2), 418.

Purnamawati, S., Indrastuti, N., Danarti, R., & Saefudin, T. (2017). The role of moisturizers in addressing various kinds of dermatitis: A review. *Clinical Medicine & Research*, *15*(3-4), 75–87.

Rosen, J., Landriscina, A., & Friedman, A. J. (2014). Principles and approaches for optimizing therapy with unique topical vehicles. *Journal of Drugs in Dermatology*, *13*(12), 1431–1435.

Saeedi, M., Morteza-Semnani, K., & Ghoreishi, M.-R. (2003). The treatment of atopic dermatitis with licorice gel. *Journal of Dermatological Treatment*, *14*(3), 153–157.

Sasseville, D. (2011). Contact dermatitis from topical antibiotics. *European Journal of Dermatology*, *21*(3), 311–322. https://doi.org/10.1684/ejd.2011.1344.

Schwartz, J., & Friedman, A. J. (2016). Exogenous factors in skin barrier repair. *Journal of Drugs in Dermatology*, *15*(11), 1289–1294.

Sheriff, T., Lin, M. J., Dubin, D., & Khorasani, H. (2019). The potential role of cannabinoids in dermatology. *The Journal of Dermatological Treatment*, 1–7. https://doi.org/10.1080/09546634.2019.1675854.

Simon, D., Nobbe, S., Nageli, M., Barysch, M., Kunz, M., Borelli, S., et al. (2018). Short- and long-term effects of two emollients on itching and skin restoration in xerotic eczema. *Dermatologic Therapy*, *31*(6), e12692. https://doi.org/10.1111/dth.12692.

Simpson, E. L., Chalmers, J. R., Hanifin, J. M., Thomas, K. S., Cork, M. J., McLean, W. H. I., et al. (2014).Emollient enhancement of the skin barrier from birth offers effective atopic dermatitis prevention. *Journal of Allergy and Clinical Immunology*, *134*(4), 818–823.

Soliman, E., Henderson, K. L., Danell, A. S., & Van Dross, R. (2016). Arachidonoyl-ethanolamide activates endoplasmic reticulum stress-apoptosis in tumorigenic keratinocytes: Role of cyclooxygenase-2 and novel J-series prostamides. *Molecular Carcinogenesis*, *55*(2), 117–130. https://doi.org/10.1002/mc.22257.

Soliman, E., & Van Dross, R. (2016). Anandamide-induced endoplasmic reticulum stress and apoptosis are mediated by oxidative stress in non-melanoma skin cancer: Receptor-independent endocannabinoid signaling. *Molecular Carcinogenesis*, *55*(11), 1807–1821. https://doi.org/10.1002/mc.22429.

Szczepanowska, J., Reich, A., & Szepietowski, J. C. (2008). Emollients improve treatment results with topical corticosteroids in childhood atopic dermatitis: A randomized comparative study. *Pediatric Allergy and Immunology*, *19*(7), 614–618. https://doi.org/10.1111/j.1399-3038.2007.00706.x.

Tan, X., Feldman, S. R., Chang, J., & Balkrishnan, R. (2012). Topical drug delivery systems in dermatology: A review of patient adherence issues. *Expert Opinion on Drug Delivery*, *9*(10), 1263–1271. https://doi.org/10.1517/17425247.2012.711756.

Tsakok, T., Woolf, R., Smith, C. H., Weidinger, S., & Flohr, C. (2019). Atopic dermatitis: The skin barrier and beyond. *British Journal of Dermatology*, *180*(3), 464–474. https://doi.org/10.1111/bjd.16934.

Verallo-Rowell, V. M., Dillague, K. M., & Syah-Tjundawan, B. S. (2008). Novel antibacterial and emollient effects of coconut and virgin olive oils in adult atopic dermatitis. *Dermatitis: Contact, Atopic, Occupational, Drug, 19*(6), 308–315.

Warner, R. R., Boissy, Y. L., Lilly, N. A., Spears, M. J., McKillop, K., Marshall, J. L., & Stone, K. J. (1999). Water disrupts stratum corneum lipid lamellae: Damage is similar to surfactants. *Journal of Investigative Dermatology, 113*(6), 960–966. https://doi.org/10.1046/j.1523-1747.1999.00774.x.

Weiss, S. C. (2011). Conventional topical delivery systems. *Dermatologic Therapy, 24*(5), 471–476. https://doi.org/10.1111/j.1529-8019.2012.01458.x.

Wilhelm, K.-P., Schölermann, A., Bohnsack, K., Wilhelm, D., & Rippke, F. (1998). Efficacy and tolerability of a topical preparation containing 10% urea in patients with atopic dermatitis. *Aktuelle Dermatologie, 24*(1), 26–30.

Wiren, K., Nohlgard, C., Nyberg, F., Holm, L., Svensson, M., Johannesson, A., et al. (2009). Treatment with a barrier-strengthening moisturizing cream delays relapse of atopic dermatitis: A prospective and randomized controlled clinical trial. *Journal of the European Academy of Dermatology and Venereology, 23*(11), 1267–1272. https://doi.org/10.1111/j.1468-3083.2009.03303.x.

Wood, B., & Wishart, J. (1997). Potent topical steroid in a Chinese herbal cream. *The New Zealand Medical Journal, 110*(1055), 420–421.

Xu, S., Immaneni, S., Hazen, G. B., Silverberg, J. I., Paller, A. S., & Lio, P. A. (2017). Cost-effectiveness of prophylactic moisturization for atopic dermatitis. *JAMA Pediatrics, 171*(2), e163909.

Ziboh, V. A., Miller, C. C., & Cho, Y. (2000). Metabolism of polyunsaturated fatty acids by skin epidermal enzymes: Generation of antiinflammatory and antiproliferative metabolites. *The American Journal of Clinical Nutrition, 71*(1 Suppl), 361S–366S. https://doi.org/10.1093/ajcn/71.1.361s.

23

Emerging Targeted Treatments

GRIFFIN R. LEE, DYLAN E. LEE, AND VIVIAN Y. SHI

KEY POINTS

- This chapter provides an overview of the pathogenesis of atopic dermatitis and the key mediators that are of therapeutic interest.
- As we acquire more knowledge into the pathogenesis of atopic dermatitis, we will be able to use more targeted treatments
- The two most recently Food and Drug Administration–approved medications are dupilumab and crisaborole.
- There are a number of topical and systemic novel and emerging targeted therapies for atopic dermatitis.
- Despite promise of these new drug therapies, potential gaps include limited head-to-head trials, lack of subgroup analysis, and high cost.

Introduction

This chapter is intended to discuss novel and emerging pharmaceutic treatments for patients affected by atopic dermatitis (AD). It will give a brief overview of the proposed mechanism of each treatment, the major side effects, and the most recent clinical data from trials and studies. We hope to provide a comprehensive overview of the new treatments available for AD and to make clinicians better informed about the particular strengths and weaknesses of each drug. It should also be noted that many of these treatments are still in development and may not be available for clinical use, and we encourage readers to follow up on the updated results of the trials and studies listed throughout each section. A summary of the medications can be found in Table 23.1.

Pathogenesis

Sustained barrier defects generated by filaggrin mutations, decreased ceramide synthesis, scratching, increased serine protease activity, and prolonged exposure to reduced environmental humidity result in epidermal dysfunction and allow for penetration of allergens found in pollen, microbes, and food (Bieber, 2008; Elias, Hatano, & Williams, 2008). In response to allergens, trauma, and inflammation, keratinocytes release inflammatory mediators such as interleukin-25

(IL25), IL33, thymic stromal lymphopoietin (TSLP), and pollen-associated lipid mediators (PALMs), which, along with presentation of allergens by dendritic cells, stimulate a T helper type 2 (Th2)-driven immune response (Bieber, 2008; Bieber & Novak, 2009; Brandt & Sivaprasad, 2011). TSLP receptor activates STAT1, STAT3, STAT5/JAK1, and JAK2, which are important for Th2 cell differentiation (O'Shea & Plenge, 2012; Wohlmann, Sebastian, Borowski, Krause, & Friedrich, 2010).

These Th2 cells subsequently produce cytokines and chemokines, including IL4, IL5, IL13, and tumor necrosis factor-α (TNF-α), which stimulate B-cell class switching, immunoglobulin E (IgE) production, and eosinophil survival; induce proliferation of leukocyte adhesion molecules; and direct circulating lymphocytes, macrophages, and eosinophils to cutaneous sites of inflammation (Leung, Jain, & Leo, 2003; Leung & Soter, 2001). IL4 has been strongly associated with AD and requires numerous agents in the JAK-STAT pathway, including JAK1, JAK3, STAT3, STAT5, and STAT6 to enact its effects (Bao, Zhang, & Chan, 2013). IgE contributes to AD pathogenesis through mast cell activation and subsequent release of preformed mediators such as histamine, IL4, and IL13, as well as through increased expression of FCεRI on Langerhans and dendritic cells, which results in further Th2 activation (Elliott, Osna, Scofield, & Khan, 2001; Liu, Goodarzi, & Chen, 2011). Mast cells also stimulate further IgE synthesis by B cells, upregulate integrins on Langerhans cells, and suppress IL12 production by dendritic cells, leading to polarization to the Th2 subtype (Liu et al., 2011). Th2 cells also release IL31, which has been associated with higher disease severity, pruritus, chemotaxis of inflammatory cells, and induction of proinflammatory molecules by eosinophils through the JAK-STAT pathway (Brandt & Sivaprasad, 2011; Cheung et al., 2010; Ohsawa & Hirasawa, 2014). Eosinophils release various cytokines and chemokines such as IL16, IL12, transforming growth factor-β (TGF-β), and IL13 (Liu et al., 2011). The JAK-STAT pathway, through STAT6-mediated gene regulation, also stimulates B-cell differentiation, IgE class switching, and major histocompatibility complex (MHC) class II production (Bao et al., 2013).

Similar to the JAK-STAT pathway, JAK-spleen tyrosine kinase (SYK) pathways have also been associated with AD pathogenesis by mediating IL17R-proximal signaling

TABLE 23.1 **List of targeted treatment options for atopic dermatitis**

Name	Topical/ systemic	Manufacturer	Result	Phase	Major adverse events
Dupilumab	Systemic	Regeneron	Favorable		Conjunctivitis, keratitis, nasopharyngitis
Tralokinumab	Systemic	AstraZeneca	Favorable	3	Upper respiratory tract infection (URTI), headache
Lebrikizumab	Systemic	Dermira/Eli Lilly	Favorable	3	URTI, headache, nasopharyngitis
Omalizumab	Systemic	Novartis	Variable	N/A	Injection site reaction, URTI, malignancies
Ligelizumab	Systemic	Novartis	Unfavorable	2	Injection site reaction, URTI
Rituximab	Systemic	Genentech Biogen	Unfavorable	N/A	
Nemolizumab	Systemic	Galderma	Favorable	3	Nasopharyngitis, URTI, asthma-related exacerbations
Tofacitinib	Systemic	Pfizer	Favorable	2	Neutropenia, lymphopenia, herpes-zoster-associated encephalitis, appendicitis, pericoronitis, skin infection
Barticitinib	Systemic	Eli Lilly	Favorable	2	Neutropenia, lymphopenia, herpes-zoster-associated encephalitis, appendicitis, pericoronitis, skin infection
Abrocitinib	Systemic	Pfizer	Favorable	3	Neutropenia, lymphopenia, herpes-zoster-associated encephalitis, appendicitis, pericoronitis, skin infection
Upadacitinib	Systemic	AbbVie	Favorable	3	Infection, neutropenia, hepatic disorder, URTI, acne, headache, nasopharyngitis, diarrhea
Gusacitinib	Systemic	Asana Biosciences	Favorable	2	Neutropenia, lymphopenia, herpes-zoster-associated encephalitis, appendicitis, pericoronitis, skin infection
Delgococitinib	Topical	LEO Pharma	Favorable	2	Infection, neutropenia, URTI, acne, nasopharyngitis, hepatic disorder
Tacrolimus	Topical	Accord Healthcare	Variable		Skin infection, application pain
Pimecrolimus	Topical	Novartis	Variable		Skin infection, application pain
Crisaborole	Systemic	Pfizer	Favorable		Application pain
Apremilast	Systemic	Celgene	Favorable	2	Diarrhea, weight loss
Ustekinumab	Systemic	Janssen Biotech Inc.	Favorable	2	Infusion reaction, nasopharyngitis, URTI, malignancies
Risankizumab	Systemic	AbbVie	Favorable	2	URTI
Secukinumab	Systemic	Novartis	Favorable	2	Nasopharyngitis, hypertension
Fezakinumab	Systemic	Pfizer	Favorable	2	URTI
Asimadoline	Systemic	Tioga Pharmaceuticals		2	N/A
Tapinarof	Topical	Dermavant Sciences	Favorable	2	Folliculitis, contact dermatitis
JNJ 39758979	Systemic	Janssen Biotech Inc.	Unfavorable	2	Neutropenia
Adriforant	Systemic	Novartis		2	N/A
DS107	Topical, Systemic	DS Biopharma	Favorable	2	N/A
Aprepitant	Systemic	Merck Ltd.	Unfavorable		Leukopenia, hypotension
Serlopitant	Systemic	Menlo Therapeutics	Unfavorable	2	Nasopharyngitis, URTI
Rosiglitazone	Systemic	GlaxoSmithKline	Favorable	N/A	Weight gain

N/A, Complete data not available yet to fully access side effect profile.

complex formation, which is responsible for upregulation of CCL20 in keratinocytes (Wu, Huang, Tsou, Lin, & Lin, 2015). CCL20 has been found to attract immature dendritic cells and effector T cells into the dermis of inflamed skin (Nakayama et al., 2001). SYK activation has also been implicated in B-cell survival, degranulation of mast cells, antigen presentation in dendritic cells, and proinflammatory cytokine production by macrophages (Singh, Masuda, & Payan, 2012).

Th17 cells have also been implicated in the pathogenesis of AD as an enhancer, and an increased percentage of Th17 in blood correlates with the severity of AD (Koga, Kabashima, Shiraishi, Kobayashi, & Tokura, 2008). Th17 cells release IL17, which enters the inflamed dermis and stimulates keratinocytes to produce proinflammatory cytokines and chemokines, including GM-CSF, TNF-α, IL8, and CXCL10 (Koga et al., 2008). Patients with chronic AD have also been found to have increased blood levels of IL22-producing T cells (Nograles et al., 2009). IL22 induces keratinocyte proliferation and epidermal proliferation, and increased levels of IL22 are correlated with AD disease severity (Nograles et al., 2008).

Phosphodiesterase (PDE) functions to hydrolyze cyclic adenosine monophosphate (cAMP), and higher levels of PDE activity have been associated with increased IgE synthesis and IL4 production (Leung, 1999). Increased PDE activity is seen in leukocytes of patients with AD and is thought to contribute to increased serum levels of IL10 and prostaglandin E2 (Hanifin et al., 1996). IL12, which is stimulated by Th2-type cells, is thought to polarize naïve T cells to Th1-type cells and terminate Th2-type cytokine patterns (Grewe et al., 1998). A switch from Th2 cells to a predominantly Th1 cell response has been associated in the chronic and late phases of AD (Thepen et al., 1996). Increased levels of IL12, mRNA, and interferon-gamma (IFN-γ) (which are produced by Th1 cells) in AD lesions have also been linked to chronic AD (Hamid et al., 1996; Thepen et al., 1996).

Pruritus in AD is caused by numerous mediators, including histamine, neuropeptides, neurotransmitters, cytokines, proteinases, and arachidonic acid derivatives (Stander & Steinhoff, 2002). Histamine induces IL13 and IL31 production and activates sensory neurons, primarily through histamine-1 receptors (H_1R) and histamine-4 receptors (H_4R) (Ohsawa & Hirasawa, 2014). Through H_4R, histamine also activates mast cells, basophils, and eosinophils (Ohsawa & Hirasawa, 2014). One potent releaser of histamine from mast cells is compound 48/80, which, upon injection, has been shown to cause itching in mice (Sugimoto, Umakoshi, Nojiri, & Kamei, 1998). Similarly, increased concentrations of substance P, a neuropeptide that induces itching through neurokinin receptors (NK1R,) and neuropeptide Y are present in patients with AD (Heimall & Spergel, 2017).

Peroxisome proliferator-activated receptor gamma (PPAR-γ) is a type of nuclear receptor that has an increased expression in the monocytes and T lymphocytes of AD patients and is responsible for keratinocyte differentiation

and permeability barrier homeostasis (Dahten, Mergemeier, & Worm, 2007; Mao-Qiang et al., 2004).

Dihomo-γ-linolenic acid (DGLA) is a fatty acid that has been found to be significantly lower in the serum of patients with AD than in healthy volunteers (Manku et al., 1982). DGLA is also metabolized into antiinflammatory eicosanoids, and oral administration of DGLA in mice prevents the development of AD by suppressing the activation of mast cells and keratinocytes (Amagai et al., 2015; Kawashima et al., 2008).

Recalcitrant and moderate to severe AD often require systemic treatment. Immunosuppressants such as methotrexate, cyclosporine A, mycophenolate mofetil, and azathioprine have traditionally been used; however, significant side effect profiles can limit their long-term use. Newer immunomodulators (i.e., biologics and small-molecule inhibitors) selectively target specific cytokines and regulators involved in AD pathogenesis and have much more desirable side effect profiles.

Currently, the only Food and Drug Administration (FDA)–approved biologic medications for AD are dupilumab and crisaborole. There are a number of new and promising treatments currently under investigation. This chapter provides a summary and review of systemic therapies that target specific mediators involved in the pathogenesis of AD and its related symptoms. Included are those therapies that have been specifically approved for AD, those undergoing clinical trials, and those that have demonstrated efficacy to a significant degree.

Treatments targeting pathogenic cytokines

Anti-IL4

Dupilumab is currently the only FDA-approved systemic immunomodulator indicated for AD. It is fully a monoclonal antibody that inhibits IL4 and IL13 receptors by binding to the α-subunit shared by these receptors (Simpson et al., 2016). In two phase 3, randomized, double-blind, placebo-controlled, parallel-group trials of identical design involving a total of 1379 adults with moderate to severe AD refractory to topical treatment, significantly more patients who received dupilumab 300 mg subcutaneously every other week for 16 weeks reached the primary endpoint of an Investigator Global Assessment (IGA) score of 0 (clear) or 1 (almost clear) (38% and 36% for the dupilumab group vs. 10% and 8% for the placebo group, $P < .001$ for both comparisons vs. placebo) (Simpson et al., 2016). Furthermore, an improvement of 75% or more on Eczema Area and Severity Index (EASI-75) (which measures erythema, induration, papulation, and edema; excoriations, and lichenification) was achieved by significantly more patients who received dupilumab compared to patients receiving placebo (51% and 44% for the dupilumab group vs. 15% and 12% for the placebo group, $P < .001$ for both groups compared to placebo). Additionally, patients who completed this trial were able to enter an ongoing maintenance trial, a phase 3, randomized, double-blind, placebo-controlled, parallel-group trial involving 422 patients who were rerandomized in a 2:1:1:1 ratio to receive their original regimen of 300 mg dupilumab weekly or every 2 weeks, a less frequent regimen of 300 mg every 4 or 8 weeks, or placebo for 36 weeks (Worm et al., 2019). More patients who continued to receive dupilumab every week or every 2 weeks maintained EASI-75 response compared to those taking dupilumab every 4 weeks, 8 weeks, or placebo (71.6%, 58.3%, 54.9%, 30.4%, respectively; $P < .001$) (Worm et al., 2019). A phase 3, non-randomized, open-label, single-group assignment of dupilumab in adult patients who have participated in previous dupilumab clinical trials is currently ongoing (Open-label Study of Dupilumab in Patients With Atopic Dermatitis, 2019). In terms of side effects, dupilumab has been associated with an increased incidence of ocular surface diseases such as conjunctivitis and keratitis (Akinlade et al., 2019; Maudinet et al., 2019).

Anti-IL13

Tralokinumab is a fully monoclonal IgG4 monoclonal antibody that binds to and neutralizes the effects of IL13 via inhibition of signal transduction (May et al., 2012). In a phase 2b, randomized, double-blinded, placebo-controlled, parallel assignment, dose-ranging study involving 204 adults with moderate to severe AD lasting longer than 1 year, participants were randomized in a 1:1:1:1 ratio to receive placebo or tralokinumab (45, 150, or 300 mg) subcutaneously every 2 weeks for 12 weeks, with a 10-week follow-up period (Wollenberg et al., 2019). At 12 weeks, more patients who were treated with 300 mg of tralokinumab were found to have a significantly improved change in EASI score compared to patients who received placebo (adjusted mean difference = -4.94, $P = .01$). Additionally, improvements in IGA response rates were associated with increasing doses of tralokinumab, with the greatest absolute percentage difference from placebo being observed in participants who received 300 mg of tralokinumab (26.7% vs. 11.8%, $P = .06$). Patients treated with 300 mg of tralokinumab also had significant improvements in SCORAD, Dermatology Life Quality Index, and pruritus numeric rating scale versus placebo. Two randomized, double-blind, placebo-controlled, parallel assignment, phase 3 clinical trials involving 780 patients being given tralokinumab and/or placebo for 52 weeks are currently ongoing or completed, but results are not yet available (Tralokinumab Monotherapy for Moderate to Severe Atopic Dermatitis - ECZTRA 1 ECZema TRAlokinumab Trial no. 1 ECZTRA 1, 2017; Tralokinumab Monotherapy for Moderate to Severe Atopic Dermatitis - ECZTRA 2 ECZema TRAlokinumab Trial no. 2 ECZTRA 2, 2017).

Lebrikizumab is a humanized monoclonal antibody that binds to IL13 and inhibits signal transduction by blocking IL13α1/IL4Rα heterodimerization (Simpson et al., 2018).

In a randomized, placebo-controlled, double-blind, phase 2 study of 209 adults with moderate to severe AD who were treated with lebrikizumab 125 mg single dose, lebrikizumab 250 mg single dose, lebrikizumab 125 mg every 4 weeks for 12 weeks, or placebo every 4 weeks for 12 weeks, significantly more patients treated with lebrikizumab 125 mg every 4 weeks achieved EASI-50 at week 12 of the study compared to patients receiving placebo every 4 weeks (82.4% vs. 62.3%, $P = .26$) (Simpson et al., 2018). Additionally, the percentage of patients who achieved an IGA of 0 or 1 and the number of patients with SCORAD-50 was higher at week 12 in all lebrikizumab groups compared with placebo. A phase 2, randomized, double-blind, placebo-controlled, dose-ranging trial for lebrikizumab in 280 adult patients with moderate to severe atopic eczema lasting longer than 1 year was completed in 2019, but results are not yet available (A Study of Lebrikizumab in Patients With Moderate-to-Severe Atopic Dermatitis, 2018). Two phase 3, randomized, double-blind, placebo-controlled, parallel-group studies involving 400 child and adult patients with moderate to severe AD being treated with lebrikizumab monotherapy are currently recruiting and are expected to be completed in 2021 (Evaluation of the Efficacy & Safety of Lebrikizumab in Moderate to Severe Atopic Dermatitis ADvocate1, 2019; Evaluation of the Efficacy & Safety of Lebrikizumab in Moderate to Severe Atopic Dermatitis ADvocate2, 2019).

Anti-IL31

Nemolizumab is a humanized monoclonal antibody against IL34 receptor A and inhibits signaling of IL31, which plays a role in pruritus (Cornelissen, Luscher-Firzlaff, Baron, & Luscher, 2012; Ruzicka & Mihara, 2017). In a phase 2, randomized, double-blind, placebo-controlled, multicenter, 12-week trial of 264 adults with moderate to severe AD refractory to topical glucocorticoids or topical calcineurin inhibitors who were given subcutaneous nemolizumab at a dose of 0.1 mg, 0.5 mg, or 2 mg per kilogram of body weight, or placebo every 4 weeks, or 2 mg nemolizumab/kg every 8 weeks with placebo given at week 4, there was significant dose-dependent reduction in pruritus from baseline as measured by the pruritus visual-analogue scale (VAS); reductions of 43.7%, 59.8%, and 63.1% were seen in the 0.1 mg/kg, 0.5 mg/kg, and 2.0 mg/kg groups, respectively, compared to a 20.9% reduction seen with the placebo ($P = .002$, $P < .001$, $P < .001$) (Ruzicka et al., 2017). Participants treated with nemolizumab also experienced significant reductions in pruritus verbal rating scale, improvements in EASI score and SCORAD, and improvements in mean percentage changes from baseline in sleep disturbance-VAS (-52.3%, -59.1%, and -62.6% for 0.1 mg/kg, 0.5 mg/kg, and 2.0 mg/kg vs. -31.9% with placebo). A follow-up study in which patients continued their previous nemolizumab dose every 4 weeks or every 8 weeks for 52 weeks in a double-blind extension found that there were maintained or decreased pruritus VAS scores from week 12 to week 64 in patients randomized to receive nemolizumab, with the greatest improvement occurring in the 0.5 mg/kg group (Kabashima et al., 2018). Mean percentage change from baseline in EASI score, SCORAD score, and sleep disturbance-VAS scores were also maintained or decreased from week 12 to week 64. Patients who received placebo in the previous study and switched to nemolizumab at week 12 experienced a favorable response to treatment in pruritus VAS score by week 16 and maintained this response through week 64. A phase 2, randomized, double-blind, multicenter, parallel-group, placebo-controlled, dose-ranging study of 351 adults with moderate to severe AD who were randomized into a nemolizumab 10 mg group, nemolizumab 30 mg group, nemolizumab 90 mg group, and a placebo group found that percent change from baseline in EASI at week 24 was −72.2%, −73.4%, −69.2%, and −58.4%, respectively, and demonstrated reductions in EASI scores that were statistically significant for nemolizumab compared to placebo for the 10 mg and 30 mg treatment groups ($P = .051$, $P = .016$), but not for the 90 mg treatment group ($P = .322$) (Dose-ranging Study of Nemolizumab in Atopic Dermatitis, 2017). A phase 2, multicenter, open-label, single-group clinical trial to assess the safety of nemolizumab in adolescents with AD is currently recruiting (A Pharmacokinetics and Safety Study of Nemolizumab in Adolescent Participants With Atopic Dermatitis (AD), 2019).

Anti-IL12/23

Ustekinumab, which is approved for the treatment of plaque psoriasis, is a fully humanized monoclonal antibody that neutralizes IL12 and IL23 by targeting the shared p40 subunit, causing regulation of Th1 and Th17/Th22 responses (Khattri et al., 2017; Leonardi et al., 2008). In a phase 2, double-blinded, placebo-controlled, crossover study of 32 adult patients with moderate to severe chronic AD who were given subcutaneous ustekinumab (45 mg and 90 mg per injection for patients weighing <100 kg or >100 kg, respectively) or placebo at weeks 0, 4, and 16 with a crossover at weeks 16, 20, and 32, for 40 weeks, the ustekinumab group achieved higher SCORAD50 response at 12 weeks, 16 weeks, and 20 weeks compared to placebo, but the difference was not statistically significant (Khattri et al., 2017). In a phase 2, randomized, double-blind, placebo-controlled, multicenter, parallel-group study of 79 adult Japanese patients with severe or very severe AD who were given 45 mg or 90 mg ustekinumab or placebo subcutaneous injections at 0 weeks and 4 weeks with a primary efficacy endpoint in percent change from baseline in EASI score at week 12, ustekinumab treatment demonstrated nonsignificant improvement in least-square mean change from baseline EASI score at week 12 (45 mg: −38.2, $P < .95$; 90 mg: −39.8%, $P < .81$; vs. placebo: −37.5%) and nonsignificant improvements in IGA, EASI-50, and EASI-75 (Saeki et al., 2017).

Risankisumab is another anti-IL23 humanized IgG monoclonal antibody that has been approved by several countries for treatment of moderate to severe plaque psoriasis (McKeage & Duggan, 2019). A phase 2, multicenter, randomized, double-blinded, placebo-controlled, parallel assignment study of 155 children and older adults with moderate to severe AD receiving double-blind placebo for 16 weeks followed by risankizumab dose 1 or 2 for 24 weeks is currently ongoing and is estimated to be completed in April 2021 (A Study to Evaluate Risankizumab in Adult & Adolescent Subjects With Moderate to Severe Atopic Dermatitis, 2018).

Anti-IL17

Secukinumab is a recombinant human monoclonal antibody that selectively targets IL17A and prevents its binding to the IL17 receptor, causing neutralization of the proinflammatory cytokine cascade (Frieder, Kivelevitch, & Menter, 2018). In a case report of an adult male with severe refractory AD, administration of subcutaneous secukinumab 300 mg caused a 66% improvement in SCORAD and marked improvement in erythema and pruritus after 16 weeks of treatment (Frieder et al., 2018). A phase 2, multicenter, randomized, double-blind, parallel-assignment pilot study of 41 adult participants with moderate to severe AD receiving secukinumab (300 mg SQ every 2 weeks) has been completed, but results are not yet available, and a phase 2, randomized, placebo-controlled, parallel-assignment, double-blind study of 45 adult participants receiving secukinumab (300 mg SQ every 2 weeks) is currently recruiting (Secukinumab for Treatment of Atopic Dermatitis, 2015; Investigation of Efficacy of Secukinumab, 2018).

Anti-IL22

Fezakinumab (ILV-094) is a fully human monoclonal antibody against IL22, which promotes keratinocyte proliferation and upregulation of antimicrobial peptides in the epidermis (Brunner et al., 2019). In a phase 2a, randomized, double-blind, placebo-controlled, multicenter clinical trial of 60 adult patients with moderate to severe AD who were given IV fezakinumab (600 mg loading dose, 300 mg every 2 weeks) or placebo for 10 weeks, patients who had severe AD and received fezakinumab experienced significant reductions in SCORAD compared to placebo at 12 weeks (21.6 vs. 9.6, $P = .029$) and at 20 weeks (27.4 vs. 11.5, $P = .010$), as well as improvements in IGA versus placebo (0.7 vs. 0.3, $P = .34$) (Guttman-Yassky et al., 2018). However, there were less significant reductions in SCORAD, BSA, and IGA observed in patients with moderate AD receiving fezakinumab compared to those with severe AD. In a phase 2a, randomized, placebo-controlled, multicenter clinical trial of 59 adult participants who were given IV fezakinumab (600 mg loading dose, 300 mg every 2 weeks) or placebo every 10 weeks, it was found that participants treated with fezakinumab experienced significantly greater reversal of the AD genomic profile versus placebo (25.3% vs. 10.5% at 4 weeks, $P = 1.7 \times 10^{-5}$; 65.5% vs. 13.9% at 12 weeks, $P = 9.5 \times 10^{-19}$) (Brunner et al., 2019).

Treatments targeting pathogenic antibodies: Anti-IgE

Omalizumab is a humanized anti-IgE IgG monoclonal antibody that prevents the binding of IgE to FCεRI and CD23 on B cells, causing a reduced number of FCεRI on basophils and reduced IgE synthesis by B cells, resulting in decreased expression of proinflammatory cytokines such as IL5, IL8, and IL13 (Chang, Wu, Hsu, & Hung, 2007; Noga, Hanf, & Kunkel, 2003; Schulman, 2001). Omalizumab has demonstrated significant efficacy in both pediatric and adult patients with AD (Andres, Belloni, Mempel, & Ring, 2008; Iyengar et al., 2013; Kim, Park, Kim, Kim, & Mun, 2013; Lane, Cheyney, Lane, Kent, & Cohen, 2006; Romano et al., 2015; Sheinkopf, Rafi, Do, Katz, & Klaustermeyer, 2008; Vigo et al., 2006). However, several studies have also demonstrated no improvement of disease with omalizumab therapy, and it is hypothesized that lack of filaggrin mutations and lower elevations of total serum IgE are associated with a favorable response to omalizumab (Heil, Maurer, Klein, Hultsch, & Stingl, 2010; Hotze et al., 2014; Thaiwat & Sangasapaviliya, 2011).

Ligelizumab is another anti-IgE monoclonal antibody that binds to the Cε3 domain of IgE and inhibits the binding of free IgE to mast cells and basophils. Two randomized, placebo-controlled, double-blind clinical trials of 183 adults with a history of atopy found that ligelizumab demonstrated greater of suppression of serum IgE and IgE bound to mast cells and basophils compared to omalizumab (Arm et al., 2014). Similarly, a double-blind, randomized, placebo-controlled, parallel-group multicenter study in 37 adult subjects with mild allergic asthma comparing the effects of ligelizumab to omalizumab found that there was a greater inhibition of skin prick test response with ligelizumab compared to omalizumab ($P < .0001$) (Gauvreau et al., 2016). A phase 2, randomized, double-blinded, placebo-controlled, parallel-group, proof of concept study of 22 adult participants with moderate to severe AD has been completed, but results have not yet been published (A study evaluating the safety and efficacy of QGE031 in atopic dermatitis patients, 2017).

Treatment targeting immune cells: Anti-CD20

Rituximab is a chimeric monoclonal anti-CD20 antibody that causes decreased immunomodulatory functions and loss of antigen presenting capability by B cells (Silverman & Weisman, 2003; Simon, Hosli, Kostylina, Yawalkar, & Simon, 2008). An open-label pilot study of four women and two men with severe AD who were refractory to topical corticosteroid and/or calcineurin inhibitor therapy were given two doses of 1000 mg of rituximab, 2 weeks apart (Simon et al., 2008). All patients experienced significant improvement of AD lesions within 4 to 8 weeks of treatment, as measured by their EASI scores (29.4 ± 4.3 at baseline vs. 8.4 ± 3.6 at 8 weeks, $P < .001$), and EASI scores remained low at weeks 16 and 24. There was also a reduction of spontaneous IL13 production by peripheral blood mononuclear cells ex vivo (25.7 ± 5.7 pg/mL vs. 5.5 ± 4.1 pg/mL, $P = .18$), indicating a reduction of activated T cells in blood. Skin histology following treatment was notable for decreased hyperkeratosis, acanthosis, spongiosis, and dermal inflammatory cells. In a case study of three adult patients with severe AD unresponsive to standard therapy, patients experienced a reduction in peripheral blood CD19+ B-cell numbers following rituximab treatment, but they did not experience significant clinical benefit as measured by EASI (McDonald, Jones, & Rustin, 2016).

Treatments targeting immune signaling: JAK-STAT/JAK-SYK

Systemic JAK inhibitors

Tofacitinib is a small-molecule janus kinase-1 (JAK1) inhibitor that inhibits cytokines directly and leads to attenuation of JAK-STAT signaling in keratinocytes (Bissonnette et al., 2016; Meyer et al., 2010). In a phase 2a, multisite, randomized, double-blind, vehicle-controlled, parallel-group study, 69 adults with mild to moderate AD were randomized 1:1 to 2% tofacitinib or vehicle ointment twice daily for 4 weeks (Bissonnette et al., 2016). Percentage change from baseline at week 4 in EASI score was significantly greater for the tofacitinib group compared to vehicle (-81.7% vs. 29.9%, $P < .001$), and a greater proportion of patients treated with tofacitinib had a Physician's Global Assessment (PGA) of clear or almost clear compared to those on placebo (73% vs. 22%, $P < .05$). In a case series of six adult patients with moderate to severe AD refractory to standard therapy, 5 mg of oral tofacitinib administered twice daily in five patients and 5 mg once daily in one patient for 29 weeks significantly decreased body surface area of dermatitis, with improvement in erythema, edema/papulation, excoriation, lichenification, pruritus, decreased sleep loss, and a decrease in the composite scoring of AD (SCORAD) index by an average of 54.8% ($P < .05$) during the initial 4 to 14 weeks (Levy, Urban, & King, 2015). This improvement was maintained with a subsequent reduction of 66.6% ($P < .05$) observed during weeks 8 to 29 of treatment.

A phase 3, multicenter, open-label study of baricitinib, a selective JAK1/2 inhibitor approved for rheumatoid arthritis treatment, in 300 adult patients with moderate to severe AD is currently recruiting (A Study of Baricitinib LY3009104 in Participants With Moderate to Severe Atopic Dermatitis BREEZE-AD6, 2018). Likewise, a phase 3, multicenter, randomized, double-blind, placebo-controlled, parallel-group, outpatient study evaluating the safety and efficacy of baricitinib in 465 pediatric patients with moderate to severe

AD is also recruiting (A Study of Baricitinib LY3009104 in Children & Adolescents With Atopic Dermatitis BREEZE-AD-PEDS, 2019).

A phase 2b, randomized, double-blind, placebo-controlled, parallel, multicenter, dose-ranging study of abrocitinib, a JAK1 inhibitor, in adults with moderate to severe AD in 267 adult patients with moderate to severe AD randomized into 10 mg, 30 mg, 100 mg, 200 mg of abrocitinib once daily, and placebo groups for 12 weeks found that a statistically significantly greater percentage of patients in the 100 mg and 200 mg treatment groups achieved grades of clear or almost clear on the IGA scale, with improvement of two grades or more compared to placebo ($P = .0184$, $P = .0032$). Patients in the 100 mg and 200 mg treatment groups also achieved more EASI-75 responses than patients in the placebo group ($P = .004$, $P < .001$) (Gooderham et al., 2019). A phase 3, randomized, double-blind, placebo-controlled, multicenter study of adolescents with moderate to severe AD treated with abrocitinib and a phase 3, randomized, double-blind, placebo-controlled, parallel group multicenter study to evaluate PF-0496582 monotherapy in participants over age 12 years with moderate to severe AD are also recruiting (JAK1 Inhibitor With Medicated, 2019; Study Evaluating Efficacy & Safety of PF-04965842 in Subjects Aged 12 Years And Older With Moderate to Severe Atopic Dermatitis JADE Mono-2, 2018).

Gusacitinib is an oral dual inhibitor of JAK and SYK kinases. In a phase 1b, randomized, double-blind, placebo-controlled multicenter study of 36 adult patients with moderate to severe AD who were given ASN002 (20 mg, 40 mg, or 80 mg) or placebo once daily for 28 days, significantly higher proportions of patients who received ASN002 (40 mg or 80 mg daily) achieved EASI-50 (100% and 83%, $P = .003$ and $P = .03$, respectively) at day 29 compared to placebo; no significant difference was seen between the 20 mg group and the placebo group (Bissonnette et al., 2019). Patients in the 40 mg group also experienced a significant decrease in change from baseline in BSA at day 29 (-21.6, $P = .03$) compared to placebo, and a significant decrease from baseline in weekly average pruritus numeric rating scale in the 80 mg group at day 29 (-4.7, $P = .01$) compared to placebo. A phase 2b, randomized, double-blind, placebo-controlled, parallel-assignment study to evaluate efficacy, safety, tolerability, and pharmacokinetics of ASN002 in adults with moderate to severe AD is ongoing (Phase 2B Study to Evaluate ASN002 in Subjects With Moderate to Severe Atopic Dermatitis RADIANT, 2018).

Upadacitinib is an oral JAK-1 inhibitor originally developed for the treatment of rheumatoid arthritis. It has a higher selectivity for JAK-1 over JAL-2 and JAK-3, and thus has a better safety profile with limited hematologic abnormalities such as cytopenia (Serhal & Edwards, 2019). In a phase 2, randomized, parallel-assignment, placebo-controlled study of 166 participants with moderate to severe AD who were randomized in a 1:1:1:1 ratio to receive upadacitinib 7.5 mg, 15 mg, 30 mg, or placebo for 16 weeks, investigators found that there was a significantly higher improvement from baseline in the upadacitinib treatment groups compared to the placebo group as measured by EASI score (39%, $P = .03$; 62%, $P < .001$; and 74%, $P < .001$ vs. placebo 23%, respectively), with a dose-response relationship (Guttman-Yassky et al., 2020). A phase 3, randomized, double-blind, parallel-group, placebo-controlled study evaluating the safety and efficacy of upadacitinib in 847 adult and adolescent participants with moderate to severe AD who were given upatacinib 15 mg, upadacitinib 30 mg, or placebo for 16 weeks found that those in the 15 mg and 30 mg treatment groups demonstrated significant improvement as measured by EASI scores (RINVOQ upadacitinib Monotherapy Shows Improvement in Skin Clearance & Itch in First Phase 3 Study for Atopic Dermatitis, 2020); 70% of participants in the 15 mg treatment group and 80% of participants in the 30 mg treatment group achieved EASI-75 at week 16, compared to 16% in the placebo group ($P < .001$). Patients in both treatment groups also experienced significantly greater improvement in Worst Pruritus Numerical Rating Scale (NRS) compared to placebo (52%, 60%, 12%, $P < .001$, respectively), and experienced significantly greater improvement in IGA-AD scores compared to patients in the placebo group (48%, 62%, 8%, $P < .001$, respectively). There is a phase 3, randomized, double-blind, active controlled study in which 692 participants will be given oral upadacitinib for 24 weeks and placebo injections for 22 weeks or dupilumab injections for 22 weeks and placebo tablets for 24 weeks (A Study to Compare Safety & Efficacy of Upadacitinib to Dupilumab in Adult Participants With Moderate to Severe Atopic Dermatitis, 2018).

JAK inhibitors have been associated with a number of adverse effects, including polyneuropathy, pancytopenia, dermatologic infections, increases in serum high-density lipoprotein, low-density lipoprotein, and total cholesterol, and gastrointestinal complaints (Shreberk-Hassidim, Ramot, & Zlotogorski, 2017).

Topical JAK inhibitors

Delgocitinib is a topical JAK inhibitor that inhibits JAK1, JAK2, JAK 3, and tyrosine kinase 2 (Tanimoto et al., 2015). A phase 2, randomized, double-blind, vehicle-controlled study of 103 pediatric patients randomized in a 1:1:1 ratio to receive 0.25% or 0.5% delgocitinib ointment or a vehicle ointment for 4 weeks demonstrated that at the end of treatment, mEASI scores in both delgocitinib groups were significantly more reduced compared to the vehicle group (0.25% group: -54.2%, $P < .001$; 0.5% group: -61.8%, $P < .001$) (Nakagawa et al., 2019). In a phase 2, randomized, vehicle-controlled, intergroup comparison study involving 327 adult patients assigned to a vehicle group, delgocitinib 0.25% group, delgocitinib 0.5% group, delgocitinib 1% group, delgocitinib 3% group, and a tacrolimus group twice daily for 4 weeks found that changes in the least-squares mean percentage from baseline in mEASI scores for the delgocitinib 0.25%, 0.5%, 1%, and 3% groups were -41.7%, $-57/1$, -72.9%, and -12%, respectively, which were signifi-cantly reduced compared to the vehicle group

($P < .001$). As of 2020 there have been no head-to-head trials comparing topical JAK inhibitors to other nonsteroidal antiinflammatory pharmaceuticals in patients with AD.

A phase 1, nonrandomized, parallel-assignment, open-label, pilot pharmacokinetic study of ruxolitinib (JAK1/2 inhibitor) phosphate cream, in 60 pediatric patients with AD is currently active (A Pharmacokinetic Study of Ruxolitinib Phosphate Cream in Pediatric Subjects With Atopic Dermatitis, 2017).

A phase 2, randomized, dose-ranging, vehicle-controlled and triamcinolone 0.1% cream-controlled study to establish safety and efficacy of ruxolitinib phosphate cream in adults with AD has also been completed, but results are not yet available (A Pharmacokinetic Study of Ruxolitinib Phosphate Cream in Pediatric Subjects With Atopic Dermatitis, 2017).

Calcineurin inhibitors

Tacrolimus and pimecrolimus are calcineurin inhibitors that bind to FK506-binding protein (FKBP), thereby inhibiting the activation of calcineurin and its downstream signaling pathway; this results in decreased production of inflammatory cytokines (Nghiem, Pearson, & Langley, 2002). Tacrolimus and pimecrolimus have the same mechanisms of action, but pimecrolimus has an altered skin penetration profile (Nghiem et al., 2002). A meta-analysis of 12 independent randomized clinical trials comparing topical calcineurin inhibitors to topical corticosteroids in the treatment of AD in pediatric and adult patients found that there were similar improvements (81% vs. 71%, $P = .01$) and treatment success (72% vs. 68%, $P = .04$) (Broeders, Ahmed Ali, & Fischer, 2016). The number of adverse events and adverse events related to treatment was higher in patients treated with calcineurin inhibitors compared to those treated with corticosteroids (adverse events: 74% vs. 64%, $P = .02$; adverse events related to treatment: 11% vs. 8%, $P = .002$).

Phosphodiesterase inhibitors

Crisaborole is a topical antiinflammatory PDE4 inhibitor that causes inhibition of proinflammatory and T-cell cytokine production (Hoy, 2017). In two identically designed, vehicle-controlled, double-blind studies (AD-301 and AD-302), 1522 patients age 2 years and older with AD were given crisaborole ointment twice daily for 28 days or a vehicle (Paller et al., 2016). Patients treated with crisaborole achieved higher Investigator's Static Global Assessment (ISGA) scores at day 29 compared to those treated with vehicle (AD-301: 32.8% vs. 25.4%, $P = .38$; AD-302: 31.4% vs. 18.0%, $P < .001$). A phase 4, multicenter, open-label safety study of crisaborole ointment in 137 children age 3 months to less than 24 months with mild to moderate AD has been completed, but results are not yet available (A Study of Crisaborole Ointment 2% in Children Aged 3-24 Months With Mild to Moderate Atopic Dermatitis, 2017).

Apremilast is an oral PDE4 inhibitor approved for the treatment of adults with moderate to severe psoriasis and psoriatic arthritis (Maloney, Zhao, Tegtmeyer, Lee, & Cheng, 2019). A phase 2, double-blind, placebo-controlled trial of 185 patients with moderate to severe AD who received apremilast 30 mg twice daily, 40 mg twice daily, or placebo for 12 weeks found that at week 12, patients who received apremilast 40 mg twice daily showed significantly greater improvement from baseline in EASI score compared to patients who received placebo (−31.6% vs. −11%, $P < .04$) (Simpson et al., 2019). Tissue biomarker data in patients taking apremilast 40 mg twice daily also showed substantial reductions in epidermal hyperplasia and inflammatory markers. Of note, those taking apremilast 30 mg twice daily did not experience statistically significant changes in EASI score versus placebo and did not have notable changes in inflammatory biomarkers. In a case series of four adults with AD since childhood who were treated with apremilast for 10 weeks to 9 months, there was clearance or reduction of eczematous papules, erythema, plaques, and pruritus (Abrouk et al., 2017).

Opioid agonists

Initially developed for treatment of irritable bowel syndrome, asimadoline is a peripherally acting κ-opioid agonist that has also been found to inhibit the itch caused by compound 48/80 (Cowan, Kehner, & Inan, 2015; Tey & Yosipovitch, 2011). A phase 2, randomized, double-blind, single-group assignment study evaluating the efficacy of asimadoline in adults with AD with pruritus is completed, but results are not yet available (Safety, Pharmacokinetics, & Preliminary Efficacy of Asimadoline in Pruritus Associated With Atopic Dermatitis, 2015).

Aryl hydrocarbon receptor (AhR) agonists

Tapinarof (5-[(E)-2-phenylethenyl]-2-[propan-2-yl] benzene-1, 3-diol) is a nonsteroidal, fully synthetic, hydroxylated stilbene compound classified as an AhR modulating agent that binds and activates the AhR, causing downregulation of proinflammatory cytokine expression and impacting barrier gene expression in human keratinocytes (Smith et al., 2017). In a phase 1, open-label, two-cohort sequential study that assessed the pharmacokinetics, safety, and efficacy of tapinarof in 11 adults with moderate to severe AD, administration of tapinarof (1% or 2%) resulted in at least 50% total EASI by day 21 and a decrease in pruritus (Bissonnette et al., 2018). In a phase 2, randomized, double-blind, vehicle-controlled, six-arm, multicenter trial of 247 adult patients with AD who were given tapinarof 1% twice daily, tapinarof 1% once daily, tapinarof 0.5% twice daily, tapinarof 0.5% once daily, vehicle twice daily, or vehicle once daily, the rate of treatment success, as measured by IGA score, with tapinarof 1% twice daily was statistically significantly higher than the rate with vehicle twice daily (53% vs. 24%, $\alpha = 0.05$ level) (Peppers et al., 2019).

Anti-H4 receptor (H4R)

JNJ 39758979 [(R)-4-(3-amino-pyrrolidin-1-yl)-6-isopropyl-pyrimidin-2-ylamine] is an H4R antagonist that has demonstrated effectiveness in reducing pruritus in healthy subjects (Kollmeier et al., 2014). In a phase 2a, randomized, double-blind, placebo-controlled, multicenter, parallel-group study of 88 Japanese adults with moderate AD who were administered one JNJ-3975879 (100 mg and 300 mg) or placebo, decreases in median EASI were observed (−3.7 and −3.0, respectively), but these changes were not significant compared to placebo (−1.30, $P = 1.672$ and 0.1992, respectively) (Murata et al., 2015). The trial was also prematurely discontinued due to side effects of neutropenia.

In a phase 2, randomized, double-blind, placebo-controlled, parallel group study, 98 adult participants with moderate to severe AD were administered adrifanant (30 mg orally daily) for 8 weeks (A Study to Determine the Efficacy of ZPL-3893787 in Subjects With Atopic Dermatitis, 2015). This study has been completed, but results are not yet available.

Dihomo-γ-linolenic acid (DGLA)

DS107 is an agent containing DGLA (DS Biopharma announces positive top-line phase IIa trial results for DS107 as an oral treatment for moderate to severe atopic dermatitis, 2018). In a phase 2a, randomized, placebo-controlled, parallel assignment trial of 102 adult participants with moderate to severe AD who received oral DS107 or placebo, patients administered DS107 experienced a statistically significant decrease in IGA compared to placebo ($P = .57$) as well as a statistically significant reduction of itch assessed by VAS compared to placebo ($P = .015$) (Oral DS107G in moderate to severe atopic dermatitis, 2017; DS Biopharma, 2016). In a phase 2b, randomized, double-blind, multicenter, vehicle-controlled study in which 326 patients with mild to moderate AD were given DS107 cream (1% and 5%) or placebo, patients receiving DS107 experienced a dose-dependent response in IGA and EASI-75, and those administered 5% DS107 cream achieved statistically significant changes in both IGA and EASI-75 ($P = .029$ and .019, respectively) (DS Biopharma announces positive top-line phase 2b trial results for DS107 as a topical treatment for mild to moderate atopic dermatitis, 2018). A phase 2, randomized, double-blind, placebo-controlled, parallel assignment study to assess efficacy and safety of oral DS107 in adult patients with moderate to severe AD is currently recruiting (Efficacy and Safety of Orally Administered DS107 in Adult Patients With Moderate to Severe Atopic Dermatitis, 2019).

Neurokinin-1 receptor (NK1-R) antagonist

NK1-R antagonists prevent the interaction between NKR-1 and substance P, which is involved in the pathogenesis of nonhistaminergic pruritus (Kulka, Sheen, Tancowny, Grammer, & Schleimer, 2008). Aprepitant is an oral NK1-R antagonist approved for treatment of nausea during chemotherapy (Lonndahl et al., 2018). In a prospective study of 20 patients with chronic pruritus refractory to therapy who were treated with aprepitant 80 mg for 3 to 13 days, patients experienced a significant decrease in pruritus intensity on the VAS (8.4 at baseline vs. 4.9 after treatment, $P < .001$) (Stander, Siepmann, Herrgott, Sunderkotter, & Luger, 2010). In an open, randomized trial of 39 patients with moderate to severe AD who were given aprepitant 80 mg daily for 7 days (n = 19) or topical treatment alone (n = 20), there were significant reductions in SCORAD (40.5–32.0, $P < .01$), mean VAS (5.5–3.8, $P < .05$), and scratching movements (77.3–48.3, $P < .05$) in the aprepitant group (Lonndahl et al., 2018). However, these reductions were not significant when compared to the control group.

Serlopitant is a NK1-R antagonist developed for chronic use in treatment of overactive bladder (Yosipovitch et al., 2018). In a phase 2, randomized, double-blind, parallel-group, placebo-controlled, multicenter, dose finding and efficacy study of 222 adult participants with pruritus lasting longer than 6 weeks refractory to antihistamines and steroids who were given serlopitant (0.25 mg, 1 mg, or 5 mg) or placebo once daily for 6 weeks, participants taking 1 mg and 5 mg of serlopitant experienced a dose-dependent decrease in VAS pruritus score compared to placebo ($P = .022$ and $P = .13$, respectively) (VPD-737 for Treatment of Chronic Pruritus, 2013; Yosipovitch et al., 2018). Mean overall Dermatology Life Quality Index (DQLI) was also lower in treatment groups, although statistically significant improvements were only seen in the 1 mg group. In a phase 2, randomized, double-blind, placebo-controlled, parallel assignment study of 484 adults and adolescents with pruritus who were given daily oral doses of serlopitant (1 mg or 5 mg) or placebo for 6 weeks, there was no significant decrease in Worst Itch Numeric Rating Scale (WI-NRS) score in either treatment group ($P = .11$ and $P = .17$, respectively) by the end of the treatment period (California: Menlo Therapeutics Inc, 2018).

In a phase 2, randomized, double-blind, placebo-controlled multicenter study of 168 adult subjects with chronic, AD-associated pruritus refractory to antihistamine and corticosteroids, participants were either given placebo or oral tradipitant (VLY-686), another NK1-R, for 8 weeks (Tradipitant in Treatment-resistant Pruritus Associated With Atopic Dermatitis, 2016). Subjects receiving trapiditant experienced significantly greater improvement on the worst itch VAS scale (−44.2 vs. −30.6, $P = .019$), the total SCORAD index (−21.3 vs. −13.6, $P = .008$), objective SCORAD (−13.3 vs. −7.2, $P = .005$), Clinician Global Impression of Change (CGI-C) (2.6 vs. 3.3, $P = .007$), Patient Global Impression of Change (PGI-C) itch (2.6 vs. 3.2, $P = .025$), and PGI-C AD (2.7 vs. 3.5, $P = .007$) compared to placebo (Evaluating the Effects of Tradipitant vs. Placebo in Atopic Dermatitis, 2018). An earlier phase 2, randomized, double-blind, placebo-controlled, proof of concept study in 69 adult participants with AD and chronic pruritus who were given oral tradipitant or placebo for 4 weeks also demonstrated significant improvement in VAS for itch from baseline for patients who received tradipitant ($P < .0001$) (Proof of concept of VLY-686 in subjects with treatment-resistant pruritus associated with atopic dermatitis, 2013; DS Biopharma, 2016). However, the change was not significant compared to placebo. A phase 3, randomized, double-blind, placebo-controlled, parallel-assignment, efficacy study of tradipitant in adult patients with chronic pruritus and AD is currently recruiting (Heitman et al., 2018).

PPAR-γ

Rosiglitazone is a PPAR-γ agonist approved for treatment of type 2 diabetes mellitus that has been shown to inhibit TLSP-induced dendritic cell maturation and reduce severity of skin lesions and scratching behavior in mice (Behshad, Cooper, & Korman, 2008; Jung et al., 2011). In a case series of six patients with severe AD, the addition of rosiglitazone (2–4 mg PO twice daily) to treatment with corticosteroids, antihistamines, and/or calcineurin inhibitors caused a BSA reduction of more than 65% in five patients and a decreased number of flares compared with baseline (Behshad et al., 2008).

Summary

Traditional therapies for AD are limited to immunosuppressants whose use can be limited by harmful and unwanted side effects. The development of targeted treatments offers safer and more specific options. Although many of the therapies mentioned in this chapter have shown much promise, only two, crisaborole and dupilumab, have been approved by the FDA for use in AD patients. Furthermore, these new treatment options are often expensive and costly. As of January 2020, the list price for Dupixent is $3019.50 for a 4-week supply (How Much Should). To usher in this new era of AD therapy, further large-scale, randomized, placebo-controlled, double-blind, multicenter trials are needed to determine efficacy and safety. More research into the specific mediators and their receptors involved in the pathogenesis of AD may also be beneficial so that further potential therapies can be developed and tested in head-to-head trials and subanalyses, and evaluated among different patient demographics. It is also necessary to conduct large-scale trials in pediatric populations due to the significantly higher prevalence of AD in this population (Bieber, 2008). Finally, trials involving a combination of target-specific treatments would be very valuable to determine drug interactions. Table 23.1 summarizes the list of currently available and emerging targeted treatment medications for AD.

Further readings

Baldo, B. A. (2016). *Safety of biologics therapy: Monoclonal antibodies, cytokines, fusion proteins, hormones, enzymes, coagulation proteins, vaccines, botulinum toxins*. Springer.

Lafaille, J. J., & Curotto de Lafaille, M. A. (Eds.), (2015). *IgE antibodies: Generation and function*. Springer.

Schneider, R., & Leonard, W. J. (Eds.), (2018). *Cytokines: From basic mechanisms of cellular control to new therapeutics (Perspectives CSHL)*. Cold Spring Harbor Laboratory Press.

References

A Pharmacokinetic Study of Ruxolitinib Phosphate Cream in Pediatric Subjects With Atopic Dermatitis. (2017). ClinicalTrials.gov.

A Pharmacokinetics and Safety Study of Nemolizumab in Adolescent Participants With Atopic Dermatitis. (2019). ClinicalTrials.gov.

A Study Evaluating the Safety and Efficacy of QGE031 in Atopic Dermatitis Patients. (2012). ClinicalTrials.gov.

A Study of Baricitinib (LY3009104) in Children and Adolescents With Atopic Dermatitis (BREEZE-AD-PEDS). (2019). ClinicalTrials.gov.

A Study of Baricitinib (LY3009104) in Participants With Moderate to Severe Atopic Dermatitis (BREEZE-AD6). (2018). ClinicalTrials.gov.

A Study of Crisaborole Ointment 2% in Children Aged 3-24 Months With Mild to Moderate Atopic Dermatitis. (2017). ClinicalTrials.gov.

A Study of Lebrikizumab in Patients With Moderate-to-Severe Atopic Dermatitis. (2018). ClinicalTrials.gov.

A Study to Compare Safety and Efficacy of Upadacitinib to Dupilumab in Adult Participants With Moderate to Severe Atopic Dermatitis. (2018). ClinicalTrials.gov.

A Study to Evaluate Risankizumab in Adult and Adolescent Subjects With Moderate to Severe Atopic Dermatitis. (2018). ClinicalTrials.gov.

A Study to Evaluate the Safety and Efficacy of Ruxolitinib Phosphate Cream Applied Topically to Adults With Atopic Dermatitis. (2017). ClinicalTrials.gov.

Abrouk, M., Farahnik, B., Zhu, T. H., Nakamura, M., Singh, R., Lee, K., et al. (2017). Apremilast treatment of atopic dermatitis and other chronic eczematous dermatoses. *Journal of the American Academy of Dermatology, 77*(1), 177–180. https://doi.org/10.1016/j.jaad.2017.03.020. https://www.ncbi.nlm.nih.gov/pubmed/28619562.

Akinlade, B., Guttman-Yassky, E., de Bruin-Weller, M., Simpson, E. L., Blauvelt, A., Cork, M. J., et al. (2019). Conjunctivitis in dupilumab clinical trials. *British Journal of Dermatology, 181*(3), 459–473. https://doi.org/10.1111/bjd.17869. https://www.ncbi.nlm.nih.gov/pubmed/30851191.

Amagai, Y., Oida, K., Matsuda, A., Jung, K., Kakutani, S., Tanaka, T., et al. (2015). Dihomo-γ-linolenic acid prevents the development of atopic dermatitis through prostaglandin D1 production in NC/Tnd mice. *Journal of Dermatological Science, 79*(1), 30–37. https://doi.org/10.1016/j.jdermsci.2015.03.010. https://www.ncbi.nlm.nih.gov/pubmed/25907057.

Andres, C., Belloni, B., Mempel, M., & Ring, J. (2008). Omalizumab for patients with severe and therapy-refractory atopic eczema? *Current Allergy and Asthma Reports, 8*(3), 179–180. https://www.ncbi.nlm.nih.gov/pubmed/18589835.

Arm, J. P., Bottoli, I., Skerjanec, A., Floch, D., Groenewegen, A., Maahs, S., et al. (2014). Pharmacokinetics, pharmacodynamics and safety of QGE031 (ligelizumab), a novel high-affinity anti-IgE antibody, in atopic subjects. *Clinical and Experimental Allergy*, *44*(11), 1371–1385. https://doi.org/10.1111/cea.12400. https://www.ncbi.nlm.nih.gov/pubmed/25200415.

Bao, L., Zhang, H., & Chan, L. S. (2013). The involvement of the JAK-STAT signaling pathway in chronic inflammatory skin disease atopic dermatitis. *JAK-STAT*, *2*(3), e24137. https://doi.org/10.4161/jkst.24137. https://www.ncbi.nlm.nih.gov/pubmed/24069552.

Behshad, R., Cooper, K. D., & Korman, N. J. (2008). A retrospective case series review of the peroxisome proliferator-activated receptor ligand rosiglitazone in the treatment of atopic dermatitis. *Archives of Dermatology*, *144*(1), 84–88. https://doi.org/10.1001/archdermatol.2007.22. https://www.ncbi.nlm.nih.gov/pubmed/18209172.

Bieber, T. (2008). Atopic dermatitis. *The New England Journal of Medicine*, *358*(14), 1483–1494. https://doi.org/10.1056/NEJMra074081. https://www.ncbi.nlm.nih.gov/pubmed/18385500.

Bieber, T., & Novak, N. (2009). Pathogenesis of atopic dermatitis: New developments. *Current Allergy and Asthma Reports*, *9*(4), 291–294. https://www.ncbi.nlm.nih.gov/pubmed/19656476.

Bissonnette, R., Maari, C., Forman, S., Bhatia, N., Lee, M., Fowler, J., et al. (2019). The oral Janus kinase/spleen tyrosine kinase inhibitor ASN002 demonstrates efficacy and improves associated systemic inflammation in patients with moderate-to-severe atopic dermatitis: Results from a Randomized double-blind placebo-controlled study. *British Journal of Dermatology*, *181*(4), 733–742. https://doi.org/10.1111/bjd.17932. https://www.ncbi.nlm.nih.gov/pubmed/30919407.

Bissonnette, R., Papp, K. A., Poulin, Y., Gooderham, M., Raman, M., Mallbris, L., et al. (2016). Topical tofacitinib for atopic dermatitis: A phase IIa randomized trial. *British Journal of Dermatology*, *175*(5), 902–911. https://doi.org/10.1111/bjd.14871. https://www.ncbi.nlm.nih.gov/pubmed/27423107.

Bissonnette, R., Vasist, L. S., Bullman, J. N., Collingwood, T., Chen, G., & Maeda-Chubachi, T. (2018). Systemic pharmacokinetics, safety, and preliminary efficacy of topical AhR agonist tapinarof: results of a phase 1 study. *Clinical Pharmacology in Drug Development*, *7*(5), 524–531. https://doi.org/10.1002/cpdd.439. https://www.ncbi.nlm.nih.gov/pubmed/29389078.

Brandt, E. B., & Sivaprasad, U. (2011). Th2 cytokines and atopic dermatitis. *Journal of Clinical and Cellular Immunology*, *2*(3). https://doi.org/10.4172/2155-9899.1000110. https://www.ncbi.nlm.nih.gov/pubmed/21994899.

Broeders, J. A., Ahmed Ali, U., & Fischer, G. (2016). Systematic review and meta-analysis of randomized clinical trials (RCTs) comparing topical calcineurin inhibitors with topical corticosteroids for atopic dermatitis: A 15-year experience. *Journal of the American Academy of Dermatology*, *75*(2), 410–419. e3. https://doi.org/10.1016/j.jaad.2016.02.1228. https://www.ncbi.nlm.nih.gov/pubmed/27177441.

Brunner, P. M., Pavel, A. B., Khattri, S., Leonard, A., Malik, K., Rose, S., et al. (2019). Baseline IL-22 expression in patients with atopic dermatitis stratifies tissue responses to fezakinumab. *The Journal of Allergy and Clinical Immunology*, *143*(1), 142–154. https://doi.org/10.1016/j.jaci.2018.07.028. https://www.ncbi.nlm.nih.gov/pubmed/30121291.

California: Menlo Therapeutics Inc. Menlo Therapeutics Announces Results From a Phase 2 Trial of Serlopitant for Pruritus Associated With Atopic Dermatitis. (2018).

Chang, T. W., Wu, P. C., Hsu, C. L., & Hung, A. F. (2007). Anti-IgE antibodies for the treatment of IgE-mediated allergic diseases. *Advances in Immunology*, *93*, 63–119. https://doi.org/10.1016/

S0065-2776(06)93002-8. https://www.ncbi.nlm.nih.gov/pubmed/17383539.

Cheung, P. F., Wong, C. K., Ho, A. W., Hu, S., Chen, D. P., & Lam, C. W. (2010). Activation of human eosinophils and epidermal keratinocytes by Th2 cytokine IL-31: Implication for the immunopathogenesis of atopic dermatitis. *International Immunology*, *22*(6), 453–467. https://doi.org/10.1093/intimm/dxq027. https://www.ncbi.nlm.nih.gov/pubmed/20410259.

Cornelissen, C., Luscher-Firzlaff, J., Baron, J. M., & Luscher, B. (2012). Signaling by IL-31 and functional consequences. *European Journal of Cell Biology*, *91*(6-7), 552–566. https://doi.org/10.1016/j.ejcb.2011.07.006. https://www.ncbi.nlm.nih.gov/pubmed/21982586.

Cowan, A., Kehner, G. B., & Inan, S. (2015). Targeting Itch with Ligands Selective for Kappa Opioid Receptors. *Pharmacology of Itch*, *226*, 291–314. https://doi.org/10.1007/978-3-662-44605-8_16. https://www.ncbi.nlm.nih.gov/pubmed/25861786.

Dahten, A., Mergemeier, S., & Worm, M. (2007). PPARγ expression profile and its cytokine driven regulation in atopic dermatitis. *Allergy*, *62*(8), 926–933. https://doi.org/10.1111/j.1398-9995.2007.01444.x. https://www.ncbi.nlm.nih.gov/pubmed/17620071.

Dose-ranging Study of Nemolizumab in Atopic Dermatitis. (2017). ClinicalTrials.gov.

DS Biopharma Announces Positive Top-Line Phase IIa Trial Results for DS107 as an Oral Treatment for Moderate to Severe Atopic Dermatitis. (2016).

DS Biopharma Announces Positive Top-Line Phase 2b Trial Results for DS107 as a Topical Treatment for Mild to Moderate Atopic Dermatitis. (2018).

Dupixent. How much should I expect to pay for Dupixent? https://www.dupixent.com/dupixent-pricing. Accessed July 2019.

Efficacy and Safety of Orally Administered DS107 in Adult Patients With Moderate to Severe Atopic Dermatitiss. (2019). ClinicalTrials.gov.

Elias, P. M., Hatano, Y., & Williams, M. L. (2008). Basis for the barrier abnormality in atopic dermatitis: outside-inside-outside pathogenic mechanisms. *The Journal of Allergy and Clinical Immunology*, *121*(6), 1337–1343. https://doi.org/10.1016/j.jaci.2008.01.022. https://www.ncbi.nlm.nih.gov/pubmed/18329087.

Elliott, K. A., Osna, N. A., Scofield, M. A., & Khan, M. M. (2001). Regulation of IL-13 production by histamine in cloned murine T helper type 2 cells. *International Immunopharmacology*, *1*(11), 1923–1937. https://www.ncbi.nlm.nih.gov/pubmed/11606024.

Evaluating the Effects of Tradipitant vs. Placebo in Atopic Dermatitis. (2018). ClinicalTrials.gov.

Evaluation of the Efficacy and Safety of Lebrikizumab in Moderate to Severe Atopic Dermatitis (ADvocate1). (2019). ClinicalTrials.gov.

Evaluation of the Efficacy and Safety of Lebrikizumab in Moderate to Severe Atopic Dermatitis (ADvocate2). (2019). ClinicalTrials.gov.

Frieder, J., Kivelevitch, D., & Menter, A. (2018). Secukinumab: A review of the anti-IL-17A biologic for the treatment of psoriasis. *Therapeutic Advances in Chronic Disease*, *9*(1), 5–21. https://doi.org/10.1177/2040622317738910. https://www.ncbi.nlm.nih.gov/pubmed/29344327.

Gauvreau, G. M., Arm, J. P., Boulet, L. P., Leigh, R., Cockcroft, D. W., Davis, B. E., et al. (2016). Efficacy and safety of multiple doses of QGE031 (ligelizumab) versus omalizumab and placebo in inhibiting allergen-induced early asthmatic responses. *The Journal of Allergy and Clinical Immunology*, *138*(4), 1051–1059. https://doi.org/10.1016/j.jaci.2016.02.027. https://www.ncbi.nlm.nih.gov/pubmed/27185571.

Gooderham, M. J., Forman, S. B., Bissonnette, R., Beebe, J. S., Zhang, W., Banfield, C., et al. (2019). Efficacy and safety of oral Janus kinase 1 inhibitor abrocitinib for patients with atopic dermatitis: A phase 2 randomized clinical trial. *JAMA Dermatology*, *155*(12), 1371–1379. https://doi.org/10.1001/jamadermatol.2019.2855. https://www.ncbi.nlm.nih.gov/pubmed/31577341.

Grewe, M., Bruijnzeel-Koomen, C. A., Schopf, E., Thepen, T., Langeveld-Wildschut, A. G., Ruzicka, T., & Krutmann, J. (1998). A role for Th1 and Th2 cells in the immunopathogenesis of atopic dermatitis. *Immunology Today*, *19*(8), 359–361. https://www.ncbi.nlm.nih.gov/pubmed/9709503.

Guttman-Yassky, E., Brunner, P. M., Neumann, A. U., Khattri, S., Pavel, A. B., Malik, K., et al. (2018). Efficacy and safety of fezakinumab (an IL-22 monoclonal antibody) in adults with moderate-to-severe atopic dermatitis inadequately controlled by conventional treatments: A randomized, double-blind, phase 2a trial. *Journal of the American Academy of Dermatology*, *78*(5), 872–881. e6. https://doi.org/10.1016/j.jaad.2018.01.016. https://www.ncbi.nlm.nih.gov/pubmed/29353025.

Guttman-Yassky, E., Thaci, D., Pangan, A. L., Hong, H. C., Papp, K. A., Reich, K., et al. (2020). Upadacitinib in adults with moderate to severe atopic dermatitis: 16-week results from a randomized, placebo-controlled trial. *The Journal of Allergy and Clinical Immunology*, *145*(3), 877–884. https://doi.org/10.1016/j.jaci.2019.11.025. https://www.ncbi.nlm.nih.gov/pubmed/31786154.

Hamid, Q., Naseer, T., Minshall, E. M., Song, Y. L., Boguniewicz, M., & Leung, D. Y. (1996). In vivo expression of IL-12 and IL-13 in atopic dermatitis. *The Journal of Allergy and Clinical Immunology*, *98*(1), 225–231. https://www.ncbi.nlm.nih.gov/pubmed/8765838.

Hanifin, J. M., Chan, S. C., Cheng, J. B., Tofte, S. J., Henderson, W. R., Jr., Kirby, D. S., & Weiner, E. S. (1996). Type 4 phosphodiesterase inhibitors have clinical and in vitro anti-inflammatory effects in atopic dermatitis. *The Journal of Investigative Dermatology*, *107*(1), 51–56. https://www.ncbi.nlm.nih.gov/pubmed/8752839.

Heil, P. M., Maurer, D., Klein, B., Hultsch, T., & Stingl, G. (2010). Omalizumab therapy in atopic dermatitis: Depletion of IgE does not improve the clinical course—a randomized, placebo-controlled and double blind pilot study. *Journal der Deutschen Dermatologischen Gesellschaft = Journal of the German Society of Dermatology*, *8*(12), 990–998. https://doi.org/10.1111/j.1610-0387.2010.07497.x. https://www.ncbi.nlm.nih.gov/pubmed/20678148.

Heimall, J., & Spergel, J. M. (2017). New pathways for itching in patients with atopic dermatitis? *The Journal of Allergy and Clinical Immunology*, *140*(2), 393–394. https://doi.org/10.1016/j.jaci.2017.06.004. https://www.ncbi.nlm.nih.gov/pubmed/28652154.

Heitman, A., Xiao, C., Cho, Y., Polymeropoulos, C., Birznieks, G., & Polymeropoulos, M. (2018). Tradipitant improves worst itch and disease severity in patients with chronic pruritus related to atopic dermatitis. *Journal of the American Academy of Dermatology*, *79*(3), AB300. https://doi.org/10.1016/j.jaad.2018.05.1184. https://doi.org/10.1016/j.jaad.2018.05.1184.

Hotze, M., Baurecht, H., Rodriguez, E., Chapman-Rothe, N., Ollert, M., Folster-Holst, R., et al. (2014). Increased efficacy of omalizumab in atopic dermatitis patients with wild-type filaggrin status and higher serum levels of phosphatidylcholines. *Allergy*, *69*(1), 132–135. https://doi.org/10.1111/all.12234. https://www.ncbi.nlm.nih.gov/pubmed/24111531.

Hoy, S. M. (2017). Crisaborole ointment 2%: A Review in mild to moderate atopic dermatitis. *American Journal of Clinical Dermatology*, *18*(6), 837–843. https://doi.org/10.1007/s40257-017-0327-4. https://www.ncbi.nlm.nih.gov/pubmed/29076116.

Investigation of Efficacy of Secukinumab in Patients With Moderate to Serve Atopic Dermatitis (Secu_in_AD). (2018). ClinicalTrials.gov.

Iyengar, S. R., Hoyte, E. G., Loza, A., Bonaccorso, S., Chiang, D., Umetsu, D. T., & Nadeau, K. C. (2013). Immunologic effects of omalizumab in children with severe refractory atopic dermatitis: a randomized, placebo-controlled clinical trial. *International Archives of Allergy and Immunology*, *162*(1), 89–93. https://doi.org/10.1159/000350486. https://www.ncbi.nlm.nih.gov/pubmed/23816920.

JAK1 Inhibitor With Medicated Topical Therapy in Adolescents With Atopic Dermatitis (JADE TEEN). (2019). ClinicalTrials.gov.

Jung, K., Tanaka, A., Fujita, H., Matsuda, A., Oida, K., Karasawa, K., et al. (2011). Peroxisome proliferator-activated receptor gamma-mediated suppression of dendritic cell function prevents the onset of atopic dermatitis in NC/Tnd mice. *The Journal of Allergy and Clinical Immunology*, *127*(2), 420–429. e1-6. https://doi.org/10.1016/j.jaci.2010.10.043. https://www.ncbi.nlm.nih.gov/pubmed/21208653.

Kabashima, K., Furue, M., Hanifin, J. M., Pulka, G., Wollenberg, A., Galus, R., et al. (2018). Nemolizumab in patients with moderate-to-severe atopic dermatitis: Randomized, phase II, long-term extension study. *The Journal of Allergy and Clinical Immunology*, *142*(4), 1121–1130. e7. https://doi.org/10.1016/j.jaci.2018.03.018. https://www.ncbi.nlm.nih.gov/pubmed/29753033.

Kawashima, H., Tateishi, N., Shiraishi, A., Teraoka, N., Tanaka, T., Tanaka, A., et al. (2008). Oral administration of dihomo-gamma-linolenic acid prevents development of atopic dermatitis in NC/Nga mice. *Lipids*, *43*(1), 37–43. https://doi.org/10.1007/s11745-007-3129-2. https://www.ncbi.nlm.nih.gov/pubmed/17985168.

Khattri, S., Brunner, P. M., Garcet, S., Finney, R., Cohen, S. R., Oliva, M., et al. (2017). Efficacy and safety of ustekinumab treatment in adults with moderate-to-severe atopic dermatitis. *Experimental Dermatology*, *26*(1), 28–35. https://doi.org/10.1111/exd.13112. https://www.ncbi.nlm.nih.gov/pubmed/27304428.

Kim, D. H., Park, K. Y., Kim, B. J., Kim, M. N., & Mun, S. K. (2013). Anti-immunoglobulin E in the treatment of refractory atopic dermatitis. *Clinical and Experimental Dermatology*, *38*(5), 496–500. https://doi.org/10.1111/j.1365-2230.2012.04438.x. https://www.ncbi.nlm.nih.gov/pubmed/23083013.

Koga, C., Kabashima, K., Shiraishi, N., Kobayashi, M., & Tokura, Y. (2008). Possible pathogenic role of Th17 cells for atopic dermatitis. *The Journal of Investigative Dermatology*, *128*(11), 2625–2630. https://doi.org/10.1038/jid.2008.111. https://www.ncbi.nlm.nih.gov/pubmed/18432274.

Kollmeier, A., Francke, K., Chen, B., Dunford, P. J., Greenspan, A. J., Xia, Y., et al. (2014). The histamine H(4) receptor antagonist, JNJ 39758979, is effective in reducing histamine-induced pruritus in a randomized clinical study in healthy subjects. *The Journal of Pharmacology and Experimental Therapeutics*, *350*(1), 181–187. https://doi.org/10.1124/jpet.114.215749. https://www.ncbi.nlm.nih.gov/pubmed/24817035.

Kulka, M., Sheen, C. H., Tancowny, B. P., Grammer, L. C., & Schleimer, R. P. (2008). Neuropeptides activate human mast cell degranulation and chemokine production. *Immunology*, *123*(3), 398–410. https://doi.org/10.1111/j.1365-2567.2007.02705.x. https://www.ncbi.nlm.nih.gov/pubmed/17922833.

Lane, J. E., Cheyney, J. M., Lane, T. N., Kent, D. E., & Cohen, D. J. (2006). Treatment of recalcitrant atopic dermatitis with omalizumab. *Journal of the American Academy of Dermatology*, *54*(1), 68–72. https://doi.org/10.1016/j.jaad.2005.09.030. https://www.ncbi.nlm.nih.gov/pubmed/16384758.

Leonardi, C. L., Kimball, A. B., Papp, K. A., Yeilding, N., Guzzo, C., Wang, Y., et al. (2008). Efficacy and safety of ustekinumab, a human interleukin-12/23 monoclonal antibody, in patients with psoriasis: 76-week results from a randomised, double-blind, placebo-controlled trial (PHOENIX 1). *Lancet, 371*(9625), 1665–1674. https://doi.org/10.1016/S0140-6736(08)60725-4. https://www.ncbi.nlm.nih.gov/pubmed/18486739.

Leung, D. Y. (1999). Pathogenesis of atopic dermatitis. *The Journal of Allergy and Clinical Immunology, 104*(3 Pt 2), S99–S108. https://www.ncbi.nlm.nih.gov/pubmed/10482860.

Leung, D. Y., Jain, N., & Leo, H. L. (2003). New concepts in the pathogenesis of atopic dermatitis. *Current Opinion in Immunology, 15*(6), 634–638. https://www.ncbi.nlm.nih.gov/pubmed/14630196.

Leung, D. Y., & Soter, N. A. (2001). Cellular and immunologic mechanisms in atopic dermatitis. *Journal of the American Academy of Dermatology, 44*(1 Suppl), S1–S12. https://www.ncbi.nlm.nih.gov/pubmed/11145790.

Levy, L. L., Urban, J., & King, B. A. (2015). Treatment of recalcitrant atopic dermatitis with the oral Janus kinase inhibitor tofacitinib citrate. *Journal of the American Academy of Dermatology, 73*(3), 395–399. https://doi.org/10.1016/j.jaad.2015.06.045. https://www.ncbi.nlm.nih.gov/pubmed/26194706.

Liu, F. T., Goodarzi, H., & Chen, H. Y. (2011). IgE, mast cells, and eosinophils in atopic dermatitis. *Clinical Reviews in Allergy & Immunology, 41*(3), 298–310. https://doi.org/10.1007/s12016-011-8252-4. https://www.ncbi.nlm.nih.gov/pubmed/21249468.

Lonndahl, L., Holst, M., Bradley, M., Killasli, H., Heilborn, J., Hall, M. A., et al. (2018). Substance P antagonist aprepitant shows no additive effect compared with standardized topical treatment alone in patients with atopic dermatitis. *Acta Dermato-Venereologica, 98*(3), 324–328. https://doi.org/10.2340/00015555-2852. https://www.ncbi.nlm.nih.gov/pubmed/29182791.

Maloney, N. J., Zhao, J., Tegtmeyer, K., Lee, E. Y., & Cheng, K. (2019). Off-label studies on apremilast in dermatology: A review. *The Journal of Dermatological Treatment*, 1–10. https://doi.org/10.1080/09546634.2019.1589641. https://www.ncbi.nlm.nih.gov/pubmed/30935262.

Manku, M. S., Horrobin, D. F., Morse, N., Kyte, V., Jenkins, K., Wright, S., & Burton, J. L. (1982). Reduced levels of prostaglandin precursors in the blood of atopic patients: Defective delta-6-desaturase function as a biochemical basis for atopy. *Prostaglandins, Leukotrienes, and Medicine, 9*(6), 615–628. https://www.ncbi.nlm.nih.gov/pubmed/6961468.

Mao-Qiang, M., Fowler, A. J., Schmuth, M., Lau, P., Chang, S., Brown, B. E., et al. (2004). Peroxisome-proliferator-activated receptor (PPAR)-gamma activation stimulates keratinocyte differentiation. *The Journal of Investigative Dermatology, 123*(2), 305–312. https://doi.org/10.1111/j.0022-202X.2004.23235.x. https://www.ncbi.nlm.nih.gov/pubmed/15245430.

Maudinet, A., Law-Koune, S., Duretz, C., Lasek, A., Modiano, P., & Tran, T. H. C. (2019). Ocular surface diseases induced by dupilumab in severe atopic dermatitis. *Ophthalmology Therapy, 8*(3), 485–490. https://doi.org/10.1007/s40123-019-0191-9. https://www.ncbi.nlm.nih.gov/pubmed/31230264.

May, R. D., Monk, P. D., Cohen, E. S., Manuel, D., Dempsey, F., Davis, N. H., et al. (2012). Preclinical development of CAT-354, an IL-13 neutralizing antibody, for the treatment of severe uncontrolled asthma. *British Journal of Pharmacology, 166*(1), 177–193. https://doi.org/10.1111/j.1476-5381.2011.01659.x. https://www.ncbi.nlm.nih.gov/pubmed/21895629.

McDonald, B. S., Jones, J., & Rustin, M. (2016). Rituximab as a treatment for severe atopic eczema: failure to improve in three consecutive patients. *Clinical and Experimental Dermatology, 41*(1), 45–47. https://doi.org/10.1111/ced.12691. https://www.ncbi.nlm.nih.gov/pubmed/26033316.

McKeage, K., & Duggan, S. (2019). Risankizumab: First global approval. *Drugs, 79*(8), 893–900. https://doi.org/10.1007/s40265-019-01136-7. https://www.ncbi.nlm.nih.gov/pubmed/31098898.

Meyer, D. M., Jesson, M. I., Li, X., Elrick, M. M., Funckes-Shippy, C. L., Warner, J. D., et al. (2010). Anti-inflammatory activity and neutrophil reductions mediated by the JAK1/JAK3 inhibitor, CP-690, 550, in rat adjuvant-induced arthritis. *Journal of Inflammation, 7*, 41. https://doi.org/10.1186/1476-9255-7-41. https://www.ncbi.nlm.nih.gov/pubmed/20701804.

Murata, Y., Song, M., Kikuchi, H., Hisamichi, K., Xu, X. L., Greenspan, A., et al. (2015). Phase 2a, randomized, double-blind, placebo-controlled, multicenter, parallel-group study of a H4 R-antagonist (JNJ-39758979) in Japanese adults with moderate atopic dermatitis. *The Journal of Dermatology, 42*(2), 129–139. https://doi.org/10.1111/1346-8138.12726. https://www.ncbi.nlm.nih.gov/pubmed/25491792.

Nakagawa, H., Nemoto, O., Igarashi, A., Saeki, H., Oda, M., Kabashima, K., & Nagata, T. (2019). Phase 2 clinical study of delgocitinib ointment in pediatric patients with atopic dermatitis. *The Journal of Allergy and Clinical Immunology, 144*(6), 1575–1583. https://doi.org/10.1016/j.jaci.2019.08.004. https://www.ncbi.nlm.nih.gov/pubmed/31425780.

Nakayama, T., Fujisawa, R., Yamada, H., Horikawa, T., Kawasaki, H., Hieshima, K., et al. (2001). Inducible expression of a CC chemokine liver- and activation-regulated chemokine (LARC)/macrophage inflammatory protein (MIP)-3 alpha/CCL20 by epidermal keratinocytes and its role in atopic dermatitis. *International Immunology, 13*(1), 95–103. https://doi.org/10.1093/intimm/13.1.95. https://www.ncbi.nlm.nih.gov/pubmed/11133838.

Nghiem, P., Pearson, G., & Langley, R. G. (2002). Tacrolimus and pimecrolimus: from clever prokaryotes to inhibiting calcineurin and treating atopic dermatitis. *Journal of the American Academy of Dermatology, 46*(2), 228–241. https://doi.org/10.1067/mjd.2002.120942. https://www.ncbi.nlm.nih.gov/pubmed/11807435.

Noga, O., Hanf, G., & Kunkel, G. (2003). Immunological and clinical changes in allergic asthmatics following treatment with omalizumab. *International Archives of Allergy and Immunology, 131*(1), 46–52. https://doi.org/10.1159/000070434. https://www.ncbi.nlm.nih.gov/pubmed/12759489.

Nograles, K. E., Zaba, L. C., Guttman-Yassky, E., Fuentes-Duculan, J., Suarez-Farinas, M., Cardinale, I., et al. (2008). Th17 cytokines interleukin (IL)-17 and IL-22 modulate distinct inflammatory and keratinocyte-response pathways. *British Journal of Dermatology, 159*(5), 1092–1102. https://doi.org/10.1111/j.1365-2133.2008.08769.x. https://www.ncbi.nlm.nih.gov/pubmed/18684158.

Nograles, K. E., Zaba, L. C., Shemer, A., Fuentes-Duculan, J., Cardinale, I., Kikuchi, T., et al. (2009). IL-22-producing "T22" T cells account for upregulated IL-22 in atopic dermatitis despite reduced IL-17-producing TH17 T cells. *The Journal of Allergy and Clinical Immunology, 123*(6), 1244–52. e2. https://doi.org/10.1016/j.jaci.2009.03.041. https://www.ncbi.nlm.nih.gov/pubmed/19439349.

Ohsawa, Y., & Hirasawa, N. (2014). The role of histamine H1 and H4 receptors in atopic dermatitis: From basic research to clinical study. *Allergology International, 63*(4), 533–542. https://doi.org/10.2332/allergolint.13-RA-0675. https://www.ncbi.nlm.nih.gov/pubmed/25249063.

Open-Label Study of Dupilumab in Patients With Atopic Dermatitis. (2019). ClinicalTrials.gov.

Oral DS107G in Moderate to Severe Atopic Dermatitis. 2017. ClinicalTrials.gov.

O'Shea, J. J., & Plenge, R. (2012). JAK and STAT signaling molecules in immunoregulation and immune-mediated disease. *Immunity*, *36*(4), 542–550. https://doi.org/10.1016/j.immuni.2012.03.014. https://www.ncbi.nlm.nih.gov/pubmed/22520847.

Paller, A. S., Tom, W. L., Lebwohl, M. G., Blumenthal, R. L., Boguniewicz, M., Call, R. S., et al. (2016). Efficacy and safety of crisaborole ointment, a novel, nonsteroidal phosphodiesterase 4 (PDE4) inhibitor for the topical treatment of atopic dermatitis (AD) in children and adults. *Journal of the American Academy of Dermatology*, *75*(3), 494–503. e6. https://doi.org/10.1016/j.jaad.2016.05.046. https://www.ncbi.nlm.nih.gov/pubmed/27417017.

Peppers, J., Paller, A. S., Maeda-Chubachi, T., Wu, S., Robbins, K., Gallagher, K., & Kraus, J. E. (2019). A phase 2, randomized dose-finding study of tapinarof (GSK2894512 cream) for the treatment of atopic dermatitis. *Journal of the American Academy of Dermatology*, *80*(1), 89–98. e3. https://doi.org/10.1016/j.jaad.2018.06.047. https://www.ncbi.nlm.nih.gov/pubmed/30554600.

Phase 2B Study to Evaluate ASN002 in Subjects With Moderate to Severe Atopic Dermatitis (RADIANT). (2018). ClinicalTrials.gov.

PR Newswire Vanda pharmaceuticals announces tradipitant phase II proof of concept study results for chronic pruritus in atopic dermatitis. Vanda pharmaceuticals announces tradipitant phase II proof of concept study results for chronic pruritus in atopic dermatitis 2015.

Proof of Concept of VLY-686 in Subjects With Treatment-Resistant Pruritus Associated With Atopic Dermatitis. (2017). ClinicalTrials.gov.

RINVOQ™ (upadacitinib) Monotherapy Shows Improvement in Skin Clearance and Itch in First Phase 3 Study for Atopic Dermatitis. (2020). Accessed June 24, 2020.

Romano, C., Sellitto, A., De Fanis, U., Balestrieri, A., Savoia, A., Abbadessa, S., et al. (2015). Omalizumab for difficult-to-treat dermatological conditions: Clinical and immunological features from a retrospective real-life experience. *Clinical Drug Investigation*, *35*(3), 159–168. https://doi.org/10.1007/s40261-015-0267-9. https://www.ncbi.nlm.nih.gov/pubmed/25578818.

Ruzicka, T., Hanifin, J. M., Furue, M., Pulka, G., Mlynarczyk, I., Wollenberg, A., et al. (2017). Anti-interleukin-31 receptor a antibody for atopic dermatitis. *The New England Journal of Medicine*, *376*(9), 826–835. https://doi.org/10.1056/NEJMoa1606490. https://www.ncbi.nlm.nih.gov/pubmed/28249150.

Ruzicka, T., & Mihara, R. (2017). Anti-interleukin-31 receptor a antibody for atopic dermatitis. *The New England Journal of Medicine*, *376*(21), 2093. https://doi.org/10.1056/NEJMc1704013. https://www.ncbi.nlm.nih.gov/pubmed/28538126.

Saeki, H., Kabashima, K., Tokura, Y., Murata, Y., Shiraishi, A., Tamamura, R., et al. (2017). Efficacy and safety of ustekinumab in Japanese patients with severe atopic dermatitis: A randomized, double-blind, placebo-controlled, phase II study. *British Journal of Dermatology*, *177*(2), 419–427. https://doi.org/10.1111/bjd.15493. https://www.ncbi.nlm.nih.gov/pubmed/28338223.

Safety and Efficacy Study of Topically Applied DS107 Cream in Mild to Moderate Atopic Dermatitis Patients. (2016). ClinicalTrials.gov.

Safety, Pharmacokinetics and Preliminary Efficacy of Asimadoline in Pruritus Associated With Atopic Dermatitis. (2015). ClinicalTrials.gov.

Schulman, E. S. (2001). Development of a monoclonal anti-immunoglobulin E antibody (omalizumab) for the treatment of allergic respiratory disorders. *American Journal of Respiratory and Critical Care Medicine*, *164*(8 Pt 2), S6–S11. https://doi.org/10.1164/ajrccm.164.supplement_1.2103025. https://www.ncbi.nlm.nih.gov/pubmed/11704611.

Secukinumab for Treatment of Atopic Dermatitis. (2015). ClinicalTrials.gov.

Serhal, L., & Edwards, C. J. (2019). Upadacitinib for the treatment of rheumatoid arthritis. *Expert Review of Clinical Immunology*, *15*(1), 13–25. https://doi.org/10.1080/1744666X.2019.1544892. https://www.ncbi.nlm.nih.gov/pubmed/30394138.

Sheinkopf, L. E., Rafi, A. W., Do, L. T., Katz, R. M., & Klaustermeyer, W. B. (2008). Efficacy of omalizumab in the treatment of atopic dermatitis: A pilot study. *Allergy and Asthma Proceedings*, *29*(5), 530–537. https://doi.org/10.2500/aap.2008.29.3160. https://www.ncbi.nlm.nih.gov/pubmed/18926061.

Shreberk-Hassidim, R., Ramot, Y., & Zlotogorski, A. (2017). Janus kinase inhibitors in dermatology: A systematic review. *Journal of the American Academy of Dermatology*, *76*(4), 745–753. e19. https://doi.org/10.1016/j.jaad.2016.12.004. https://www.ncbi.nlm.nih.gov/pubmed/28169015.

Silverman, G. J., & Weisman, S. (2003). Rituximab therapy and autoimmune disorders: Prospects for anti-B cell therapy. *Arthritis and Rheumatism*, *48*(6), 1484–1492. https://doi.org/10.1002/art.10947. https://www.ncbi.nlm.nih.gov/pubmed/12794814.

Simon, D., Hosli, S., Kostylina, G., Yawalkar, N., & Simon, H. U. (2008). Anti-CD20 (rituximab) treatment improves atopic eczema. *The Journal of Allergy and Clinical Immunology*, *121*(1), 122–128. https://doi.org/10.1016/j.jaci.2007.11.016. https://www.ncbi.nlm.nih.gov/pubmed/18206507.

Simpson, E. L., Bieber, T., Guttman-Yassky, E., Beck, L. A., Blauvelt, A., Cork, M. J., et al. (2016). Two phase 3 trials of dupilumab versus placebo in atopic dermatitis. *The New England Journal of Medicine*, *375*(24), 2335–2348. https://doi.org/10.1056/NEJMoa1610020. https://www.ncbi.nlm.nih.gov/pubmed/27690741.

Simpson, E. L., Flohr, C., Eichenfield, L. F., Bieber, T., Sofen, H., Taieb, A., et al. (2018). Efficacy and safety of lebrikizumab (an anti-IL-13 monoclonal antibody) in adults with moderate-to-severe atopic dermatitis inadequately controlled by topical corticosteroids: A randomized, placebo-controlled phase II trial (TREBLE). *Journal of the American Academy of Dermatology*, *78*(5), 863–871 e11. https://doi.org/10.1016/j.jaad.2018.01.017. https://www.ncbi.nlm.nih.gov/pubmed/29353026.

Simpson, E. L., Imafuku, S., Poulin, Y., Ungar, B., Zhou, L., Malik, K., et al. (2019). A phase 2 randomized trial of apremilast in patients with atopic dermatitis. *The Journal of Investigative Dermatology*, *139*(5), 1063–1072. https://doi.org/10.1016/j.jid.2018.10.043. https://www.ncbi.nlm.nih.gov/pubmed/30528828.

Singh, R., Masuda, E. S., & Payan, D. G. (2012). Discovery and development of spleen tyrosine kinase (SYK) inhibitors. *Journal of Medicinal Chemistry*, *55*(8), 3614–3643. https://doi.org/10.1021/jm201271b. https://www.ncbi.nlm.nih.gov/pubmed/22257213.

Smith, S. H., Jayawickreme, C., Rickard, D. J., Nicodeme, E., Bui, T., Simmons, C., et al. (2017). Tapinarof is a natural AhR agonist that resolves skin inflammation in mice and humans. *The Journal of Investigative Dermatology*, *137*(10), 2110–2119. https://doi.org/10.1016/j.jid.2017.05.004. https://www.ncbi.nlm.nih.gov/pubmed/28595996.

Stander, S., Siepmann, D., Herrgott, I., Sunderkotter, C., & Luger, T. A. (2010). Targeting the neurokinin receptor 1 with aprepitant: a novel antipruritic strategy. *PLoS One*, *5*(6), e10968. https://doi.org/10.1371/journal.pone.0010968. https://www.ncbi.nlm.nih.gov/pubmed/20532044.

Stander, S., & Steinhoff, M. (2002). Pathophysiology of pruritus in atopic dermatitis: An overview. *Experimental Dermatology, 11*(1), 12–24. https://www.ncbi.nlm.nih.gov/pubmed/11952824.

Study Evaluating Efficacy and Safety of PF-04965842 in Subjects Aged 12 Years And Older With Moderate to Severe Atopic Dermatitis (JADE Mono-2). (2018). ClinicalTrials.gov.

Sugimoto, Y., Umakoshi, K., Nojiri, N., & Kamei, C. (1998). Effects of histamine H1 receptor antagonists on compound 48/80-induced scratching behavior in mice. *European Journal of Pharmacology, 351*(1), 1–5. https://www.ncbi.nlm.nih.gov/pubmed/9698198.

Tanimoto, A., Ogawa, Y., Oki, C., Kimoto, Y., Nozawa, K., Amano, W., et al. (2015). Pharmacological properties of JTE-052: A novel potent JAK inhibitor that suppresses various inflammatory responses in vitro and in vivo. *Inflammation Research 64*(1), 41–51. https://doi.org/10.1007/s00011-014-0782-9. https://www.ncbi.nlm.nih.gov/pubmed/25387665.

Tey, H. L., & Yosipovitch, G. (2011). Targeted treatment of pruritus: a look into the future. *British Journal of Dermatology, 165*(1), 5–17. https://doi.org/10.1111/j.1365-2133.2011.10217.x. https://www.ncbi.nlm.nih.gov/pubmed/21219293.

Thaiwat, S., & Sangasapaviliya, A. (2011). Omalizumab treatment in severe adult atopic dermatitis. *Asian Pacific Journal of Allergy and Immunology / Launched by the Allergy and Immunology Society of Thailand, 29*(4), 357–360. https://www.ncbi.nlm.nih.gov/pubmed/22299316.

Thepen, T., Langeveld-Wildschut, E. G., Bihari, I. C., van Wichen, D. F., van Reijsen, F. C., Mudde, G. C., & Bruijnzeel-Koomen, C. A. (1996). Biphasic response against aeroallergen in atopic dermatitis showing a switch from an initial TH2 response to a TH1 response in situ: An immunocytochemical study. *The Journal of Allergy and Clinical Immunology, 97*(3), 828–837. https://www.ncbi.nlm.nih.gov/pubmed/8613640.

Tradipitant in Treatment-resistant Pruritus Associated With Atopic Dermatitis. (2016). ClinicalTrials.gov.

Tralokinumab Monotherapy for Moderate to Severe Atopic Dermatitis - ECZTRA 1 (ECZema TRAlokinumab Trial no. 1) (ECZTRA 1). (2017). ClinicalTrials.gov.

Tralokinumab Monotherapy for Moderate to Severe Atopic Dermatitis - ECZTRA 2 (ECZema TRAlokinumab Trial no. 2) (ECZTRA 2). (2017). ClinicalTrials.gov.

Vigo, P. G., Girgis, K. R., Pfuetze, B. L., Critchlow, M. E., Fisher, J., & Hussain, I. (2006). Efficacy of anti-IgE therapy in patients with atopic dermatitis. *Journal of the American Academy of Dermatology, 55*(1), 168–170. https://doi.org/10.1016/j.jaad.2005.12.045. https://www.ncbi.nlm.nih.gov/pubmed/16781320.

VPD-737 for Treatment of Chronic Pruritus. (2013). ClinicalTrials.gov.

Wohlmann, A., Sebastian, K., Borowski, A., Krause, S., & Friedrich, K. (2010). Signal transduction by the atopy-associated human thymic stromal lymphopoietin (TSLP) receptor depends on Janus kinase function. *Biological Chemistry, 391*(2-3), 181–186. https://doi.org/10.1515/BC.2010.029. https://www.ncbi.nlm.nih.gov/pubmed/20128689.

Wollenberg, A., Howell, M. D., Guttman-Yassky, E., Silverberg, J. I., Kell, C., Ranade, K., et al. (2019). Treatment of atopic dermatitis with tralokinumab, an anti-IL-13 mAb. *The Journal of Allergy and Clinical Immunology, 143*(1), 135–141. https://doi.org/10.1016/j.jaci.2018.05.029. https://www.ncbi.nlm.nih.gov/pubmed/29906525.

Worm, M., Simpson, E. L., Thaçi, D., et al. (2020). Efficacy and Safety of Multiple Dupilumab Dose Regimens after Initial Successful Treatment in Patients with Atopic Dermatitis: A Randomized Clinical Trial. *Journal of the American Academy of Dermatology, 156*(2), 131–143. doi:10.1001/jamadermatol.2019.3617.

Wu, N. L., Huang, D. Y., Tsou, H. N., Lin, Y. C., & Lin, W. W. (2015). Syk mediates IL-17-induced CCL20 expression by targeting Act1-dependent K63-linked ubiquitination of TRAF6. *The Journal of Investigative Dermatology, 135*(2), 490–498. https://doi.org/10.1038/jid.2014.383. https://www.ncbi.nlm.nih.gov/pubmed/25202827.

Yosipovitch, G., Stander, S., Kerby, M. B., Larrick, J. W., Perlman, A. J., Schnipper, E. F., et al. (2018). Serlopitant for the treatment of chronic pruritus: Results of a randomized, multicenter, placebo-controlled phase 2 clinical trial. *Journal of the American Academy of Dermatology, 78*(5), 882–891. e10. https://doi.org/10.1016/j.jaad.2018.02.030. https://www.ncbi.nlm.nih.gov/pubmed/29462657.

24

Microbiome Modulation

PAUL BLACKCLOUD AND JENNIFER HSIAO

KEY POINTS

- The use of probiotics to promote a healthy state has been widely studied.
- Oral probiotics have been shown to aid in the prevention of atopic dermatitis in select populations.
- Oral probiotics may also help in the treatment of atopic dermatitis, though data to support this are less clear.
- Details on specific probiotic strain, dose, and duration of treatment for efficacy are lacking.
- Multiple topical modalities to alter the skin microbiome are being explored, many with promising results.

Introduction

As disruption of the healthy microbiome, referred to as dysbiosis, has been recognized as a risk factor for the development and exacerbation of atopic dermatitis (AD), treatments aimed at restoring balance in the microbiome have been explored. Over the past few decades, numerous studies and subsequent reviews and meta-analyses have been conducted, investigating the use of oral probiotics for both treatment and prevention of AD. Though results are mixed, and study methodologies varied, certain populations appear to benefit from their use. Probiotics are considered generally safe, though they should be used with caution in select populations. More recently, topical preparations have been explored in small studies with varying results.

Oral probiotics

As defined by the International Scientific Association for Probiotics and Prebiotics, probiotics refers to "live microorganisms that, when administered in adequate amounts, confer a health benefit on the host" (Hill et al., 2014), while a prebiotic is defined as "a substrate that is selectively utilized by host microorganisms conferring a health benefit" (Gibson et al., 2017). In short, probiotics are active bacterial cultures, and prebiotics are what feed them. Synbiotics are a combination of probiotics and prebiotics. The term *postbiotics* refers to metabolic byproducts of live bacteria (either secreted or released through lysis) that, like probiotics, provide a health benefit to the host (Gao et al., 2019) (Fig. 24.1).

Gut commensals in the microbiome aid human health through a variety of mechanisms, including competitive inhibition of pathogenic organisms, protection of the gut epithelial barrier, assisting in nutrient metabolism, and immunomodulation (Jandhyala et al., 2015). For example, intake of macronutrients such as complex carbohydrates are metabolized by gut bacteria through fermentation into end products used by humans for energy, such as short-chain fatty acids (SCFAs) (Oliphant & Allen-Vercoe, 2019). To be effective, bacterial strains used in oral probiotics should be able to survive passage through the acidic environment and digestive enzymes of the upper gastrointestinal (GI) tract, adhere to intestinal epithelial cells, colonize the lower GI tract, and be safe for use (i.e., nonvirulent, nontoxin producing) (de Melo Pereira, de Oliveira Coelho, Magalhães Júnior, Thomaz-Soccol, & Soccol, 2018).

Dosage of probiotics is measured in colony-forming units (CFU), which indicate the number of live or viable organisms per serving (i.e., capsule or gram). Probiotic dosage typically ranges from 1 to 10 billion CFU, and in guidelines from the World Gastroenterology Organisation (WGO), due to variation in dosage and strains used in studies, there is no one recommended dose; instead, dosage should be based on the studies of the disorder treated (World Gastroenterology Organisation, 2017). Though probiotics and prebiotics are readily available as supplements in drugstores and supermarkets, several common foods contain live microbes and prebiotics as well (Table 24.1).

Dysbiosis has been purported to play a role in the development and exacerbation of AD, and as such, probiotic use has been explored in both the prevention and treatment of the disease. The exact mechanism of action of probiotics is unclear, though likely through influencing both the microbiome and the immune system (Fig. 24.2). Like commensals, probiotics aid in barrier function, compete for nutrients or displace pathogenic organisms, produce AMPs, and stimulate the immune system to target pathogenic organisms (Dargahi, Johnson, Donkor, Vasiljevic, & Apostolopoulos, 2019). *Lactobacillus*, a genus of commensal bacteria in the phylum Firmicutes (a predominant gut phylum), is commonly used in probiotics. Studies have shown a range of benefits by different species within *Lactobacillus*. For example, *Lactobacillus rhamnosus* GG can protect the gut barrier

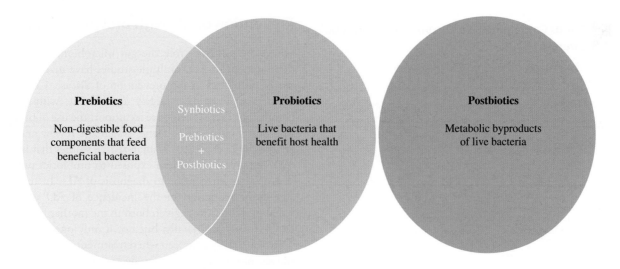

• **Fig. 24.1** Prebiotics, probiotics, synbiotics, and post-biotics.

by minimizing mucosal lining permeability and protecting against oxidative stress-induced damage to tight junctions, the intercellular connections that prevent the passage of molecules (Rao & Samak, 2013). Another *Lactobacillus* species, *Lactobacillus reuteri*, produces reuterin, an antimicrobial compound with broad coverage against gram-positive bacteria, gram-negative bacteria, fungi, yeasts, and protozoa (Spinler et al., 2008).

Both the innate and adaptive immune systems are influenced by probiotic administration. Depending on the strain, this is accomplished through different mechanisms. *L. reuteri* and *Lactobacillus casei*, for example, induce increased inhibitory regulatory T-cell (Treg) differentiation after detection by tolerogenic dendritic cells, while *Lactobacillus acidophilus*, *Lactobacillus bulgaricus*, and *Bifidobacterium bifidum* increase protective immunoglobulin G (IgG) and IgA antibodies (Dargahi et al., 2019). Regardless of species and strain differences, probiotics can inhibit the differentiation of naïve T cells to T helper type 2 (Th2) cells and stimulate the production of antiinflammatory cytokines such as interferon-gamma and interleukin-10 (IL10) (Dargahi et al., 2019; Rather et al., 2016). Prebiotics also play a role by increasing production of SCFAs, byproducts of fermentation by gut commensals, which have antiinflammatory effects and decrease pH, creating a more favorable environment for commensal over pathogenic bacteria and promoting gut homeostasis (Tan et al., 2014).

Treatment of AD with oral probiotics

Numerous studies, systematic reviews, and meta-analyses on the use of probiotics for the treatment of AD have been published, with conflicting results and conclusions. The most recent Cochrane review published by Makrgeorgou et al. (2018) analyzed 39 randomized clinical trials (RCT) on the use of probiotics (specifically *Lactobacillus* and *Bifidobacteria*) in 2599 participants with at least mild AD

of all ages. Key findings from the review were that the use of probiotics as treatment did not help with AD symptoms or quality of life, concluding that the "use of probiotics for the treatment of eczema is currently not evidence-based" (Makrgeorgou et al., 2018). This review was an update to the 2008 Cochrane review of 12 RCTs with 781 participants (pediatric patients only), which also found lack of benefit with probiotic use as treatment for AD (Boyle, Leonardi-Bee, Bath-Hextall, & Tang, 2009).

A meta-analysis specifically investigating improvements in the scoring of AD (SCORAD) measure following probiotic therapy was conducted by Kim et al. (2014) and identified 25 RCTs with 1599 participants. Results from this analysis conflict with the Cochrane reviews and showed a benefit in the use of probiotics in children at least 1 year of age (–5.74-point difference in SCORAD compared to controls) and adults (–9.69-point difference in SCORAD compared to controls), though this benefit was not seen in infants less than 1 year old. Differences in benefit were influenced by type of probiotic and severity of AD, with greater benefits seen in those supplemented with *Lactobacillus* or a mixture of bacteria rather than *Bifidobacterium* alone (Kim et al., 2014). In subgroup analysis, this benefit from probiotics was limited to those with moderate to severe AD rather than those with mild disease (Kim et al., 2014). However, some studies included in the meta-analysis allowed patients to continue using topical emollients and medications in addition to probiotics, making these results challenging to interpret. Similar results were seen in a more recent meta-analysis focused on infantile AD, which identified a significant benefit of probiotic supplementation (specifically with *Lactobacillus*) in children ages 1 to 18 years with moderate to severe AD (Zhao, Shen, & Ma, 2018).

The benefits of probiotics also vary dependent upon the population studied. A meta-analysis conducted by Huang et al. (2017) found that only certain strains of *Lactobacillus* improved SCORAD in children, showing that *Lactobacillus*

| TABLE 24.1 | Foods Containing Live Microbes and Prebiotic Sources |

Foods Contaning Live Microbes (Rezac, Kok, Heermann, & Hutkins, 2018)

Dairy Products

Yogurt

Frozen yogurt

Kefir

Cultured buttermilk

Select cheeses

Fermented Vegetables

Sauerkraut

Olives

Pickles

Kimchi

Other Fermented Products

Miso

Tempeh (fermented soy beans)

Fish sauce

Fermented meats (i.e., sausage, salami)

Fermented tea (kombucha)

Select beer (i.e., sour beer)

Select cereals (i.e., fermented porridge)

Foods Containing Prebiotics (Florowska, Krygier, Florowski, & Dłużewska, 2016)

Asparagus

Garlic

Leeks

Onions

Bananas

Jerusalem artichoke

Chicory root

Wheat (bran, flour)

Barley

fermentum and *Lactobacillus salivarius* (as well as probiotics of varying combinations of *Lactobacillus* and *Bifidobacterium* strains) led to significant improvement, while single strain treatment with *L. rhamnosus* GG or *L. plantarum* did not. Differences in benefit were also age dependent, and even geography dependent, with significant improvements in SCORAD only seen in children age greater than 1 year and in those in Asia, though not in Europe (Huang et al., 2017). This suggests that there may be different phenotypes of AD that respond more favorably to probiotics than others.

Prevention of AD with oral probiotics

Given the potential role the gut microbiome plays in the development of AD, multiple studies have investigated the use of probiotics in the prevention of disease. Conclusions of meta-analyses have largely agreed that, within certain parameters, there is evidence to support the use of probiotics in a preventative role. A large systematic review and meta-analysis by Li et al. (2019) analyzed 28 studies that included 6907 infants and children exposed to probiotics prenatally and/or after birth prior to diagnosis of AD. In this study, significant reduction in the incidence of AD was found when probiotics were given both to the mother in utero and to the infant postnatally, but not if only one or the other. This benefit was only seen when treatment occurred through the age of 6 months, with no decreased risk in the development of AD in those treated for more than 1 year. Contrary to studies on treatment of AD, this benefit of disease prevention was seen across strains, including *Bifidobacterium*, *Propionibacterium*, and *Lactobacillus* strains, with certain *Lactobacillus* strains (*L. rhamnosus* and *Lactobacillus paracasei*) showing greater efficacy (Li et al., 2019). This benefit continued to be sustained on long-term, at least 5-year, follow-up (Cao et al., 2015). Multiple other systematic reviews and meta-analyses have also concluded that early probiotic use decreases risk of AD development (Cuello-Garcia et al., 2015; Elazab et al., 2013; Mansfield, Bergin, Cooper, & Olsen, 2014; Panduru, Panduru, Sălăvăstru, & Tiplica, 2015; Pelucchi et al., 2012; Zuccotti et al., 2015).

The use of prebiotics, given as oligosaccharides (i.e., fructo- and galactooligosaccharide) for prevention of AD has also been evaluated. A Cochrane review published in 2013 by Osborn and Sinn investigated the role of prebiotics in infants for the prevention of allergic disease. A significant risk reduction was observed in the development of AD (four studies, 1218 infants), though not in the development of allergy or asthma (Osborn & Sinn, 2013). A strength of this review is that there was no significant heterogeneity among AD studies. Contradictory to these findings, a meta-analysis published that same year included subgroup analysis of three RCTs investigating prebiotic use and found no benefit in the prevention of AD, though heterogeneity among the included studies was moderate (I^2 of 48%) (Dang et al., 2013).

The use of synbiotics for both the prevention and treatment of AD has also been investigated. In a meta-analysis published in 2016, Chang et al. included six studies on the treatment and two studies on the prevention of AD in children and found that use of synbiotics were shown to help in the treatment but not the prevention of AD. In this meta-analysis, significant improvements in SCORAD were seen in those ages 1 to 18 years treated for 8 weeks, and when treated with mixed bacterial strains rather than a single strain. Synbiotics were associated with lower incidence of AD in the two individual studies used in the meta-analysis; however, when combined, the pooled relative risk was not significant (Chang et al., 2016; Kukkonen et al., 2007; Rozé et al., 2012). Theoretically, synbiotics should perform

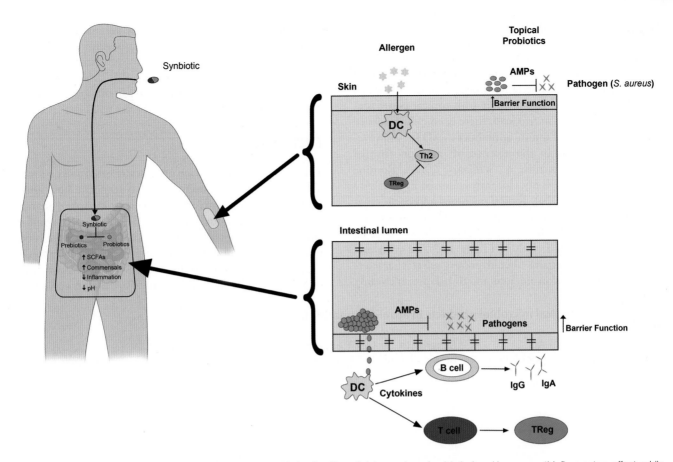

• **Fig. 24.2** Synbiotic and topical probiotic mechanisms. Prebiotics feed beneficial organisms (probiotics) and have an anti-inflammatory effect, while the probiotic organisms compete with pathogenic organisms in the gut, improve barrier function and modulate the immune system. In the skin, increased regulatory T cells decrease the Th2 response elicited from allergen exposure. Topical probiotics applied to skin can limit levels of *S. aureus* and improve barrier function. *AMPs*, Antimicrobial peptides. *DC*, Dendritic cell. *IgG*, Immunoglobulin G. *IgA*, Immunoglobulin A. *SCFA*, Short-chain fatty acids. *TReg*, Regulatory T cell. *Th2*, T helper type 2 cell.

as well as or better than either separate component; however, to date, there are no studies specifically comparing probiotics to synbiotics in the prevention and treatment of AD, and comparisons of separate meta-analyses is challenging in the setting of study heterogeneity (Chang et al., 2016).

Recommendations

Translating current meta-analyses into evidence-based recommendations is challenging given the heterogeneity among studies, particularly in strains used, doses used, timing and duration of supplementation, concomitant treatments, and outcome assessment. Though recognizing the low quality of evidence, the World Allergy Organization (WAO) currently recommends considering supplementation in the following scenarios:

a. "using probiotics in pregnant women at high risk for having an allergic child;

b. using probiotics in women who breastfeed infants at high risk of developing allergy; and

c. using probiotics in infants at high risk of developing allergy" (Fiocchi et al., 2015).

The WAO also recommends use of prebiotics specifically in "not-exclusively breastfed infants" (Cuello-Garcia et al., 2016), though no specific strains or regimens are provided. A follow-up meta-analysis to these recommendations, specifically

evaluating use of *L. rhamnosus* GG (LGG) in the abovementioned three groups, found that LGG supplementation did not reduce the risk of AD (Szajewska & Horvath, 2018). In their guidelines on the management of AD, the American Academy of Dermatology (AAD) acknowledges the current interest in the study of probiotics but does not currently recommend the use of probiotics or prebiotics for treatment of established AD based on the available evidence (Sidbury et al., 2014). Other expert groups have not endorsed the use of probiotics, prebiotics, or synbiotics for the prevention of allergic disease, including the American Academy of Pediatrics, National Institute of Allergy and Infectious Diseases, European Academy of Allergy and Clinical Immunology, European Society of Paediatric Gastroenterology, Hepatology, and Nutrition, and the Food and Agriculture Organization of the United Nations/World Health Organization (West, Dzidic, Prescott, & Jenmalm, 2017).

Though oral probiotics have been studied in other cutaneous diseases as well, such as psoriasis (Navarro-López et al., 2019) and acne (Jung, Tse, Guiha, & Rao, 2013), many questions remain regarding their mechanism of action. In addition to unanswered questions already discussed, there are questions regarding how long probiotics need to stay in the gut to work, how many CFU are needed to make a compositional change, and whether a transient encounter in the gut is enough to change the immune milieu or behavior of the microbial community.

Topical microbial therapy

As skin dysbiosis, particularly overgrowth of *Staphylococcus aureus*, is associated with AD, topical approaches to return the skin to a balanced state have been studied. Although topical antibiotics in conjunction with topical corticosteroids can decrease *S. aureus* load, there is no clear evidence supporting the use of topical antibiotics in AD for improvement in symptoms in the absence of infection (Birnie, Bath-Hextall, Ravenscroft, & Williams, 2008). Routine topical antibiotic use is not currently endorsed by the AAD (Eichenfield et al., 2014). Topical microbial approaches that have recently been studied include topical probiotics (live organisms), bacterial lysates (products of lysed bacterial cells), endolysins, and clothing (Table 24.2). As with oral probiotics, topical strains should possess select characteristics to return the skin microbiome to balance, including

the ability to adhere to skin, decrease adhesion of potential skin pathogens, compete against pathogens, decrease biofilm formation by pathogens, and in some cases even break down mature biofilms (Lopes et al., 2017). Topical autologous microbial transplant using the patient's own protective commensals has also been studied (Nakatsuji et al., 2017).

Lactobacillus

Lactobacillus johnsonii (even once heat-treated and no longer able to replicate) has been shown to stimulate host innate immune response, with expression of antimicrobial peptides (AMPs) such as cathelicidin and β-defensin (Rosignoli et al., 2018). Blanchet-Réthoré et al. (2017) studied the effects of a lotion containing a strain of heat-treated *L. johnsonii* on 21 patients with mild to moderate AD and positive swabs of *S. aureus* at the start of the study. Participants applied the

TABLE 24.2 Use of topical microbial products in atopic dermatitis (AD)

Microbial agent	AD population	Severity of atopic disease	Treatment duration	Treatment results	Reference
Lactobacillus johnsonii	Adults (N = 21)	Mild to moderate	3 weeks	Reduction in *Staphylococcus aureus* load, improvement in SCORAD	Blanchet-Réthoré et al. (2017)
Rosemonas mucosa	Adults (N = 10) Children (N = 5)	Minimum SCORAD of 10	Adults: 6 weeks Children: 16 weeks	Adults: reduction in intensity, pruritus, antecubital SCORAD Children: improvement in SCORAD, pruritus, steroid usage	Myles et al. (2018)
Vitreoscilla filiformis	Age not disclosed (N =1 0)	Slight to moderate	4 weeks	Improvement in AD	Guéniche, Dahel, et al. (2008)
V. filiformis	Age ≥14 years (N = 13)	Slight to moderate	4 weeks	Improvement in mEASI, EASI, and pruritus	Guéniche et al. (2006)
V. filiformis	Adults and children (N = 75)	Mild	30 days	Improvement in SCORAD, pruritus, sleep, transepidermal water loss Reduction in *S. aureus*	Gueniche, Knaudt, et al. (2008)
V. filiformis	Adults and children (N = 60)	Moderate	4 weeks	Improvement in SCORAD Increase in *Xanthomonas*	Seité et al. (2017)
CoNS (autologous microbiome transplant with *Staphylococcus epidermidis* or *Staphylococcus hominis*)	Adults (N = 5)	Severity not defined	1 day	Reduction in *S. aureus* load	Nakatsuji et al. (2017)
Streptococcus thermophilus	Adults (N = 11)	Average SCORAD of 39	2 weeks	Increase in ceramides Reduction in erythema, scaling, and pruritus	Di Marzio et al. (2003)
Endolysins	Adults (N = 100)	Moderate to severe	12 weeks	No difference in TCS use or *S. aureus* reduction	de Wit et al. (2019)

TCS, topical corticosteroid.

lotion to a target lesion twice daily for 3 weeks and reevaluated using SCORAD. Results showed a significant decrease of *S. aureus* in treated skin, with significant clinical improvement in SCORAD, in a well-tolerated lotion (Blanchet-Réthoré et al., 2017).

Topical use of *L. reuteri* has also been investigated, though not yet in human in vivo application. Khmaladze, Butler, Fabre, and Gillbro (2019) conducted in vitro and ex vivo studies on human epidermal explants evaluating both live *L. reuteri* and lysate products of the bacteria. Both the live bacteria and bacterial lysate reduced inflammatory cytokines IL6 and IL8, and both improved skin barrier function through multiple mechanisms, including upregulation of aquaporin-3 (live bacteria) and laminin A/B expression (lysate). Microbial inhibition was also observed with use of the live culture, but not the lysate, with increased antimicrobial activity against pathogens *Pseudomonas aeruginosa* and *Streptococcus pyogenes* compared to commensals *Staphylococcus epidermidis* and *Cutibacterium acnes* (Khmaladze et al., 2019).

Roseomonas

Myles et al. (2016) investigated culturable gram-negative (CGN) bacteria from patients with AD (N = 17) and healthy volunteers (N = 26), and found that *Roseomonas mucosa* was the predominant species in the healthy volunteers. CGNs from healthy controls can limit *S. aureus* growth, improve barrier function through reduced transepidermal water loss, and induce an innate immune response (Myles et al., 2016). In a single arm follow-up study, 15 patients with AD were treated with a topical solution containing *R. mucosa* (10 adults treated twice weekly for 6 weeks; 5 pediatric patients treated twice weekly for 16 weeks) (Myles et al., 2018). Combined, 10 of the 15 patients achieved a greater than 50% improvement in SCORAD, with no reported adverse events. Lack of response was associated with a family history of AD that continued through adulthood.

Vitreoscilla

Vitreoscilla filiformis is a filamentous gram-negative bacterium found in thermal springs. It has been shown to have immune-modulating effects through induction of dendritic cells, production of IL10 (an antiinflammatory cytokine), and subsequent priming of regulatory T cells (Tr1 cells) (Guéniche et al., 2006; Volz et al., 2014). Two double-blind, randomized, placebo-controlled studies investigating its use topically, one with participants with mild AD (Gueniche, Knaudt et al., 2008), the other with participants with moderate AD (Seité, Zelenkova, & Martin, 2017), found significant decreases in SCORAD in the treated group after 4 weeks, compared to the vehicle-only control group. Changes in participant microbiome were also noted in both studies. Gueniche, Knaudt et al. (2008) observed a nonsignificant decrease in bacterial colonization in the treated group. Seité et al. (2017) observed a significant increase in *Xanthomonas* in the treated group, while the control group had a nonsignificant increase in *Staphylococcus*. Additional

human studies have also observed clinical improvement in AD with topical application of *Vitreoscilla* (Guéniche et al., 2006; Guéniche, Dahel et al., 2008).

Bifidobacterium

A cream containing the lysate of *Bifidobacterium longum*, a gram-positive anaerobe, was tested by Guéniche et al. (2010) in a randomized, double-blind, placebo-controlled trial of 66 female participants with reactive skin, as determined by report of sensitive skin, leg dryness, and face roughness. Patients were instructed to apply either the lysate cream (N = 33) or control cream (N = 33) twice daily for 2 months, with evaluation at baseline, 1-month, and 2-month follow-up, assessing skin sensitivity, skin barrier function, and skin hydration. A decrease in skin sensitivity at 2 months, improvement in skin barrier function at 2 months, and a reduction in facial roughness and leg dryness at 1 month in the study group were observed. Although not tested in AD, authors suggest that topical *B. longum* can improve skin barrier function (Guéniche et al., 2010).

Staphylococcus

Skin dysbiosis in patients with AD is marked by changes in the abundance of different species of *Staphylococcus* bacteria. Select species of coagulase-negative *Staphylococcus* (CoNS) are known to produce AMPs that limit the growth of *S. aureus*. Nakatsuji et al. (2017) used this concept to test autologous transplant of CoNS onto five *S. aureus*–positive participants with AD. In this double-blind study, a cream containing antimicrobial strains of *S. epidermidis* and/or *Staphylococcus hominis* isolated from each of the five patients was applied back to the originating subject on one forearm, while vehicle was applied to the other forearm as control. Assessment of bacterial composition 1 day after application showed a significant decrease in *S. aureus* abundance on the area that received treatment with the antimicrobial CoNS, with no change in the abundance of *S. aureus* on untreated and vehicle areas (Nakatsuji et al., 2017). Clinical assessment of AD was not measured in this study, but results indicate a potential effective topical approach to treating skin dysbiosis. Additional investigation into autologous transplant is still underway (ClinicalTrials.gov. NCT01959113, NCT02144142).

Streptococcus

Streptococcus thermophilus is a gram-positive facultative anaerobe that has been shown to increase ceramide levels both in vitro and in vivo (Di Marzio, Cinque, De Simone, & Cifone, 1999). On the premise that topical application of ceramides can improve barrier function, and thus potentially benefit patients with AD, Di Marzio et al. (2003) investigated use of a cream containing *S. thermophilus* on 11 patients with AD, with participants treating one forearm with the formulation and the other with the vehicle as control. Evaluation of participants in this study at 2 weeks showed significant improvement in *S. thermophilus*-treated areas with regard to erythema, scaling, pruritus, and vesiculation. A statistically significant increase was also seen in the ceramide levels of the stratum corneum of treated skin, further supporting the importance of having a functioning skin barrier in control of AD. It should be noted that all study participants stopped application with the vehicle within 5 days due to lack of efficacy (Di Marzio et al., 2003).

Endolysins

Endolysins are enzymes produced by bacteriophages (viruses that infect bacteria) that break down the peptidoglycan cell wall of the bacteria, resulting in cell lysis (Toyofuku, Nomura, & Eberl, 2019). Staphefekt SA.100 is a recombinant phage endolysin that specifically targets *S. aureus*, including both methicillin-sensitive and resistant (MRSA) strains (Herpers & Leeson, 2015). Its use as a targeted topical therapy was theorized to decrease *S. aureus* levels without indiscriminately affecting skin commensals, as would be seen with a topical antibiotic or antiseptic (Totté et al., 2017). However, such efficacy was not demonstrated in clinical application. In a recent double-blind, vehicle-controlled study, 100 adult patients with clinically noninfected moderate to severe AD were given either Staphefekt SA.100 or vehicle to apply topically twice daily for 12 weeks (de Wit et al., 2019). The primary outcome was the difference in topical corticosteroid use with patients using the topical endolysin versus placebo. At the end of the 12-week intervention, no statistically significant difference in use of topical corticosteroids was observed between the two groups, nor were significant reductions in *S. aureus* seen, as measured by culture and qPCR (de Wit et al., 2019).

Antimicrobial-embedded clothing

The use of chitosan, a biopolymer found in nature as a component of the exoskeleton of shellfish, has been explored in multiple products, including cosmetics, medical products, and agriculture, due to its antimicrobial activity (Raafat & Sahl, 2009). Its use in clothing has also been studied and shown to have antimicrobial activity against *S. aureus* (Tavaria et al., 2012). In a study of 78 adults with AD, the use of chitosan-coated pajamas improved SCORAD values from patient baseline; however, this improvement was not statistically significant when compared to controls (Lopes et al., 2015). A systematic review of 13 studies investigating the use of other antimicrobial clothing items (silver-coated, silk, borage oil) found that these were generally safe and may improve disease severity (Lopes, Silva, Delgado, Correia, & Moreira, 2013).

Safety and Food and Drug Administration regulations

Use of probiotics is considered generally safe and well tolerated. A systematic review and meta-analysis evaluating the safety of *Lactobacillus* and *Bifidobacterium* in pregnancy (eight RCTs, 1546 patients) found that their use had no effect on cesarean section rate, birthweight, or gestational age (Dugoua et al., 2009). The most recent Cochrane review (see Oral Probiotics, earlier) included this review as well as two other reviews of probiotic safety and found no increased risk or adverse effects with their use (Makrgeorgou et al., 2018). The meta-analysis conducted by Kim et al. (2014) on the use of probiotics in treating AD reviewed safety data in 9 of the 25 included randomized trials and found no significant differences in adverse events in treatment versus control groups, with GI symptoms being the most common. Thus probiotic use in the treatment and prevention of AD is generally considered safe.

However, caution may be prudent in specific patient populations. There have been reports of serious adverse events such as sepsis, fungemia, and bowel ischemia in at-risk patients, including the critically ill in the intensive care unit, critically sick infants, postoperative and hospitalized patients, and immunocompromised patients (Didari, Solki, Mozaffari, Nikfar, & Abdollahi, 2014). There is also emerging concern that probiotics may alter the metabolism of anticancer drugs, altering their effects (Sotoudegan, Daniali, Hassani, Nikfar, & Abdollahi, 2019).

The US Food and Drug Administration (FDA) allows probiotics to be regulated as a dietary supplement, food, or drug, which is dependent upon the intended use (U.S. Food & Drug Administration, 2006). Food is defined as "articles used for food or drink for man or other animals," while a dietary supplement is defined as "a product intended to supplement the diet" and includes vitamins, minerals, herbs, and other nonconventional food items intended for ingestion (Federal Food, Drug, & Cosmetic Act, 2016). To be categorized as a drug, the intended use of the product is for "diagnosis, cure, mitigation, treatment, or prevention of disease" (Federal Food, Drug, & Cosmetic Act, 2016). Therefore, for a probiotic to market health benefits like a drug, it would need to go through the FDA approval process. If a probiotic is categorized as a food, it needs to be generally recognized as safe (GRAS), and if not, then it would need to have premarket clearance. A dietary supplement can go direct to market, and even make claims regarding its effect on a body structure or function (i.e., supports the immune system), provided it does not make specific health claims as related to a disease, which would then change its intended use to that of a drug (Degnan, 2008). Currently, a variety of probiotics have been categorized as dietary supplements and foods; however, to date, none have been approved to prevent or treat health problems under the category of drug (U.S. Food & Drug Administration, 2018, 2019).

Treatments on the horizon

Studies on the use of oral probiotics for the treatment and prevention of AD have shown mixed results. Though conclusions in meta-analyses are limited by study heterogeneity, investigators are now also examining how differences in individual microbiomes play a role in their effectiveness. Zmora et al. (2018) studied gut microbiome changes following administration of an 11-strain probiotic (predominantly *Lactobacillus* and *Bifidobacterium* strains) and found that the gut microbiome of study participants varied at baseline, and subsequently only a portion were colonized by the administered strains ("permissive"), while others were not ("resistant"), as measured by samples collected via colonoscopy and deep enteroscopy (representing gut mucosal colonization) following 3 weeks of treatment. This was independent from those bacteria shed in participant stool (Zmora et al., 2018). In a separate study by Suez et al. (2018), changes in the gut microbiome were investigated following oral antibiotics, with participant intervention being probiotics, autologous fecal microbiome transplant (aFMT), or no intervention ("watchful waiting"). Results showed that the gut microbiome of those receiving aFMT returned to baseline in as quickly as 1 day, while those taking probiotics did not return to baseline by 5 months after completion of probiotics course; those in the watchful waiting group returned to baseline at a time in between interventions (around 3 weeks) (Suez et al., 2018).

Microbiome precision editing, or modifying a person's microbiome for treatment of disease, is also being explored as a future investigative direction (Petrosino, 2018). Zhu et al. (2018) studied the impact of tungsten administration (a metal that can inactivate an *Enterobacteriacea* cofactor) on mice with chemically induced colitis. In the study, mice were colonized with bacteria (*Escherichia coli*, Family: *Enterobacteriaceae*) from human patients with inflammatory bowel disease, treated with oral tungstate, and reported to have a selective decrease of *Enterobacteriaceae* with subsequent decrease in inflammation, without observed changes to the microbiome in homeostasis (Zhu et al., 2018). Together, these examples suggest that the effects of probiotics vary by person, dependent on individual microbiomes, and that a tailored approach may produce better results.

New insights into the impact on the microbiome of already existing treatments are emerging. A recent investigation into the effects of dupilumab, an IL4a receptor antagonist that is FDA approved for the treatment of moderate to severe AD, demonstrated that treatment with dupilumab not only resulted in clinical improvement but also in microbiome changes (Callewaert et al., 2020). Prior to treatment, higher levels of *S. aureus* and lower microbial diversity were seen in lesional skin, consistent with other studies. Following 16 weeks of treatment with dupilumab, significant decreases in *S. aureus* and increases in microbial diversity were observed (Callewaert et al., 2020). Further investigation into topical therapies that alter the microbiome and lead to improvement in AD are also underway. The safety and efficacy of a targeted microbiome transplant (TMT) lotion on adult patients with moderate to severe AD and positive *S. aureus* skin lesions is ongoing (ClinicalTrials.gov. NCT03151148).

Summary

Interest in the use of probiotics for the prevention and treatment of AD has increased as our understanding of the microbiome has expanded. However, evidence gathered on the benefits of use of oral probiotics from systematic reviews and meta-analyses has been less convincing. As of now, a promising new avenue for treatment is the topical use of products geared toward altering the cutaneous microbiome. However, studies to date remain small and limited.

In the United States, currently no probiotics have gone through the rigorous testing for approval as a drug, and so cannot be sold for the purpose of treatment or prevention of disease. Thus they remain largely unregulated in regard to strain, dosage, and validity of health claims. Recognizing that the microbiome of each individual is unique and may contribute to the heterogenous clinical response to treatment with probiotics, future work may investigate and utilize a more personalized approach to treatment.

Further readings

Baldassarre, M. E., Palladino, V., Amoruso, A., Pindinelli, S., Mastromarino, P., Fanelli, M., et al. (2018). Rationale of probiotic supplementation during pregnancy and neonatal period. *Nutrients, 10*(11). https://doi.org/10.3390/nu10111693.

Chang, Y. S., Trivedi, M. K., Jha, A., Lin, Y. F., Dimaano, L., & García-Romero, M. T. (2016). Synbiotics for prevention and treatment of atopic dermatitis: A meta-analysis of randomized clinical trials. *JAMA Pediatrics, 170*(3), 236–242. https://doi.org/10.1001/jamapediatrics.2015.3943.

Forsberg, A., West, C. E., Prescott, S. L., & Jenmalm, M. C. (2016). Pre- and probiotics for allergy prevention: Time to revisit recommendations? *Clinical & Experimental Allergy, 46*(12), 1506–1521. https://doi.org/10.1111/cea.12838.

Hulshof, L., Van't Land, B., Sprikkelman, A. B., & Garssen, J. (2017). Role of microbial modulation in management of atopic dermatitis in children. *Nutrients, 9*(8), 854. https://doi.org/10.3390/nu9080854.

Lopes, E. G., Moreira, D. A., Gullón, P., Gullón, B., Cardelle-Cobas, A., & Tavaria, F. K. (2017). Topical application of probiotics in skin: Adhesion, antimicrobial and antibiofilm invitro assays. *Journal of Applied Microbiology, 122*(2), 450–461. https://doi.org/10.1111/jam.1334.

Makrgeorgou, A., Leonardi-Bee, J., Bath-Hextall, F. J., Murrell, D. F., Tang, M. L., Roberts, A., & Boyle, R. J. (2018). Probiotics for treating eczema. *Cochrane Database of Systematic Reviews, 11* https://doi.org/10.1002/14651858.CD006135.pub3. CD006135.

Nakatsuji, T., Chen, T. H., Narala, S., Chun, K. A., Two, A. M., Yun, T., et al. (2017). Antimicrobials from human skin commensal bacteria protect against *Staphylococcus aureus* and are deficient in atopic dermatitis. *Science Translational Medicine, 9*(378). https://doi.org/10.1126/scitranslmed.aah4680.

Rather, I. A., Bajpai, V. K., Kumar, S., Lim, J., Paek, W. K., & Park, Y. H. (2016). Probiotics and atopic dermatitis: An overview. *Frontiers in Microbiology, 7*, 507. https://doi.org/10.3389/fmicb.2016.00507.

West, C. E., Dzidic, M., Prescott, S. L., & Jenmalm, M. C. (2017). Bugging allergy; role of pre-, pro- and synbiotics in allergy prevention. *Allergology International, 66*(4), 529–538. https://doi.org/10.1016/j.alit.2017.08.001.

References

Birnie, A. J., Bath-Hextall, F. J., Ravenscroft, J. C., & Williams, H. C. (2008). Interventions to reduce *Staphylococcus aureus* in the management of atopic eczema. *Cochrane Database of Systematic Reviews, 16*(3), CD003871. https://doi.org/10.1002/14651858. CD003871.pub2.

Blanchet-Réthoré, S., Bourdès, V., Mercenier, A., Haddar, C. H., Verhoeven, P. O., & Andres, P. (2017). Effect of a lotion containing the heat-treated probiotic strain *Lactobacillus johnsonii* NCC 533 on *Staphylococcus aureus* colonization in atopic dermatitis. *Clinical, Cosmetic and Investigational Dermatology, 10*, 249–257. https://doi.org/10.2147/CCID.S135529.

Boyle, R. J., Leonardi-Bee, J., Bath-Hextall, F. J., & Tang, M. L. (2009). Probiotics for the treatment or prevention of eczema. *The Journal of Allergy and Clinical Immunology, 123*(1), 266–267. https://doi.org/10.1016/j.jaci.2008.07.042.

Callewaert, C., Nakatsuji, T., Knight, R., Kosciolek, T., Vrbanac, A., Kotol, P., et al. (2020). IL 4a blockade by dupilumab decreases *Staphylococcus aureus* colonization and increases microbial diversity in atopic dermatitis. *Journal of Investigative Dermatology, 140*(1), 191–202.E7. https://doi.org/10.1016/j.jid.2019.05.024.

Cao, L., Wang, L., Yang, L. J., Tao, S. Q., Xia, R. S., & Fan, W. X. (2015). Long-term effect of early-life supplementation with probiotics on preventing atopic dermatitis: A meta-analysis. *Journal of Dermatological Treatment, 26*(6), 537–540. https://doi.org/10.31 09/09546634.2015.1027168.

Chang, Y. S., Trivedi, M. K., Jha, A., Lin, Y. F., Dimaano, L., & García-Romero, M. T. (2016). Synbiotics for prevention and treatment of atopic dermatitis: A meta-analysis of randomized clinical trials. *JAMA Pediatrics, 170*(3), 236–242. https://doi.org/10.1001/jamapediatrics.2015.3943.

ClinicalTrials.gov. NCT01959113. Phase 1 Study of the Short-term Antimicrobial Action of Transplanted Bacteria in Adult Patients With Atopic Dermatitis. "Actual Study Completion Date" listed as June 2016 (https://clinicaltrials.gov/ct2/show/NCT01959113? term=nct01959113&draw=2&rank=1).

ClinicalTrials.gov. NCT02144142. Phase 2 Study Evaluating the Kinetic Properties of an Autologous Microbiome Transplant in Adult Atopic Dermatitis Patients. "Estimated Study Completion Date" of July 2022 (https://clinicaltrials.gov/ct2/show/study/NCT 02144142?term=nct02144142&draw=2&rank=1).

ClinicalTrials.gov. NCT03151148. A First in Man Evaluation of the Safety and Efficacy of an Allogeneic Targeted Microbiome Transplant in Adults With Moderate-to-Severe Atopic Dermatitis (ADRN-08). "Actual Study Completion Date" listed as June 7, 2019 (from https://clinicaltrials.gov/ct2/show/NCT03151148?ter m=nct03151148&draw=2&rank=1).

Cuello-Garcia, C. A., Brożek, J. L., Fiocchi, A., Pawankar, R., Yepes-Nuñez, J. J., Terracciano, L., et al. (2015). Probiotics for the prevention of allergy: A systematic review and meta-analysis of randomized controlled trials. *The Journal of Allergy and Clinical Immunology, 136*(4), 952–961. https://doi.org/10.1016/j. jaci.2015.04.031.

Cuello-Garcia, C. A., Fiocchi, A., Pawankar, R., Yepes-Nuñez, J. J., Morgano, G. P., Zhang, Y., et al. (2016). World Allergy Organization—McMaster University Guidelines for Allergic Disease Prevention (GLAD-P): Prebiotics. *The World Allergy Organization Journal, 9*, 10. https://doi.org/10.1186/s40413-016-0102-7.

Dang, D., Zhou, W., Lun, Z. J., Mu, X., Wang, D. X., & Wu, H. (2013). Meta-analysis of probiotics and/or prebiotics for the prevention of eczema. *Journal of International Medical Research, 41*(5), 1426–1436. https://doi.org/10.1177/0300060513493692.

Dargahi, N., Johnson, J., Donkor, O., Vasiljevic, T., & Apostolopoulos, V. (2019). Immunomodulatory effects of probiotics: Can they be used to treat allergies and autoimmune diseases? *Maturitas, 119*, 25–38. https://doi.org/10.1016/j.maturitas.2018.11.002.

de Wit, J., Totté, J. E. E., van Mierlo, M. M. F., van Veldhuizen, J., van Doorn, M. B. A., Schuren, F. H. J., et al. (2019). Endolysin treatment against *Staphylococcus aureus* in adults with atopic dermatitis: A randomized controlled trial. *The Journal of Allergy and Clinical Immunology, 144*(3), 860–863. https://doi.org/10.1016/j. jaci.2019.05.020.

Degnan, F. H. (2008). The US Food and Drug Administration and probiotics: Regulatory categorization. *Clinical Infectious Diseases, 46*(Suppl 2), S133–S136. https://doi.org/10.1086/523324. discussion S144–51.

Di Marzio, L., Centi, C., Cinque, B., Masci, S., Giuliani, M., Arcieri, A., et al. (2003). Effect of the lactic acid bacterium *Streptococcus thermophilus* on stratum corneum ceramide levels and signs and symptoms of atopic dermatitis patients. *Experimental Dermatology, 12*(5), 615–620. https://doi. org/10.1034/j.1600-0625.2003.00051.x.

Di Marzio, L., Cinque, B., De Simone, C., & Cifone, M. G. (1999). Effect of the lactic acid bacterium *Streptococcus thermophilus* on ceramide levels in human keratinocytes in vitro and stratum corneum in vivo. *Journal of Investigative Dermatology, 113*(1), 98–106. https://doi.org/10.1046/j.1523-1747.1999.00633.x.

Didari, T., Solki, S., Mozaffari, S., Nikfar, S., & Abdollahi, M. (2014). A systematic review of the safety of probiotics. *Expert Opinion on Drug Safety, 13*(2), 227–239. https://doi.org/10.1517/14740338 .2014.872627.

Dugoua, J. J., Machado, M., Zhu, X., Chen, X., Koren, G., & Einarson, T. R. (2009). Probiotic safety in pregnancy: A systematic review and meta-analysis of randomized controlled trials of *Lactobacillus, Bifidobacterium,* and *Saccharomyces* spp. *Journal of Obstetrics and Gynaecology Canada, 31*(6), 542–552. https://doi. org/10.1016/S1701-2163(16)34218-9.

Eichenfield, L. F., Tom, W. L., Berger, T. G., Krol, A., Paller, A. S., Schwarzenberger, K., et al. (2014). Guidelines of care for the management of atopic dermatitis Section 2. Management and treatment of atopic dermatitis with topical therapies. *Journal of the American Academy of Dermatology, 71*(1), 116–132. https://doi. org/10.1016/j.jaad.2014.03.023.

Elazab, N., Mendy, A., Gasana, J., Vieira, E. R., Quizon, A., & Forno, E. (2013). Probiotic administration in early life, atopy, and asthma: A meta-analysis of clinical trials. *Pediatrics, 132*(3), e666–e676. https://doi.org/10.1542/peds.2013-0246.

Federal Food, Drug, and Cosmetic Act. (2016). 21 USC 321: Definitions; generally.

Fiocchi, A., Pawankar, R., Cuello-Garcia, C., Ahn, K., Al-Hammadi, S., Agarwal, A., et al. (2015). World Allergy Organization–McMaster University Guidelines for Allergic Disease Prevention (GLAD-P): Probiotics. *The World Allergy Organization Journal, 8*(1), 4.https://doi.org/10.1186/s40413-015-0055-2.

Florowska, A., Krygier, K., Florowski, T., & Dłużewska, E. (2016). Prebiotics as functional food ingredients preventing diet-related diseases. *Food and Function, 7*(5), 2147–2155. https://doi. org/10.1039/c5fo01459j.

Gao, J., Li, Y., Wan, Y., Hu, T., Liu, L., Yang, S., et al. (2019). A novel postbiotic from *Lactobacillus rhamnosus* GG with a beneficial effect on intestinal barrier function. *Frontiers in Microbiology, 10*, 477. https://doi.org/10.3389/fmicb.2019.00477.

Gibson, G. R., Hutkins, R., Sanders, M. E., Prescott, S. L., Reimer, R. A., Salminen, S. J., et al. (2017). Expert consensus document: The International Scientific Association for Probiotics and Prebiotics (ISAPP) consensus statement on the definition and scope of prebiotics. *Nature Reviews Gastroenterology & Hepatology, 14*(8), 491–502. https://doi.org/10.1038/nrgastro.2017.75.

Guéniche, A., Bastien, P., Ovigne, J. M., Kermici, M., Courchay, G., Chevalier, V., et al. (2010). *Bifidobacterium longum* lysate, a new ingredient for reactive skin. *Experimental Dermatology, 19*(8), e1–e8. https://doi.org/10.1111/j.1600-0625.2009.00932.x.

Guéniche, A., Dahel, K., Bastien, P., Martin, R., Nicolas, J. F., & Breton, L. (2008). *Vitreoscilla filiformis* bacterial extract to improve the efficacy of emollient used in atopic dermatitis symptoms. *Journal of the European Academy of Dermatology and Venereology, 22*(6), 746–747. https://doi.org/10.1111/j.1468-3083.2007.02428.x.

Guéniche, A., Hennino, A., Goujon, C., Dahel, K., Bastien, P., Martin, R., et al. (2006). Improvement of atopic dermatitis skin symptoms by *Vitreoscilla filiformis* bacterial extract. *European Journal of Dermatology, 16*(4), 380–384.

Gueniche, A., Knaudt, B., Schuck, E., Volz, T., Bastien, P., Martin, R., et al. (2008). Effects of nonpathogenic gram-negative bacterium *Vitreoscilla filiformis* lysate on atopic dermatitis: A prospective, randomized, double-blind, placebo-controlled clinical study. *British Journal of Dermatology, 159*(6), 1357–1363. https://doi.org/10.1111/j.1365-2133.2008.08836.x.

Herpers, B. L., & Leeson, N. (2015). Endolysins: Redefining antibacterial therapy. *Future Microbiology, 10*(3), 309–311. https://doi.org/10.2217/fmb.14.142.

Hill, C., Guarner, F., Reid, G., Gibson, G. R., Merenstein, D. J., Pot, B., et al. (2014). Expert consensus document. The International Scientific Association for Probiotics and Prebiotics consensus statement on the scope and appropriate use of the term probiotic. *Nature Reviews Gastroenterology & Hepatology, 11*(8), 506–514. https://doi.org/10.1038/nrgastro.2014.66.

Huang, R., Ning, H., Shen, M., Li, J., Zhang, J., & Chen, X. (2017). Probiotics for the treatment of atopic dermatitis in children: A systematic review and meta-analysis of randomized controlled trials. *Frontiers in Cellular and Infection Microbiology, 7*, 392. https://doi.org/10.3389/fcimb.2017.00392.

Jandhyala, S. M., Talukdar, R., Subramanyam, C., Vuyyuru, H., Sasikala, M., & Nageshwar Reddy, D. (2015). Role of the normal gut microbiota. *World Journal of Gastroenterology, 21*(29), 8787–8803. https://doi.org/10.3748/wjg.v21.i29.8787.

Jung, G. W., Tse, J. E., Guiha, I., & Rao, J. (2013). Prospective, randomized, open-label trial comparing the safety, efficacy, and tolerability of an acne treatment regimen with and without a probiotic supplement and minocycline in subjects with mild to moderate acne. *Journal of Cutaneous Medicine and Surgery, 17*(2), 114–122. https://doi.org/10.2310/7750.2012.12026.

Khmaladze, I., Butler, É., Fabre, S., & Gillbro, J. M. (2019). *Lactobacillus reuteri* DSM 17938–A comparative study on the effect of probiotics and lysates on human skin. *Experimental Dermatology, 28*(7), 822–828. https://doi.org/10.1111/exd.13950.

Kim, S. O., Ah, Y. M., Yu, Y. M., Choi, K. H., Shin, W. G., & Lee, J. Y. (2014). Effects of probiotics for the treatment of atopic dermatitis: A meta-analysis of randomized controlled trials. *Annals of Allergy, Asthma and Immunology, 113*(2), 217–226. https://doi.org/10.1016/j.anai.2014.05.021.

Kukkonen, K., Savilahti, E., Haahtela, T., Juntunen-Backman, K., Korpela, R., Poussa, T., et al. (2007). Probiotics and prebiotic galacto-oligosaccharides in the prevention of allergic diseases: A randomized, double-blind, placebo-controlled trial. *The Journal of Allergy and Clinical Immunology, 119*(1), 192–198. https://doi.org/10.1016/j.jaci.2006.09.009.

Li, L., Han, Z., Niu, X. P., Zhang, G. Z., Jia, Y. L., Zhang, S. G., & He, C. Y. (2019). Probiotic supplementation for prevention of atopic dermatitis in infants and children: A systematic review and meta-analysis. *American Journal of Clinical Dermatology, 20*(3), 367–377. https://doi.org/10.1007/s40257-018-0404-3.

Lopes, C., Silva, D., Delgado, L., Correia, O., & Moreira, A. (2013). Functional textiles for atopic dermatitis: A systematic review and meta-analysis. *Pediatric Allergy and Immunology, 24*(6), 603–613. https://doi.org/10.1111/pai.12111.

Lopes, C., Soares, J., Tavaria, F., Duarte, A., Correia, O., Sokhatska, O., et al. (2015). Chitosan coated textiles may improve atopic dermatitis severity by modulating skin staphylococcal profile: A randomized controlled trial. *PLoS One, 10*(11), e0142844. https://doi.org/10.1371/journal.pone.0142844.

Lopes, E. G., Moreira, D. A., Gullón, P., Gullón, B., Cardelle-Cobas, A., & Tavaria, F. K. (2017). Topical application of probiotics in skin: Adhesion, antimicrobial and antibiofilm in vitro assays. *Journal of Applied Microbiology, 122*(2), 450–461. https://doi.org/10.1111/jam.13349.

Makrgeorgou, A., Leonardi-Bee, J., Bath-Hextall, F. J., Murrell, D. F., Tang, M. L., Roberts, A., & Boyle, R. J. (2018). Probiotics for treating eczema. *Cochrane Database of Systematic Reviews, 11*, CD006135. https://doi.org/10.1002/14651858.CD006135.pub3.

Mansfield, J. A., Bergin, S. W., Cooper, J. R., & Olsen, C. H. (2014). Comparative probiotic strain efficacy in the prevention of eczema in infants and children: A systematic review and meta-analysis. *Military Medicine, 179*(6), 580–592. https://doi.org/10.7205/Milmed-D-13-00546.

Myles, I. A., Earland, N. J., Anderson, E. D., Moore, I. N., Kieh, M. D., Williams, K. W., et al. (2018). First-in-human topical microbiome transplantation with *Roseomonas mucosa* for atopic dermatitis. *JCI Insight, 3*(9). https://doi.org/10.1172/jci.insight.120608.

Myles, I. A., Williams, K. W., Reckhow, J. D., Jammeh, M. L., Pincus, N. B., Sastalla, I., et al. (2016). Transplantation of human skin microbiota in models of atopic dermatitis. *JCI Insight, 1*(10). https://doi.org/10.1172/jci.insight.86955.

Nakatsuji, T., Chen, T. H., Narala, S., Chun, K. A., Two, A. M., Yun, T., et al. (2017). Antimicrobials from human skin commensal bacteria protect against *Staphylococcus aureus* and are deficient in atopic dermatitis. *Science Translational Medicine, 9*(378). https://doi.org/10.1126/scitranslmed.aah4680.

Navarro-López, V., Martínez-Andrés, A., Ramírez-Boscá, A., Ruzafa-Costas, B., Núñez-Delegido, E., Carrión-Gutiérrez, M. A., et al. (2019). Efficacy and safety of oral administration of a mixture of probiotic strains in patients with psoriasis: A randomized controlled clinical trial. *Acta Dermato-Venereologica, 99*(12), 1078–1084. https://doi.org/10.2340/00015555-3305.

Oliphant, K., & Allen-Vercoe, E. (2019). Macronutrient metabolism by the human gut microbiome: Major fermentation by-products and their impact on host health. *Microbiome, 7*(1), 91. https://doi.org/10.1186/s40168-019-0704-8.

Osborn, D. A., & Sinn, J. K. (2013). Prebiotics in infants for prevention of allergy. *Cochrane Database of Systematic Reviews, 3*, CD006474. https://doi.org/10.1002/14651858.CD006474.pub3.

Panduru, M., Panduru, N. M., Sălăvăstru, C. M., & Tiplica, G. S. (2015). Probiotics and primary prevention of atopic dermatitis: A meta-analysis of randomized controlled studies. *Journal of the*

European Academy of Dermatology and Venereology, 29(2), 232–242. https://doi.org/10.1111/jdv.12496.

Pelucchi, C., Chatenoud, L., Turati, F., Galeone, C., Moja, L., Bach, J. F., & La Vecchia, C. (2012). Probiotics supplementation during pregnancy or infancy for the prevention of atopic dermatitis a meta-analysis. *Epidemiology, 23*(3), 402–414. https://doi.org/10.1097/EDE.0b013e31824d5da2.

de Melo Pereira, G. V., de Oliveira Coelho, B., Magalhães Júnior, A. I., Thomaz-Soccol, V., & Soccol, C. R. (2018). How to select a probiotic? A review and update of methods and criteria. *Biotechnology Advances, 36*(8), 2060–2076. https://doi.org/10.1016/j.biotechadv.2018.09.003.

Petrosino. J. F. (2018). The microbiome in precision medicine: The way forward. *Genome Medicine, 10*(1), 12. https://doi.org/10.1186/s13073-018-0525-6.

Raafat, D., & Sahl, H. G. (2009). Chitosan and its antimicrobial potential—A critical literature survey. *Microbial Biotechnology, 2*(2), 186–201. https://doi.org/10.1111/j.1751-7915.2008.00080.x.

Rao, R. K., & Samak, G. (2013). Protection and restitution of gut barrier by probiotics: Nutritional and clinical implications. *Current Nutrition & Food Science, 9*(2), 99–107. https://doi.org/10.2174/1573401311309020004.

Rather, I. A., Bajpai, V. K., Kumar, S., Lim, J., Paek, W. K., & Park, Y. H. (2016). Probiotics and atopic dermatitis: An overview. *Frontiers in Microbiology, 7*, 507. https://doi.org/10.3389/fmicb.2016.00507.

Rezac, S., Kok, C. R., Heermann, M., & Hutkins, R. (2018). Fermented foods as a dietary source of live organisms. *Frontiers in Microbiology, 9*, 1785. https://doi.org/10.3389/fmicb.2018.01785.

Rosignoli, C., Thibaut de Ménonville, S., Orfila, D., Béal, M., Bertino, B., Aubert, J., et al. (2018). A topical treatment containing heat-treated *Lactobacillus johnsonii* NCC 533 reduces *Staphylococcus aureus* adhesion and induces antimicrobial peptide expression in an in vitro reconstructed human epidermis model. *Experimental Dermatology, 27*(4), 358–365. https://doi.org/10.1111/exd.13504.

Rozé, J. C., Barbarot, S., Butel, M. J., Kapel, N., Waligora-Dupriet, A. J., De Montgolfier, I., et al. (2012). An alpha-lactalbumin-enriched and symbiotic-supplemented v. a standard infant formula: A multicentre, double-blind, randomised trial. *The British Journal of Nutrition, 107*(11), 1616–1622. https://doi.org/10.1017/S000711451100479X.

Seité, S., Zelenkova, H., & Martin, R. (2017). Clinical efficacy of emollients in atopic dermatitis patients—relationship with the skin microbiota modification. *Clinical, Cosmetic and Investigational Dermatology, 10*, 25–33. https://doi.org/10.2147/CCID.S121910.

Sidbury, R., Tom, W. L., Bergman, J. N., Cooper, K. D., Silverman, R. A., Berger, T. G., et al. (2014). Guidelines of care for the management of atopic dermatitis: Section 4. Prevention of disease flares and use of adjunctive therapies and approaches. *Journal of the American Academy of Dermatology, 71*(6), 1218–1233. https://doi.org/10.1016/j.jaad.2014.08.038.

Sotoudegan, F., Daniali, M., Hassani, S., Nikfar, S., & Abdollahi, M. (2019). Reappraisal of probiotics' safety in human. *Food and Chemical Toxicology, 129*, 22–29. https://doi.org/10.1016/j.fct.2019.04.032.

Spinler, J. K., Taweechotipatr, M., Rognerud, C. L., Ou, C. N., Tumwasorn, S., & Versalovic, J. (2008). Human-derived probiotic *Lactobacillus reuteri* demonstrate antimicrobial activities targeting diverse enteric bacterial pathogens. *Anaerobe, 14*(3), 166–171. https://doi.org/10.1016/j.anaerobe.2008.02.001.

Suez, J., Zmora, N., Zilberman-Schapira, G., Mor, U., Dori-Bachash, M., Bashiardes, S., et al. (2018). Post-antibiotic gut mucosal microbiome reconstitution is impaired by probiotics and improved by autologous FMT. *Cell, 174*(6), 1406–1423. https://doi.org/10.1016/j.cell.2018.08.047. e16.

Szajewska, H., & Horvath, A. (2018). *Lactobacillus rhamnosus* GG in the primary prevention of eczema in children: A systematic review and meta-analysis. *Nutrients, 10*(9). https://doi.org/10.3390/nu10091319.

Tan, J., McKenzie, C., Potamitis, M., Thorburn, A. N., Mackay, C. R., & Macia, L. (2014). The role of short-chain fatty acids in health and disease. *Advances in Immunology, 121*, 91–119. https://doi.org/10.1016/B978-0-12-800100-4.00003-9.

Tavaria, F. K., Soares, J. C., Reis, I. L., Paulo, M. H., Malcata, F. X., & Pintado, M. E. (2012). Chitosan: Antimicrobial action upon staphylococci after impregnation onto cotton fabric. *Journal of Applied Microbiology, 112*(5), 1034–1041. https://doi.org/10.1111/j.1365-2672.2012.05274.x.

Totté, J., de Wit, J., Pardo, L., Schuren, F., van Doorn, M., & Pasmans, S. (2017). Targeted anti-staphylococcal therapy with endolysins in atopic dermatitis and the effect on steroid use, disease severity and the microbiome: Study protocol for a randomized controlled trial (MAAS trial). *Trials, 18*(1), 404. https://doi.org/10.1186/s13063-017-2118-x.

Toyofuku, M., Nomura, N., & Eberl, L. (2019). Types and origins of bacterial membrane vesicles. *Nature Reviews Microbiology, 17*(1), 13–24. https://doi.org/10.1038/s41579-018-0112-2.

U.S. Food and Drug Administration. (2019) Microorganisms & Microbial-Derived Ingredients Used in Food (Partial List). https://www.fda.gov/food/generally-recognized-safe-gras/microorganisms-microbial-derived-ingredients-used-food-partial-list. Accessed September 9, 2019.

U.S. Food and Drug Administration. (2006). "Complementary and Alternative Medicine Products and Their Regulation by the Food and Drug Administration: Guidance for Industry. https://www.fda.gov/regulatory-information/search-fda-guidance-documents/complementary-and-alternative-medicine-products-and-their-regulation-food-and-drug-administration. Accessed September 9, 2019.

U.S. Food and Drug Administration. (2018). Statement from FDA Commissioner Scott Gottlieb, M.D. on advancing the science and regulation of live microbiome-based products used to prevent, treat, or cure diseases in humans. Accessed September 9, 2019.

Volz, T., Skabytska, Y., Guenova, E., Chen, K. M., Frick, J. S., Kirschning, C. J., et al. (2014). Nonpathogenic bacteria alleviating atopic dermatitis inflammation induce IL-10-producing dendritic cells and regulatory Tr1 cells. *Journal of Investigative Dermatology, 134*(1), 96–104. https://doi.org/10.1038/jid.2013.291.

West, C. E., Dzidic, M., Prescott, S. L., & Jenmalm, M. C. (2017). Bugging allergy; role of pre-, pro- and synbiotics in allergy prevention. *Allergology International, 66*(4), 529–538. https://doi.org/10.1016/j.alit.2017.08.001.

World Gastroenterology Organisation. (2017). Prebiotics and probiotics. https://www.worldgastroenterology.org/UserFiles/file/guidelines/probiotics-and-prebiotics-english-2017.pdf.

Zhao, M., Shen, C., & Ma, L. (2018). Treatment efficacy of probiotics on atopic dermatitis, zooming in on infants: A systematic review and meta-analysis. *International Journal of Dermatology, 57*(6), 635–641. https://doi.org/10.1111/ijd.13873.

Zhu, W., Winter, M. G., Byndloss, M. X., Spiga, L., Duerkop, B. A., Hughes, E. R., et al. (2018). Precision editing of the gut microbiota ameliorates colitis. *Nature, 553*(7687), 208–211. https://doi.org/10.1038/nature25172.

Zmora, N., Zilberman-Schapira, G., Suez, J., Mor, U., Dori-Bachash, M., Bashiardes, S., et al. (2018). Personalized gut mucosal colonization resistance to empiric probiotics is associated with unique host and microbiome features. *Cell, 174*(6), 1388–1405. https://doi.org/10.1016/j.cell.2018.08.041. e21.

Zuccotti, G., Meneghin, F., Aceti, A., Barone, G., Callegari, M. L., Di Mauro, A., et al. (2015). Probiotics for prevention of atopic diseases in infants: Systematic review and meta-analysis. *Allergy, 70*(11), 1356–1371. https://doi.org/10.1111/all.12700.

25

Itch and Pain Treatments

CHRISTINA KURSEWICZ, KAYLA FOURZALI, AND GIL YOSIPOVITCH

KEY POINTS

- Itch and pain are key symptoms of atopic dermatitis (AD) that significantly affect quality of life; various classes of treatment aim to reduce these symptoms.
- Nonpharmacologic and topical therapies are effective for mild or moderate itch or pain symptoms and for maintenance therapy of AD.
- Systemic therapies that target the immune system are effective as antipruritics, but many have side effects that limit their use.
- Newer biologic and small-molecule therapies have been developed to target itch-mediated signaling pathways and have shown exciting results in AD patients.
- Several experimental therapies are on the horizon that target nonhistaminergic itch pathways and show promise in clinical trials.

Introduction

Pruritus, or itch, is the predominant feature of atopic dermatitis (AD) and it is an essential diagnostic feature of the disease (Eichenfield, Tom, Chamlin et al., 2014). The underlying mechanism of AD and the itch that it causes is multifactorial due to a complex interplay of genetic, environmental, and immunologic factors. A key aspect of AD pathogenesis and target of many first-line interventions is dysfunction of the physical epidermal barrier that contributes to transepidermal water loss (TEWL). TEWL has been shown to be associated with itch intensity in AD patients (Lee et al., 2006). Barrier disruption allows for entry of irritants, allergens, and pruritogens from the external environment, leading to immune activation and inflammation, and pruritus. Defects in the barrier also lead to alkalization of the skin pH, promoting protease activation and upregulation of pruritogenic receptors and proinflammatory neuropeptides. The type 2 immunologic response, also key to pathogenesis of this disease, is mediated by cytokines such as interleulin-4 (IL4) and IL13, which are targets of newer AD medications. Other key immune mediators in AD are IL2, IL31, and IL33. Itch in AD is known to be nonhistaminergic in nature and not responsive to antihistamine medications. Emerging evidence shows that hypersensitivity of the neural pathways that conduct nonhistaminergic itch sensation in the peripheral and central nervous system may play a role in pathogenesis of this and other chronic pruritic diseases (Mollanazar, Smith, & Yosipovitch, 2016; Stander & Steinhoff, 2002).

Itch experienced in AD may vary from patient to patient, but surveys have shown that people with AD tend to experience itch more frequently at night, have high pleasurability with scratching, and have itch accompanied by a sensation of heat (Dawn et al., 2009). Aggravating factors commonly reported by AD patients include stress, perspiration, and skin dryness (Yosipovitch et al., 2002). Skin pain is often reported in patients with AD, and while this is at least partially explained by scratching or excoriated lesions, a subset of AD patients experience painlike itch independent of scratching that is similar to neuropathic pain (Rosen, Fostini, Chan, Nattkemper, & Yosipovitch, 2018; Vakharia et al., 2017). Pain is most often described by patients as burning, stinging, soreness, or tightness of the skin and is most likely to accompany lesions on the hands, feet, and around the mouth. AD-related pain has similar triggers to those associated with itch (i.e., sweat, stress, and warm temperatures) (Maarouf et al., 2018). Skin pain is not often directly measured as part of standardized AD disease scores but has been shown to strongly correlate with measures of AD severity and symptoms (e.g., Patient Oriented Eczema Measure [POEM] and Eczema Area and Severity Index [EASI]) as well as poorer sleep and increased itch on numeric rating scales (Maarouf et al., 2018; Vakharia et al., 2017). Quality of life is reported by patients to be greatly affected by their symptoms, as is seen in chronic itch of various etiologies (Kini et al., 2011; Yosipovitch et al. 2001; Yosipovitch, Goon, Wee, Chan, & Goh, 2000). The neurosensory mechanisms underlying pruritus in general and involving AD in particular are discussed in greater detail in Chapter 16.

The goal of therapy in AD is to significantly reduce or eliminate the patient's symptoms, namely pruritus and pain, while also reducing the burden of skin lesions and preventing infection. Itch is not only a bothersome symptom but also leads to scratching, which promotes further inflammation of the skin, excoriations, and the potential for infection and chronic skin changes. This itch-scratch cycle must be interrupted to prevent these complications. Numerous treatment methods have been proposed for reducing symptoms of itch and pain in AD, ranging from at-home skin care techniques to systemic medications to integrative medicine approaches. This chapter aims to review those techniques that have demonstrated efficacy in reducing the burden of these symptoms.

Nonpharmacologic therapies: Moisturization and bathing practices reducing itch

The goal of moisturization is to improve the epidermal barrier, so to limit TEWL and prevent exposure to irritants and allergens causing itch. Moisturizing agents are readily available over the counter (OTC) and are integral to the daily therapy of AD and can be used as an adjuvant to topical or systemic treatments. While moisturization has been shown to effectively reduce xerotic and pruritic symptoms of AD, systematic review has not shown a specific topical moisturizer to be most effective in AD (Boralevi et al., 2014; Tiplica et al., 2018; van Zuuren, Fedorowicz, & Arents, 2017). Considering there are minimal adverse effects to moisturizer application, patients are recommended to reapply frequently and in liberal amounts. Additional moisturization and skin barrier repair recommendations are discussed in Chapter 22.

There is limited evidence informing the recommended frequency or duration of bathing for individuals with AD, but many practitioners recommend warm water bathing up to once daily for no longer than 10 minutes. Bar soaps used while bathing are often alkaline in pH (~pH 10), which can lead to increased activity of proteases in the epidermis and subsequent degradation of the barrier function and activation of itch receptors (Ali & Yosipovitch, 2013; Hachem et al., 2005). To reduce the potential for exacerbation of pruritus, nonsoap cleansers (synthetic detergents or syndets) with a neutral or low pH (~pH 5–7) are recommended. Additional bathing recommendations are discussed in Chapter 26.

Oatmeal-based products derived from the plant *Avena sativa* have been used for many years as an additive to bathing products and moisturizers. Colloid oatmeal agents have been shown to help with restoring normal skin pH, improve barrier integrity, reduce itch, and act as an antioxidant and antiinflammatory (Kurtz & Wallo, 2007). Formulations used as moisturizers or bathing products have been shown to improve AD-related symptoms, including pruritus, with regular use and are generally well tolerated (Fowler, Nebus, Wallo, & Eichenfield, 2012; Lisante, Nunez, Zhang, & Mathes, 2017). Additional complementary and alternative modalities are discussed in Chapter 26.

Topical pharmacologic treatments

Topical corticosteroids

Topical corticosteroids (TCS) are the first-line pharmacologic treatment for AD, often introduced for maintenance therapy and use in the treatment of acute flares (Eichenfield, Tom, Berger et al., 2014). While TCS do not have a direct antipruritic effect, multiple studies have shown that routine use reduces AD symptoms, including itch and pain due to their antiinflammatory properties and reduction in itch-related cytokines such as IL31 (Hoare, Li Wan Po, & Williams, 2000). TCS are available in various potencies that range from very low (class VII; e.g., hydrocortisone 0.25%) to very high (class I; e.g., clobetasol 0.05%). In general, the lowest potency to achieve control of disease for that patient should be used so to minimize adverse effects. Some evidence shows that moderate-to-high potency TCS offer a greater antipruritic effect than low potency (Yarbrough, Neuhaus, & Simpson, 2013). Side effects of TCS on the skin are dependent on the potency, frequency, and location of application of the agent and include atrophic changes of the skin, telangiectasias, striae, and easy bruising (Hengge, Ruzicka, Schwartz, & Cork, 2006). Skin atrophy is more likely to occur in older patients and with use of higher potency TCS in areas of the body where the skin is thin (e.g., face, neck, intertriginous areas) or with occlusive therapies. Systemic side effects such as suppression of the hypothalamic pituitary axis are possible when using high-potency dosages or with extensive body surface usage.

Topical calcineurin inhibitors

Topical calcineurin inhibitors (TCIs) are a more recently introduced class of nonsteroid antiinflammatory treatments for AD. The antipruritic effectiveness of TCIs may be due in part to their stimulatory effect of the transient receptor potential ion channel member 1 (TRPV1) in cutaneous nerves (Pereira et al., 2010). These topicals (e.g., tacrolimus 0.03% or 0.1%, pimecrolimus 1%) have been shown to reduce pruritus scores in AD and may be as effective as midpotency TCs (El-Batawy, Bosseila, Mashaly, & Hafez, 2009; Sher, Chang, Patel, Balkrishnan, & Fleischer, 2012). In a randomized trial, pruritus scores with pimecrolimus 1% were significantly improved by 56% versus only 34% with vehicle alone, and benefit was noted within 48 hours of treatment (Kaufmann et al., 2006). Similar reduction of pruritus scores and maintenance of the antipruritic effect was also demonstrated in a 26-week study (Langley et al., 2008). Because these agents are nonsteroidal they are preferred for areas prone to steroid-induced atrophy (i.e., face). TCIs have the notable adverse effect of burning of the skin upon application, but this effect typically diminishes after several days of use (Stander, Reinhardt, & Luger, 2006; Stander, Schurmeyer-Horst, Luger, & Weisshaar, 2006). The US Food and Drug Administration (FDA) placed a black box warning on TCIs, based on animal studies and case reports showing an increased incidence of malignancy, particularly lymphoma and skin cancers, in patients with AD using this medication (Chia & Tey, 2015) but recent meta-analyses have not confirmed this association (Legendre et al., 2015; Siegfried, Jaworski, Kaiser, & Hebert, 2016).

Topical phosphodiesterase-4 inhibitors

Crisaborole is a phosphodiesterase-4 (PDE4) inhibitor that reduces the release of proinflammatory cytokines (Hanifin et al., 1996). This nonsteroidal topical is used for the treatment of mild to moderate AD and has shown effectiveness in phase 3 studies in reducing itch in AD (Paller et al., 2016). In a post hoc analysis of randomized controlled trials (RCTs), crisaborole has been demonstrated to have a rapid effect on pruritus score reduction, evident within 2 to 6 days of use (Yosipovitch, Gold et al., 2018). Reduction of pruritus while using this topical medication has been shown to lead to significant improvements in quality of life scores among patients (Simpson et al., 2019; Ständer, Spellman, Kwon, & Yosipovitch, 2019; Stander, Yosipovitch et al., 2019; Yosipovitch, Gold et al., 2018). Crisaborole is generally well tolerated with use in thin or sensitive skin areas for which TCS are not appropriate (Zane, Hughes, & Shakib, 2016). The drug has a favorable safety profile and is generally well tolerated with adverse effects such as application site burning reported infrequently.

Topical anesthetics, analgesics, and cooling agents

Topical anesthetics, analgesics, and cooling agents work by activating the nociceptors, thermoreceptors, or otherwise modulating cutaneous neural pathways. Capsaicin's antipruritic properties are due to activation of the transient receptor potential 1 (TRPV1) receptors in keratinocytes and nociceptive C-nerve fibers. Application of topical capsaicin (0.025%–0.1% or 8% patch) has been shown to be effective in pain and itch relief of various etiologies (Papoiu & Yosipovitch, 2010). Of note, topical capsaicin has an initial burning effect that can be avoided with pretreatment with topical anesthetics (i.e., lidocaine or EMLA). The topical anesthetic pramoxine 1% is available in formulations with ceramide moisturizers and has been shown to have antipruritic properties and provide relief in patients with AD-related itch (Yosipovitch & Maibach, 1997; Young et al., 2009; Zirwas & Barkovic, 2017). Menthol activates thermosensitive TRPM8 ion channels present on sensory nerves to induce a cooling effect on the skin. As an antipruritic in 1% concentration, menthol is particularly useful for patients with AD who report that cooling of the skin (e.g., cold showers) improves their pruritic symptoms (Patel, Ishiuji, & Yosipovitch, 2007). Menthol also has analgesic properties at low concentrations (e.g., ≤1%) but may cause irritation and cold-induced pain at higher concentrations. Polidocanol 3% concentration is another topical anesthetic with antipruritic efficacy demonstrated in a large observational study with few adverse effects noted (Freitag & Hoppner, 1997; Simon et al., 2018).

Topical ketamine blocks N-methyl-D-aspartate receptors (NMDA) and sodium channels to reduce the sensitivity of peripheral nerves. A combination cream of ketamine 5% to 10%, amitriptyline 5%, and lidocaine 5% (KAL) has been used in the treatment of chronic pruritus, and in one study, including patients with AD, pruritus scores were significantly improved with relief achieved within a few minutes on average (Lee et al., 2017). KAL has been reported to be well tolerated in limited clinical studies, with burning sensation and redness reported in a minority of patients (Lee et al., 2017). Ketamine is a controlled substance with potential for psychoactive effects if ingested, and therefore patients should be advised to not ingest the product and to limit use to prescribed areas only (<20% body surface area).

Topical cannabinoids

Endocannabinoids such as N-palmitoylethanolamine (PEA), an agonist of the cannabinoid 2 receptor, have been demonstrated to have antiinflammatory and antipruritic properties (Stander, Reinhardt et al., 2006; Stander, Schurmeyer-Horst et al., 2006; Szepietowski, Szepietowski, & Reich, 2005). An open-label, noncontrolled, prospective cohort study in a group of nearly 2500 subjects with AD demonstrated that a cream containing PEA decreased pruritic symptoms by 47% within 6 days and by 60% after 4 to 6 weeks, improved sleep quality reported by patients, and was well tolerated (Eberlein, Eicke, Reinhardt, & Ring, 2008).

Wet wrap treatment

Wet wrap treatment (WWT) consists of a topical agent (i.e., TCS) applied to the skin and then covering the area with a wetted layer of bandages or nonirritant fabric (i.e., cotton) followed by an overlying layer of dry fabric. WWT may be left on for several hours and is typically continued for several days up to 2 weeks. WWT is often recommended for severe flares or recalcitrant disease to attain a relatively rapid reduction in symptoms, including itch. This method reduces itch through various mechanisms, including cooling of the skin, improving penetration of topical medications, and providing a physical barrier to prevent excoriation. The presence of a physical barrier may also prevent stimulation of cutaneous nerve fibers that are in close proximity to the damaged skin barrier (Barham & Yosipovitch, 2005). WWT has been shown to be efficacious in reducing objective and subjective AD symptoms, including pruritus, as well as improvement in quality of life measures (Janmohamed et al., 2014; Pei, Chan, & Ho, 2001; Schnopp et al., 2002). Because of the enhanced effect of the topical agents being applied it is recommended that low to medium potency corticosteroids be used or they be diluted to 5% to 10% of their original strength (Devillers & Oranje, 2012; Wolkerstorfer, Visser, De Waard van der Spek, Mulder, & Oranje, 2000).

Oral immunosuppressants

Cyclosporine A

Cyclosporine A, an immunosuppressant targeting T cells and IL2, has the strongest body of evidence among the systemic immunosuppressants as a first-line systemic agent for short-term use in moderate to severe AD (Sidbury et al., 2014). In RCTs, cyclosporine has demonstrated significant reduction in pruritus and improvement of quality of life measures among those with AD (Harper et al., 2000; Hoare et al., 2000; Roekevisch, Spuls, Kuester, Limpens, & Schmitt, 2014). The use of cyclosporine in AD is limited by its numerous potential adverse effects, including opportunistic infection secondary to immunosuppression, nephrotoxicity, hypertension, and increased risk of certain malignancies (Madan & Griffiths, 2007). In addition to these effects, rapid discontinuation of cyclosporine may cause a rebound flare of AD symptoms. This effect can be mitigated by tapering and coadministration of other systemic agents (Sidbury et al., 2014).

Azathioprine

Azathioprine is a purine analog that interferes with DNA production and therefore B- and T-cell proliferation that has been shown to be efficacious in AD and is used off-label for treatment of refractory disease (Roekevisch et al., 2014). In RCTs, azathioprine has demonstrated significant antipruritic effects and quality of life improvements in AD patients in comparison to placebo (Meggitt, Gray, & Reynolds, 2006). In a comparison trial with methotrexate, comparable reductions in pruritus measures and quality of life improvement were achieved with each treatment (Schram et al., 2011). Azathioprine has apparent antipruritic effects aside from its use in AD, as it has been shown to be effective in patients with itch of unknown etiology (Elmariah, 2017). Its adverse effect profile includes the potential for lymphocytopenia, for which laboratory monitoring may be considered, as well as a hypersensitivity reaction that occurs in a subset of patients within the first few weeks of treatment (Patel, Swerlick, & McCall, 2006). Of particular concern is the apparent increased risk of nonmelanoma skin cancer, associated with increased dosage, duration of use, and sun exposure (Patel et al., 2006). Reduced activity of the thiopurine methyltransferase (TPMT) due to genetic polymorphisms is common in the general population and affects the toxicity of azathioprine. Thus baseline TPMT levels should be obtained prior to initiating therapy, with dosage adjustments accordingly.

Methotrexate

Methotrexate is an oral medication that inhibits dihydrofolate reductase, inhibiting the synthesis of purines and limiting T-cell proliferation. The off-label use of methotrexate in AD is typically limited to refractory AD, and it has been shown to be effective in improving AD symptoms, including itch (Lyakhovitsky et al., 2010; Weatherhead, Wahie, Reynolds, & Meggitt, 2007). In a comparison trial with azathioprine, similar efficacy in reducing pruritus was noted between the two agents (Schram et al., 2011). Low-dose methotrexate (up to 15 mg weekly) can be effective for itch

caused by inflammatory skin diseases (Pavlis & Yosipovitch, 2018; Qureshi, Azam, Laura, Yosipovitch, & Adam, 2019; Stull, Grossman, & Yosipovitch, 2016; Stull, Lavery, & Yosipovitch, 2016). Adverse effects of methotrexate are well described as nausea and gastrointestinal upset. Although they are uncommonly seen at low doses, hepatoxicity and bone marrow suppression are concerns with use of this medication, and laboratory monitoring may be considered. Because of its antifolate mechanism of action, concurrent folate supplementation (skipping folate on the day of methotrexate intake) is recommended to reduce the potential for hematologic effects.

Mycophenolate

Mycophenolate mofetil is an immunosuppressant that inhibits B- and T-cell proliferation by blocking de novo purine synthesis. Multiple studies have demonstrated its efficacy in reducing AD symptoms, including pruritus, and it is considered an alternative systemic therapy for refractory AD (Prussick, Plotnikova, & Gottlieb, 2016; Sidbury et al., 2014). A single-blinded RCT showed mycophenolate mofetil may be as effective as cyclosporine for AD maintenance therapy and showed comparable antipruritic effect, but it requires a longer treatment time to show benefit (Haeck et al., 2011). Gastrointestinal complaints are common with use of this medication, which can be mitigated by use of the enteric-coated formulation. Also hematologic adverse effects are a concern, warranting laboratory monitoring for cytopenia (Sidbury et al., 2014).

Biologic therapies

Dupilumab is a monoclonal antibody targeting the receptor for IL4 that blocks Th2-mediated inflammatory signaling, and has demonstrated in large RCTs to be an effective treatment for moderate to severe AD (Blauvelt et al., 2017; Simpson, Akinlade, & Ardeleanu, 2017). Significant improvement in pruritus scores was seen within 2 weeks of initiating therapy in these trials along with improvements in quality of life and sleep (Simpson et al., 2017). A longer term study showed significant improvements in pruritus scores maintained through 52 weeks with a significant reduction in peak pruritus rating of up to 56.2% versus 28.6% for placebo (Blauvelt et al., 2017). Adverse effects known to be associated with dupilumab include conjunctivitis and injection site reactions. Considering its dramatic effects on AD symptoms and favorable safety profile, dupilumab may be considered for first-line treatment of severe AD or AD-related pruritus.

Additional biologic therapies that target the AD inflammatory signaling pathways show promise with respect to their antipruritic effects in early phase RCTs. Nemolizumab is an IL31 inhibitor that has demonstrated antiitch efficacy in phase 2 trials for patients with moderate to severe AD (Kabashima et al., 2018; Ruzicka et al., 2017). IL13 is a cytokine produced by Th2 lymphocytes, which can induce

IgE production. Similar to IL4, IL13 is an important player in AD pathogenesis, and IL13 mRNA expression is elevated in patients with AD and increases with disease severity (Metwally et al., 2004). Lebrikizumab is a monoclonal antibody against IL13 that was tested in a phase 2 trial in AD patients and was used in combination with topical corticosteroid therapy. It showed significant improvement in EASI scores, along with a reduction in pruritus scores, and improvements in sleep loss (Simpson et al., 2018). IL17, an inflammatory cytokine produced by Th17 cells, is elevated in AD patients (particularly in Asian patients) (Batista et al., 2015). Secukinumab, a monoclonal antibody directed against IL17A, is currently approved for plaque psoriasis, and a place 2 trial for adults with moderate to severe AD is currently in its recruitment phase (Yosipovitch, Berger, & Fassett, 2019).

The Janus kinase (JAK) inhibitors are small-molecule agents that target the JAK-STAT pathway activated by cytokine signaling. Tofacitinib has FDA approval for use in rheumatologic conditions and has demonstrated antipruritic effects in case series of patients with AD (Fowler & Yosipovitch, 2019; Levy, Urban, & King, 2015). Other agents—baricitinib, abrocitinib, and upadacitinib—show promise for rapid antipruritic effects in AD in phase 2 and 3 trials (Erickson, Nahmias, Rosman, & Kim, 2018; Fowler & Yosipovitch, 2020). Emerging immunomodulators and targeted treatments are further discussed in Chapter 23.

Miscellaneous therapies

Phototherapy

Phototherapy (ultraviolet A [UVA] and UVB) has long been used for treating inflammatory skin conditions such as AD and psoriasis. It has a local immunosuppressive effect by targeting activated T cells (Kemény, Varga, & Novak, 2019). Low reactive level laser therapy was also shown to reduce itch sensation in AD patients (Morita, Kohno, Hori, & Kitano, 1993). However, compliance and feasibility of obtaining regular phototherapy is a challenge for patients and physicians.

Complementary therapies

Interventions to reduce stress and anxiety can be beneficial in patients with chronic itch, who suffer from significant emotional and psychological distress. Habit reversal training, relaxation training, and cognitive behavioral therapy can be offered to patients in addition to medical therapy if they are open-minded to alternative therapies (Schut, Mollanazar, Kupfer, Gieler, & Yosipovitch, 2016). In patients with AD, psychological interventions can reduce disease severity, itch intensity, and scratching behavior (Chida, Steptoe, Hirakawa, Sudo, & Kubo, 2007). Acupuncture, as well as progressive muscle relaxation techniques, can significantly reduce pruritus in patients with AD (Bae et al., 2012; Napadow et al., 2014). Complementary and alternative modalities are further discussed in Chapter 26 and 27.

Drugs targeting neural sensitization

Anticonvulsants

Neural hypersensitization plays an important role in chronic pruritus and in AD-related itch, and it may be reduced by certain treatments (Stull et al. 2016; Stull et al. 2016). Gabapentinoid anticonvulsant medications such as gabapentin and pregabalin can be used to manage pruritus as well as chronic pain. Although not yet tested in studies for AD, this class of medications has been shown to be effective in treating different types of itch and to reduce neural sensitization (Yosipovitch et al., 2019). Weight gain, drowsiness, and lower extremity edema are side effects (Pavlis & Yosipovitch, 2018).

Kappa agonists and mu antagonists

Butorphanol is a mixed κ-opioid receptor agonist and μ-opioid receptor antagonist that reduces itch sensation transmission in the central nervous system (Papoiu, Kraft, Coghill, & Yosipovitch, 2015). It is administered intranasally and has been shown to be effective in patients with intractable pruritus of different types, including inflammatory skin conditions such as atopic eczema (Dawn & Yosipovitch, 2006). μ-Antagonists such as naltrexone have also been reported to reduce the itch of AD (Phan, Bernhard, Luger, & Ständer, 2010).

Mirtazapine

Mirtazapine, a serotonergic antidepressant, can be used in low dosages to decrease nocturnal pruritus, which is a common problem in patients suffering from AD (Hundley & Yosipovitch, 2004). It also has been shown to increase the nociceptive threshold in healthy subjects (Arnold, Vuadens, Kuntzer, Gobelet, & Deriaz., 2008). Furthermore, it may indirectly reduce itch through its anxiolytic properties. The most common side effects of mirtazapine are somnolence, appetite stimulation, and weight gain (Hundley & Yosipovitch, 2004). Therefore mirtazapine is a good option in AD patients who are anxious, thin, itchy, and need to sleep better.

Experimental treatments

TRP inhibitors

Chronic pruritus is mediated mainly through the non-histaminergic pathway (Yosipovitch & Bernhard, 2013). Transient receptor potential ankyrin (TRPA) and transient receptor potential vanilloid (TRPV) channels are cation channels involved in generating action potentials in response to certain pruritogens via unmyelinated C fibers (Kittaka & Tominaga, 2017). Therefore TRP channel inhibitors are potential targets for itch management. The long-term antipruritic effect of botulinum neurotoxin A in mice is thought to be associated with the downregulation of TRPA1 and

TABLE 25.1   Topical antipruritic agents

Name	Mechanism of action	Recommended dosing	Side effects	Other notable points
Topical corticosteroids	Antiinflammatory, reduces itch-related cytokines	Available in very low potency (i.e., hydrocortisone 0.25%) to very high potency (i.e., clobetasol 0.05%)	Atrophic skin changes, telangiectasias, striae, easy bruising potential for systemic effects (i.e., HPA suppression) with high potency or large surface area use	Not recommended for areas of thin skin (face, neck, intertriginous areas) Used for WWT with dilution
Topical calcineurin inhibitors (tacrolimus, pimecrolimus)	Immunomodulation of T cells and inhibition of cytokine release, activation of TRPV1 ion channels	Tacrolimus 0.03%, 0.1% ointment Pimecrolimus 1% cream	Application site burning upon application	Suitable for areas of thin skin and face FDA black box warning for lymphoma and skin cancer risks
Crisaborole	PDE4 inhibition, inhibition of inflammatory cytokines	2% ointment	Well tolerated, reports of mild application site burning	
Capsaicin	TRPV1 receptor activation	0.025%–0.1% formulations	Burning, erythema at application site in first 2 weeks of use (reduced by application of topical anesthetic such as lidocaine)	Avoid mucosal areas and eyes
Pramoxine	Inhibition of voltage-gated sodium channels	1% formulations	Well tolerated, reports of contact dermatitis and application site irritation	
Menthol	Activates TRPM8 ion channels, cooling effect	1%–5% formulations	May cause cold-induced pain or irritation at higher concentrations	Recommended for patients that report relief of symptoms with cooling of the skin
Polidocanol	Anesthetic with antipruritic properties	3% formulations	Well tolerated, reports of mild application site irritation	
Ketamine-amitriptyline-lidocaine	NMDA receptor and sodium channel blockade	10% ketamine, 5%, amitriptyline, 5% lidocaine cream	Mild application site burning, erythema; potential for psychoactive effects if ingested; case report of systemic effects from topical overuse	Contains controlled substance (ketamine) Limit use to <20% body surface area
Topical cannabinoids (i.e., PEA)	Increases activity of endogenous cannabinoids and agonism of cannabinoid receptors	PEA 0.3%	Well tolerated, reports of mild application site irritation	

HPA, Hypothalamic pituitary axis; *NMDA*, N-methyl-D-aspartate; *PDE4*, phosphodiesterase 4; *PEA*, N-palmitoylethanolamine; *TRPM8*, transient receptor potential melastatin 8; *TRPV1*, transient receptor potential ion channel member 1; *WWT*, wet wrap therapy.

Adapted from Pavlis, J., & Yosipovitch, G. (2018). Management of itch in atopic dermatitis. *American Journal of Clinical Dermatology, 19*(3), 319–332. https://doi.org/10.1007/s40257-017-0335-4. https://www.ncbi.nlm.nih.gov/pubmed/29285724; Yosipovitch, G., & Bernhard, J. D. (2013). Clinical practice. Chronic pruritus. *New England Journal of Medicine, 368*(17), 1625–1634. https://doi.org/10.1056/NEJMcp1208814. https://www.ncbi.nlm.nih.gov/pubmed/23614588.

TRPV1 (Cao et al., 2017). Furthermore, RNA sequencing has shown that overexpression of TRPV1 in itchy skin correlates with itch intensity in AD patients, and TRPA1 gene expression was increased in itchy atopic skin (Nattkemper et al., 2018).

Nav 1.7 inhibitors

Voltage-gated sodium (Nav) channels are activated by TRPV1 and TRPA, and control action potentials involved in itch propagation (Kittaka & Tominaga, 2017). In animal models, a Nav 1.7 monoclonal antibody provided pain relief and neuropathic and inflammatory itch reduction (Lee et al., 2014). Furthermore, a Nav 1.7 antagonist reduced pain and itch in rodent models, suggesting Nav 1.7 to be a promising therapeutic target for both itch and pain

in AD (Roecker et al., 2017). Neu-P12, an investigational drug that is a combination of a TRPV1 antagonist with a Nav 1.7 inhibitor, has been recently developed for the treatment of itch (Shefer et al., 2019).

Topical nonsteroidal antiinflammatory agents

Tapinarof is a new topical nonsteroidal agent that has shown efficacy in patients with AD and psoriasis. Its antiinflammatory properties are mediated through the activation of the aryl hydrocarbon receptor (AhR), which is expressed in various cell types, including human skin. Tapinarof induces barrier gene expression in keratinocytes and reduces Th17 cytokine responses, which are beneficial in treating AD symptoms (Smith et al., 2017). A phase 2 trial was conducted for tapinarof in AD patients, which showed

TABLE 25.2 Systemic antipruritic agents

Name	Mechanism of action	Recommended dosing	Side effects	Other notable points
Cyclosporine	Inhibits transcription of interleukin-2 (IL2)	2.5–5 mg/kg daily	Nephrotoxicity, hypertension, hirsutism, increased risk of certain malignancies	Rapid discontinuation of cyclosporine may cause a rebound flare of atopic dermatitis (AD) symptoms
Azathioprine	Purine analog	25–275 mg daily	Transaminitis, gastrointestinal (GI) symptoms, lymphocytopenia, hypersensitivity drug reaction, increased risk of nonmelanoma skin cancer	Baseline TPMT levels should be obtained prior to initiating therapy
Methotrexate	Purine synthesis inhibitor	Up to 15 mg weekly	GI symptoms, hepatotoxicity, bone marrow suppression	Concurrent folate supplementation recommended
Mycophenolate	Purine synthesis inhibitor	2 g daily	GI symptoms, leukopenia	
Dupilumab	Anti-IL4 receptor subunit-α antibody	600 mg, followed by 300 mg biweekly	Conjunctivitis, injection site reaction	
Tofacitinib	JAK inhibitor	5–10 mg daily	Upper respiratory tract infection, systemic bacterial and fungal infections, increased risk of malignancy	
Gabapentin Pregabalin	Reduction in central neural hypersensitization	300–1200 mg TID 25–225 mg BID	Somnolence, insomnia, GI symptoms, weight gain, lower extremity swelling	Can be used to manage chronic pain, neuropathic forms of itch
Butorphanol	κ-opioid receptor agonist, μ-opioid receptor antagonist	1–4 mg/mL nightly	Somnolence, disorientation, bizarre dreams, GI symptoms	Use for severe intractable pruritus
Naltrexone	μ-opioid receptor antagonist	25–50 mg daily	Skin reaction, GI symptoms	
Mirtazapine	Serotonergic antidepressant	7.5–15 mg nightly	Somnolence, weight gain	Can have antinociceptive effects

BID, Twice a day; *JAK*, Janus kinase; *TID*, three times a day; *TPMT*, thiopurine methyltransferase.
Adapted from Yosipovitch, G., Rosen, J. D., & Hashimoto, T. (2018). Itch: From mechanism to (novel) therapeutic approaches. *The Journal of Allergy and Clinical Immunology, 142*(5), 1375–1390. https://doi.org/10.1016/j.jaci.2018.09.005.

treatment efficacy with minimal adverse events (Peppers et al., 2019).

NK-1 inhibitors

Substance P activates the neurokinin-1 (NK-1) receptor, which is involved in nonhistaminergic itch signaling; gene transcripts of substance P and NK-1 are elevated in atopic patients (Nattkemper et al., 2018). An oral NK-1 receptor antagonist, serlopitant, improved pruritus scores in patients suffering from chronic pruritus in a phase 2 clinical trial with no significant safety concerns (Yosipovitch, Stander, et al., 2018). Serlopitant also reduced pruritus scores in AD patients in a phase 2 clinical trial; however, the differences were not statistically significant. Overall, with serlopitant meeting the primary endpoint in three of four studies assessing its efficacy in chronic pruritus, NK-1 antagonism is a promising mechanism for itch reduction across a range of patient populations (Ständer et al., 2019). Tradipitant is another NK-1 inhibitor undergoing a phase 2 trial, which has shown preliminary improvements in itch of AD patients (Yosipovitch et al., 2019).

Summary

Patients with AD suffer from itch and pain, which can severely affect their quality of life. There are many different treatment options available aimed at combatting these symptoms, summarized in Tables 25.1 and 25.2. For mild AD and maintenance therapy, nonpharmacologic therapies, such as moisturization and bathing practices, can improve itch and pain. For mild to moderate AD, topical therapies, including corticosteroids, calcineurin inhibitors, PDE4 inhibitors, and various analgesics and anesthetics, are helpful. For moderate to severe AD, systemic therapies that suppress the immune system can be effective; however, these have a multitude of side effects that limit their use as a long-term therapy. For moderate to severe AD, biologic agents that specifically target itch-mediated signaling pathways have been very effective with few known side effects. There are also a variety of drugs that decrease neural sensitization, which can be helpful in reducing chronic itch and pain. These drugs targeting neural sensitization have been shown to decrease pain. The analgesic effects of the other antipruritic agents have not been specifically studied but could be a potential avenue for future investigation. Complementary therapies intended to reduce stress and anxiety can be beneficial when used in conjunction with other therapies. Furthermore, several experimental therapies that specifically target nonhistaminergic itch pathways are currently being tested in clinical trials and have shown promising results.

Further reading

Eichenfield, L. F., Tom, W. L., Berger, T. G., Krol, A., Paller, A. S., Schwarzenberger, K., et al. (2014). Guidelines of care for the management of atopic dermatitis: section 2. *Management and treatment of atopic dermatitis with topical therapies. Journal of the American Academy of Dermatology, 71*(1), 116–132.

Fowler, E. & Yosipovitch, G. A new generation of treatments for itch. *Acta Dermato-Venereologica, 100*(2):adv00027.

Mollanazar, N. K., Smith, P. K., & Yosipovitch, G. (2016). Mediators of chronic pruritus in atopic dermatitis: getting the itch out? *Clinical Reviews in Allergy and Immunology, 51*(3), 263–292.

Yosipovitch, G., Berger, T., & Fassett, M. S. (2020). Neuroimmune interactions in chronic itch of atopic dermatitis. *Journal of the European Academy of Dermatology and Venereology, 34*(2), 239–250.

Yosipovitch, G., Rosen, J. D., & Hashimoto, T. (2018). Itch: From mechanism to (novel) therapeutic approaches. *Journal of Allergy and Clinical Immunology, 142*(5), 1375–1390.

References

Ali, S. M., & Yosipovitch, G. (2013). Skin pH: From basic science to basic skin care. *Acta Dermato-Venereologica, 93*(3), 261–267. https://doi.org/10.2340/00015555-1531. https://www.ncbi.nlm.nih.gov/pubmed/23322028.

Arnold, P., Vuadens, P., Kuntzer, T., Gobelet, C., & Deriaz, O. (2008). Mirtazapine decreases the pain feeling in healthy participants. *The Clinical Journal of Pain, 24*(2), 116–119. https://doi.org/10.1097/AJP.0b013e318159f94a. https://www.ncbi.nlm.nih.gov/pubmed/18209516.

Bae, B. G., Oh, S. H., Park, C. O., Noh, S., Noh, J. Y., Kim, K. R., & Lee, K. H. (2012). Progressive muscle relaxation therapy for atopic dermatitis: Objective assessment of efficacy. *Acta Dermato-Venereologica, 92*(1), 57–61. https://doi.org/10.2340/00015555-1189. https://www.ncbi.nlm.nih.gov/pubmed/21879233.

Barham, K. L., & Yosipovitch, G. (2005). It's a wrap: The use of wet pajamas in wet-wrap dressings for atopic dermatitis. *Dermatology Nursing/Dermatology Nurses' Association, 17*(5), 365–367. https://www.ncbi.nlm.nih.gov/pubmed/16294940.

Batista, D. I., Perez, L., Orfali, R. L., Zaniboni, M. C., Samorano, L. P., Pereira, N. V., et al. (2015). Profile of skin barrier proteins (filaggrin, claudins 1 and 4) and Th1/Th2/Th17 cytokines in adults with atopic dermatitis. *Journal of the European Academy of Dermatology and Venereology, 29*(6), 1091–1095. https://doi.org/10.1111/jdv.12753. https://www.ncbi.nlm.nih.gov/pubmed/25271795.

Blauvelt, A., de Bruin-Weller, M., Gooderham, M., Cather, J. C., Weisman, J., Pariser, D., et al. (2017). Long-term management of moderate-to-severe atopic dermatitis with dupilumab and concomitant topical corticosteroids (LIBERTY AD CHRONOS): A 1-year, randomised, double-blinded, placebo-controlled, phase 3 trial. *Lancet, 389*(10086), 2287–2303. https://doi.org/10.1016/s0140-6736(17)31191-1.

Boralevi, F., Saint Aroman, M., Delarue, A., Raudsepp, H., Kaszuba, A., Bylaite, M., & Tiplica, G. S. (2014). Long-term emollient therapy improves xerosis in children with atopic dermatitis. *Journal of the European Academy of Dermatology and Venereology, 28*(11), 1456–1462. https://doi.org/10.1111/jdv.12314.

Cao, L. F., Si, M., Huang, Y., Chen, L. H., Peng, X. Y., Qin, Y. Q., et al. (2017). Long-term anti-itch effect of botulinum neurotoxin A is associated with downregulation of TRPV1 and TRPA1 in the dorsal root ganglia in mice. *Neuroreport, 28*(9), 518–526. https://doi.org/10.1097/WNR.0000000000000779. https://www.ncbi.nlm.nih.gov/pubmed/28410268.

Chia, B. K., & Tey, H. L. (2015). Systematic review on the efficacy, safety, and cost-effectiveness of topical calcineurin inhibitors in atopic dermatitis. *Dermatitis: Contact, Atopic, Occupational, Drug, 26*(3), 122–132. https://doi.org/10.1097/der.0000000000000118.

Chida, Y., Steptoe, A., Hirakawa, N., Sudo, N., & Kubo, C. (2007). The effects of psychological intervention on atopic dermatitis. A systematic review and meta-analysis. *International Archives of Allergy and Immunology, 144*(1), 1–9. https://doi.org/10.1159/000101940.https://www.ncbi.nlm.nih.gov/pubmed/17449959.

Dawn, A. G., & Yosipovitch, G. (2006). Butorphanol for treatment of intractable pruritus. *Journal of the American Academy of Dermatology, 54*(3), 527–531. https://doi.org/10.1016/j.jaad.2005.12.010. https://www.ncbi.nlm.nih.gov/pubmed/16488311.

Dawn, A., Papoiu, A. D., Chan, Y. H., Rapp, S. R., Rassette, N., & Yosipovitch, G. (2009). Itch characteristics in atopic dermatitis: Results of a web-based questionnaire. *British Journal of Dermatology, 160*(3), 642–644. https://doi.org/10.1111/j.1365-2133.2008.08941.x. https://www.ncbi.nlm.nih.gov/pubmed/19067703.

Devillers, A. C., & Oranje, A. P. (2012). Wet-wrap treatment in children with atopic dermatitis: A practical guideline. *Pediatric Dermatology, 29*(1), 24–27. https://doi.org/10.1111/j.1525-1470.2011.01691.x.

Eberlein, B., Eicke, C., Reinhardt, H. W., & Ring, J. (2008). Adjuvant treatment of atopic eczema: Assessment of an emollient containing N-palmitoylethanolamine (ATOPA study). *Journal of the European Academy of Dermatology and Venereology, 22*(1), 73–82. https://doi.org/10.1111/j.1468-3083.2007.02351.x.

Eichenfield, L. F., Tom, W. L., Berger, T. G., Krol, A., Paller, A. S., Schwarzenberger, K., et al. (2014). Guidelines of care for the management of atopic dermatitis: Section 2. Management and treatment of atopic dermatitis with topical therapies. *Journal of the American Academy of Dermatology, 71*(1), 116–132. https://doi.org/10.1016/j.jaad.2014.03.023.

Eichenfield, L. F., Tom, W. L., Chamlin, S. L., Feldman, S. R., Hanifin, J. M., Simpson, E. L., et al. (2014). Guidelines of care for the management of atopic dermatitis: Section 1. Diagnosis and assessment of atopic dermatitis. *Journal of the American Academy of Dermatology, 70*(2), 338–351. https://doi.org/10.1016/j.jaad.2013.10.010.

El-Batawy, M. M., Bosseila, M. A., Mashaly, H. M., & Hafez, V. S. (2009). Topical calcineurin inhibitors in atopic dermatitis: A systematic review and meta-analysis. *Journal of Dermatological Science, 54*(2), 76–87. https://doi.org/10.1016/j.jdermsci.2009.02.002.

Elmariah. S. B. (2017). Adjunctive management of itch in atopic dermatitis. *Dermatologic Clinics, 35*(3), 373–394. https://doi.org/10.1016/j.det.2017.02.011.

Erickson, S., Nahmias, Z., Rosman, I. S., & Kim, B. S. (2018). Immunomodulating agents as antipruritics. *Dermatologic Clinics, 36*(3), 325–334. https://doi.org/10.1016/j.det.2018.02.014.

Fowler, E., & Yosipovitch, G. (2019). Chronic itch management: Therapies beyond those targeting the immune system. *Annals of Allergy, Asthma & Immunology, 123*(2), 158–165. https://doi.org/10.1016/j.anai.2019.01.016. https://www.ncbi.nlm.nih.gov/pubmed/30685562.

Fowler, E., & Yosipovitch, G. (2020). A New Generation of Treatments for Itch. *Acta Dermato-Venereologica, 100*, advo0027.

Fowler, J. F., Nebus, J., Wallo, W., & Eichenfield, L. F. (2012). Colloidal oatmeal formulations as adjunct treatments in atopic dermatitis. *Journal of Drugs in Dermatology, 11*(7), 804–807.

Freitag, G., & Hoppner, T. (1997). Results of a postmarketing drug monitoring survey with a polidocanol-urea preparation for dry, itching skin. *Current Medical Research and Opinion, 13*(9), 529–537. https://doi.org/10.1185/03007999709113326.

Hachem, J. P., Man, M. Q., Crumrine, D., Uchida, Y., Brown, B. E., Rogiers, V., et al. (2005). Sustained serine proteases activity by prolonged increase in pH leads to degradation of lipid processing enzymes and profound alterations of barrier function and stratum corneum integrity. *The Journal of Investigative Dermatology, 125*(3), 510–520. https://doi.org/10.1111/j.0022-202X.2005.23838.x.

Haeck, I. M., Knol, M. J., Ten Berge, O., van Velsen, S. G., de Bruin-Weller, M. S., & Bruijnzeel-Koomen, C. A. (2011). Enteric-coated mycophenolate sodium versus cyclosporin A as long-term treatment in adult patients with severe atopic dermatitis: A randomized controlled trial. *Journal of the American Academy of Dermatology, 64*(6), 1074–1084. https://doi.org/10.1016/j.jaad.2010.04.027.

Hanifin, J. M., Chan, S. C., Cheng, J. B., Tofte, S. J., Henderson, W. R., Jr., Kirby, D. S., & Weiner, E. S. (1996). Type 4 phosphodiesterase inhibitors have clinical and in vitro anti-inflammatory effects in atopic dermatitis. *The Journal of Investigative Dermatology, 107*(1), 51–56. https://doi.org/10.1111/1523-1747.ep12297888.

Harper, J. I., Ahmed, I., Barclay, G., Lacour, M., Hoeger, P., Cork, M. J., et al. (2000). Cyclosporin for severe childhood atopic dermatitis: Short course versus continuous therapy. *British Journal of Dermatology, 142*(1), 52–58. https://doi.org/10.1046/j.1365-2133.2000.03241.x.

Hengge, U. R., Ruzicka, T., Schwartz, R. A., & Cork, M. J. (2006). Adverse effects of topical glucocorticosteroids. *Journal of the American Academy of Dermatology, 54*(1), 1–15, quiz 16-8. https://doi.org/10.1016/j.jaad.2005.01.010.

Hoare, C., Li Wan Po, A., & Williams, H. (2000). Systematic review of treatments for atopic eczema. *Health Technology Assessment (Winchester, England), 4*(37), 1–191.

Hundley, J. L., & Yosipovitch, G. (2004). Mirtazapine for reducing nocturnal itch in patients with chronic pruritus: A pilot study. *Journal of the American Academy of Dermatology, 50*(6), 889–891. https://doi.org/10.1016/j.jaad.2004.01.045. https://www.ncbi.nlm.nih.gov/pubmed/15153889.

Janmohamed, S. R., Oranje, A. P., Devillers, A. C., Rizopoulos, D., van Praag, M. C., Van Gysel, D., et al. (2014). The proactive wet-wrap method with diluted corticosteroids versus emollients in children with atopic dermatitis: A prospective, randomized, double-blind, placebo-controlled trial. *Journal of the American Academy of Dermatology, 70*(6), 1076–1082. https://doi.org/10.1016/j.jaad.2014.01.898.

Kabashima, K., Furue, M., Hanifin, J. M., Pulka, G., Wollenberg, A., Galus, R., et al. (2018). Nemolizumab in patients with moderate-to-severe atopic dermatitis: Randomized, phase II, long-term extension study. *The Journal of Allergy and Clinical Immunology, 142*(4). https://doi.org/10.1016/j.jaci.2018.03.018. 1121–1130.e7.

Kaufmann, R., Bieber, T., Helgesen, A. L., Andersen, B. L., Luger, T., Poulin, Y., et al. (2006). Onset of pruritus relief with pimecrolimus cream 1% in adult patients with atopic dermatitis: A randomized trial. *Allergy, 61*(3), 375–381. https://doi.org/10.1111/j.1398-9995.2005.00977.x.

Kemény, L., Varga, E., & Novak, Z. (2019). Advances in phototherapy for psoriasis and atopic dermatitis. *Expert Review of Clinical Immunology, 15*(11), 1205–1214. https://doi.org/10.1080/1744666X.2020.1672537. https://www.ncbi.nlm.nih.gov/pubmed/31575297.

Kini, S. P., DeLong, L. K., Veledar, E., McKenzie-Brown, A. M., Schaufele, M., & Chen, S. C. (2011). The impact of pruritus on quality of life: The skin equivalent of pain. *Archives of Dermatology, 147*(10), 1153–1156. https://doi.org/10.1001/archdermatol.2011.178.

Kittaka, H., & Tominaga, M. (2017). The molecular and cellular mechanisms of itch and the involvement of TRP channels in the peripheral sensory nervous system and skin. *Allergology*

International, 66(1), 22–30. https://doi.org/10.1016/j.alit.2016.10.003. https://www.ncbi.nlm.nih.gov/pubmed/28012781.

Kurtz, E. S., & Wallo, W. (2007). Colloidal oatmeal: History, chemistry and clinical properties. *Journal of Drugs in Dermatology, 6*(2), 167–170.

Langley, R. G., Eichenfield, L. F., Lucky, A. W., Boguniewicz, M., Barbier, N., & Cherill, R. (2008). Sustained efficacy and safety of pimecrolimus cream 1% when used long-term (up to 26 weeks) to treat children with atopic dermatitis. *Pediatric Dermatology, 25*(3), 301–307. https://doi.org/10.1111/j.1525-1470.2008.00671.x.

Lee, C. H., Chuang, H. Y., Shih, C. C., Jong, S. B., Chang, C. H., & Yu, H. S. (2006). Transepidermal water loss, serum IgE and beta-endorphin as important and independent biological markers for development of itch intensity in atopic dermatitis. *British Journal of Dermatology, 154*(6), 1100–1107. https://doi.org/10.1111/j.1365-2133.2006.07191.x.

Lee, H. G., Grossman, S. K., Valdes-Rodriguez, R., Berenato, F., Korbutov, J., Chan, Y. H., et al. (2017). Topical ketamine-amitriptyline-lidocaine for chronic pruritus: A retrospective study assessing efficacy and tolerability. *Journal of the American Academy of Dermatology, 76*(4), 760–761. https://doi.org/10.1016/j.jaad.2016.10.030. https://www.ncbi.nlm.nih.gov/pubmed/28325395.

Lee, J. H., Park, C. K., Chen, G., Han, Q., Xie, R. G., Liu, T., et al. (2014). A monoclonal antibody that targets a NaV1.7 channel voltage sensor for pain and itch relief. *Cell, 157*(6), 1393–1404. https://doi.org/10.1016/j.cell.2014.03.064. https://www.ncbi.nlm.nih.gov/pubmed/24856969.

Legendre, L., Barnetche, T., Mazereeuw-Hautier, J., Meyer, N., Murrell, D., & Paul, C. (2015). Risk of lymphoma in patients with atopic dermatitis and the role of topical treatment: A systematic review and meta-analysis. *Journal of the American Academy of Dermatology, 72*(6), 992–1002. https://doi.org/10.1016/j.jaad.2015.02.1116.

Levy, L. L., Urban, J., & King, B. A. (2015). Treatment of recalcitrant atopic dermatitis with the oral Janus kinase inhibitor tofacitinib citrate. *Journal of the American Academy of Dermatology, 73*(3), 395–399. https://doi.org/10.1016/j.jaad.2015.06.045.

Lisante, T. A., Nunez, C., Zhang, P., & Mathes, B. M. (2017). A 1% colloidal oatmeal cream alone is effective in reducing symptoms of mild to moderate atopic dermatitis: Results from two clinical studies. *Journal of Drugs in Dermatology, 16*(7), 671–676.

Lyakhovitsky, A., Barzilai, A., Heyman, R., Baum, S., Amichai, B., Solomon, M., et al. (2010). Low-dose methotrexate treatment for moderate-to-severe atopic dermatitis in adults. *Journal of the European Academy of Dermatology and Venereology, 24*(1), 43–49. https://doi.org/10.1111/j.1468-3083.2009.03351.x.

Maarouf, M., Kromenacker, B., Capozza, K. L., Kempton, D., Hendricks, A., Tran, K., & Shi, V. Y. (2018). Pain and itch are dual burdens in atopic dermatitis. *Dermatitis: Contact, Atopic, Occupational, Drug, 29*(5), 278–281. https://doi.org/10.1097/der.0000000000000406.

Madan, V., & Griffiths, C. E. (2007). Systemic ciclosporin and tacrolimus in dermatology. *Dermatologic Therapy, 20*(4), 239–250. https://doi.org/10.1111/j.1529-8019.2007.00137.x.

Meggitt, S. J., Gray, J. C., & Reynolds, N. J. (2006). Azathioprine dosed by thiopurine methyltransferase activity for moderate-to-severe atopic eczema: A double-blind, randomised controlled trial. *The Lancet, 367*(9513), 839–846.

Metwally, S. S., Mosaad, Y. M., Abdel-Samee, E. R., El-Gayyar, M. A., Abdel-Aziz, A. M., & El-Chennawi, F. A. (2004). IL-13 gene expression in patients with atopic dermatitis: Relation to IgE level and to disease severity. *The Egyptian Journal of Immunology/Egyptian Association of Immunologists, 11*(2), 171–177. https://www.ncbi.nlm.nih.gov/pubmed/16734130.

Mollanazar, N. K., Smith, P. K., & Yosipovitch, G. (2016). Mediators of chronic pruritus in atopic dermatitis: Getting the itch out? *Clinical Reviews in Allergy & Immunology, 51*(3), 263–292. https://doi.org/10.1007/s12016-015-8488-5. https://www.ncbi.nlm.nih.gov/pubmed/25931325.

Morita, H., Kohno, J., Hori, M., & Kitano, Y. (1993). Clinical application of low reactive level laser therapy (LLLT) for atopic dermatitis. *The Keio Journal of Medicine, 42*(4), 174–176. https://doi.org/10.2302/kjm.42.174. https://www.ncbi.nlm.nih.gov/pubmed/7907380.

Napadow, V., Li, A., Loggia, M. L., Kim, J., Schalock, P. C., Lerner, E., et al. (2014). The brain circuitry mediating antipruritic effects of acupuncture. *Cerebral Cortex, 24*(4), 873–882. https://doi.org/10.1093/cercor/bhs363. https://www.ncbi.nlm.nih.gov/pubmed/23222890.

Nattkemper, L. A., Tey, H. L., Valdes-Rodriguez, R., Lee, H., Mollanazar, N. K., Albornoz, C., et al. (2018). The genetics of chronic itch: Gene expression in the skin of patients with atopic dermatitis and psoriasis with severe itch. *The Journal of Investigative Dermatology, 138*(6), 1311–1317. https://doi.org/10.1016/j.jid.2017.12.029. https://www.ncbi.nlm.nih.gov/pubmed/29317264.

Paller, A. S., Tom, W. L., Lebwohl, M. G., Blumenthal, R. L., Boguniewicz, M., Call, R. S., et al. (2016). Efficacy and safety of crisaborole ointment, a novel, nonsteroidal phosphodiesterase 4 (PDE4) inhibitor for the topical treatment of atopic dermatitis (AD) in children and adults. *Journal of the American Academy of Dermatology, 75*(3), 494–503.e6. https://doi.org/10.1016/j.jaad.2016.05.046.

Papoiu, A. D., & Yosipovitch, G. (2010). Topical capsaicin. The fire of a 'hot' medicine is reignited. *Expert Opinion on Pharmacotherapy, 11*(8), 1359–1371. https://doi.org/10.1517/14656566.2010.481670. https://www.ncbi.nlm.nih.gov/pubmed/20446852.

Papoiu, A. D. P., Kraft, R. A., Coghill, R. C., & Yosipovitch, G. (2015). Butorphanol suppression of histamine itch is mediated by nucleus accumbens and septal nuclei: A pharmacological fMRI study. *The Journal of Investigative Dermatology, 135*(2), 560–568. https://doi.org/10.1038/jid.2014.398. https://www.ncbi.nlm.nih.gov/pubmed/25211175.

Patel, A. A., Swerlick, R. A., & McCall, C. O. (2006). Azathioprine in dermatology: The past, the present, and the future. *Journal of the American Academy of Dermatology, 55*(3), 369–389. https://doi.org/10.1016/j.jaad.2005.07.059.

Patel, T., Ishiuji, Y., & Yosipovitch, G. (2007). Menthol: A refreshing look at this ancient compound. *Journal of the American Academy of Dermatology, 57*(5), 873–878. https://doi.org/10.1016/j.jaad.2007.04.008. https://www.ncbi.nlm.nih.gov/pubmed/17498839.

Pavlis, J., & Yosipovitch, G. (2018). Management of itch in atopic dermatitis. *American Journal of Clinical Dermatology, 19*(3), 319–332. https://doi.org/10.1007/s40257-017-0335-4. https://www.ncbi.nlm.nih.gov/pubmed/29285724.

Pei, A. Y., Chan, H. H., & Ho, K. M. (2001). The effectiveness of wet wrap dressings using 0.1% mometasone furoate and 0.005% fluticasone proprionate ointments in the treatment of moderate to severe atopic dermatitis in children. *Pediatric Dermatology, 18*(4), 343–348. https://doi.org/10.1046/j.1525-1470.2001.01952.x.

Peppers, J., Paller, A. S., Maeda-Chubachi, T., Wu, S., Robbins, K., Gallagher, K., & Kraus, J. E. (2019). A phase 2, randomized dose-finding study of tapinarof (GSK2894512 cream) for the treatment of atopic dermatitis. *Journal of the American Academy of*

Dermatology, 80(1). https://doi.org/10.1016/j.jaad.2018.06.047. 89-98.e3. https://www.ncbi.nlm.nih.gov/pubmed/30554600.

Pereira, U., Boulais, N., Lebonvallet, N., Pennec, J. P., Dorange, G., & Misery, L. (2010). Mechanisms of the sensory effects of tacrolimus on the skin. *British Journal of Dermatology, 163*(1), 70–77. https://doi.org/10.1111/j.1365-2133.2010.09757.x.

Phan, N. Q., Bernhard, J. D., Luger, T. A., & Stände, S. (2010). Antipruritic treatment with systemic μ-opioid receptor antagonists: A review. *Journal of the American Academy of Dermatology, 63*(4), 680–688. https://doi.org/10.1016/j.jaad.2009.08.052. https://www.ncbi.nlm.nih.gov/pubmed/20462660.

Prussick, L., Plotnikova, N., & Gottlieb, A. (2016). Mycophenolate mofetil in severe atopic dermatitis: A Review. *Journal of Drugs in Dermatology, 15*(6), 715–718.

Qureshi, Azam, A., Laura, E. A., Yosipovitch, G., & Adam, J. F. (2019). A systematic review of evidence-based treatments for prurigo nodularis. *Journal of the American Academy of Dermatology, 80*(3), 756–764. https://doi.org/10.1016/j.jaad.2018.09.020. http://www.sciencedirect.com/science/article/pii/S0190962218326288.

Roecker, A. J., Egbertson, M., Jones, K. L. G., Gomez, R., Kraus, R. L., Li, Y., et al. (2017). Discovery of selective, orally bioavailable, N-linked arylsulfonamide Na. *Bioorganic & Medicinal Chemistry Letters, 27*(10), 2087–2093. https://doi.org/10.1016/j.bmcl.2017.03.085. https://www.ncbi.nlm.nih.gov/pubmed/28389149.

Roekevisch, E., Spuls, P. I., Kuester, D., Limpens, J., & Schmitt, J. (2014). Efficacy and safety of systemic treatments for moderate-to-severe atopic dermatitis: A systematic review. *The Journal of Allergy and Clinical Immunology, 133*(2), 429–438. https://doi.org/10.1016/j.jaci.2013.07.049.

Rosen, J. D., Fostini, A. C., Chan, Y. H., Nattkemper, L. A., & Yosipovitch, G. (2018). Cross-sectional study of clinical distinctions between neuropathic and inflammatory pruritus. *Journal of the American Academy of Dermatology, 79*(6), 1143–1144. https://doi.org/10.1016/j.jaad.2018.05.1236. https://www.ncbi.nlm.nih.gov/pubmed/29864468.

Ruzicka, T., Hanifin, J. M., Furue, M., Pulka, G., Mlynarczyk, I., Wollenberg, A., et al. (2017). Anti-interleukin-31 receptor a antibody for atopic dermatitis. *The New England Journal of Medicine, 376*(9), 826–835. https://doi.org/10.1056/NEJMoa1606490.

Schnopp, C., Holtmann, C., Stock, S., Remling, R., Folster-Holst, R., Ring, J., & Abeck, D. (2002). Topical steroids under wet-wrap dressings in atopic dermatitis—A vehicle-controlled trial. *Dermatology, 204*(1), 56–59. https://doi.org/10.1159/000051811.

Schram, M. E., Roekevisch, E., Leeflang, M. M., Bos, J. D., Schmitt, J., & Spuls, P. I. (2011). A randomized trial of methotrexate versus azathioprine for severe atopic eczema. *The Journal of Allergy and Clinical Immunology, 128*(2), 353–359. https://doi.org/10.1016/j.jaci.2011.03.024.

Schut, C., Mollanazar, N. K., Kupfer, J., Gieler, U., & Yosipovitch, G. (2016). Psychological interventions in the treatment of chronic itch. *Acta Dermato-Venereologica, 96*(2), 157–161. https://doi.org/10.2340/00015555-2177. https://www.ncbi.nlm.nih.gov/pubmed/26073701.

Shefer, Y Katz, A Mircheva, L Zisapel, N Yosipovitch, G Nankova, V. 2019. Multiple dose study of safety, tolerability, pharmacokinetics, and pharmacodynamic activity of Neu-P12, a novel drug candidate developed for the treatment of itch, in subjects with scalp pruritus. *Itch, 4*, 1-62.

Sher, L. G., Chang, J., Patel, I. B., Balkrishnan, R., & Fleischer, A. B., Jr. (2012). Relieving the pruritus of atopic dermatitis: A meta-analysis. *Acta Dermato-Venereologica, 92*(5), 455–461. https://doi.org/10.2340/00015555-1360.

Sidbury, R., Davis, D. M., Cohen, D. E., Cordoro, K. M., Berger, T. G., Bergman, J. N., et al. (2014). Guidelines of care for the management of atopic dermatitis: Section 3. Management and treatment with phototherapy and systemic agents. *Journal of the American Academy of Dermatology, 71*(2), 327–349. https://doi.org/10.1016/j.jaad.2014.03.030.

Siegfried, E. C., Jaworski, J. C., Kaiser, J. D., & Hebert, A. A. (2016). Systematic review of published trials: Long-term safety of topical corticosteroids and topical calcineurin inhibitors in pediatric patients with atopic dermatitis. *BMC Pediatrics, 16*, 75. https://doi.org/10.1186/s12887-016-0607-9.

Simon, D., Nobbe, S., Nageli, M., Barysch, M., Kunz, M., Borelli, S., et al. (2018). Short- and long-term effects of two emollients on itching and skin restoration in xerotic eczema. *Dermatologic Therapy, 31*(6), e12692. https://doi.org/10.1111/dth.12692.

Simpson, E. L., Akinlade, B., & Ardeleanu, M. (2017). Two phase 3 trials of dupilumab versus placebo in atopic dermatitis. *The New England Journal of Medicine, 376*(11), 1090–1091. https://doi.org/10.1056/NEJMc1700366. https://www.ncbi.nlm.nih.gov/pubmed/28296614.

Simpson, E. L., Flohr, C., Eichenfield, L. F., Bieber, T., Sofen, H., Taieb, A., et al. (2018). Efficacy and safety of lebrikizumab (an anti-IL-13 monoclonal antibody) in adults with moderate-to-severe atopic dermatitis inadequately controlled by topical corticosteroids: A randomized, placebo-controlled phase II trial (TREBLE). *Journal of the American Academy of Dermatology, 78*(5), 863–871. https://doi.org/10.1016/j.jaad.2018.01.017. e11.

Simpson, E. L., Yosipovitch, G., Bushmakin, A. G., Cappelleri, J. C., Luger, T., et al. (2019). Direct and indirect effects of crisaborole ointment on quality of life in patients with atopic dermatitis: A mediation analysis. *Acta Dermato-Venereologica, 99*(9), 756–761. https://doi.org/10.2340/00015555-3181. https://www.ncbi.nlm.nih.gov/pubmed/30896779.

Smith, S. H., Jayawickreme, C., Rickard, D. J., Nicodeme, E., Bui, T., Simmons, C., et al. (2017). Tapinarof is a natural AhR agonist that resolves skin inflammation in mice and humans. *The Journal of Investigative Dermatology, 137*(10), 2110–2119. https://doi.org/10.1016/j.jid.2017.05.004. https://www.ncbi.nlm.nih.gov/pubmed/28595996.

Stander, S., Reinhardt, H. W., & Luger, T. A. (2006). [Topical cannabinoid agonists. An effective new possibility for treating chronic pruritus]. *Der Hautarzt; Zeitschrift fur Dermatologie, Venerologie, und Verwandte Gebiete, 57*(9), 801–807. https://doi.org/10.1007/s00105-006-1180-1.

Stander, S., Schurmeyer-Horst, F., Luger, T. A., & Weisshaar, E. (2006). Treatment of pruritic diseases with topical calcineurin inhibitors. *Therapeutics and Clinical Risk Management, 2*(2), 213–218. https://doi.org/10.2147/tcrm.2006.2.2.213.

Stände, S., Spellman, M. C., Kwon, P., & Yosipovitch, G. (2019). The NK1 receptor antagonist serlopitant for treatment of chronic pruritus. *Expert Opinion on Investigational Drugs, 28*(8), 659–666. https://doi.org/10.1080/13543784.2019.1638910. https://www.ncbi.nlm.nih.gov/pubmed/31272246.

Stander, S., & Steinhoff, M. (2002). Pathophysiology of pruritus in atopic dermatitis: An overview. *Experimental Dermatology, 11*(1), 12–24.

Stander, S., Yosipovitch, G., Bushmakin, A. G., Cappelleri, J. C., Luger, T., Tom, W. L., et al. (2019). Examining the association between pruritus and quality of life in patients with atopic dermatitis treated with crisaborole. *Journal of the European Academy of Dermatology and Venereology, 33*(9), 1742–1746. https://doi.org/10.1111/jdv.15712. https://www.ncbi.nlm.nih.gov/pubmed/31132182.

Stull, C., Grossman, S., & Yosipovitch, G. (2016). Current and emerging therapies for itch management in psoriasis. *American Journal of Clinical Dermatology, 17*(6), 617–624. https://doi.org/10.1007/s40257-016-0213-5. https://www.ncbi.nlm.nih.gov/pubmed/27460912.

Stull, C., Lavery, M. J., & Yosipovitch, G. (2016). Advances in therapeutic strategies for the treatment of pruritus. *Expert Opinion on Pharmacotherapy, 17*(5), 671–687. https://doi.org/10.1517/14656566.2016.1127355. https://www.ncbi.nlm.nih.gov/pubmed/26630350.

Szepietowski, J. C., Szepietowski, T., & Reich, A. (2005). Efficacy and tolerance of the cream containing structured physiological lipids with endocannabinoids in the treatment of uremic pruritus: A preliminary study. *Acta Dermatovenerologica Croatica, 13*(2), 97–103.

Tiplica, G. S., Boralevi, F., Konno, P., Malinauskiene, L., Kaszuba, A., Laurens, C., et al. (2018). The regular use of an emollient improves symptoms of atopic dermatitis in children: A randomized controlled study. *Journal of the European Academy of Dermatology and Venereology, 32*(7), 1180–1187. https://doi.org/10.1111/jdv.14849.

Vakharia, P. P., Chopra, R., Sacotte, R., Patel, K. R., Singam, V., Patel, N., et al. (2017). Burden of skin pain in atopic dermatitis. *Annals of Allergy, Asthma & Immunology, 119*(6), 548–552.e3. https://doi.org/10.1016/j.anai.2017.09.076.

van Zuuren, E. J., Fedorowicz, Z., & Arents, B. W. M. (2017). Emollients and moisturizers for eczema: Abridged Cochrane systematic review including GRADE assessments. *British Journal of Dermatology, 177*(5), 1256–1271. https://doi.org/10.1111/bjd.15602.

Weatherhead, S. C., Wahie, S., Reynolds, N. J., & Meggitt, S. J. (2007). An open-label, dose-ranging study of methotrexate for moderate-to-severe adult atopic eczema. *British Journal of Dermatology, 156*(2), 346–351. https://doi.org/10.1111/j.1365-2133.2006.07686.x.

Wolkerstorfer, A., Visser, R. L., De Waard van der Spek, F. B., Mulder, P. G., & Oranje, A. P. (2000). Efficacy and safety of wet-wrap dressings in children with severe atopic dermatitis: Influence of corticosteroid dilution. *British Journal of Dermatology, 143*(5), 999–1004. https://doi.org/10.1046/j.1365-2133.2000.03833.x.

Yarbrough, K. B., Neuhaus, K. J., & Simpson, E. L. (2013). The effects of treatment on itch in atopic dermatitis. *Dermatologic Therapy, 26*(2), 110–119. https://doi.org/10.1111/dth.12032.

Yosipovitch, G., Berger, T., & Fassett, M. S. (2019). Neuroimmune interactions in chronic itch of atopic dermatitis. *Journal of the European Academy of Dermatology and Venereology, 34*(2), 239–250. https://doi.org/10.1111/jdv.15973. https://www.ncbi.nlm.nih.gov/pubmed/31566796.

Yosipovitch, G., & Bernhard, J. D. (2013). Clinical practice. Chronic pruritus. *The New England Journal of Medicine, 368*(17), 1625–1634. https://doi.org/10.1056/NEJMcp1208814. https://www.ncbi.nlm.nih.gov/pubmed/23614588.

Yosipovitch, G., Gold, L. F., Lebwohl, M. G., Silverberg, J. I., Tallman, A. M., & Zane, L. T. (2018). Early relief of pruritus in atopic dermatitis with crisaborole ointment, a non-steroidal, phosphodiesterase 4 inhibitor. *Acta Dermato-Venereologica, 98*(5), 484–489. https://doi.org/10.2340/00015555-2893. https://www.ncbi.nlm.nih.gov/pubmed/29363715.

Yosipovitch, G., Goon, A., Wee, J., Chan, Y. H., & Goh, C. L. (2000). The prevalence and clinical characteristics of pruritus among patients with extensive psoriasis. *British Journal of Dermatology, 143*(5), 969–973. https://doi.org/10.1046/j.1365-2133.2000.03829.x. https://www.ncbi.nlm.nih.gov/pubmed/11069504.

Yosipovitch, G., Goon, A. T., Wee, J., Chan, Y. H., Zucker, I., & Goh, C. L. (2002). Itch characteristics in Chinese patients with atopic dermatitis using a new questionnaire for the assessment of pruritus. *International Journal of Dermatology, 41*(4), 212–216. https://pubmed.ncbi.nlm.nih.gov/12031029/.

Yosipovitch, G., & Maibach, H. I. (1997). Effect of topical pramoxine on experimentally induced pruritus in humans. *Journal of the American Academy of Dermatology, 37*(2 Pt 1), 278–280. https://doi.org/10.1016/s0190-9622(97)80143-0. https://www.ncbi.nlm.nih.gov/pubmed/9270522.

Yosipovitch, G., Stander, S., Kerby, M. B., Larrick, J. W., Perlman, A. J., Schnipper, E. F., et al. (2018). Serlopitant for the treatment of chronic pruritus: Results of a randomized, multicenter, placebo-controlled phase 2 clinical trial. *Journal of the American Academy of Dermatology, 78*(5), 882–891.E10. https://doi.org/10.1016/j.jaad.2018.02.030. https://www.ncbi.nlm.nih.gov/pubmed/29462657.

Yosipovitch, G., Zucker, I., Boner, G., Gafter, U., Shapira, Y., & David, M. (2001). A questionnaire for the assessment of pruritus: Validation in uremic patients. *Acta Dermato-Venereologica, 81*(2), 108–111. https://doi.org/10.1080/00015550152384236. https://www.ncbi.nlm.nih.gov/pubmed/11501646.

Young, T. A., Patel, T. S., Camacho, F., Clark, A., Freedman, B. I., Kaur, M., et al. (2009). A pramoxine-based anti-itch lotion is more effective than a control lotion for the treatment of uremic pruritus in adult hemodialysis patients. *The Journal of Dermatological Treatment, 20*(2), 76–81. https://doi.org/10.1080/09546630802441218. https://www.ncbi.nlm.nih.gov/pubmed/18821119.

Zane, L. T., Hughes, M. H., & Shakib, S. (2016). Tolerability of crisaborole ointment for application on sensitive skin areas: A randomized, double-blind, vehicle-controlled study in healthy volunteers. *American Journal of Clinical Dermatology, 17*(5), 519–526. https://doi.org/10.1007/s40257-016-0204-6.

Zirwas, M. J., & Barkovic, S. (2017). Anti-pruritic efficacy of itch relief lotion and cream in patients with atopic history: Comparison with hydrocortisone cream. *Journal of Drugs in Dermatology, 16*(3), 243–247.

26

Complementary and Alternative Approaches I

CLAIRE WILSON, JOANNA JAROS, AND VIVIAN Y. SHI

KEY POINTS

- Current first-line conventional treatments for atopic dermatitis include topical corticosteroids, emollients, and topical and/or systemic immunomodulators (e.g., dupilumab).
- However, a majority of patients with atopic dermatitis are interested in or have tried complementary and alternative medicine (CAM) approaches.
- CAM approaches with clinical evidence in atopic dermatitis include topical and oral oils, topical and oral micronutrients, bathing additives, fabric selection, and topical endocannabinoids.
- Treatment of atopic dermatitis can be augmented with CAM and can be strategically integrated with conventional therapies in appropriate cases.

Introduction

The goals of atopic dermatitis (AD) treatment are to (1) dampen skin inflammation, (2) decrease itch and pain, (3) repair the skin barrier, and (4) restore the microbiome. Conventional treatment of AD is therefore multitiered and includes a combination of emollients, topical antiinflammatory medications, and in more severe cases systemic immunosuppressants and immunomodulators. Conventionally, such immunosuppressants were not target specific and could be poorly tolerated due to their side effect profiles, thus limiting their value in long-term usage. There has not been a safe and efficacious immunosuppressive medication for moderate to severe AD until the recent introduction of dupilumab in 2017. Dupilumab is a monoclonal antibody targeting interleukin-4 (IL4) production approved for use in teens ages 12 to 17 and adults (Thaci et al., 2019).

While research has made great strides in AD treatment over the last 5 years, a recent survey found that more than half of patients with AD use complementary and alternative medicine (CAM) in addition to their conventional treatments (Darmstadt, 2004). Factors contributing to this staggering number may include treatment resistance or partial response to conventional therapy, safety concerns in infants and children, and the undesirable side effects of long-term topical steroids and systemic agents.

The National Center for Complementary and Alternative Medicine (NCCAM) of the National Insitutes of Health defines CAM as "a group of diverse medical and health care systems, practices, and products that are not presently considered to be part of conventional medicine" (Clearinghouse, 2018). Complementary therapies typically refer to modalities used in tandem with conventional therapies, while alternative therapies are modalities used in place of conventional therapies. We believe that evidence-based CAM modalities may be integrated into conventional treatment plans to improve overall treatment outcomes and/ or to limit side effects. For example, certain topical CAM products may reduce topical corticosteroid use and limit skin atrophy and hypopigmentation side effects.

This chapter discusses the existing scientific evidence for CAM in AD, including topical and oral oils, micronutrients, bathing additives, topical endocannabinoids, fabric selection, and cryotherapy. We specifically examine the role of these modalities in augmenting conventional AD treatment. Additional CAM modalities, including acupuncture, acupressure, cupping, herbal supplements, sleep hygiene, and mind-body techniques, will be discussed in Chapter 27.

Topical natural oils

Natural oils are an attractive treatment modality due to their high free fatty acid (FFA) and triglyceride (TG) content. Long-chain fatty acids, particularly linoleic acid, are components of a healthy skin barrier that are deficient in AD patients (Zhu, Zhu, Tran, Sivamani, & Shi, 2018). Replacement of these FFAs with topical oils is a potential treatment strategy.

One thing to note is that each topical oil has a unique ratio of FFAs and TGs, which in turn dictates efficacy in AD (Mack Correa et al., 2014). For example, oils composed mainly of monounsaturated oleic acid increase skin permeability more than oils containing an even mix of both mono- and polyunsaturated fatty acids. Topical oils also come in various forms and concentrations. When recommending a natural oil to patients, we recommend that patients look for a cold-pressed and/or, virgin natural oil product. Essential oils, which are highly concentrated, and fragranced oils are known triggers of irritant and allergic contact dermatitis and should be avoided in AD patients (de Groot & Schmidt, 2016). A list of topical and oral oils used for AD is summarized in Table 26.1.

Sunflower seed oil

Sunflower seed oil (SSO) contains linoleic acid, an omega-6 FFA, which is a major fatty acid component of the skin barrier. Linoleic acid exerts positive effects through potent activation of peroxisome proliferator-activated receptor-α (PPAR-α)—a nuclear receptor found in skin cells that plays a role in regulating keratinocyte proliferation, maintaining skin barrier homeostasis, and dampening inflammation (Hanley et al., 1997). PPAR-α has significantly reduced gene expression in both the skin of lesional and nonlesional AD patients, and its loss likely contributes to the dysregulated inflammatory cascade in AD (Plager et al., 2007).

Daily SSO application for 4 weeks has been shown to improve skin erythema and transepidermal water loss (TEWL) in AD patients. Long-term usage is likely needed to maintain its beneficial benefits (Eichenfield, McCollum, & Msika, 2009). Studies in children also suggest that SSO may reduce rates of cutaneous infections. A randomized controlled trial (RCT) of preterm infants in Egypt found that topical application of SSO three times daily significantly reduced rates of invasive nosocomial infections compared with infants who did not receive SSO (Darmstadt et al., 2004). Another trial found that topical application of SSO significantly reduced mortality rates in preterm hospitalized infants, likely due to enhanced skin barrier integrity (Darmstadt et al., 2002). Given its low cost and efficacy, SSO application has a role in skin barrier repair and can potentially be a lifesaving topical treatment for preterm infants in developing countries.

Sunflower oleodistillate

Sunflower oleodistillate (SOD), a derivative of SSO, is produced through a mineral distillation process resulting in a lipid-rich oil composed largely of oleic and linoleic acids.

TABLE 26.1	Summary of topical and oral oils for atopic dermatitis	
Oil	Treatment regimen	Studied effect
Topical oils		
Sunflower seed oil	1. 2×/day for 4 weeks 2. 3×/day	1. Decreased erythema and transepidermal water loss (TEWL) (Eichenfield et al., 2009) 2. Reduced rates of invasive nosocomial infections and reduced mortality in neonates (Darmstadt et al., 2002; Darmstadt et al., 2004)
Sunflower oleodistillate	2% cream every other day in combo with/topical corticosteroid	Improved lichenification, excoriation, and quality of life (Eichenfield et al., 2009)
Virgin coconut oil	2×/day for 8 week	Reduced SCORAD and TEWL (Evangelista et al., 2014)
Manuka honey	Daily overnight application for 1 week	Improved atopic dermatitis (AD) lesions (Alangari et al., 2017)
Menthol	3% cream daily for 1 month	Reduced itch (Tey et al., 2017)
Tea-tree oil (in acne)	5% tea-tree oil gel for 3 months	Decrease in mean acne lesions (both open and closed comedones) (Bassett et al., 1990) Note: This is an essential oil and should be avoided in AD patients.
Olive oil	6 drops 2×/day for 5 weeks	Reduction in the integrity of stratum corneum and induced mild erythema in participants with and without AD (Danby et al., 2013)
Combination oils	100,000 IU of superoxide dismutase and 4% of a combination of plant extracts (blackcurrant seed oil, sunflower oil concentrate, balloon vine extract)	Reduced SCORAD and pruritus as well as improved quality of life (Sgouros et al., 2018)
Oral oils		
Hempseed oil	2 tbsp for 8 weeks	Improved plasma fatty acid levels and reduced dryness and pruritus at 2 weeks (Callaway et al., 2005)

Compared with naturally occurring SSO, the physical processing of SOD results in a product with a 10-fold higher concentration of phytosterols and vitamins (Msika et al., 2008). This phytosterol content confers additional antiinflammatory and barrier-promoting promoting properties (Eichenfield et al., 2009). A RCT of 86 pediatric patients with moderate AD found that the addition of 2% SOD to conventional topical corticosteroid therapy led to statistically significant improvements in lichenification, excoriation, and quality of life when compared to once- or twice-daily application of steroids alone (Eichenfield et al., 2009). SOD appears to decrease steroid requirements and thus may be a safe alternative in patients who cannot tolerate topical corticosteroids (Eichenfield et al., 2009).

Virgin coconut oil

Virgin coconut oil (VCO) is produced by a wet-milling and cold-press process that does not involve heat or chemical processing (Evangelista, Abad-Casintahan, & Lopez-Villafuerte, 2014). VCO contains monolaurin, a medium-chain fatty acid that demonstrates broad-spectrum antibacterial activity against *Staphylococcus aureus* (Verallo-Rowell, Dillague, & Syah-Tjundawan, 2008). Patients with AD are frequently and disproportionately colonized by *S. aureus* when compared to healthy counterparts. A meta-analysis of 95 observational studies in AD patients reported a pooled prevalence of *S. aureus* colonization of 70% in lesional skin, 39% in nonlesional skin, and 62% in the nares (Kong et al., 2012; Totte et al., 2016). A double-blind, controlled trial of 52 patients with AD found that VCO significantly reduced the objective-SCORAD severity index (O-SSI) through its antibacterial activity against *S. aureus* (based on its culture results) and overall antimicrobial activity as compared to virgin olive oil (Verallo-Rowell et al., 2008).

In a RCT of 117 pediatric patients with AD, twice-daily application of VCO for 8 weeks led to significant improvements in SCORAD and TEWL as compared to mineral oil (Evangelista et al., 2014). In preterm very low-birthweight neonates who have an immature stratum corneum, VCO has been used to reduce TEWL eventuating in improved barrier function (Nangia et al., 2015). The efficacy of VCO is theorized to be due to its superior ability to penetrate the skin and reduce inflammation (Escobar, Achenbach, Iannantuono, & Torem, 1992; Tollesson & Frithz, 1993). Due to its safety and efficacy in both adults and children, VCO is a great alternative daily moisturizer for AD patients or an adjunct to current therapy.

Borage seed oil

Patients with AD are thought to have a reduced rate of conversion from linoleic acid to γ-linolenic acid (GLA), dihomo-γ-linolenic acid, or arachidonic acid as compared with healthy subjects (Levin & Maibach, 2002). Thus AD patients are deficient in the barrier-forming FFA GLA. Borage seed oil (BSO), which contains 23%

GLA, one of the highest concentrations found in a plant, may be helpful in replenishing barrier GLA (Henz et al., 1999). To date, topical BSO has not been studied in AD patients. Sparse investigations of oral BSO supplementation and BSO-containing clothing have had mixed results in improving AD symptomatology and severity (Henz et al., 1999; Kanehara, Ohtani, Uede, & Furukawa, 2007). Additional studies are needed to elucidate the role of BSO in AD.

Menthol

Cooling baths have been shown to be beneficial in AD patients (Fruhstorfer, Hermanns, & Latzke, 1986), and cooling may be one strategy for combating itching sensations. Menthol is a naturally occurring cyclic terpene alcohol that has a cooling and antipruritic effect when applied to the skin. Menthol's antipruritic properties are due to its activity on the TRMP8 receptor in C fibers (unmyelinated pain fibers) (Patel, Ishiuji, & Yosipovitch, 2007; Peier et al., 2002), direct stimulation of A-delta fibers (myelinated pain fibers) (Bromm, Scharein, Darsow, & Ring, 1995), and selective activation of κ-opioid fibers (Galeotti, Di Cesare Mannelli, Mazzanti, Bartolini, & Ghelardini, 2002).

An itch-relieving moisturizing cream containing 3% menthol and ceramides significantly reduced itch in healthy individuals and AD patients; however, 1/60 participants reported stinging sensations (Tey, Tay, & Tan, 2017). Menthol has also been shown to cause allergic contact dermatitis (Wilkinson & Beck, 1994), and high concentration (40%) products may cause erythema and burning (Hatem, Attal, Willer, & Bouhassira, 2006). Moreover, menthol promotes TEWL at a level higher than regular rubbing alcohol, so it should be used with caution in xerotic skin, and should not substitute a proper emollient (Hong, Buddenkotte, Berger, & Steinhoff, 2011; Patel et al., 2007). Larger RCTs are needed to investigate the positive and negative effects of menthol in AD patients. A 3% menthol is the appropriate concentration to recommend to patients with AD who are interested in menthol products.

Tea-tree oil

Tea-tree oil (TTO) is an essential oil derived from the leaves of the Australian plant *Melaleuca alternifolia* (Bassett, Pannowitz, & Barnetson, 1990). TTO contains terpinen-4-ol, a potent antibacterial agent against methicillin-resistant *S. aureus* (MRSA) and was shown to be as effective as topical mupirocin against *S. aureus* in vivo (Loughlin, Gilmore, McCarron, & Tunney, 2008). TTO has been studied in acne vulgaris, and topical application was shown to have a statistically significant effect on mean total acne lesions (Bassett et al., 1990). However, to date, no RCTs have been conducted in AD patients. We suggest avoiding all essential oils, including TTO, in AD patients due to their potential for triggering contact dermatitis (de Groot & Schmidt, 2016).

Olive oil

Despite the perceived safety and benefit of most natural oils in AD, olive oil promotes and exacerbates AD. The negative effects of olive oil are due to its high ratio of short-chain oleic to linoleic acid (7:1), which increases TEWL (Darmstadt et al., 2002; Schliemann-Willers, Wigger-Alberti, Kleesz, Grieshaber, & Elsner, 2002). Oleic acid also disrupts cutaneous homeostasis through its activation of NMDA cell surface receptors, resulting in delayed barrier repair and epidermal hyperplasia (Katsuta, Iida, Hasegawa, Inomata, & Denda, 2009). In a RCT, six drops of oil twice daily for 5 weeks led to a significant reduction in the integrity of stratum corneum and induced mild erythema in participants with and without AD, when compared to SSO. These negative effects of olive oil were more prominent in AD patients when compared to healthy counterparts (Danby et al., 2013). A clinical trial of 115 healthy neonates found that olive oil is especially damaging to the immature stratum corneum of infants because it disrupts crucial neonatal lipid organization in the skin (Cooke et al., 2016). Olive oil and related products should be discouraged in AD patients.

Combination topicals

Superoxide dismutase is an antioxidant enzyme that reduces oxidative stress and inflammation and has antipruritic properties in AD. Superoxide dismutase reduces production of nitrogen oxide and inflammatory cytokines such as tumor necrosis factor-α (TNF-α), IL1, and IL6, thereby decreasing itch (Sgouros, Katoulis, & Rigopoulos, 2018). A RCT of 20 AD patients (from 8 months to 72 years old) trialed a novel topical agent containing 100,000 IU of superoxide dismutase and 4% of a combination of plant extracts (blackcurrant seed oil, sunflower oil concentrate, balloon vine extract) and found that the topical preparation significantly reduced SCORAD and pruritus as well as improved quality of life (Sgouros et al., 2018). No adverse events were reported. Larger, single-ingredient, placebo-controlled trials of superoxide dismutase are needed before it can be recommended in AD.

Oral oils

Oral hempseed oil

Omega-6 and omega-3 polyunsaturated fatty acids (PUFAs) such as GLA and stearidonic acid (SDA) account for 80% of the composition of hempseed oil. PUFAs are skin barrier building blocks that play a role in regulating permeability and decreasing TEWL (Wu et al., 1999). In a RCT of 20 patients with chronic AD, oral hempseed oil significantly improved plasma fatty acid levels and reduced dryness and pruritus at 2 weeks when compared to oral olive oil. While PUFAs are abundant in hempseed oil, olive oil has low levels of PUFAs, which may contribute to its lack of efficacy in AD (Callaway et al., 2005). The trial reported no adverse events with the use of hempseed oil supplements. Larger, longitudinal (>2 weeks), placebo-controlled studies are needed before oral hempseed oil can be recommended to patients.

Borage seed oil and evening primrose

Two additional oral oils that contain large amounts of PUFAs are evening primrose oil (EPO) and BSO. EPO contains 8% to 10% GLA; BSO contains at least 23% GLA (Bamford et al., 2013). A 2013 Cochrane review of 27 studies with a total of 1596 patients found that neither oral BSO nor EPO are efficacious in improving global AD symptoms or quality of life. Adverse effects included mild gastrointestinal upset (Bamford et al., 2013). One case report found an increased risk of inflammation, thrombosis, and immunosuppression with prolonged use of EPO; another study found an increased risk of bleeding with patients on concomitant warfarin therapy (Bamford et al., 2013). To date, there does not appear to be convincing evidence for either oral EPO and BSO in the treatment of AD. One alarming case report in 2011 found that 1 week of BSO use was associated with development of status epilepticus in a 41-year-old woman (Al-Khamees, Schwartz, Alrashdi, Algren, & Morgan, 2011).

Topical micronutrients

Vitamin B$_{12}$

Vitamin B$_{12}$ is a water-soluble vitamin found in several cobalt-bound forms collectively known as the cobalamins. The most common commercial forms of B$_{12}$ are cyanocobalamin and methylcobalamin. Vitamin B$_{12}$ is crucial for red blood cell production (lack of B$_{12}$ leads to megaloblastic anemias), DNA synthesis, and neurologic function. Animal meat from animals that ingest dirt through feeding (e.g., chickens, cattle) are common sources of dietary B$_{12}$. One major action of vitamin B$_{12}$ is its inhibition of nitric oxide synthase, attenuating nitric oxide synthesis. Nitric oxide is a small molecule that induces microvascular vasodilation, which manifests as erythema in the skin. Additionally, nitric oxide activates components of the inflammatory response such as T-cell proliferation (Stucker et al., 2004). In a RCT of 49 adults with AD, topical 0.07% vitamin B$_{12}$ applied twice daily resulted in significant improvement of AD symptoms as compared to placebo after 8 weeks. A similarly designed RCT of 21 children with AD found the same results by week 2 of treatment with topical B$_{12}$ (Januchowski, 2009). Due to its low side effect profile, vitamin B$_{12}$ may be recommended following treatment with high-potency glucocorticoids to prevent relapse and is considered safe to use in children (Stucker et al., 2004). Vitamin B$_{12}$ topical cream can be made by a compounding pharmacy using the following ingredients: 0.07 g cyanocobalamin (vitamin B$_{12}$), 46 g persea gratissima oil (avocado oil), 45.42 g water, 8 g TEGO Care PS or methyl glucose stearate (an emulsifier),

0.26 g potassium sorbate (a preservative), and 0.25 g citric acid. The cream is pink in color due to its B_{12} content and has even been referred to as "Pink Magic."

Oral micronutrients

Vitamin D

Vitamin D or calciferol is a fat-soluble vitamin that exerts its effects on cutaneous homeostasis via regulation of calcium, magnesium, and phosphate levels. The two major forms of vitamin D are D_2 and D_3 (ergo- and cholecalciferol) and are found in dietary supplements and fortified foods. D_2 (ergocalciferol) is human made and added to foods, whereas D_3 (cholecalciferol) is synthesized within the skin from 7-dehydrocholesterol. Vitamin D deficiency has been associated with AD severity. Serum levels of 25-hydroxycholecalciferol of 40 to 60 ng/mL are recommended for proper immune function (Bikle, Pillai, Gee, & Hincenbergs, 1989; Borzutzky & Camargo, 2013; Grant, 2009; Vaughn, Foolad, Maarouf, Tran, & Shi, 2019). A 2019 systematic review concluded that vitamin D oral supplements decrease eczema severity in adults and children with AD (Vaughn et al., 2019). In two similarly designed RCTs, daily vitamin D_3 supplementation at 1000 IU improved global investigator scores (IGA) and eczema severity (EASI) after just 1 month (Borzutzky & Camargo, 2013; Camargo et al., 2014). Another RCT found that daily supplementation for 60 days with 1600 IU vitamin D_3 led to significant improvements in SCORAD and Three-Item Severity Score (TIS) when compared to healthy controls (Amestejani et al., 2012). Although largely positive effects have been reported, mixed efficacy of vitamin D in AD patients was reported in two small RCTs (Vaughn et al., 2019). Given the positive results in AD patients, safety, and low cost, vitamin D should be considered as an adjunct in both adult and pediatric patients.

Vitamin E

Vitamin E, also known as tocopherol, is an antioxidant that has been shown to decrease levels of serum immunoglobulin E (IgE) in AD patients (Thiele, Hsieh, & Ekanayake-Mudiyanselage, 2005; Tsoureli-Nikita, Hercogova, Lotti, & Menchini, 2002; Vaughn et al., 2019). A RCT of 70 adults with AD found that supplementation with oral vitamin E (400 IU/day for 4 months) significantly improved AD symptoms as compared to placebo, and these effects were sustained for 3 months after treatment (Jaffary, Faghihi, Mokhtarian, & Hosseini, 2015). A similar single-blinded RCT of 96 patients with AD showed that oral vitamin E (400 IU/day for 8 months) led to significant improvements in AD symptoms and a decrease in serum IgE in 50% of patients. A RCT of 44 patients examined the effects of combination vitamin E with additional emollients and antioxidants into a nonsteroidal cream (MD 2011001) and found significant reductions in AD symptoms (Patrizi et al., 2016).

In a randomized, double-blind, placebo-controlled trial of 45 patients, an association between vitamin E plasma levels and SCORAD was noted after supplementation, but no correlation was found between vitamin D plasma levels and SCORAD. However, the greatest SCORAD reduction was observed in a third, combination treatment arm receiving both vitamins D and E, which suggests a potential synergistic relationship (Javanbakht et al., 2011). A RCT of 58 adults and children with AD supplemented with either vitamin D_3 at 5000 IU/day or placebo for 3 months found that serum levels of vitamin D_3 greater than 20 ng/mL in conjunction with standard therapy reduced SCORAD (Sanchez-Armendariz et al., 2018). Regardless of treatment group, a lower SCORAD correlated with serum levels of 25(OH)D 20 ng/mL and above, and no significant differences were noted between patients with serum levels of 20 ng/mL and above versus 30 ng/mL and above (Sanchez-Armendariz et al., 2018).

Low-dose vitamin E supplementation may be an effective adjunctive therapy for AD patients (Jaffary et al., 2015). Research has not found any adverse events with consumption of vitamin E in food products; however, vitamin E supplementation has a known potential to disrupt the clotting cascade and platelet activation. It should be used with caution and/or avoided in patients on anticoagulants (e.g., warfarin, novel oral anticoagulants [NOACs]) or those with hemophilia.

L-histidine

L-histidine is an amino acid that supports the skin barrier formation. Filaggrin, an important protein that contributes to barrier function, relies on histidine for enhanced processing (Tan, Brown, Griffiths, Weller, & Gibbs, 2017). Both filaggrin mutations and L-histidine deficiency in the skin have been linked with the development of AD in adults and infants (Kopple & Swendseid, 1975). In a double-blind, randomized pilot study of 24 adult AD patients, 4 g of oral L-histidine supplements significantly reduced AD severity after 4 weeks of treatment as compared to placebo with no reported adverse effects. The clinical effects of L-histidine were similar to that of midpotency topical corticosteroids, suggesting that L-histidine may be a safe, nonsteroidal approach to AD (Tan et al., 2017). However, larger RCTs are needed to confirm these findings before further recommendations can be made.

Bathing additives

Bathing additives and oils are substances added to bath water for their antiinflammatory, skin barrier repair, antimicrobial, and antioxidative properties. They are most useful as an adjunct treatment for inflammatory dermatoses affecting a large body surface area. Patients using bathing oils should be reminded of the potential for falls due to oily skin after product use. Clinicians should recommend that patients gently towel off excess oil from the skin after bathing before stepping out of the tub or shower. A list of bathing additives used for AD is depicted in Table 26.2.

Dead Sea therapy

Balneotherapy (*balneum*, "bath" in Latin) is the practice of bathing, usually in minerals and other additives, as a therapeutic modality. One popular form of balneotherapy involves bathing in Dead Sea water and/or water with Dead Sea salt. The Dead Sea is a body of water located between Jordan and Israel and is known for its high concentrations of magnesium (Mg^{2+}), calcium (Ca^{2+}), potassium, and bromine ions. The incredibly high content of magnesium ions (30× normal ocean water) is thought to play a curative role in inflammatory skin diseases, namely AD and psoriasis (Proksch, Nissen, Bremgartner, & Urquhart, 2005). Magnesium exerts its effects by (1) maintaining skin ionic homeostasis through regulation of other ions (Lee et al., 1992) and (2) suppression of inflammatory cytokine such as TNF-α and IL12 (Schempp et al., 2000).

Combination therapy of Dead Sea saltwater and UVB phototherapy decreases the capacity of cutaneous Langerhans cells to present antigens and trigger an inflammatory cascade (Schempp et al., 2000). A split-arm, controlled study of a Dead Sea salt solution in AD patients found that submerging the forearm for 15 minutes in 5% bathing solution (Mavena Dermaline Mg Dead Sea salt) daily for 6 weeks improved skin barrier function and reduced roughness and erythema compared to the contralateral forearm, which was submerged in tap water. Additionally, patients with elevated TEWL at the start of the study experienced a significant reduction in TEWL (Proksch et al., 2005).

Ultimately, Dead Sea salt solution appears to indirectly reduce inflammation and does not irritate skin (Proksch et al., 2005). Spas and rehabilitation facilities have modalities that mimic the ionic composition of the Dead Sea, but the high cost and access to these centers may not be realistic for all patients. An in-home Dead Sea salt bathing additive is a reasonable alternative.

Water softeners

Hard water, defined as water with calcium and chlorine concentrations greater than 120 parts per million (ppm) (Quality, 2012) is a known risk factor for the development of AD (Perkin et al., 2016). High calcium and chlorine content is also thought to exacerbate AD, though the exact mechanism remains unclear. Studies evaluating the effect of hardened water using ion-exchange machines have yielded mixed results in AD patients (Danby et al., 2018; Thomas et al., 2011; Togawa et al., 2014). For example, one small trial showed that ion-exchange softened water baths for 6 weeks led to improvements in pruritus scores, but not severity of the AD (Togawa et al., 2014). Although there have been no reported adverse effects of water softening, several authors mentioned the prohibitive cost of the ion-exchange machines (average price: $3000 USD) for patients and research teams.

TABLE 26.2 Summary of bathing additives for atopic dermatitis

Additive	Treatment regimen	Studied effect
Bleach	1/2 cup of 6% common household bleach in a bathtub (150L) full of water (Shi et al., 2016)	Decrease in atopic dermatitis severity (Chopra, Vakharia, Sacotte, & Silverberg, 2017)
Dead Sea salt	Mavena Dermaline Mg Dead Sea Salt Use 15min/day for 6 weeks	Improved skin barrier function, decreased roughness and erythema of skin; decreased transepidermal water loss (TEWL) if high at baseline (Proksch et al., 2005)
Water softeners	Ion exchange softened water for 6 weeks	Potential decrease in pruritus (Togawa et al., 2014)
Colloidal oatmeal	Colloidal oat powder daily for 1–3 weeks	Improvement of active lesions in up to 41% of patients (Sompayrac & Ross, 1959)
Rice starch Rice bran	1. 10g/L, 15min 2x/daily for 4 consecutive days 2. 5g/L, daily for 2 weeks	1. Decreased TEWL (De Paepe et al., 2002) 2. Decreased itching, lichenification, erythema, papule formation (Fujiwaki & Furusho, 1992) 50% patients decreased topical corticosteroid use
Natural oils	1. Balneum Hermal (85% soybean oil) 2. Balmandol (almond/paraffin) 3. Alpha Keri Bath Oil (mineral/lanolin)	1. Decreased TEWL and improved skin hydration scores (Kottner et al., 2017), nonsignificant change in dryness symptoms 2. Decreased TEWL (Hill & Edwards, 2002) 3. Patient-reported improvements in skin dryness (Stanfield, 1981)

Colloidal oatmeal

Colloidal oatmeal (*Avena sativa*, Latin) is made from finely ground oats, which are boiled to form a small-sized particulate suspension. Oats contain compounds that enhance moisturization of the skin, rid the skin of oils and dirt, and perform antioxidant, antiinflammatory, and skin barrier repair functions (Fowler, Nebus, Wallo, & Eichenfield 2012). Colloidal oatmeal has been shown to be both safe and beneficial in AD patients. A study of pediatric patients with mild to severe AD examined the addition of colloidal oatmeal powder (46% oat starch, 24% oat protein, 9% oat oil, 0.03% crude fiber, 8% moisture) to baths. At 1 to 3 weeks, there was complete clearance and great improvement of active lesions in half of patients, respectively, and some improvement in two-fifths. In total, over 90% of patients had at least some improvement occurring within 1 to 3 weeks (Sompayrac & Ross, 1959).

Rice (starch and bran) bath

Rice bran and starch bathing is a popular medicinal treatment in Japanese folk culture. Little is known about rice's impact on skin pathology, but several studies have proposed that its chemical constituents (e.g., γ-oryzanol) may have positive antiinflammatory, antiaging, microcirculatory, and skin barrier maintenance effects (Fujiwaki & Furusho, 1992; Islam et al., 2009). Two small studies (n = 13, 16) found evidence for the efficacy of rice starch baths (10 g/L, 15 minutes 2×/day for 4 consecutive days) on improving TEWL, reducing eczema severity, and TCS use (De Paepe, Hachem, Vanpee, Roseeuw, & Rogiers, 2002; Fujiwaki & Furusho, 1992). Of note, one patient experienced cutaneous itching and erythema after treatment and discontinued the protocol (Fujiwaki & Furusho, 1992). Given the scarcity of literature on this topic and promising results, additional, larger trials are needed to further verify the benefits of rice baths.

Bathing oils

Bathing oils have been used since the 1960s in patients with eczema to aid in moisturization of the skin. After bathing in an oil, a lipid-rich residue remains on the skin surface, thus preventing water loss and promoting cutaneous moisturization (Kottner et al., 2017). Any topically applied oil can easily be used as a bathing oil; however, patients should be cautioned about falls and slipping after bathing in oil.

Soybean oil is a common commercially available oil that was trialed as a lipid barrier on the skin.

A RCT of 60 children and adults with dry skin (xerosis cutis) bathed with a commercially available bath oil (Balneum Hermal: 85% refined soy bean oil, 20 minutes every other day) found that the experimental group had significantly lower TEWL and improved skin hydration compared to controls. Given the strong roles of TEWL and xerosis in AD pathogenesis, the absence of reported adverse events, and relative low cost, a trial of soy bean oil in AD

may be used on a case-by-case basis (Kottner et al., 2017). A second, small study of eight patients with moderate to severe xerosis of the legs found that bathing with mineral and lanolin oil (Alpha Keri Bath Oil, Westwood Pharmaceuticals Inc., ~$10–15/16 oz) for 10 minutes daily for 17 days led to significant patient-reported improvements in dry skin as early as 2 hours after bathing, when compared to a control group using commercial soap. There appeared to be a cumulative improvement over the 17-day period (Stanfield, 1981). However, lanolin can stimulate an allergic contact dermatitis and may not be suitable for patients with sensitive skin (Fransen, Overgaard, Johansen, & Thyssen, 2018).

Cannabinoids

The endocannabinoid system (ECS) is comprised of an extensive network of G protein–coupled cannabinoid receptors and lipid messengers that mediate proliferation and differentiation of a myriad of skin cell types, immune function, and sensory transmission (Biro, Toth, Hasko, Paus, & Pacher, 2009). Endocannabinoids are known to decrease inflammation and transmission of itch and pain in the skin (Trusler, Clark, Sivamani, & Shi, 2017). Topical N-palmitoylethanolamine (PEA), a synthetic cannabinoid with no psychoactive properties, has been shown to decrease the hyperproliferation of keratinocytes that usually results in thick, lichenified skin in AD patients (Trusler et al., 2017). A PEA-containing cream significantly improved itching, lichenification, and AD severity in one study of 18 AD patients as compared to hydrocortisone 1% cream with reduced skin dryness after 1 week of treatment (Kemeny, 2005). A multicenter, prospective cohort study of 2456 patients found significant reductions in erythema, pruritus, excoriation, scaling, lichenification, and dryness in patients using a PEA-containing cream for 6 weeks (Eberlein, Eicke, Reinhardt, & Ring, 2008). Although the role of PEA cream as a stand-alone treatment in AD requires more evidence, PEA can be recommended as an adjunct to topical corticosteroids (Del Rosso, 2007).

Manuka honey

Manuka honey is derived from the manuka tree *(Leptospermum scoparium)* and has been used for centuries for its healing and antimicrobial properties (Adams et al., 2008). All honey products contain hydrogen peroxide, which is responsible for its antimicrobial action. However, manuka honey also contains high levels of methylglyoxal (Allen, Molan, & Reid, 1991), an antimicrobial organic compound resistant to inactivation by catalase-positive bacteria such as *S. aureus*, *Escherichia coli*, *Salmonella*, and *Pseudomonas aeruginosa* (Adams et al., 2008). Specifically, methylglyoxal is known to inhibit bacterial cell cycle progression and biofilm production eventuating in decreases in cutaneous inflammation and colonization by catalase-positive organisms when applied topically (Adams et al., 2008; Lee, Sinno, & Khachemoune, 2011; Sherlock et al., 2010). In a clinical trial of 20 adults, 1 week of daily overnight manuka honey treatment significantly improved AD lesions. Authors found that manuka honey application was associated with a downregulation in IL4-induced CCL26 release from keratinocytes, an eosinophil chemoattractant, and subsequent mast cell degranulation (Alangari et al., 2017).

While manuka honey is a promising and ancient antimicrobial, patients should be informed that honey products should be avoided in children younger than 1 year of age due to the risk of infantile botulism caused by *Clostridium botulinum* spores, often found in raw honey. Recently, this risk has been largely mitigated with the introduction of γ-irradiation in honey manufacturing, which has been shown to effectively prevent botulism without attenuating antibacterial effects (Molan & Allen, 1996). However, the authors prefer to avoid honey in children less than 1 year of age given the severe consequences of infantile botulism. In adults and older children, manuka honey is a promising topical treatment.

Fabrics and clothing considerations

Traditionally, cotton and silk have been recommended for AD patients based on comfort preferences. However, the evidence for these fabrics in AD patients is sparse, and high variability in fiber processing and dyeing confounds any existing evidence. Wool was historically considered a potent itch activator; however, it is now manufactured at super- and ultrafine diameters (<30 μm in diameter), which does not stimulate itch receptors and may be beneficial in reducing AD severity when worn consistently (Fowler, Fowler, & Lorenz, 2019). Bioactive textiles such as silver-coated cellulose, BSO-coated and zinc-coated cottons, polyurethane, and chitosan are currently underway and have anti-*S. aureus* and antimicrobial properties that could be applied in AD. Study design for these fabrics is variable; results need to be replicated in randomized, placebo-controlled trials with adequate sample sizes prior to recommendation.

Summary

Many CAM modalities have been used anecdotally for centuries, and the scientific community is beginning to formally validate these therapies due to patient interest. Given the existing evidence, SSO and VCO are likely safe and efficacious add-on topical therapies. Patients should be counseled to avoid olive oil and olive oil-containing products. Oral oils have limited evidence; however, hempseed oil is the most promising oral oil. Vegetable oils such as sunflower, safflower, corn, and sea buckthorn are also rich in fatty acids and/or δ-linoleic acid and may be considered for future investigations. Topical and oral micronutrients that may have efficacy include topical B_{12} and oral L-histidine, and vitamins D and E. Several bathing additives are promising in AD treatment, including Dead Sea salt, colloidal oatmeal, rice, and natural oils (see Table 26.1). To our knowledge, no major adverse reactions were associated with consistent use of these bathing additives, and their use may be recommended in clinical practice.

Cotton and silk fabrics have been anecdotally recommended for AD and are generally safe, although data supporting their use in AD are lacking. Promising new fabrics for AD patients include silver-coated, chitosan-coated, and cellulose-based materials, but these require larger scale studies to validate their efficacy. Endocannabinoid-containing topical formulation (i.e., PEA) has been shown to reduce the symptoms of AD with a low risk of adverse events and may be chosen for add-on therapy.

On the whole, current evidence for CAM modalities is limited by trial size and design. However, as CAM modalities continue to be validated, they will be increasingly integrated into conventional management guidelines.

Acknowledgments

We would like to thank Dr. Peter Lio for generously contributing his recipe for topical B_{12} cream "Pink Magic" for the readership.

References

Adams, C. J., Boult, C. H., Deadman, B. J., Farr, J. M., Grainger, M. N., Manley-Harris, M., & Snow, M. J. (2008). Isolation by HPLC and characterisation of the bioactive fraction of New Zealand manuka (*Leptospermum scoparium*) honey. *Carbohydrate Research*, *343*(4), 651–659.

Al-Khamees, W. A., Schwartz, M. D., Alrashdi, S., Algren, A. D., & Morgan, B. W. (2011). Status epilepticus associated with borage oil ingestion. *Journal of Medical Toxicology*, *7*(2), 154–157.

Alangari, A. A., Morris, K., Lwaleed, B. A., Lau, L., Jones, K., Cooper, R., & Jenkins, R. (2017). Honey is potentially effective in the treatment of atopic dermatitis: Clinical and mechanistic studies. *Immunity, Inflammation and Disease*, *5*(2), 190–199.

Allen, K. L., Molan, P. C., & Reid, G. M. (1991). A survey of the antibacterial activity of some New Zealand honeys. *The Journal of Pharmacy and Pharmacology*, *43*(12), 817–822.

Amestejani, M., Salehi, B. S., Vasigh, M., Sobhkhiz, A., Karami, M., Alinia, H., et al. (2012). Vitamin D supplementation in the treatment of atopic dermatitis: A clinical trial study. *Journal of Drugs in Dermatology*, *11*(3), 327–330.

Bamford, J. T., Ray, S., Musekiwa, A., van Gool, C., Humphreys, R., & Ernst, E. (2013). Oral evening primrose oil and borage oil for eczema. *Cochrane Database of Systematic Reviews*, *4*, Cd004416.

Bassett, I. B., Pannowitz, D. L., & Barnetson, R. S. (1990). A comparative study of tea-tree oil versus benzoylperoxide in the treatment of acne. *The Medical Journal of Australia*, *153*(8), 455–458.

Bikle, D. D., Pillai, S., Gee, E., & Hincenbergs, M. (1989). Regulation of 1,25-dihydroxyvitamin D production in human keratinocytes by interferon-gamma. *Endocrinology*, *124*(2), 655–660.

Biro, T., Toth, B. I., Hasko, G., Paus, R., & Pacher, P. (2009). The endocannabinoid system of the skin in health and disease: Novel perspectives and therapeutic opportunities. *Trends in Pharmacological Sciences*, *30*(8), 411–420.

Borzutzky, A., & Camargo, C. A., Jr. (2013). Role of vitamin D in the pathogenesis and treatment of atopic dermatitis. *Expert Review of Clinical Immunology*, *9*(8), 751–760.

Bromm, B., Scharein, E., Darsow, U., & Ring, J. (1995). Effects of menthol and cold on histamine-induced itch and skin reactions in man. *Neuroscience Letters*, *187*(3), 157–160.

Callaway, J., Schwab, U., Harvima, I., Halonen, P., Mykkanen, O., Hyvonen, P., & Jarvinen, T. (2005). Efficacy of dietary hempseed oil in patients with atopic dermatitis. *The Journal of Dermatological Treatment*, *16*(2), 87–94.

Camargo, C. A., Jr, Ganmaa, D., Sidbury, R., Erdenedelger, K., Radnaakhand, N., & Khandsuren, B. (2014). Randomized trial of vitamin D supplementation for winter-related atopic dermatitis in children. *The Journal of Allergy and Clinical Immunology*, *134*(4), 831–835.e831.

Chopra, R., Vakharia, P. P., Sacotte, R., & Silverberg, J. I. (2017). Efficacy of bleach baths in reducing severity of atopic dermatitis: A systematic review and meta-analysis. *Annals of Allergy, Asthma and Immunology*, *119*(5), 435–440.

Clearinghouse, N. (2018). Complementary, Alternative, or Integrative Health: What's In a Name? https://nccih.nih.gov/health/integrative-health. Accessed January 20, 2021.

Cooke, A., Cork, M. J., Victor, S., Campbell, M., Danby, S., Chittock, J., & Lavender, T. (2016). Olive oil, sunflower oil or no oil for baby dry skin or massage: A pilot, assessor-blinded, randomized controlled trial (the Oil in Baby SkincaRE [OBSeRvE] Study). *Acta Dermato-Venereologica*, *96*(3), 323–330.

Danby, S. G., AlEnezi, T., Sultan, A., Lavender, T., Chittock, J., Brown, K., & Cork, M. J. (2013). Effect of olive and sunflower seed oil on the adult skin barrier: Implications for neonatal skin care. *Pediatric Dermatology*, *30*(1), 42–50.

Danby, S. G., Brown, K., Wigley, A. M., Chittock, J., Pyae, P. K., Flohr, C., & Cork, M. J. (2018). The effect of water hardness on surfactant deposition after washing and subsequent skin irritation in atopic dermatitis patients and healthy control subjects. *The Journal of Investigative Dermatology*, *138*(1), 68–77.

Darmstadt, G. L., Badrawi, N., Law, P. A., Ahmed, S., Bashir, M., Iskander, I., et al. (2004). Topically applied sunflower seed oil prevents invasive bacterial infections in preterm infants in Egypt: A randomized, controlled clinical trial. *The Pediatric Infectious Disease Journal*, *23*(8), 719–725.

Darmstadt, G. L., Mao-Qiang, M., Chi, E., Saha, S. K., Ziboh, V. A., Black, R. E., et al. (2002). Impact of topical oils on the skin barrier: Possible implications for neonatal health in developing countries. *Acta Paediatrica*, *91*(5), 546–554.

de Groot, A. C., & Schmidt, E. (2016). Essential oils, part I: Introduction. *Dermatitis: Contact, Atopic, Occupational, Drug*, *27*(2), 39–42.

De Paepe, K., Hachem, J. P., Vanpee, E., Roseeuw, D., & Rogiers, V. (2002). Effect of rice starch as a bath additive on the barrier function of healthy but SLS-damaged skin and skin of atopic patients. *Acta Dermato-Venereologica*, *82*(3), 184–186.

Del Rosso. J. Q. (2007). Use of a palmitoylethanolamide- containing nonsteroidal cream for treating atopic dermatitis: Impact on the duration of response and time between flares. *Cosmetic Dermatology*, *20*, 208–211.

Eberlein, B., Eicke, C., Reinhardt, H. W., & Ring, J. (2008). Adjuvant treatment of atopic eczema: Assessment of an emollient containing N-palmitoylethanolamine (ATOPA study). *Journal of the European Academy of Dermatology and Venereology*, *22*(1), 73–82.

Eichenfield, L. F., McCollum, A., & Msika, P. (2009). The benefits of sunflower oleodistillate (SOD) in pediatric dermatology. *Pediatric Dermatology*, *26*(6), 669–675.

Escobar, S. O., Achenbach, R., Iannantuono, R., & Torem, V. (1992). Topical fish oil in psoriasis--A controlled and blind study. *Clinical and Experimental Dermatology*, *17*(3), 159–162.

Evangelista, M. T., Abad-Casintahan, F., & Lopez-Villafuerte, L. (2014). The effect of topical virgin coconut oil on SCORAD index, transepidermal water loss, and skin capacitance in mild to moderate pediatric atopic dermatitis: A randomized, double-blind, clinical trial. *International Journal of Dermatology*, *53*(1), 100–108.

Fowler, J. F., Nebus, J., Wallo, W., & Eichenfield, L. F. (2012). Colloidal oatmeal formulations as adjunct treatments in atopic dermatitis. *Journal of Drugs in Dermatology*, *11*(7), 804–807. https://pubmed.ncbi.nlm.nih.gov/22777219/.

Fowler, J. F., Jr., Fowler, L. M., & Lorenz, D. (2019). Effects of merino wool on atopic dermatitis using clinical, quality of life, and physiological outcome measures. *Dermatitis: Contact, Atopic, Occupational, Drug*, *30*(3), 198–206.

Fransen, M., Overgaard, L. E. K., Johansen, J. D., & Thyssen, J. P. (2018). Contact allergy to lanolin: Temporal changes in prevalence and association with atopic dermatitis. *Contact Dermatitis*, *78*(1), 70–75.

Fruhstorfer, H., Hermanns, M., & Latzke, L. (1986). The effects of thermal stimulation on clinical and experimental itch. *Pain*, *24*(2), 259–269.

Fujiwaki, T., & Furusho, K. (1992). The effects of rice bran broth bathing in patients with atopic dermatitis. *Pediatrics International*, *34*(5), 505–510.

Galeotti, N., Di Cesare Mannelli, L., Mazzanti, G., Bartolini, A., & Ghelardini, C. (2002). Menthol: A natural analgesic compound. *Neuroscience Letters*, *322*(3), 145–148.

Grant. W. B. (2009). Critique of the U-shaped serum 25-hydroxyvitamin D level-disease response relation. *Dermatoendocrinol*, *1*(6), 289–293.

Hanley, K., Jiang, Y., Crumrine, D., Bass, N. M., Appel, R., Elias, P. M., et al. (1997). Activators of the nuclear hormone receptors PPARα and FXR accelerate the development of the fetal epidermal permeability barrier. *The Journal of Clinical Investigation*, *100*(3), 705–712.

Hatem, S., Attal, N., Willer, J. C., & Bouhassira, D. (2006). Psychophysical study of the effects of topical application of menthol in healthy volunteers. *Pain*, *122*(1-2), 190–196.

Henz, B. M., Jablonska, S., van de Kerkhof, P. C., Stingl, G., Blaszczyk, M., Vandervalk, P. G., et al. (1999). Double-blind, multicentre analysis of the efficacy of borage oil in patients with atopic eczema. *British Journal of Dermatology*, *140*(4), 685–688.

Hill, S., & Edwards, C. (2002). A comparison of the effects of bath additives on the barrier function of skin in normal volunteer subjects. *The Journal of Dermatological Treatment*, *13*(1), 15–18.

Hong, J., Buddenkotte, J., Berger, T. G., & Steinhoff, M. (2011). Management of itch in atopic dermatitis. *Seminars in Cutaneous Medicine and Surgery*, *30*(2), 71–86.

Islam, M. S., Yoshida, H., Matsuki, N., Ono, K., Nagasaka, R., Ushio, H., et al. (2009). Antioxidant, free radical–scavenging, and NF-κB–inhibitory activities of phytosteryl ferulates: Structure–activity studies. *Journal of Pharmacological Sciences*, *111*(4), 328–337.

Jaffary, F., Faghihi, G., Mokhtarian, A., & Hosseini, S. M. (2015). Effects of oral vitamin E on treatment of atopic dermatitis: A randomized controlled trial. *Journal of Research in Medical Sciences*, *20*(11), 1053–1057.

Januchowski. R. (2009). Evaluation of topical vitamin B(12) for the treatment of childhood eczema. *Journal of Alternative and Complementary Medicine*, *15*(4), 387–389.

Javanbakht, M. H., Keshavarz, S. A., Djalali, M., Siassi, F., Eshraghian, M. R., Firooz, A., et al. (2011). Randomized controlled trial using vitamins E and D supplementation in atopic dermatitis. *The Journal of Dermatological Treatment*, *22*(3), 144–150.

Kanehara, S., Ohtani, T., Uede, K., & Furukawa, F. (2007). Clinical effects of undershirts coated with borage oil on children with atopic dermatitis: A double-blind, placebo-controlled clinical trial. *The Journal of Dermatology*, 34(12), 811–815.

Katsuta, Y., Iida, T., Hasegawa, K., Inomata, S., & Denda, M. (2009). Function of oleic acid on epidermal barrier and calcium influx into keratinocytes is associated with N-methyl D-aspartate-type glutamate receptors. *British Journal of Dermatology*, 160(1), 69–74.

Kemeny. L. (2005). Comparative study of S236 cream and hydrocortisone 1% in patients with atopic dermatitis. *Journal of the American Academy of Dermatology*, 52(3, Supplement), P68. ISSN 0190-9622, https://doi.org/10.1016/j.jaad.2004.10.282. https://www.jaad.org/article/S0190-9622(04)03054-3/fulltext.

Kong, H. H., Oh, J., Deming, C., Conlan, S., Grice, E. A., Beatson, M. A., et al. (2012). Temporal shifts in the skin microbiome associated with disease flares and treatment in children with atopic dermatitis. *Genome Research*, 22(5), 850–859.

Kopple, J. D., & Swendseid, M. E. (1975). Evidence that histidine is an essential amino acid in normal and chronically uremic man. *The Journal of Clinical Investigation*, 55(5), 881–891.

Kottner, J., Kanti, V., Dobos, G., Hahnel, E., Lichterfeld-Kottner, A., Richter, C., et al. (2017). The effectiveness of using a bath oil to reduce signs of dry skin: A randomized controlled pragmatic study. *International Journal of Nursing Studies*, 65, 17–24.

Lee, D. S., Sinno, S., & Khachemoune, A. (2011). Honey and wound healing: An overview. *American Journal of Clinical Dermatology*, 12(3), 181–190.

Lee, S. H., Elias, P. M., Proksch, E., Menon, G. K., Mao-Quiang, M., & Feingold, K. R. (1992). Calcium and potassium are important regulators of barrier homeostasis in murine epidermis. *The Journal of Clinical Investigation*, 89(2), 530–538.

Levin, C., & Maibach, H. (2002). Exploration of "alternative" and "natural" drugs in dermatology. *Archives of Dermatology*, 138(2), 207–211.

Loughlin, R., Gilmore, B. F., McCarron, P. A., & Tunney, M. M. (2008). Comparison of the cidal activity of tea tree oil and terpinen-4-ol against clinical bacterial skin isolates and human fibroblast cells. *Letters in Applied Microbiology*, 46(4), 428–433.

Mack Correa, M. C., Mao, G., Saad, P., Flach, C. R., Mendelsohn, R., & Walters, R. M. (2014). Molecular interactions of plant oil components with stratum corneum lipids correlate with clinical measures of skin barrier function. *Experimental Dermatology*, 23(1), 39–44.

Molan, P. C., & Allen, K. L. (1996). The effect of gamma-irradiation on the antibacterial activity of honey.". *The Journal of Pharmacy and Pharmacology*, 48(11), 1206–1209.

Msika, P., De Belilovsky, C., Piccardi, N., Chebassier, N., Baudouin, C., & Chadoutaud, B. (2008). New emollient with topical corticosteroid-sparing effect in treatment of childhood atopic dermatitis: SCORAD and quality of life improvement. *Pediatric Dermatology*, 25(6), 606–612.

Nangia, S., Paul, V. K., Deorari, A. K., Sreenivas, V., Agarwal, R., & Chawla, D. (2015). Topical oil application and trans-epidermal water loss in preterm very low birth weight infants—A randomized trial. *Journal of Tropical Pediatrics*, 61(6), 414–420.

Patel, T., Ishiuji, Y., & Yosipovitch, G. (2007). Menthol: A refreshing look at this ancient compound. *Journal of the American Academy of Dermatology*, 57(5), 873–878.

Patrizi, A., Raone, B., Neri, I., Gurioli, C., Carbonara, M., Cassano, N., & Vena, G. A. (2016). Randomized, controlled, double-blind clinical study evaluating the safety and efficacy of MD2011001 cream in mild-to-moderate atopic dermatitis of the face and neck in children, adolescents and adults. *The Journal of Dermatological Treatment*, 27(4), 346–350.

Peier, A. M., Moqrich, A., Hergarden, A. C., Reeve, A. J., Andersson, D. A., Story, G. M., et al. (2002). A TRP channel that senses cold stimuli and menthol. *Cell*, 108(5), 705–715.

Perkin, M. R., Craven, J., Logan, K., Strachan, D., Marrs, T., Radulovic, S., et al. (2016). Association between domestic water hardness, chlorine, and atopic dermatitis risk in early life: A population-based cross-sectional study. *The Journal of Allergy and Clinical Immunology*, 138(2), 509–516.

Plager, D. A., Leontovich, A. A., Henke, S. A., Davis, M. D. P., McEvoy, M. T., Sciallis, G. F., 2nd, & Pittelkow, M. R. (2007). Early cutaneous gene transcription changes in adult atopic dermatitis and potential clinical implications. *Experimental Dermatology*, 16(1), 28–36.

Proksch, E., Nissen, H. P., Bremgartner, M., & Urquhart, C. (2005). Bathing in a magnesium-rich Dead Sea salt solution improves skin barrier function, enhances skin hydration, and reduces inflammation in atopic dry skin. *International Journal of Dermatology*, 44(2), 151–157.

Quality, U. O. o. W. (2012, December 28, 2016). Water Hardness and Alkalinity. http://water.usgs.gov/owq/hardness-alkalinity.html. Accessed January 14, 2019.

Sanchez-Armendariz, K., Garcia-Gil, A., Romero, C. A., Contreras-Ruiz, J., Karam-Orante, M., Balcazar-Antonio, D., & Dominguez-Cherit, J. (2018). Oral vitamin D3 5000 IU/day as an adjuvant in the treatment of atopic dermatitis: A randomized control trial. *International Journal of Dermatology*, 57(12), 1516–1520.

Schempp, C. M., Dittmar, H. C., Hummler, D., Simon-Haarhaus, B., Schulte-Monting, J., Schopf, E., & Simon, J. C. (2000). Magnesium ions inhibit the antigen-presenting function of human epidermal Langerhans cells in vivo and in vitro. Involvement of ATPase, HLA-DR, B7 molecules, and cytokines. *The Journal of Investigative Dermatology*, 115(4), 680–686.

Schliemann-Willers, S., Wigger-Alberti, W., Kleesz, P., Grieshaber, R., & Elsner, P. (2002). Natural vegetable fats in the prevention of irritant contact dermatitis. *Contact Dermatitis*, 46(1), 6–12.

Sgouros, D., Katoulis, A., & Rigopoulos, D. (2018). Novel topical agent containing superoxide dismutase 100 000 IU and 4% of plant extracts as a mono-therapy for atopic dermatitis. *Journal of Cosmetic Dermatology*, 17(6), 1069–1072.

Sherlock, O., Dolan, A., Athman, R., Power, A., Gethin, G., Cowman, S., & Humphreys, H. (2010). Comparison of the antimicrobial activity of Ulmo honey from Chile and Manuka honey against methicillin-resistant *Staphylococcus aureus*, *Escherichia coli* and *Pseudomonas aeruginosa*. *BMC Complementary and Alternative Medicine*, 10, 47.

Shi, V. Y., Foolad, N., Ornelas, J. N., Hassoun, L. A., Monico, G., Takeda, N., et al. (2016). Comparing the effect of bleach and water baths on skin barrier function in atopic dermatitis: A split-body randomized controlled trial. *The British Journal of Dermatology*, 175(1), 212–214.

Sompayrac, L., & Ross, C. (1959). Colloidal oatmeal in atopic dermatitis of the young. *Journal of the Florida Medical Association*, 45(12), 1411–1412.

Stanfield. J. W. (1981). A new technique for evaluating bath oil in the treatment of dry skin. *Cutis*, 28(4), 458–460.

Stucker, M., Pieck, C., Stoerb, C., Niedner, R., Hartung, J., & Altmeyer, P. (2004). Topical vitamin B12—A new therapeutic approach in atopic dermatitis-evaluation of efficacy and tolerability in a randomized placebo-controlled multicentre clinical trial. *The British Journal of Dermatology*, 150(5), 977–983.

Tan, S. P., Brown, S. B., Griffiths, C. E., Weller, R. B., & Gibbs, N. K. (2017). Feeding filaggrin: Effects of l-histidine supplementation in atopic dermatitis. *Clinical, Cosmetic and Investigational Dermatology, 10*, 403–411.

Tey, H. L., Tay, E. Y., & Tan, W. D. (2017). Safety and antipruritic efficacy of a menthol-containing moisturizing cream. *Skinmed, 15*(6), 437–439.

Thaci, D. L. S. E., Deleuran, M., Kataoka, Y., Chen, Z., Gadkari, A., Eckert, L., et al. (2019). Efficacy and safety of dupilumab monotherapy in adults with moderate-to-severe atopic dermatitis: A pooled analysis of two phase 3 randomized trials (LIBERTY AD SOLO 1 and LIBERTY AD SOLO 2). *Journal of Dermatological Science, 94*(2), 266–275.

Thiele, J. J., Hsieh, S. N., & Ekanayake-Mudiyanselage, S. (2005). Vitamin E: Critical review of its current use in cosmetic and clinical dermatology. *Dermatologic Surgery, 31*(7 Pt 2), 805–813. discussion 813.

Thomas, K. S., Koller, K., Dean, T., O'Leary, C. J., Sach, T. H., Frost, A., et al. (2011). A multicentre randomised controlled trial and economic evaluation of ion-exchange water softeners for the treatment of eczema in children: The Softened Water Eczema Trial (SWET). *Health Technology Assessment, 15*(8), v–vi. 1–156.

Togawa, Y., Kambe, N., Shimojo, N., Nakano, T., Sato, Y., Mochizuki, H., et al. (2014). Ultra-pure soft water improves skin barrier function in children with atopic dermatitis: A randomized, double-blind, placebo-controlled, crossover pilot study. *Journal of Dermatological Science, 76*(3), 269–271.

Tollesson, A., & Frithz, A. (1993). Borage oil, an effective new treatment for infantile seborrhoeic dermatitis. *British Journal of Dermatology, 129*(1), 95.

Totte, J. E., van der Feltz, W. T., Hennekam, M., van Belkum, A., van Zuuren, E. J., & Pasmans, S. G. (2016). Prevalence and odds of *Staphylococcus aureus* carriage in atopic dermatitis: A systematic review and meta-analysis. *British Journal of Dermatology, 175*(4), 687–695.

Trusler, A. R., Clark, A. K., Sivamani, R. K., & Shi, V. Y. (2017). The endocannabinoid system and its role in eczematous dermatoses. *Dermatitis: Contact, Atopic, Occupational, Drug, 28*(1), 22–32.

Tsoureli-Nikita, E., Hercogova, J., Lotti, T., & Menchini, G. (2002). Evaluation of dietary intake of vitamin E in the treatment of atopic dermatitis: A study of the clinical course and evaluation of the immunoglobulin E serum levels. *International Journal of Dermatology, 41*(3), 146–150.

Vaughn, A. R., Foolad, N., Maarouf, M., Tran, K. A., & Shi, V. Y. (2019). Micronutrients in atopic dermatitis: A systematic review. *Journal of Alternative and Complementary Medicine, 25*(6), 567–577.

Verallo-Rowell, V. M., Dillague, K. M., & Syah-Tjundawan, B. S. (2008). Novel antibacterial and emollient effects of coconut and virgin olive oils in adult atopic dermatitis. *Dermatitis: Contact, Atopic, Occupational, Drug, 19*(6), 308–315.

Wilkinson, S. M., & Beck, M. H. (1994). Allergic contact dermatitis from menthol in peppermint. *Contact Dermatitis, 30*(1), 42–43.

Wu, D., Meydani, M., Leka, L. S., Nightingale, Z., Handelman, G. J., Blumberg, J. B., & Meydani, S. N. (1999). Effect of dietary supplementation with black currant seed oil on the immune response of healthy elderly subjects. *The American Journal of Clinical Nutrition, 70*(4), 536–543.

Zhu, T. H., Zhu, T. R., Tran, K. A., Sivamani, R. K., & Shi, V. Y. (2018). Epithelial barrier dysfunctions in atopic dermatitis: A skin-gut-lung model linking microbiome alteration and immune dysregulation. *British Journal of Dermatology, 179*(3), 570–581.

Further readings

Clearinghouse, N. (2020). Complementary, alternative, or integrative health: What's in a name? National Center for Complementary and Integrative Health. https://nccih.nih.gov/health/integrative-health.

Goddard, A. L., & Lio, P. A. (2015). Alternative, complementary, and forgotten remedies for atopic dermatitis. *Evidence-Based Complementary and Alternative Medicine, 2015*, 676897.

Levin, C., & Maibach, H. (2002). Exploration of "alternative" and "natural" drugs in dermatology. *Archives of Dermatology, 138*(2), 207–211.

27

Complementary and Alternative Approaches II

JONWEI HWANG, MARTA TUROWSKI, JOANNA JAROS, AND VIVIAN Y. SHI

KEY POINTS

- A review of a variety of alternative therapies for atopic dermatitis (AD) is the focus of this chapter. Among those reviewed are acupuncture, cupping, and herbal therapies, which are common traditional Chinese therapies used by AD patients.
- We discuss the limited, but compelling research surrounding acupuncture and its subtypes' success in treating AD symptoms such as itch.
- Cupping has less clear evidence for its use. We review the positive as well as the negative effects it may produce.
- We consider ancient Chinese herbal remedies, as well as teas and caffeine, their efficacy, and how their use translates into modern treatment of AD.

Introduction

According to some experts in traditional Chinese medicine, atopic dermatitis (AD) is caused by "a congenitally weak constitution, resulting in a predisposition toward atopic diseases and susceptibility toward external or internal pathogenic factors, such as wind, dampness, and heat. Its recurrent and chronic nature can injure Yin (as in Yin/Yang) and blood and generate dryness" (Tan, Zhang, Chen, Xue, & Lenon, 2013). Traditional Chinese medicine is an alternative medicine practice that includes using many herbs that are specifically formulated for the needs of each individual patient (Koo & Desai, 2003). Since this ancient definition of AD, science has come a long way in understanding the mechanism behind AD. As research moves to unveil the mechanisms responsible for the pathogenesis of AD, there will be more opportunity to understand the reasons for different treatment modalities' efficacy or lack thereof. Until a comprehensive pathophysiology is uncovered about AD, patients may continue to seek other nonconventional practices that have succeeded in managing symptoms of many diseases for centuries. Thus patients may look to those ancient Chinese remedies such as herbal extracts for healing their diseased skin.

The current data suggest that approximately one-third of AD patients will use complementary or alternative therapies in the lifetime of their disease. This is at least in part due to the chronicity of AD, its predilection for development in pediatric populations, and treatment resistance (Holm, Clausen, Agner, & Thomsen, 2019).

In the instances where patients look for alternative therapies for management of their AD, the goal should be to confirm safety of the treatment rather than move to stop its practice. The high level of patients seeking to use complementary and alternative treatment therapies may suggest that conventional health treatments are not providing high levels of satisfactory results (Holm et al., 2019).

This chapter focuses on existing evidence and gaps in research for complementary therapies in AD, including acupuncture, cupping, and herbal therapies. We explore the human and animal trials that are starting to uncover evidence for therapies that in some cultures have been used for centuries for the treatment of dermatologic disease. Additional complementary and alternative therapies, including supplementary oils, bathing additives, topical endocannabinoids, and fabric selection, are discussed in Chapter 26.

Physical treatments

Acupuncture

In acupuncture, thin caliber (20-40 gauge) needles are placed at specific target locations on the body to modulate neurosensory transmission. A randomized, sham-controlled, single-blinded preliminary trial with 30 adult participants with mild to moderate AD administered verum acupuncture three times weekly for 4 weeks, twice weekly for 4 weeks, and sham acupuncture twice weekly for 4 weeks. Both acupuncture groups had a significant reduction in eczema severity when compared to sham. However, there were no significant improvements in insomnia, pruritus, or EASI scoring of eczema severity (Kang et al., 2018). A randomized, double-blinded, placebo-controlled, crossover trial with 20 adult patients with AD found higher reductions in itch intensity between acupuncture and antihistamine itch therapy and significantly higher reductions of itch when compared to placebo (Pfab et al., 2012). A 2016 review stated that acupuncture treatment for symptoms of itch seems promising, but larger, randomized, placebo-controlled studies needed to be done before conclusions can be made (Vieira, Lim, Lohman, & Lio, 2016).

Electroacupuncture

An alternative form of acupuncture is electroacupuncture in which an electrical current is passed between acupuncture needles. There are no studies on electroacupuncture treatment in human patients with AD. A study on a model of AD in rats suggests high-frequency electroacupuncture alleviates pruritus through causing dynorphin neurotransmitter release, which acts on opioid receptors to decrease itch. Paradoxically, there was no significant difference in pain scores in rats even though pain and itch share many of the same neurologic pathways (Jung, Lee, Choi, Na, & Hong, 2014). Lack of human clinical trials precludes the possibility of concluding electroacupuncture can be used to treat AD until further studies are completed.

Acupressure

Acupressure uses a small titanium bead to massage an acupoint on the skin. Most promising is a randomized, controlled pilot study of 15 adults with AD by Lio et al., which applies acupressure for 3 minutes three times per week for 4 weeks. They found significant improvements in pruritus and lichenification in the treatment group but also conclude that larger scale studies will be needed to confirm efficacy (Lee et al., 2012). Current treatment guidelines for AD by Sidbury et al. state that there is insufficient evidence to support acupressure in the management of AD (Sidbury et al., 2014). Acupressure may be a good alternative for pediatric patients who are less likely to tolerate traditional acupuncture.

Cupping therapy

Cupping therapy is an ancient Chinese modality in which partial, local suctioning is created on the skin by placing inverted cups and sealing with heat or suction. Cupping creates temporary bruises and microtrauma and is believed to dispel stagnation of blood and lymph and therefore improve energy (qi) flow (Cui & Cui, 2012). There is very little published on the subject of cupping and AD.

One study of 88 patients compared blood-letting puncturing and cupping with a placebo of Claritin and Pairuisong Ointment. The study concluded there was a definite therapeutic effect on acute eczema, which is better than Western medicine. However, this study has limited scientific data included in its references and was not able to

be examined in detail because it is written in Chinese (Cui & Cui, 2012). Notably, the only other literature referencing cupping and AD is a case report of an 11-year-old girl with AD who developed blisters and oozing after cupping therapy, which rapidly evolved into purulent ulcerations (Hon, Luk, Leong, & Leung, 2013).

Currently there is very limited evidence that supports the use of cupping for treating AD, and there is concern for patient harm. Therefore more data on the safety and efficacy of cupping in patients with AD are needed before it can be recommended.

Herbal therapy

Traditional Chinese medicine is historically a popular complementary medicine in many Asian societies. PentaHerbs Formula (PHF) is based on a widely used ancestral Chinese concoction of five herbs: Flos Lonicerae (Jinyinhua), Herba Menthae (Bohe), Cortex Moutan (Mudanpi), Rhizoma Atractylodis (Cangzhu), and Cortex Phellodendri (Huangbai). In a randomized, double-blind, placebo-controlled study in children with AD, oral PHF was well tolerated and significantly improved symptoms and quality of life; there was also a reduction in topical corticosteroid requirement (Hon et al., 2004, 2007, 2012).

Cardiospermum (balloon vine) extract contains flavonoids with antiinflammatory and antipruritic effects. Balloon vine was a minor ingredient in an open-label, forearm-controlled pilot study, which found that balloon vine-containing ointment applied twice daily led to significant improvements in transepidermal water loss (TEWL), hydration, skin elasticity and firmness, erythema. Skin roughness and smoothness were assessed via Visioscan VC98 which uses special illumination to capture high-resolution images of the skin (Wakeman, 2017). However, balloon vine was among many ingredients contained in the ointment, therefore efficacy of balloon vine extract cannot be discerned. A review article described a double-blind, placebo-controlled study of an ointment containing balloon vine leaf extract and found it to be slightly superior when compared to placebo in patients with mild eczema. We cannot confirm the study design, ingredients, or any other details due to the study being written in German (Merklinger, Messemer, & Niederle, 1995; Reuter, Wolfle, Weckesser, & Schempp, 2010). At this time there is insufficient evidence for the use of balloon vine extract in AD.

Tea and caffeine

Black tea

Black tea compresses have anecdotally been used by German dermatologists to treat eczema and dermatitis for decades. The mechanism for black tea's efficacy in skin disorders has not been fully elucidated. Some researchers theorize that tannins, polyphenol organic molecules, and flavonoids act as astringents and antiinflammatories.

In a prospective, open, uncontrolled study of 22 patients with atopic or contact facial dermatitis, black tea dressings and an emollient cream were administered four to five times daily to the face for 6 days. A significant reduction of eczema severity occurred within the first 3 days of treatment, with continued improvement through day 6. The study suggests that black tea is not only rapidly effective for the treatment of facial dermatitis, but it is also easy to use and low cost compared to many typically prescribed medication options. Of note, the process of the applications does require a patient willing to follow a strict compress regiment in order to see results (Witte, Krause, Zillikens, & Shimanovich, 2019).

Animal models have shown efficacy in using tea to suppress type I and type IV allergic skin reactions (Ohmori et al., 1995). In a study of 121 patients with recalcitrant AD, a 10-g oolong teabag placed in 1000 mL of boiling water steeped for 5 minutes was divided into three equal servings, and one serving was consumed daily after three regular meals. The study assessed severity of pruritus using a 6-point Likert-like scale and assessed visual morphology and observed marked to moderate improvement of AD severity. Benefits were first after 1 to 2 weeks of treatment. There were no reported clinical side effects found during the study (Uehara, Sugiura, & Sakurai, 2001). Due to a lack of adverse effects, treatment of AD with regularly ingested tea appears to be a safe and reasonable addition to a patient's current regimen.

Green tea

Oral green tea efficacy for AD-like lesions has been recently studied in a murine model, and significant reductions in skin inflammation and TEWL were observed (Hwang, Chang, Kim, & Kim, 2019). A nonblinded, nonrandomized pilot study of green tea extract bathing additive treatment three times weekly for 4 weeks in four patients found improvement in eczema severity, visual lesion severity, and decreased mean serum eosinophil counts in four patients with *Malassezia*-associated AD (Kim et al., 2012). Larger, randomized, and blinded trials of topical and oral tea in AD need to be conducted before formal, evidence-based recommendations can be delineated. However, due to safety and affordability, black tea compresses, oral oolong tea, and oral green tea may be useful adjunctive therapies in AD.

Caffeine

Caffeine's action is thought to be due to elevation of local cyclic adenosine monophosphate (cAMP) by inhibiting phosphodiesterase (PDE). PDE4 is an important regulator for inflammatory cytokine production in AD. Its mechanism of action depends on degrading cAMP. The inhibition of PDE4 has been shown to reduce the release of proinflammatory cytokines (Paller et al., 2016). This similar mechanism has thought to suppress histamine release during acute inflammatory skin reactions (Kaplan, Daman, Rosenberg, &

Feigenbaum, 1978). There have been oral medications such as apremilast (a PDE inhibitor), used for other dermatologic conditions such as psoriasis (Paller et al., 2016). A topical version of such a drug may help limit its effect on nontarget tissue. In theory, topical caffeine application could provide this desired effect.

A double-blind trial of 83 patients with AD found that topically applied caffeine 30%-hydrocortisone 0.5% in hydrophilic ointment and betamethasone valerate 0.1% cream performed significantly better than a control of hydrocortisone 0.5% in hydrophilic ointment when looking at metrics such as lichenification, excoriation, and global impression. The study results suggest that caffeine-hydrocortisone combinations could be useful in the treatment of AD and could reduce the need for topical steroids and associated cutaneous side effects such as hypopigmentation or cutaneous atrophy (Kaplan et al., 1978).

Summary

As patients look to complementary and alternative therapies for the management of AD, it is important that the dermatologic community moves to understand the evidence behind these therapies' efficacy as well as their limitations, including their potentially harmful side effects. Although there are few studies with limited trial sizes, given the available evidence we believe that evidence-based complementary and alternative treatment modalities may be integrated into conventional treatment plans for AD to improve overall patient treatment outcomes.

A few randomized controlled trials investigating the use of acupuncture and acupressure have shown promising results with regard to eczema severity in AD (Kang et al., 2018; Lee et al., 2012; Pfab et al., 2012). Current evidence supports that these practices are likely safe adjunct or supplementary treatments for patients seeking alternative therapy for AD. Acupressure may be particularly well suited for nervous or pediatric patients who prefer to avoid traditional acupuncture. Electroacupuncture has only been studied in rats thus far and should not be recommended to patients.

Therapies adapted from ancient Chinese medicine, including herbal therapies and teas, have sparse but positive evidence. Oral PHF, balloon vine-containing ointment, and caffeine have been shown to improve AD symptoms (Hon et al., 2004, 2007, 2012; Kaplan et al., 1978; Wakeman, 2017). However, these studies are very small with confounding variables (e.g., other ingredients tested simultaneously), and the results need to be interpreted accordingly. Due to the lack of negative side effects reported, these herbal remedies can be used cautiously if requested by the patient. However, patients should be made aware that there is limited evidence for efficacy.

Tea modalities have limited clinical trials supporting their use; nevertheless, they have been studied more closely than other herbal supplements. Black tea dressings, oral administration of oolong, as well as green tea bathing

TABLE 27.1	Summary of alternative treatments for atopic dermatitis	
Method	**Treatment regiment**	**Studied effect**
Acupuncture	a. Verum acupuncture three times weekly for 4 weeks, twice weekly for 4 weeks, and sham acupuncture twice weekly for 4 weeks b. Verum acupuncture both preventative and abortive with 1-week break between session c. High-frequency electroacupuncture d. Acupressure for 3 min three times weekly for 4 weeks	a. Significant reduction in eczema severity (Kang et al., 2018) b. Reduced itch intensity compared to antihistamines and statistically significant itch reduction compared to placebo (Pfab et al., 2012) c. Reduction in itch in a rat model (Jung et al., 2014) d. Significant improvement in pruritus and lichenification (Lee et al., 2012)
Cupping	Cupping—no specified regiment	Definite therapeutic effect (Cui & Cui, 2012)
Herbal therapy	a. Oral PentaHerbs b. Cardiospermum (balloon vine-containing ointment)	a. Significantly improved quality of life and reduced topical corticosteroid requirements (Hon et al., 2004, 2007, 2012) b. Significant improvements in transepidermal water loss (TEWL), hydration, skin elasticity and firmness, erythema, and skin roughness and smoothness (Wakeman, 2017)

Tea	1. Black tea
	  a. Black tea dressings and an emollient cream were administered four to five times daily to the face for 6 days
	  b. 10-g oolong teabag placed in 1000 mL of boiling water steeped for 5 minutes was divided into three equal servings and one serving was consumed daily after three regular meals
	2. Green tea
	  a. Oral green tea
	  b. Green tea extract bathing additive treatment three times weekly for 4 weeks
		1. Black tea
		  a. Significant reduction of eczema severity (Witte et al., 2019)
		  b. Marked to moderate improvement of atopic dermatitis severity in terms of pruritis and visual morphology (Uehara et al., 2001)
		2. Green tea
		  a. Significant reductions in skin inflammation and TEWL (Hwang et al., 2019)
		  b. Improvement in eczema severity, visual lesion severity, and decreased mean serum eosinophil counts (Kim et al., 2012)

Caffeine	Caffeine 30%-hydrocortisone 0.5% in hydrophilic ointment and betamethasone valerate 0.1% cream	Significant improvement in lichenification, excoriation, and global impression (Kaplan et al., 1978)

additives have shown promise in improving eczema severity (Kim et al., 2012; Uehara et al., 2001; Witte et al., 2019). To our knowledge no major adverse reactions were associated with using tea orally and topically, and its use may be recommended in clinical practice.

Overall, the data for traditional Chinese medicine in AD is sparse. The existing research is limited by small sample size, confounding variables, language barriers, and study design flaws. However, there continues to be a large interest among patients for these supplementary treatment methods, which should serve as an impetus to test their safety and efficacy. Several modalities are safe and may be trialed on a case-by-case basis. As the evidence evolves, physicians will likely begin to integrate alternative therapies into everyday practice.

Table 27.1 summarizes alternative treatments for AD discussed in this chapter.

Practical pearls

Table 27.2 provides clinical pearls for the integrative management of AD discussed in this chapter and in Chapter 26. We have included links to scoring tools and lists that we have found useful in our clinical practice.

TABLE 27.2	Clinical pearls for integrative treatment of atopic dermatitis	
Practical suggestions	**Comments**	
1. Recommend patients engage in practices that can improve or prevent symptoms.	a. Wear hypoallergenic fabrics	
	b. Use HEPA filters to decrease dust mite exposure	
	c. Use wet wrap therapy	
	d. Practice massage therapy prior to sleep to increase moisturizer penetration for 20 min/day	
	e. Drink green, black, or oolong tea with regular frequency	
2. Discuss complementary and alternative therapies with patients. Manage their expectations and explain the limited research behind their efficacy.	a. Consider bathing with additives such as bleach, Dead Sea salt, water softeners, colloidal oatmeal, rice starch, rice bran, or natural oils	
	b. Consider using certain topical oils such as sunflower seed oil, sunflower oleodistillate, and virgin coconut oil	
	c. Consider use of topical and oral micronutrients such as topical B_{12} and oral L-histidine	
	d. Consider engaging in acupuncture or acupressure therapy with a licensed provider	
3. Counsel patients to avoid certain triggers that can make symptoms worse.	a. Extreme temperatures, maintain cooler temperatures whenever possible	
	b. Caffeine/nicotine 6 h before bed	
	c. Avoid excessive use of blankets and layers of clothing	
4. Counsel patients to avoid certain potentially harmful and irritating complementary and alternative practices.	a. Fragrances and aromatherapy	
	b. Essential oils	
	c. Olive oil	
	d. Cupping	
5. If the patient is unable to manage their symptoms through other means, recommend medication treatment.	Antihistamine therapy for 1–3 months maximum	

HEPA, High efficiency particulate air filter.

Further readings

Dinicola, C., Kekevian, A., & Chang, C. (2012). Integrative medicine as adjunct therapy in the treatment of atopic dermatitis—the role of traditional Chinese medicine, dietary supplements, and other modalities. *Clinical Reviews in Allergy & Immunology, 44*(3), 242–253. https://doi.org/10.1007/s12016-012-8315-1.

Tan, H. Y., Lenon, G. B., Zhang, A. L., & Xue, C. C. (2015). Efficacy of acupuncture in the management of atopic dermatitis: A systematic review. *Clinical and Experimental Dermatology, 40*(7), 711–716. https://doi.org/10.1111/ced.12732.

Zink, A., & Traidl-Hoffmann, C. (2015). Green tea in dermatology—myths and facts. *Journal Der Deutschen Dermatologischen Gesellschaft, 13*(8), 768–775. https://doi.org/10.1111/ddg.12737.

References

Cui, S., & Cui, J. (2012). Progress of researches on the mechanism of cupping therapy. *Zhen ci yan jiu, 37*(6), 506–510.

Holm, J. G., Clausen, M.-L., Agner, T., & Thomsen, S. F. (2019). Use of complementary and alternative therapies in outpatients with atopic dermatitis from a dermatological university department. *Dermatology (Basel, Switzerland), 235*(3), 189–195. https://doi.org/10.1159/000496274.

Hon, K. L., Leung, T. F., Ng, P. C., Lam, M. C., Kam, W. Y., Wong, K. Y., et al. (2007). Efficacy and tolerability of a Chinese herbal medicine concoction for treatment of atopic dermatitis: A randomized, double-blind, placebo-controlled study. *The British Journal of Dermatology, 157*(2), 357–363. https://doi.org/10.1111/j.1365-2133.2007.07941.x. https://www.ncbi.nlm.nih.gov/pubmed/17501956.

Hon, K. L., Leung, T. F., Wong, Y., Lam, W. K., Guan, D. Q., Ma, K. C., et al. (2004). A pentaherbs capsule as a treatment option for atopic dermatitis in children: An open-labeled case series. *The American Journal of Chinese Medicine, 32*(6), 941–950. https://doi.org/10.1142/S0192415X04002545. https://www.ncbi.nlm.nih.gov/pubmed/15673199.

Hon, K. L., Lo, W., Cheng, W. K., Leung, T. F., Chow, C. M., Lau, C. B., et al. (2012). Prospective self-controlled trial of the efficacy and tolerability of a herbal syrup for young children with eczema. *The Journal of Dermatological Treatment, 23*(2), 116–121. https://doi.org/10.3109/09546634.2010.514893. https://www.ncbi.nlm.nih.gov/pubmed/21294644.

Hon, K. L., Luk, D. C., Leong, K. F., & Leung, A. K. (2013). Cupping therapy may be harmful for eczema: A PubMed search. *Case Reports in Pediatrics, 2013*, 605829. https://doi.org/10.1155/2013/605829.

Hwang, Y., Chang, B., Kim, T., & Kim, S. (2019). Ameliorative effects of green tea extract from tannase digests on house dust mite antigen-induced atopic dermatitis-like lesions in NC/Nga mice. *Archives of Dermatological Research, 311*(2), 109–120. https://doi.org/10.1007/s00403-018-01886-6.

Jung, D. L., Lee, S. D., Choi, I. H., Na, H. S., & Hong, S. U. (2014). Effects of electroacupuncture on capsaicin-induced model of atopic dermatitis in rats. *Journal of Dermatological Science*, *74*(1), 23–30. https://doi.org/10.1016/j.jdermsci.2013.11.015.

Kang, S., Kim, Y. K., Yeom, M., Lee, H., Jang, H., Park, H. J., & Kim, K. (2018). Acupuncture improves symptoms in patients with mild-to-moderate atopic dermatitis: A randomized, sham-controlled preliminary trial. *Complementary Therapies in Medicine*, *41*, 90–98. https://doi.org/10.1016/j.ctim.2018.08.013.

Kaplan, R. J., Daman, L., Rosenberg, E. W., & Feigenbaum, S. (1978). Topical use of caffeine with hydrocortisone in the treatment of atopic dermatitis. *Archives of Dermatology*, *114*(1), 60–62.

Kim, H. K., Chang, H. K., Baek, S. Y., Chung, J. O., Rha, C. S., Kim, S. Y., et al. (2012). Treatment of atopic dermatitis associated with malassezia sympodialis by green tea extracts bath therapy: A pilot study. *Mycobiology*, *40*(2), 124–128. https://doi.org/10.5941/myco.2012.40.2.124.

Koo, J., & Desai, R. (2003). Traditional Chinese medicine in dermatology. *Dermatologic Therapy*, *16*(2), 98–105. https://doi.org/10.1046/j.1529-8019.2003.01617.x.

Lee, K. C., Keyes, A., Hensley, J. R., Gordon, J. R., Kwasny, M. J., West, D. P., & Lio, P. A. (2012). Effectiveness of acupressure on pruritus and lichenification associated with atopic dermatitis: A pilot trial. *Acupuncture in Medicine*, *30*(1), 8–11. https://doi.org/10.1136/acupmed-2011-010088.

Merklinger, S., Messemer, C., & Niederle, S. (1995). Ekzembehandlung mit Cardiospermum halicacabum. *Zeitschrift für Phytotherapie*, *16*, 263.

Ohmori, Y., Ito, M., Kishi, M., Mizutani, H., Katada, T., & Konishi, H. (1995). Antiallergic constituents from oolong tea stem. *Biological and Pharmaceutical Bulletin*, *18*(5), 683–686. https://doi.org/10.1248/bpb.18.683.

Paller, A. S., Wynnis, L. T., Lebwohl, M. G., Blumenthal, R. L., Boguniewicz, M., Call, R. S., et al. (2016). Efficacy and safety of crisaborole ointment, a novel, nonsteroidal phosphodiesterase 4 (PDE4) inhibitor for the topical treatment of atopic dermatitis (AD) in children and adults. *Journal of the American Academy of Dermatology*, *75*(3). https://doi.org/10.1016/j.jaad.2016.05.046.

Pfab, F., Kirchner, M. T., Huss-Marp, J., Schuster, T., Schalock, P. C., Fuqin, J., et al. (2012). Acupuncture compared with oral antihistamine for type I hypersensitivity itch and skin response in adults with atopic dermatitis: A patient- and examiner-blinded, randomized, placebo-controlled, crossover trial. *Allergy*, *67*(4), 566–573. https://doi.org/10.1111/j.1398-9995.2012.02789.x. https://www.ncbi.nlm.nih.gov/pubmed/22313287.

Reuter, J., Wolfle, U., Weckesser, S., & Schempp, C. (2010). Which plant for which skin disease? Part 1: Atopic dermatitis, psoriasis, acne, condyloma and herpes simplex. *Journal der Deutschen Dermatologischen Gesellschaft = Journal of the German Society of Dermatology*, *8*(10), 788–796. https://doi.org/10.1111/j.1610-0387.2010.07496.x. https://www.ncbi.nlm.nih.gov/pubmed/20707875.

Sidbury, R., Tom, W. L., Bergman, J. N., Cooper, K. D., Silverman, R. A., Berger, T. G., et al. (2014). Guidelines of care for the management of atopic dermatitis: Section 4. Prevention of disease flares and use of adjunctive therapies and approaches. *Journal of the American Academy of Dermatology*, *71*(6), 1218–1233. https://doi.org/10.1016/j.jaad.2014.08.038. https://www.ncbi.nlm.nih.gov/pubmed/25264237.

Tan, H. Y., Zhang, A. L., Chen, D., Xue, C. C., & Lenon, G. B. (2013). Chinese herbal medicine for atopic dermatitis: A systematic review. *Journal of the American Academy of Dermatology*, *69*(2), 295–304. https://doi.org/10.1016/j.jaad.2013.01.019.

Uehara, M., Sugiura, H., & Sakurai, K. (2001). A trial of oolong tea in the management of recalcitrant atopic dermatitis. *Archives of Dermatology*, *137*(1), 42–43. https://doi.org/10.1001/archderm.137.1.42.

Vieira, B. L., Lim, N. R., Lohman, M. E., & Lio, P. A. (2016). Complementary and alternative medicine for atopic dermatitis: An evidence-based review. *American Journal of Clinical Dermatology*, *17*(6), 557–581. https://doi.org/10.1007/s40257-016-0209-1. https://www.ncbi.nlm.nih.gov/pubmed/27388911.

Wakeman, M. P. (2017). An open-label forearm-controlled pilot study to assess the effect of a proprietary emollient formulation on objective parameters of skin function of eczema-prone individuals over 14 days. *Clinical, Cosmetic and Investigational Dermatology*, *10*, 275–283. https://doi.org/10.2147/ccid.S135841.

Witte, M., Krause, L., Zillikens, D., & Shimanovich, I. (2019). Black tea dressings—A rapidly effective treatment for facial dermatitis. *The Journal of Dermatological Treatment*, *30*(8), 785–789. https://doi.org/10.1080/09546634.2019.1573306.

Glossary

A

Abrocitinib: An inhibitor for Janus kinase 1 (JAK1), a signaling molecule. It has been tested in clinical trial for patients with atopic dermatitis.

Adaptive immunity: A part of the immune system that requires a prior exposure to "learn" and "memorize" invaders, so subsequent encounters would trigger enhanced immune responses. Vaccination is a good example of medicine that takes advantage of this adaptive immunity to allow the immune system to "pre-learn" and "remember" the pretended invaders (the altered pathogen-containing vaccine). When the "pre-learned" real invaders are encountered in the future, the immune system is ready to mount a robust response, thus preventing disease to occur. The major components of this system include T lymphocytes (T cells), B cells, and antibodies.

AhR (Acryl hydrocarbon receptor): A receptor on the surface of keratinocytes that is critical for regulating the body's physiologic responses to major environmental pollutants. AhR expression is highly upregulated in skin of atopic dermatitis patients.

Allergic contact dermatitis: Allergen-mediated skin inflammation, characterized as an antigen presenting cell/T-cell–mediated process. It is a delayed type of hypersensitivity reaction, requiring preexposure to the same allergen to induce skin inflammation during subsequent reexposures.

Alloknesis: A neurologic phenomena in which normal or nonpruritic stimuli are perceived as such by the central nervous system.

Angiogenesis: The initiation, development, and differentiation of new blood or lymphatic vessels. In an animal model of atopic dermatitis (the keratin-14/interleukin-4–transgenic model), dermal angiogenesis is associated with upregulation of VEGF-A and VEGFR2, and the degree of angiogenesis paralleled the degree of disease progression, supporting a notion that angiogenesis process may play a role in atopic dermatitis pathogenesis.

Antigen presenting cells: A group of cells that function to process and carry forward antigen to stimulate T-cell activation. These cell types include dendritic cells, Langerhans cells, macrophages, and B cells. Antigen presenting cells are functionally characterized by their cell surface molecular marker, MHC class I or II, which interact with T-cell receptors.

Antimicrobial-embedded clothing: Chitosan, a biopolymer found in nature as a component of the exoskeleton of shellfish, has been studied as an embedded antimicrobial in textiles for patients with atopic dermatitis.

Antimicrobial peptides: Fondly called "body's own antibiotics," these are a group of small molecular weight proteins that have wide-ranging antimicrobial properties against bacteria, fungi, and viruses. Some of these peptides are located on the surface of the skin: β-defensins and cathelicidins. The skin of atopic dermatitis patients has decreased expression of antimicrobial peptides, rendering them more susceptible to skin infections and colonization by pathogens, especially by *Staphylococcus aureus* bacteria.

Apremilast: A phosphodiesterase type 4 inhibitor approved by the Food and Drug Administration for the treatment of moderate to severe psoriasis and psoriatic arthritis in adults. Clinical trials for treatment of atopic dermatitis are ongoing.

Atopic march: The phenomenon of sequential development and progression of multiple allergic conditions, where patients with early childhood atopic dermatitis develop asthma, allergic rhinitis (hay fever), or other allergic conditions later on in life.

Atopiform dermatitis: This term has been proposed by some academicians to classify a group of patients affected by a chronic inflammatory skin disease just like "atopic dermatitis," but in the absence of total serum IgE elevation. This group of patients has also been classified as an "intrinsic" subset of atopic dermatitis.

Atopy: A term that describe a set of allergic diseases or conditions that usually includes atopic dermatitis, allergic rhinitis, and asthma.

α-toxin: A toxin produced by *Staphylococcus aureus* that causes damage to keratinocytes, leading to inflammatory responses.

Autocrine: A term describing a self-stimulating loop in which a cytokine released from a cell binds to and activates or inactivates its own cellular receptor.

B

β-defensin: An important skin antimicrobial peptide in humans, particularly β-defensin-1, β-defensin-2 (both monomers), and β-defensin-3 (a dimer).

C

Cathelicidin: A family of conserved, cationic, antimicrobial peptides in living organisms, primarily stored in the lysosomes of macrophages and neutrophils but also in epithelial cells. As a part of the innate immune system, these molecules have broad activity against bacterial, fungi, and enveloped viruses. In humans, only one cathelicidin, LL-37, is known to exist. Cathelicidin levels are decreased in the skin of atopic dermatitis patients.

Chemokine: A large family of small size cell-produced proteins that function to attract certain immune cells, such as in the case that interleukin-8 attracts neutrophils and in the case that eotaxin attracts eosinophils. While chemokines are usually classified as a special class of cytokines, they are sometimes regarded as a separated class from cytokines.

Circadian rhythms: The physical, mental, hormonal, and behavioral changes that follow a recurrent cycle. Disruption of circadian rhythms can disrupt physiologic homeostasis and lead to disorders of physical, mental, or both aspects.

Claudin-1: An important protein component of epidermal tight junction (between epidermal keratinocytes). Its expression is suppressed by the actions of Th2 cytokines, including IL4, IL13, and IL31.

Coagulase-negative *Staphylococcus* (CoNS): This group of bacteria includes commensal bacteria such as *Staphylococcus epidermidis* and *Staphylococcus hominis*, known to produce antimicrobial peptides that limit the growth of pathogenic strain *Staphylococcus aureus*. Application of autologous CoNS to skin of atopic dermatitis patients leads to reduction of pathogenic strain *S. aureus*.

Crisaborole: A topical agent approved by the Food and Drug Administration since 2016 for mild to moderate atopic dermatitis. Mechanistically it is a small molecule phosphodiesterase-4 inhibitor that results in a downstream decrease in the production of proinflammatory cytokines. Currently the commercially available product by prescription-only is crisaborole 2% topical ointment.

Cutaneous microcirculation: A group of related circulatory vessels, including arterioles (minute arteries), capillaries, venules (minute veins), and lymphatic vessels, that function together to deliver oxygen and nutrition and returning return excessive fluid to the venous system. The cutaneous microcirculation is well known to play an important role in inflammation dermatoses, such as in psoriasis and atopic dermatitis.

Cytokine: A large number of small size cell-produced proteins that can influence the functions of other cells by providing signals for growth stimulation, proliferation, regulation, differentiation, and other biologic functions. Some major groups of cytokines include interferon (IFN), interleukin (IL), colony-stimulating factor (CSF), and tumor necrosis factor (TNF). Cytokines of the Th2 family, such as IL4, IL13, IL31, play significant roles in the inflammatory process of atopic dermatitis. Transgenic over-expression of IL4 in mice epidermis results in an animal model of atopic dermatitis. Treatment with antibody blocking the α cellular receptor for IL4 leads to significant clinical improvement of atopic dermatitis.

D

Dead Sea therapy: A complementary and alternative treatment option for atopic dermatitis, by bathing patients with Dead Sea–like water (i.e., water containing high concentrations of minerals such as magnesium, calcium, potassium, and bromine ions).

Delgocitinib: A topically applied pan-Janus kinase (JAK) inhibitor that inhibits JAK1, JAK2, JAK 3, and tyrosine kinase 2. It has been tested in clinical trial for treatment of atopic dermatitis and hand dermatitis.

Desmosome: A protein structure that connects keratinocytes in the middle and lower levels of epithelium to maintain intraepidermal structural integrity. Bacterial toxin or autoantibodies that target desmosomes leads to epidermal cell-cell separation, forming blisters clinically and acantholysis on histopathology.

Dihomo-gamma-linolenic acid (DGLA): A 20-carbon long-chain omega-6 fatty acid with antiproliferative property. Its breakdown product contributes to the lipid component of the skin barrier.

Diluted bleach bath: Bath water that is made up of approximately 0.005% sodium hypochlorite, recommended for patients with atopic dermatitis. Usually, 0.25 cup of household bleach (typically 6% sodium hypochlorite) is added to a regular-sized bathtub half-full of warm water in which the patient bathes for 5 to 10 minutes daily to every other day.

δ-Toxin: A toxin produced by *Staphylococcus aureus*, capable of stimulating mast cells leading to inflammatory cytokine release.

Dupilumab: A biologic drug that is a humanized monoclonal antibody that blocks the interleukin-4 receptor α, a cellular receptor for both IL4 and IL13; inhibition by dupilumab eliminates the stimulatory functions of both IL4 and IL13, the key cytokines involved in the pathogenesis of atopic dermatitis.

Dysbiosis: A phenomenon describing alteration of normal homeostasis of commensal and pathogenic microorganisms. Dysbiosis is present on the skin of atopic dermatitis patients, with decreased overall microbial diversity and commensal bacteria, and an increase in pathogenic *Staphylococcus aureus* bacteria.

E

Eczema Area and Severity Index (EASI): A commonly used clinical severity assessment tool for atopic dermatitis that accounts for the lesional morphologic severity and area of involvement.

Eczema coxsackium: A condition that occurs in patients with a history of atopic dermatitis when the skin is exposed to *Coxsackie* viruses. It is clinically characterized by extensive skin eruptions of papules and blisters, and can occur even in patients without active atopic dermatitis lesions.

Eczema herpeticum: A condition that occurs in patients who have clinical manifestion of atopic dermatitis overlapping with localized to disseminated herpes virus infection.

Eczema vaccinatum: A condition that occurs in patients with atopic dermatitis after natural infection by the smallpox virus or after smallpox vaccination, resulting in a widespread and severe dissemination of smallpox infection. This is a life-threatening medical emergency that requires hospitalization.

Enterotoxin B: A toxin produced by *Staphylococcus aureus* that induces leukocyte production of IL31, a pruritus-inducing cytokine.

Epidermal stem cell: A population of epidermal cells located at the lowest level of epidermis and are usually called basal epidermal cells. These basal epidermal cells are capable of dividing and providing populations of epidermal cells for their continuing replacement of the upper epidermal cell layers.

Epidermal tight junction: An intercellular junction formed between adjacent keratinocytes at the stratum granulosum layer of the epidermis, just below stratum corneum. It is essential for skin barrier function and structure.

Extrinsic atopic dermatitis: A major subset of atopic dermatitis characterized by elevation of total serum IgE.

F

FcεRI: High-affinity IgE receptor (IgER), a tetrameric (α, β, γ, γ) immunoreceptor with tyrosine-based activation motif, expressed on mast cells and basophils. Upon activation by IgE binding, it mediates degranulation, eicosanoid production, and cytokine production by these leukocytes.

FcεRII: A low-affinity IgE receptor (or CD23) that is a C-type lectin, expressed on B cells. It regulates IgE production, and antigen processing and presentation.

Filaggrin: A skin barrier protein located in the stratum corneum with an apparent molecular weight of 37 kD and is derived from a high molecular weight profilaggrin protein (>220 kD). Filaggrin expression is suppressed by Th2 cytokines IL4 and IL13. Up to 50% of European patients affected by atopic dermatitis have a loss-of-function mutation of the gene *(FLG)* encoding filaggrin.

G

Guanylate-binding protein 1 (GBP1): A large GTPase of the dynamin superfamily that regulates membrane, cytoskeleton, and cell cycle progression dynamics. In endothelial cells and monocytes, GBP1 expression is strongly induced by IFN-γ and acts to inhibit inflammatory cell proliferation.

Gusacitinib: A dual inhibitor of Janus kinase (JAK) and spleen tyrosine kinase (SYK) that is under investigation for the treatment of atopic dermatitis.

H

"Hygiene hypothesis": First proposed by Strachan in 1989, who speculates that the arising prevalence of atopic dermatitis is largely due to the modern family practice of keeping young children in extremely clean (hygiene) condition so children grow up lacking exposure to certain pathogens. Underexposure to common pathogens is thought to skew immune maturation toward Th2, which favors allergic immune responses such as occurred in atopy.

Hyperknesis: A neurologic phenomenon in which a pruritic stimulus triggers excessive itch perception.

I

Ichthyosis vulgaris: A genetic skin condition characterized by fish-scale appearance. Most patients have loss-of-function genetic mutation of a stratum corneum protein filaggrin. Some, but not all, patients with ichthyosis vulgaris also develop atopic dermatitis.

Immunoglobulin E (IgE): A class of immuno-globulin produced by B cells through IL4 stimulation. It plays an important role in the pathogenesis of atopic dermatitis.

Innate lymphoid cells (ILC): A type of immune cells that are phenotypically similar to Th subsets, but without T- or B-cell antigen receptors. ILCs are characterized by their immune plasticity; their phenotypes and functions can be modified by their microenvironments.

Innate immunity: A part of the immune system that acts as the front-line defense by recognizing and fighting foreign invaders. Prior exposure is not needed for the activation of innate immune response. Some of the innate immune system components are antimicrobial peptides, neutrophils, and natural killer cells.

Interleukin-4: An important T-cell cytokine produced by Th2 cells and is essential for IgE production; it is the key driver for atopic dermatitis. A transgenic mouse line where IL4 is overexpressed in the epidermis develops chronic, itchy, inflammatory skin disease that fulfills the diagnostic criteria of atopic dermatitis in humans.

Interleukin-13: An important Th2 cytokine that plays a role in the pathogenesis of atopic dermatitis. IL13 shares the same cellular receptor, IL4Rα, with IL4. The commercially available biologic treatment for atopic dermatitis, dupilumab blocks the IL4Rα and improves the clinical condition of atopic dermatitis.

Interleukin-31: A cytokine characterized as a member of the Th2 cytokine family, and plays an important role in inflammatory and itch signaling pathways. IL31 is produced by Th2 cells, mast cells, macrophages, dendritic cells, and eosinophils. Receptors (α-chain) for IL31 are identified in peripheral nerves and epidermal keratinocytes.

Intrinsic atopic dermatitis: A minor subset of atopic dermatitis characterized by the absence of elevation of total serum IgE. Some academicians have proposed to rename this subset "atopiform dermatitis."

Involucrin: A 65-kD skin barrier protein within the stratum corneum that contributes to cellular envelope formation that protects corneocytes. Involucrin expressions are suppressed by Th2 cytokine IL4.

Irritant contact dermatitis: A type of skin inflammation resulting from irritation due to contacting substances of nonimmune-mediated nature. Since it does not require preexposure to the irritating substance, its onset is not delayed as seen in allergic contact dermatitis.

J

Janus kinase (JAK): A signaling molecule. JAK usually forms JAK-STAT signaling pathway to regulate the production and action of cytokines and growth factors. JAK-STAT signaling has been implicated in the pathogenesis of atopic dermatitis. Importantly, IL4 signals via JAK-STAT6 pathway to regulate Th2-related target genes in lymphocytes.

L

***Lactobacillus johnsonii*:** A bacterium strain that has been shown to stimulate host innate immune response for expression of antimicrobial peptides (AMPs) such as cathelicidin and β-defensin. Topical application of lotion containing heat-treated *L. johnsonii* results in reduction of pathogenic *Staphylococcus aureus* in the skin of atopic dermatitis patients.

Langerhans cells: First discovered by Paul Langerhans, a German pathologist, Langerhans cells are professional antigen presenting cells located in the epidermis. They have an important role in diseases involving T-cell–mediated immune responses such as allergic contact dermatitis. Immunologically, Langerhans cells are characterized by positive and functional cell surface markers of CD1a and CD207 (Langerin).

Lebrikizumab: A biologic medication that is a humanized monoclonal antibody binding to IL13 to prevent IL13α1/IL4Rα heterodimerization and inhibits its signal transduction.

Loricrin: A skin barrier protein located at the stratum corneum with a molecular weight of 26 kD. It is a terminally differentiated protein comprising more than 70% of cornified envelope, thus a major cornified envelope protein. Loricrin is expressed in all stratified epithelia, and its expression is highest in humid epithelial surfaces such as mucous membranes. Loricrin expression is suppressed by Th2 cytokine IL4.

Lymphangiogenesis: The process of making and differentiating new lymphatic vessels. Dermal lymphangiogenesis is a prominent feature in a mouse model of atopic dermatitis (keratin-14/IL4–transgenic mice) and is documented to be driven by CD11b+ macrophages and cytokine VEGF-C.

Lymphatic vessel endothelial hyaluronan receptor 1 (LYVE-1): A CD44 homolog resided primarily on lymphatic endothelial cells, with potential roles in hyaluronan transport and turnover. It is a marker for lymphoid tissues and lymphangiogenesis.

M

Microbiome: The genetic material of a community of microorganisms, including bacteria, fungi, and viruses, that inhabit the body both inside and on the skin surface.

N

Nemolizumab: A biologic medication that is a humanized monoclonal antibody targeting IL31Rα. It inhibits IL31 signaling, which dampens pruritus signaling.

P

Pericyte: A special kind of perivascular cell surrounding the endothelial cells in capillaries and venules of microcirculation, such as those present in the skin. Pericyte's contractile property may function to regulate circulation and maintain homeostasis.

Phenol-soluble modulin: A *Staphylococcus aureus* protein that can stimulate cytokine release by keratinocytes.

Pimecrolimus: A calcineurin inhibitor that binds to FK506-binding protein (FKBP), which inhibits the activation of calcineurin and its downstream signaling pathway leading to decreased production of inflammatory cytokines. A topical pimecrolimus formulation is approved for the treatment of atopic dermatitis.

Probiotics: Live microorganism-containing products that can be administered to humans and confers health benefits to human hosts. Probiotics can be administered either orally or topically.

Protein A: *Staphylococcus aureus* product that can trigger keratinocyte-driven inflammatory responses.

R

Roseomonas mucosa: A strain of culturable gram-negative bacteria and a predominant commensal species of healthy skin. *R. mucosa* derived from healthy individuals shows ability to limit *Staphylococcus aureus* growth, improve barrier function through reduced transepidermal water loss, and induce an innate immune response in atopic dermatitis patients.

Rosiglitazone: An activator for peroxisome proliferator-activated receptor-gamma (PPAR-γ) that is approved for the treatment of type 2 diabetes mellitus. Since it inhibits TLSP-induced dendritic cell maturation, it has been studied for treatment of atopic dermatitis.

S

SCORAD (SCORing Atopic Dermatitis): A widely used clinical assessment tool to measure the extent and severity of atopic dermatitis.

Serlopitant: A neurokinin 1 receptor (NK1-R) antagonist developed for chronic use in overactive bladder, and has antipruritic property. It has been tested to treat pruritus in patients with atopic dermatitis.

Staphylococcus aureus: *Staphylo* means "bunch of grapes" in Greek; *coccus* means "sphere" and is derived from "berry" in Greek. *Staphylococcus* is a spherically shaped gram positive catalase positive bacteria that commonly groups like a cluster of grapes. *Staphylococcus aureus* colonizes the skin and plays a significant role in the pathophysiology of atopic dermatitis. It can become resistant to the methicillin family of antibiotics (methicillin, amoxicillin, penicillin, and oxacillin) and even newer antibiotics (vancomycin, linezolid, teicoplanin, daptomycin) and is then termed methicillin-resistant *S. aureus* (MRSA).

Staphylococcus epidermidis: A common skin-commensal bacterium. On the skin of atopic dermatitis patients, it is decreased in density while pathogenic bacteria such as *Staphylococcus aureus* are increased in density.

STAT (Signal transduction and activator of transcription): There are seven known STATs. STAT proteins are critical mediators of cytokine signaling. Importantly, STAT6 is activated by Th2-type cytokines IL4 and IL13 and thus plays an important role in atopic dermatitis pathogenesis.

Stratum corneum: The outermost layer of the epidermis made of nonnucleated dead keratinocytes. The stratum corneum is mostly made of keratin and skin barrier proteins, such as filaggrin, involucrin, and loricrin, as well as barrier lipids and antimicrobial peptides. Stratum corneum has important physical and immunologic skin barrier functions.

Streptococcus thermophilus: A gram-positive facultative anaerobic bacterium that has been shown to increase ceramide levels both in vitro and in vivo. Application of a moisturizer containing *S. thermophilus* led to increased ceramide levels and improved skin conditions in patients with atopic dermatitis.

Suprachiasmatic nucleus (SCN): A brain structure located in the hypothalamus that is composed of 20,000 neurons. The SCN receives signals directly from the eyes and is responsible for coordinating the body's circadian rhythm, which in turn regulates a multitude of physiologic functions including that of the skin.

T

Tacrolimus: A calcineurin inhibitor that binds to FK506-binding protein (FKBP), which inhibits the activation of calcineurin and its downstream signaling pathway, resulting in decreased production of inflammatory cytokines.

Tfh cells (T follicular helper cells): These leukocytes exhibit a unique CXCR5+ CXCL13+ ICOS+ PD-1+ BCL6+ BTLA+ SAP+ immune phenotype. These cells are specialized to support B-cell response, including extrafollicular response of short-lived PC production and GC formation essential for class switching recombination and somatic hypermutation for high-affinity antibody PC and memory generation.

Th2 (Helper T-cell subset 2): Important cells for immune functions relating to parasitic infection and allergic responses, with IL4 as its signature cytokine. Th2 cells antagonize the functions of helper T cell subset 1 (Th1).

Th17 (Helper T cell subset 17): A unique helper T cell characterized by its production of IL17, a highly proinflammatory cytokine. Studies have indicated that Th17 cells are important in the pathogenesis of rheumatoid arthritis, inflammatory bowel disease, asthma, and some skin diseases such as psoriasis and allergic contact dermatitis.

Th22 (Helper T cell subset 22): A distinct subset of Th cells derived from a lineage of Th17 cells and plays a role in allergic diseases such as allergic contact dermatitis. Th22 cells are characterized by their secretion of IL22 and their absence of production of IFN-γ, IL4, and IL17 under general condition, thus distinguishing it from Th1, Th2, and Th17 subsets, respectively. Under special conditions, however, Th22 cells can be induced to produce IL13 and IFN-γ, signature cytokines for Th2 and Th1 subsets, respectively.

Tofacitinib: A small-molecule JAK1 inhibitor medication. It inhibits the effect of inflammatory cytokines by attenuation of JAK-STAT signaling in keratinocytes and inflammatory cells.

Topical calcineurin inhibitors (TCIs): Introduced in the 2000s, TCIs are approved for the treatment of atopic dermatitis. TCIs inhibit calcineurin-dependent T-cell activation, thus preventing production of proinflammatory cytokines and mediators. Two agents, tacrolimus ointment (0.03% and 0.1%) and pimecrolimus cream (1%) are currently available commercially.

Topical corticosteroid (TCS): A group of topically applied corticosteroids with a variety of strength and vehicles. The TCS strength is classified by the World Health Organization (WHO), ranging from class I (ultrahigh potency; e.g., clobetasol propionate 0.05%) to class VII (lowest potency; e.g., hydrocortisone acetate 1%). TCS can be made with a variety of vehicles ranging from gel, solution, spray, lotion, cream, to ointment. TCS is one of the most commonly used topical medications for inflammatory skin diseases.

Tralokinumab: A biologic medication and a monoclonal IgG4 antibody that binds to and neutralizes the effects of IL13. It is under investigation for treatment of atopic dermatitis and other allergic diseases.

Transepidermal water loss (TEWL): A measurement of amount of water loss through the epidermis to the surrounding atmosphere by either diffusion or evaporation process. The average overall TEWL in humans is approximately 300 to 400 mL/day. The amount of water loss is influenced by environmental humidity, temperature, ventilation, skin barrier intactness, skin irritation, and other environmental factors.

Tregs (Regulatory T cells): These leukocytes are marked by CD4+ CD25hi Foxp3+. They establish and maintain immune homeostasis by suppressing immune responses. Tregs are derived during thymic T-cell development as a subset of self-reactive T cells under transcription factor Foxp3 regulation.

Thymic stromal lymphopoietin (TSLP): A cytokine closely related to IL7. Originally identified as secreting cytokine from thymic stromal cell line, TSLP has been linked to the pathogenesis of allergic diseases, including atopic dermatitis.

V

VEGF (Vascular endothelial growth factor): A factor that is essential for initiating new blood vessel and lymphatic vessel generation.

VEGF-A120: An isoform 120 of the vascular endothelial growth factor type that has been shown to be upregulated in a mouse model of atopic dermatitis and it is experimentally inducible by IL6 and IFN-γ.

VEGF-C (Vascular endothelial cell growth factor type C): A growth factor involved in lymphangiogenesis and has been shown to be upregulated in a mouse model of atopic dermatitis.

VEGFR (Vascular endothelial growth factor receptor): Receptors on endothelial cells and are responsible for receiving signals from VEGF to trigger angiogenesis process. The upregulation of its expressions in a mouse model of atopic dermatitis suggests angiogenesis plays a role in the pathogenesis of atopic dermatitis.

Bibliography

Burks, A., Wesley, S. I., Holgate, R. E., O'Hehir, D. H., Broide, L. B., Bacharier, G. K., et al. (Eds.), (2019). *Middleton's allergy: Principles and practice* (10th ed.). Elsevier.

Elias, P. M., & Feingold, K. R. (Eds.), (2005). *Skin barrier*. CRC Press.

Fromm, M., & Schulzke, J.-D. (Eds.), (2012). *Barriers and channels formed by tight junction proteins II* (1st ed.). *Annals of the New York Academy of Science, 1258*. Wiley-Blackwell.

Ji, Y. (2020). *Methicillin-resistant Staphylococcus aureus (MRSA) protocols: Cutting edge technologies and advancements (methods in molecular biology)*. Humana Publishing.

Katashima, K. (2016). *Immunology of the skin: Basic and clinical sciences in skin immune responses* (1st ed.). Springer.

Matsuzaki, K. (2019). *Antimicrobial peptides: Basics for clinical application (advances in experimental medicine and biology book 1117)* (1st ed.). Springer.

Wahn, H. U., & Sampson, H. A. (Eds.), (2015). *Allergy, immunity and tolerance in early childhood: The first steps of atopic march*. Academic Press.

Index

Note: Page numbers followed by '*f*' indicate figures and those followed by '*t*' indicate tables.

Junctional adhesion molecules (JAMs), 107–108
Junctional defects, 152–153

K

Kallikreins, skin barrier, 40
Kaposi varicelliform eruption, 183
Kappa agonists and mu antagonists, 268
κ-opioid receptors (KORs), 162
Keratin-14/IL4 transgenic mice
    cutaneous blood vessels, 108–111, 109*f*
    lymphatic vessels, cutaneous in, 115–119
Keratinocytes
    in adaptive immune responses, 95–96
    barrier proteins, 96
        roles, 92
    combined IL4/IL13 reduces filaggrin
        expression, 97–98
    cutaneous sensation, 93–94, 94*f*
    epidermal-dermal adhesion, 93
    epidermal structure roles
        epidermal tight junction, 92–93
        stratum corneum, 91–92
    in immune regulation, 94–95
    inflamed human skin, 91*f*
    in innate immune responses, 95
    microbiome, 45
    physical barrier proteins, 97
    roles of, 90
    in skin structure and integrity, 90–91
    in wound healing, 94
KIF3A gene, 28, 171

L

Lactobacillus johnsonii, 256–257
Lamellar granules, 226
Lamellar lipids, 226
Langerhans cells (LCs), 18, 135–136
Lanolin, 228–229
Leaky gut, microbiome, 50–51, 50*f*
Lebrikizumab, 195, 240
Leukotriene B-4 (LTB4), 164
Leukotrienes (LTs), 162
L-histidine, 280
Ligelizumab, 242
Linoleic acid, 278
Lipid alterations, 146–147
Lipid mediators, 162
Lipopolysaccharide (LPS), 49
Lipoteichoic acid (LTA), 119, 212
Loricrin, 97, 98*f*
Lotions, 228
Lung
    changes in atopic dermatitis, 153*t*
    permeability, 151
Lymphangiogenesis, 119
Lymphatic vessels, cutaneous
    in cancer, 114
    capillaries of arterial and, 113*t*, 114*f*
    functions, 113–115
    immunofluorescence microscopy, 118*f*
    in keratin-14/IL4 transgenic mice, 115–119
    lymphatic hyperproliferation parallel
        progression of skin inflammation, 116*f*
    roles in atopic dermatitis, 115
    structures, 113
Lymphoepithelial Kazal-type 5 (LETK1), 28

M

Macrophage inflammatory protein 3 alpha
    (MIP-3α), 183
Macrophage migration inhibitory factor (MIF),
    213

Major histocompatibility complex (MHC)
    molecules, 134–135
Malnutrition, 71–72
Manuka honey, 282–283
Mast cells, 18, 139, 212
Maternal diet, intrapartum, 67–68
Medical comorbidities, 30
Mediterranean diet, 68
Melatonin, sleep disturbance and, 19–20
Mental health, 30–31
Menthol, 278
Methotrexate, 267
Microbiome, 44–46
    AD with oral probiotics
        prevention, 254–255
        treatment, 253–254
    bacterial composition, 46
    characteristics, 46*t*
    dysbiosis, skin barrier, 40–41
    establishment of, 48
    factors influencing, 45*t*
        infant, 49*t*
    gut dysbiosis, 47, 47*f*
    implications, 47–48
    leaky gut, 50–51, 50*f*
    modulation
        antimicrobial-embedded clothing, 258
        Bifidobacterium, 257
        endolysins, 258
        Lactobacillus, 256–257
        oral probiotics, 252–253
        recommendations, 255
        Roseomonas, 257
        safety and food and drug administration
            regulations, 258
        Staphylococcus, 257
        Streptococcus, 257–258
        topical microbial therapy, 256, 256*t*
        treatments on horizon, 258–259
        Vitreoscilla, 257
    risk factors, skin dysbiosis, 46
    role, wound care, 212
    skin dysbiosis, 46
    Staphylococcus aureus importance, 46–47
Microcirculation, cutaneous, 106–107, 107*f*
Micronutrients, 72–73
    iron, 73
    selenium, 73
    topical, 279–280
    vitamin C, 72
    vitamin D, 72
    vitamin E, 72
    zinc, 72
MicroRNAs (miRNAs), 168, 170–171, 170*t*
Microvasculature, cutaneous, 106
Mimyx cream, 231–232
miR-10a-5p, 174
Mirtazapine, 268
Moisturization
    and bathing practices, 265
    therapeutic guidelines, 191
Moisturizers, 226
    alternative and natural, 231–232
    definition, 227
    delivery systems, 227, 227*t*
    vs. emollient, 227
    ingredients, 228–231, 229*t*
    proactive use of, 232–233
    therapeutic guidelines, 191
mRNA
    and protein expressions of factors, 117*f*
    and protein levels, 111*f*

mRNA *(Continued)*
    and protein levels downregulation, loricrin,
        97, 98*f*
    and protein production, involucrin, 97, 98*f*
Mycobacterium leprae, 181
Mycophenolate mofetil, 267
Myelin basic protein (MBP) peptide, 95–96

N

National Center for Complementary and
    Alternative Medicine (NCCAM), 276
National Institute of General Medical Services
    (NIGMS), 19
Natural oils, 276–277
Nav 1.7 inhibitors, 270
Nemolizumab, 240–241
Nerve growth factor (NGF), 160
Neural hypersensitization, 268
Neural sensitization, drugs targeting, 268
Neurokinin receptor-1 (NK-1), 162
    inhibitors, 271
Neurokinin-1 receptor (NK1-R) antagonist,
    245–246
Neurologic control, of circadian rhythm, 20*f*
Neuronal sensitization
    barrier dysfunction, 160
    cytokines, 162
    epidermis, 160
    itch and pain, 160, 161*f*
        association of, 165
        mediators in skin, 160–163
        pathogenesis, 163–164
    itch processing in spinal cord and, 162–163
    nerve growth factor (NGF), 160
    pain, 164
        amines, 164
        cytokines, 164
        ion channels, 164
        lipid mediators, 164
        mediators in skin and neuronal sensitiza-
            tion, 164–165
        neuropeptides, 164
        processing in brain, 165
        processing in spinal cord, 164–165
    neuropeptides, 164
Neurosensory mechanisms, itch, 159–160
Neurotic eczema, 4
NK-1. *See* Neurokinin receptor-1 (NK-1)
NLRP2, 172
N-methyl-D-aspartate receptors (NMDA), 266
NOD-like receptors (NLR), 58
Nonpharmaceutic agents, therapeutic guidelines,
    191
Nonpharmacologic therapies, 265
Nonsteroidal antiinflammatory agents, topical,
    270–271
Nonuniform clinical responses to immune
    modulatory therapeutics, 13
North American Contact Dermatitis Group
    (NACDG) members, 62, 62*t*
Nutrition
    randomized controlled trials (RCTs), 67
    recommendations, 73*t*, 74*t*
    wound care
        adequate, 215
        role in, 215

O

Oatmeal
    colloidal, 282
    and rice bran, bathing, 200
Occlusive topical agents, 227